Green & Richmond

# PEDIATRIC DIAGNOSIS

**Interpretation of Symptoms**
**and Signs in Different Age Periods**

3RD EDITION

## MORRIS GREEN, M.D.

Perry W. Lesh Professor and Chairman,
Department of Pediatrics,
Indiana University School of Medicine;
Physician-in-Chief,
James Whitcomb Riley Hospital for Children,
Indianapolis, Indiana

1980
W. B. SAUNDERS COMPANY
PHILADELPHIA • LONDON • TORONTO

W. B. Saunders Company:   West Washington Square
Philadelphia, Pa. 19105

1 St. Anne's Road
Eastbourne, East Sussex BN21 3UN, England

1 Goldthorne Avenue
Toronto, Ontario M8Z 5T9, Canada

Pediatric Diagnosis

ISBN 0-7216-4242-X

Last digit is the print number:   9     8     7     6     5     4     3     2     1

*This book is affectionately dedicated to my wife, JANICE,*

*and to our children,*

*DAVID, ALAN, CAROLYN, SUSAN, MARCIA and SYLVIA*

# PREFACE

This book was written to fill a need in pediatric practice and education not fully met by encyclopedic textbooks of pediatrics, synopses, handbooks or the monographs on specific diseases, organ systems and age periods. The text is based on the simple fact that children are brought to the doctor because of symptoms, signs and problems, or for health promotion. I am pleased that the kind of problem-oriented approach introduced in the previous editions appears to have been helpful in serving as a guide to pediatric diagnosis for medical students, pediatric residents, pediatricians, family practitioners, pediatric nurses and allied health professionals who care for children.

A number of new chapters have been added. These include discussions of encopresis, enuresis, hyperactivity, chest pain, recurrent infections, fatigue, school failure, depression, sleep disorders and psychologic symptoms. Dr. Sally A. Provence has extensively revised her chapter on the development of young children.

Although there was a temptation to introduce multiple authorship in this edition, it was finally decided to make this book an individual effort. Single authorship remains valid for an effort of this kind because the clinician must be prepared to deal effectively with whatever symptom or sign that a child may present. If an academic clinician with considerable clinical experience could not integrate the relevant information, the approach utilized in this book would seem contrived.

I deeply regret that Dr. Julius B. Richmond's duties as Assistant Secretary for Health and Surgeon General of the United States have precluded his participation as a co-author in this edition. I greatly appreciate his steady encouragement and support.

I am indebted to hundreds of persons who have contributed to my knowledge of pediatric diagnosis. Space does not permit their individual recognition. I do however wish to make public acknowledgment of the full support that I have received at many levels from Indiana University and from the James Whitcomb Riley Memorial Association. Mr. Al Meier, Vice President and Editor of the W. B. Saunders Company, has been generous in his time and advice. Dr. Richard Schreiner kindly provided the photographs on pages 16 and 17. Mrs. Glenna Downton, who typed the manuscript through many drafts, deserves special commendation. I appreciate deeply her dedication and skill.

MORRIS GREEN, M.D.

v

# CONTENTS

vii

To provide the reader with a quick point of reference, major chapters in Part II, Signs and Symptoms, include an outline of the etiologic classifications.

PART I

# THE INTERVIEW AND PHYSICAL EXAMINATION

# CHAPTER 1

# THE PEDIATRIC INTERVIEW AND HISTORY

## INTRODUCTION

Discussion of the pediatric history here differs from the traditional presentation (chief complaints, present illness, past medical history, developmental and feeding history, family history and review of systems) in dealing principally with the process of interviewing. This approach is taken not to devalue the customary practice — indeed, the entire volume is concerned with the presenting complaint, development and other traditional content — but to emphasize the importance of the interview as the basic tool for pediatric diagnosis. For many symptoms, the interview is the quickest and often the only key to diagnosis, whether the problem is biomedical, biosocial or both. Both biomedical and psychosocial diagnostic possibilities need to be integrated into the initial interview since it provides not only an opportunity for obtaining data but also a way to help the patient* psychologically. Certainly, the doctor's demonstration of diagnostic thoroughness and skill in eliciting a comprehensive history is, in itself, supportive psychologically.

This discussion of the technique of interviewing seeks to provide some general principles, recognizing that the process is highly dependent upon the personality and experience of the doctor. The interview is unique for every patient and for every clinician — no two people can be interviewed in exactly the same way; no two patients with the same disorder present the same history; and no two physicians who interview skillfully do it the same way.

## BEGINNING THE INTERVIEW

The pediatric history involves a triangular relationship among physician, child and parents. Pediatric diagnosis and management generally requires a family focus. Whether the physician interviews parents and child together or separately depends upon the presenting complaints. In many instances the physician may initially interview the parents and child together and later interview them separately. Interviewing the family as a unit, including children above the age of eight years, has a place in pediatric diagnosis. In other cases, the physician may first interview the parents and then see the child. Generally, children who are old enough to express themselves verbally may profitably be interviewed separately by the physician if there is an emotional problem present. If the parent seems

---

*The term *patient* will be used to refer either to the child or to the parents as appropriate in the text.

3

hesitant to talk in front of the child, the doctor may stand and say, "I think Johnny may be more comfortable with my secretary (or nurse) until we finish talking." The manner in which the family members communicate during the interview and who does most of the talking is of interest. Although it is usually helpful to interview the parents together and thus gain some impression of their interaction, separate interviews with each parent may be indicated in some cases. When interviews are to extend over several sessions, the physician may wish to utilize the help of a social worker in elaboration of the history.

As happens so frequently, first impressions may have a significant influence on both immediate and subsequent interactions. To promote communication, one creates the kind of warm and encouraging atmosphere that facilitates openness. Each patient should feel the doctor's interest. This is conveyed by the courteous way in which appointments are arranged, by the cordiality of the receptionist ("oh, yes, Mrs. _____, Dr. Smith is expecting you"), by the doctor's friendliness and, importantly, by the doctor's prompt beginning of the appointment at the time set. The doctor should have the parents' and child's names in mind as he prepares to meet them. If the name is an unfamiliar one, his nurse or secretary should introduce the family, using the correct pronunciation.

The pediatric interview should not add to the patient's stress. An abiding rule is for the interviewer to be genuine, gracious and encouraging. Privacy is, of course, essential. Careful attention must be given to assure that the interviewing room is relatively soundproof, that the chairs are comfortable, that the lighting is not too bright and that the furnishings are "nonclinical"; that is, the room is obviously one intended for an interview, not just for physical examination or procedures. Interviews should be conducted with both patient and doctor able to see each other without strain and sitting down, rather than with the doctor standing over the patient or cocktail party style with both standing.

Lewin has stated appropriately that "the patient comes to the doctor with an attitude that has a history." This attitude may condition the outcome of diagnostic and therapeutic efforts. That most patients come to the physician with the attitude that they will be helped usually provides them some relief, at least for the first visit. They want the doctor to care. They also come with questions. Whether or not considered relevant by the doctor, the patient's questions must be answered and his or her expectations dealt with in some manner; otherwise, the patient may leave dissatisfied. Of course, the needs and expectations of some patients may be so great or unrealistic that no physician can satisfy them.

To help place patients at ease and give them a moment to become comfortable, the interview should begin with a social comment or two unrelated to the patient's chief problem and then proceed to the main purpose of the visit. One may begin with a question such as, "Would you tell me what has been concerning you about Johnny?" and then later, "What are the other problems?" The chief complaint initially given by a parent may not be the most important reason for bringing the child to the physician. The real problem may not become apparent to either the parent or the physician until later. Some patients on their own may not have thought about the situation in a sufficiently concentrated or pointed fashion; on the other hand, the parent may not feel free to disclose the primary reason for coming until he or she has decided that the physician is receptive and understanding. Experienced clinicians recognize that patients often initially present a facade at variance with reality.

Most patients come to the doctor with the wish and the expectation to be helped, but often with some reservation about both. They have their own agenda of concerns and notions of what would be helpful. The chief complaint, however, reflects the problem with which the patient is most concerned or feels most comfortable in presenting. Even though the physician recognizes or suspects that this is not the real problem, the central focus of the consultation should remain the chief complaint. The discussion should always be brought back to this topic before the interview is brought to a close. If not, the parent, rendered unduly anxious by the physician's interest in sensitive areas, may fail to return.

## STRENGTHS AND RESOURCES; PROBLEMS AND VULNERABILITIES

The effective pediatric interview is based on a conceptual scheme, illustrated in Figure 1–1, that permits a balanced integration of (1) biomedical and biosocial considerations; (2) the child, the family and the community; and (3) health and disease. While most pediatric interviews deal with squares D, C and H, the extended interview involves all squares. This clarifying approach permits a comprehensive view of the situation, identifies what needs to be done by whom and the strengths and resources available and permits the patient and the parents to reveal to themselves and to the doctor many positive factors instead of being limited to a recital of their weaknesses and vulnerabilities. This kind of balanced interview helps preserve the patient's self-esteem and promotes his or her active participation and therapeutic alliance.

## BEING FACILITATIVE

There are a number of considerations that permit patients to talk freely. The physical distance between the physician and the patient affects communications. Sitting too close, too far away or behind a large desk may impede openness.

THE SCOPE OF CHILD HEALTH SERVICES

Figure 1–1 The child-, family- and community-oriented record. From Green, M. and Haggerty, R.J. (eds.): Ambulatory Pediatrics II. Philadelphia, W. B. Saunders, 1977, p. 1.

| COMPONENTS OF CHILD HEALTH | CHILD HEALTH CONSTITUENCIES | | |
| --- | --- | --- | --- |
| | CHILD | FAMILY | COMMUNITY |
| STRENGTHS | A | E | I |
| RESOURCES | B | F | J |
| VULNERABILITIES | C | G | K |
| ILLNESS AND PROBLEMS | D | H | L |

Some clinicians are most at ease when interviewing patients from a background similar to their own; others have different preferences. The interview is facilitated if the physician is a warm, friendly, nonjudgmental, responsive and courteous person who sincerely wants to understand the problem. The successful interviewer projects acceptance of the patient through the alertness with which he follows what the patient is saying, his facial expression and the tone of his voice. Optimally, the patient can sense that the physician knows how he feels. The more empathetic the interviewer, the greater the likelihood he can identify and perhaps express for the patient what he is feeling. Empathy is a blend of intuition, a feel for what one's own responses would be in a similar situation and the experience of having listened thoughtfully to large numbers of persons with similar problems.

The physician is a person with special status who is able to promote confidence and rapport. He has knowledge that gives relief, and an understanding of people without a need to moralize, judge or reprove. Although doctors tend sometimes to undervalue the effectiveness of this process, it is therapeutic for the patient to ventilate feelings, to sort out thoughts, to be encouraged and enabled to communicate fears and worries and to discharge feelings with a physician who is interested and listens actively. The physician's capacity to listen and to facilitate the patient's expression of feelings depends on his personal experiences and training. The patient who feels that the doctor understands him will usually share his real concerns and problems. Secure in his relationship with a physician who appears unhurried and personally concerned and in whom he has confidence, the patient is able to bring up and discuss feelings and problems that ordinarily might be embarrassing much more easily than if the physician is perceived as austere, judgmental and impersonal. Since for many patients it is helpful if the physician is not too smoothly articulate, he should avoid giving the impression that he has all the answers. A more tentative, slightly halting approach may overcome the patient's hesitancy in talking. The patient may be helped in bringing up pertinent associations if the physician indicates his understanding by a statement such as, "These things are hard to talk about."

Patients will generally talk freely about their problems if given a chance. If not, it is important to determine why. Is the patient comfortable? Did the interviewer do anything verbally or nonverbally to interfere with rapport? Did the patient come against his own wishes? Is the patient angry, depressed or psychotic? Is the patient reluctant to talk in front of another family member? Is the patient in the process of evaluating the doctor and therefore not ready to talk freely on this initial visit? Is there a basic mismatch between the clinician and this specific patient?

Care needs to be taken lest one pass by the patient who does not comfortably or adequately articulate his problems or feelings or who tends to remain quiet in a family group, especially when the conversation is dominated by someone else. The periods of silence that may occasionally occur during a patient's narrative should not be hurriedly interrupted. The patient may be trying to remember some elusive detail or to verbalize a troublesome experience. If the pause is prolonged and the patient is waiting for a cue, the examiner can say, "Now, you've been telling me about _____. Could you tell me something about _____?" or "Won't you go on?"

An interval between interviews may be helpful in making the patient aware of new associations. At the end of the interview the patient can be asked to think further about some of the things that have been discussed. It may also be suggested that other pertinent ideas will probably come to mind before the next visit.

## INTERVIEWING CHILDREN

The manner in which children are interviewed varies considerably with their age. The doctor introduces himself to the child and may explain what kind of physician he is: "I'm Doctor Smith. I'm a doctor who is interested in helping children." Friendliness helps to put the child at ease. Some pediatricians find casualness useful; others do not. It is best to behave as you feel most comfortable.

Although some children talk more readily than others, getting them to talk generally presents no problem. In talking with a child, the physician should use simple words, but language that a child expects from an adult. Very young children are commonly "interviewed" for a few minutes by informal, casual games that the physician and the child enjoy as a way of getting to know each other. There are no set rules or ideas for this. With young children the interview may be facilitated if a few toys are available, such as a ball, crayons and pad of paper, picture books or a doll and bottle. The older child may be able to add a great deal of factual material to the history and will benefit from being encouraged to talk about himself.

Although it may take some time before adolescent patients bring up their most worrisome problems, they usually discuss their thoughts readily, especially when their parents are not present and confidentiality is assured. The adolescent should be advised that he is free to discuss the interview with his parents but that the doctor will not unless the patient concurs, or the information is so potentially harmful to the patient that the parents need to know. In that event, the doctor will share with the adolescent his intention to do so. If the adolescent denies that there is a problem, it may be that he is angry and offended about coming to see the doctor. Some may be shy, embarrassed and unaccustomed to talking to adults. Others may be depressed or anxious. When the adolescent does not respond, it is generally fruitless to continue the interview beyond a short time. The abbreviated session may be ended graciously with an appointment made to see him again. One might also try a statement such as, "I can appreciate that you weren't wild about coming and that you don't feel there's any reason to be here, but since we have some time, I'd just like to talk with you about how things are going." With this approach one would hope to talk about neutral items that may be of interest to the patient and that may lead to a more open relationship. The interviewer need not feel challenged to make the patient talk, nor should he press about subjects the adolescent obviously at that time has ruled out of bounds.

After the introductory amenities, the physician might ask, "I wonder if you would tell me why you came to see me (or why your parents brought you to see me)?" If the child denies knowing the reason for the referral, the physician might mention what the parents have indicated as the problem or ask what the child thinks this might be. The child who says that he doesn't know can be encouraged to come up with his best guess as to the reason. In seeing an adolescent at his parents' request, it's generally advisable to tell him or her what you have heard the problem to be: "I understand you're having a problem at school. . . ."

When a child does not talk spontaneously, the physician can be more directive.

Topics for discussion with children include members of the family, school experiences, friendships, recreational interests, career aspirations, television programs, heroes and dreams. Other questions might include, "What kinds of things do you do for fun?" "Do you have a special friend?" "How are the other children in your room (neighborhood)?" "What do you and mother (father) do together for fun?" "What would you like to do when you are finished with school?" "Do you think you'll get married?" "Would you like to have children?" "What do you do when someone makes you angry?" "How could I tell that you were angry?" "If you could turn the calendar back, to what date would you turn it?"

In order that the child not feel especially different from others, it may be well to preface some of the questions by a statement such as, "Most girls your age are concerned about _____. I imagine that you may be also." Other topics that may be appropriate to question about include things that make the child angry, sad, worried or happy, and what he does under these circumstances. The question as to three wishes the child would most like to have fulfilled is often very informative of his emotional life. Other suggestions include, "If I had a million dollars, I would _____," or "If I were calling someone long distance, writing a postcard or sending a telegram about my problems, I would say or write _____." Or the doctor might say, "Let's imagine that you're the doctor, and a boy (or girl) your age tells you that he has _____ (the child's symptom). What would you think might be causing his trouble? What do you think would help him?"

## LISTENING TO THE PATIENT

Successful interviews consist mainly of the interviewer's listening with few interruptions or much physical activity. He should talk sparingly. The doctor does not probe, prod, interrogate aggressively or attempt to extract data but rather creates an atmosphere in which the patient is encouraged to talk openly and to be an active participant in the interview.

Although experienced clinicians obviously have a "game plan" for an interview derived from such considerations as the complaint, the purpose of the visit and the characteristics of the patient and his family, they are prepared to make use of unanticipated opportunities as these arise. Flexibility is a key characteristic of the accomplished interviewer. Another is the ability to get the patient to talk about material needed for understanding and management. The patient's narrative may be interrupted to have the patient elaborate upon some detail, to help him go on with the history or to lead the discussion into more productive channels. Pertinent interruptions are not sensed as intrusions but serve to show that the physician is listening carefully and that he is interested in obtaining an accurate understanding of the problem. The interview can continue during the physical examination since patients may talk more freely at this time than before. They may also recall facts that did not come to mind while the main body of the history was being elicited.

In listening to the patient's narrative, especially if the chief complaint seems not to justify the visit, the physician needs to identify the real reason for the patient's coming. Particularly in the case of psychologic complaints, one learns to regard as tentative the history as first given and not to rule out other possibilities by accepting the initial story as complete. The sequence in which the patient presents the problems may reflect his ordering of their importance and may suggest which ones bother him the most. The physician listens for recurrent references, important omissions and association of ideas and events. The patient's first statement and the one at the very end of the interview (when the interview is "over") are of special interest. It is useful to pause at the end of the visit to allow the patient to slip in a phrase such as, "Oh, yes, Doctor, I forgot, but. . . ." Sometimes this is the most useful statement of the entire visit.

## SOME USEFUL QUESTIONS

The parent's or child's narrative may be supplemented by questions phrased to obtain certain specific items of information or to permit a more generalized discussion. For the latter purpose, open-ended or leading questions may be asked that permit more meaningful answers than simply yes or no. Usually, patients with problems want to talk to someone about them. An indication from the physician that he believes such discussion would be helpful in determining the cause of the patient's problems and possibly their solution is usually productive. With the request for information presented in this light, cooperation is usually excellent, and the patient is helped to understand the importance of certain questions.

A number of techniques may be employed to have the patient supply desired additional information: repetition with a changed inflection of a significant word or phrase from the patient's preceding statement; asking "Why do you say that?" in response to a statement; replying to a patient's question with "Why do you ask?" or "How do *you* feel about it?"; and the use of gestures that encourage the patient to go on.

Questions or statements that permit an evaluation of a patient include "How are things going?" "You seem kind of sad today." "How have you felt lately?" "How would you describe yourself (your usual mood) (your feelings)?" "How do others feel toward you?" "How would you describe your father (mother, husband, wife, child)?" "Often our children remind us of someone. Whom does John remind you of?" "Would you tell me what has really been worrying you about your child?" "Why do you think that is?" "What do you think would be helpful?" "That must get you sort of angry." "How do you think all this has affected Bobby?" "Tell me how Johnny spends his day." When one is reviewing the pregnancy or early infancy, the question "Did you have anyone help you during this time?" may provide some information on the mother's concept of her relation to others.

## CLARIFICATION

When it is difficult to determine just what the chief problem is, or the patient is discursive or self-contradictory, it is often appropriate to shift one's posture, scratch one's head or look puzzled and to interject, "You know, I'm a little puzzled about what you consider your main problem to be. . . ." If the patient disclaims an opinion on what the problem is ("I don't know" or "I have no idea"), the physician can encourage a response by a statement such as, "I recognize that you don't know, but since it's been going on some time, I'm sure you've had some notions about it . . . and it would be helpful to know your ideas." When the physician has cause to believe that the child's symptoms are due to parental problems, a properly phrased question may bring out the underlying difficulty that the physician's experience has shown is likely pertinent.

This associative exploration is useful, of course, in the diagnosis of both biomedical and biosocial disorders. If a mother consults a physician because her child is "nervous," the question, "Who else in the family would you say is nervous?" may be productive of much significant information about the mother's or father's "nervousness." The terms "sensitive" or "blue" may be easier for the patient to talk about than "nervous" or "depressed." The physician is interested in the presence of marital conflicts, symptoms or illnesses of the parents and other members of the family (especially those illnesses similar to the patient's), recent deaths in the family and their cause, the father's and mother's employment and who lives in the house. Since the kind of relationship that a parent had with his own parents as a child may color the attitude that he now directs toward the physician, this historical information is often clarifying. Usually it is also important to know the way in which a patient has coped with major vicissitudes in his life: "That must have been a trying time for you. . . . What did you do?"

Since words often carry unintended meanings or inferences, the physician may wish to rephrase an important question several times if he believes that the patient has not understood. It is helpful to know what the parent or child means by terms such as *mental retardation, mental illness, spoiled, nervous, high-strung, slow* and *reasonably well*. The child should be asked what a specific disease or symptom means to him and what he has been told about it. What the parents have been doing about the problem, why they come in now, whose idea it was to come and what they expect the physician to do are pertinent items of information. To a certain extent, knowledge of what the parents expect permits the physician to present his evaluation in a meaningful way. The physician must determine what the patient really wants and whether he is ready to accept help. Obviously the patient's cultural, social, educational and intellectual background conditions his expectations of the physician.

Discretion and tact are indicated when inquiring about matters that the patient may be hesitant to discuss. The pace of the interview, generally set by the interviewer, should not exceed that at which the patient is prepared to move. It is unwise to push the patient to reveal more than he is prepared to disclose; otherwise, the interview is needlessly unsettling. The patient's defenses should be respected. It may be suggested to the patient, however, that further interviews would be helpful in getting to know the child and family better. As rapport develops in subsequent visits, problems may be dealt with more fully.

Secret worries related to the child — such as those about the possibility of malignancy, vulnerability to serious illness, inheritance of familial disorders, ability of a handicapped child to lead a normal life or the possibility of institutionalization — are difficult for parents to bring up. As long as these concerns are conscious, it may be appropriate for them to be brought up by the physician if the parent does not do so. This could be preceded by a statement such as, "I know that many parents in this situation have this sort of question. . . ." The parents may be made more comfortable and feel more "normal" if the physician points out that other persons in a similar situation have like concerns or fears. If patients do not bring out clarifying information when there is a good physician-patient relationship, they are probably not consciously aware of it.

## DEVELOPMENTAL QUESTIONS

Questions about the developmental history of the child, especially during infancy, permit an appraisal of the child's neuromuscular progress. Some estimation of the child's role in the family, parental attitudes and practices and the response of the child to such expectations may be obtained by talking with the parents about breast feeding, sleeping, bowel and bladder training, play, discipline and socialization of the child.

It is important to know about the child's interactions with other children and adults in the home, at school and at play. The parents may make comparisons, favorable or unfavorable, between the patient and other siblings. Their ideas of what constitutes normal progress may be too demanding, while the overprotective mother may be afraid to let her child do more. Parental disagreements about child-rearing practices may be noted. The physician has an interest in housing and sleeping arrangements, separation experiences, parental illness and history of severe illnesses in the child. Questions concerning the father's participation in the family are often productive. Inquiry as to whether the mother has time away from the children or whether she and the father have joint or individual social interests outside the home gives clues as to whether the family members are isolated or the family is one in which the mother never separates from the children. Asking the parent to describe the child's day (a "good" day, a "bad" day) is often informative. Some mothers can give only a poor description of the day or they give a report devoid of personalization or warmth. When a parent has made many statements about how troublesome a child has been, it may be well to ask her what she considers the child's strengths or likeable traits to be.

Questions asked of parents related to the presence of psychologic problems in their children are generally accepted if the doctor is comfortable and not defensive or apologetic in posing them. Some parents are, however, simply not psychologically minded. An opportunity should be provided that makes it relatively easy for parents to ask such questions themselves. Such an invitation may be made during the visit by asking the parents whether they have other questions. If the physician is perceived as a relaxed, understanding and supportive professional, this approach will often be productive of questions about enuresis, anorexia, sleep disturbances, school problems and other difficulties such as marital stress.

## NONVERBAL BEHAVIOR

The physician's observation of the behavior of the patient during the interview and the understanding of such behavior augment the meaning and significance of what is expressed verbally. For the clinician, interviewing is like watching a movie: the message and the feelings transmitted are tremendously enhanced by sight as well as hearing. One not only listens attentively to the words but also observes those nuances of behavior that are communicated through facial expression, gesture and posture. For example, changes in behavior, activity and appearance in patients during the interview may include perspiration; controlled, uneven or blocked speech; blushing or paling; increased prominence of a tic; frequent swallowing movements; tenseness; restlessness and fidgetiness; increased alertness; preoccupation; avoidance of eye contact; and a mendicant posture.

That a second adult other than the father accompanies the mother, e.g., a woman friend or relative, may imply that the mother feels uncertain of her competence, that she is very dependent or that she expects bad news. On the other hand, it may simply be that she is able to turn to friends for support and companionship or that she does not drive. Reddening of the eyes or crying is an indication that the interview has touched upon an experience or feeling of special emotional significance. One can be supportive at this time by waiting, offering some facial tissues, or by quietly remarking that this is a difficult subject to think about or saying, "This seems to upset you." Though it may be helpful in these situations to provide the patient with verbal support or to change the point of discussion, at times it may be desirable to approach a problem more directly. This can be done by a statement such as, "This seems to be bothering you somewhat, and I am wondering if you would like to tell me about it."

## HELPING THE PATIENT FEEL BETTER

Since the doctor's job is to make people feel better, he should take the opportunity, present in every visit, to commend the patient in some way. The physician sees many persons, both children and parents, who have low self-esteem. Such patients may be especially helped by the skillful interviewer. The patient must believe that the physician values him as a person, accepts him with whatever feelings he has and understands him. This feeling of acceptance may permit an otherwise insecure person to function more effectively. Although it may be necessary for the patient to share with the doctor his weaknesses and failures, the discomfort or embarrassment that may be engendered by this recital may be lessened by the nonjudgmental acceptance of an empathetic interviewer who skillfully helps the patient also to identify and report his strengths and successes.

Since physicians generally have high self-esteem, it may be difficult for many to understand those who do not. Such persons are often considered weak or poorly motivated. Mothers who felt positively evaluated by their physicians ("I think he likes me" or "he thinks I'm a good mother") were found to be more compliant in a program for rheumatic fever prophylaxis in children than those who felt negatively evaluated ("the doctor thinks I'm stupid").

The supportive relationship between a skilled physician and his patient that involves the sharing of successes and assets as well as worries, feelings and puzzlements, promotes an understanding of the patient's problems and helps establish a health-promoting bond between doctor and parent or child. Through the interview, this relationship helps to achieve the kind of constructive assessment that leads to a diminution of anxiety. Apart from reassurance, when indicated, active, empathetic listening is often much more important therapeutically than what the physician has to say. Incidentally, explanations to a very anxious person should be brief and touch on one item at a time, because of the patient's difficulty in concentration.

Parents often feel better if they have a diagnosis applied to their child's problem and an idea as to its cause, what can be done and the outlook. This can usually be provided in acute situations. When this is not possible, the parents may think that the doctor is minimizing the problem. On the other hand, direct confrontation of the parents with an interpretation of psychosocial etiologic relationships, even though obvious to the physician, is usually undesirable. Such an approach may arouse further anxiety and give rise to resistance to the interpretation and possibly the failure of the parents to return.

## THE "DIFFICULT" PATIENT

It is well for the physician to have a useful understanding of the dynamics of adult relationships; some knowledge of his own blind spots and prejudices; awareness of those situations that tend to make him anxious, sad or angry; and a sensitivity to those upsetting feelings that may arise within himself during the interview. Understanding the basis for "objectionable" and "inappropriate" patient attitudes or behavior helps the physician to accept the patient and his problem and work productively with those whom he might otherwise find disturbing and frustrating. Thus, the patient's anger may be recognized by the experienced observer as a manifestation of anxiety, cocky self-assurance as a compensation for tense insecurity, and "sweetness and light" as a reflection of hostility. The nonchalance of adolescence may indicate anxiety and not sophistication. Difficult behavior may reflect the patient's previous relationships with authority figures.

There are a number of ways in which the interviewer may respond when a patient is angry, uncooperative, belittling or challenging. "I'm sure that you must be very worried about your child's condition. . . ." Above all, the doctor should not respond with anger, defensiveness or apparent loss of equanimity. The physician who expects from prior information that the patient will be hostile or challenging can frequently disarm the patient at the onset. Rather than permit the patient's anger or antagonism to dominate the interview, the doctor demonstrates immediately that he understands how the patient feels. He can do this by taking the opportunity to make some complimentary or positive remark about how he admires the parent's interest in his child or his conscientiousness and accomplishments as a parent.

## THE "UNRELIABLE" INFORMANT

The history may be unreliable because of the informant's limited memory, intelligence or education. The psychologically disturbed patient may also, unconsciously or consciously, be an unreliable informant, omitting significant details, altering others and resisting efforts of the interviewer to learn additional facts. When the presentation is extremely diffuse, the problem may lie in the patient's anxiety or other psychiatric difficulty. Parents of children who are acutely ill are especially likely, because of their anxiety, to give a confused and often inadequate history. As their anxiety lessens, the accuracy of the history increases. A parent may not give a factual history because he or she is afraid of what the physician will find out or because he or she was referred by the school or other agency against his or her wishes. In the latter event, it is especially difficult to obtain accurate or unbiased information. When the interviewer suspects this, he should clarify the situation by asking how the parent feels about coming to see the doctor.

## SOME PRACTICAL MATTERS

Printed forms are often used for medical history taking. Such forms are undoubtedly helpful in the organization of data important for many diagnoses and, perhaps, in saving time. Their major disadvantage lies in their impersonality. Forms and outlines may be a convenient way for the student to learn the questions necessary for eliciting the history of a pathologic process and for obtaining background information (e.g., dates of immunization), and for review of symptoms. While useful for screening in generally healthy populations (well-child visits or in some acute illnesses), they have definite limitations, however, and may even be antitherapeutic and antidiagnostic in complex and long-term problems. Interviews centered only on data collection have a limited psychotherapeutic effect, with the important exception that they may underline the doctor's interest, competence and thoroughness.

Interviewers differ in their attitudes toward note-taking. In general, it is proper to jot down pertinent dates and names. Too vigorous recording, however, may suppress significant portions of the history, especially if the problem is a psychologic one. In addition, it is difficult both to write and to observe the patient as the story unfolds, and observation may be more important than what is said. If adequate notes are not made during the interview, a summary should be prepared promptly after the session.

## THE LENGTH OF THE INTERVIEW

When the physician has a continuing relationship with a child and a family in health and illness, the interview is a progressive, cumulative process that requires relatively few minutes at any one visit. In other instances, especially in the case of consultations, with new patients, the interview requires more time, depending upon the nature, complexity and duration of the problem. There is no "complete" history, especially the initial one. Rather, the interview is a longitudinal process. In emergency situations and when seeing children who are acutely ill, the interview is limited to data essential for immediate management.

Occasionally, parents do not recognize the diagnostic importance of a thorough history. Believing that by examining the child the physician can find "the answer," they wonder why so much time is taken up with questions and why the physician does not check the child immediately. When one senses this attitude, the initial history should be brief, obtaining just enough information to permit an intelligently directed physical examination. The history may be continued during this time. After completion of the physical examination the parent may then be ready to complete the details of the history.

Adequate time should be permitted for the history, but the interview should be kept within limits that are fruitful. Since the interview is a disciplined, goal-directed process rather than an aimless social discourse, the data obtained must be relevant so that the physician does not waste his time or that of the patient. The physician who does not set time limits tends to depreciate himself and reduces his effectiveness. An excessive amount of time spent with the patient may also promote undesirable dependency.

The interview may be brought to a close by standing, by walking to the door, or by a statement such as, "Well, I guess that our time is up."

## GENERAL REFERENCES

Engel, G.L. and Morgan, W.L., Jr.: *Interviewing the Patient.* Philadelphia, W. B. Saunders Co., 1973.
Korsch, B.M. and Alvey, E.F.: Pediatric interviewing techniques. *Cur. Prob. Pediatr. 3*:3, 1973.
Senn, M.J.E.: The contribution of psychiatry to child health services. *Am. J. Orthopsychiatry 21*:138, 1951.
Senn, M.J.E.: Emotions and symptoms in pediatric practice. *Adv. Pediatr. 3*:69, 1948.
Senn, M.J.E.: The psychotherapeutic role of the pediatrician. *Pediatrics 2*:147, 1948.
Simmons, J.E.: Interviewing. *In* Green, M. and Haggerty, R.J. (eds.): *Ambulatory Pediatrics.* 1st ed. Philadelphia, W. B. Saunders Co., 1968, p. 110.
Simmons, J.E.: *Psychiatric Examination of Children.* 2nd ed. Philadelphia, Lea and Febiger, 1974.

CHAPTER 2

# APPROACH TO THE PEDIATRIC PHYSICAL EXAMINATION

In addition to providing information as to the status of the physical findings, a comprehensive and skillful physical examination provides considerable reassurance for the patient and his family. Parents are favorably impressed by the physician who does a complete physical appraisal and dissatisfied with the doctor whose examination is hurried and incomplete. Once the parents are confident of the thoroughness of the examination, they are able to accept the findings. The infant or the child also senses the physician's confidence and tends to respond with cooperation. To fulfill this role the physician must be highly skilled. There is no substitute for intensive training and practice in order to develop the required self-confidence and competence.

The evaluation begins the moment the physician sees the child and the parents. These initial impressions help direct the subsequent interview and physical examination. These observations are not intended to encourage "snap" diagnoses but rather to explain the ability of the experienced clinician to gather information quickly and to make his time with the patient productive. The diagnostic value of impressions based on inspection is often not fully appreciated by the beginning clinician. Experience in quickly assessing the total picture is of great value in the rapid and accurate formulation of provisional diagnoses and therapeutic possibilities and prognostic outlook to be substantiated, modified or discarded at the completion of more detailed examination, history-taking, laboratory tests and observation of the course of the illness.

The appraisal of the physical and psychologic status of the patient is an important part of this impression. This assessment is largely based on an inspection of the facies, physical development, activity, affect and the behavior that the patient and his parents demonstrate.

Characteristic facies or facial appearance has been described for patients with numerous disorders. Because a number of excellent atlases are available that illustrate and describe a wide variety of facies (see references on pp. 20–21), this edition includes only a few selected photographs (Figs. 2–1 through 2–10).

The position and activity of the patient may be informative. Thus the older child

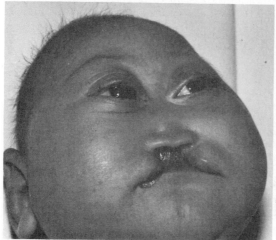

Figure 2–1  Holoprosencephaly.

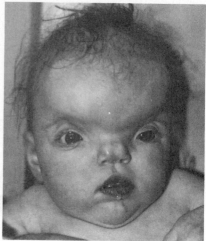

Figure 2–2  Frontonasal dysplasia.

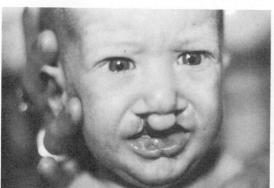

Figure 2–3  Popliteal pterygium syndrome.

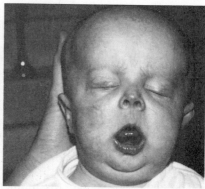

Figure 2–4  Halermann–Streiff syndrome.

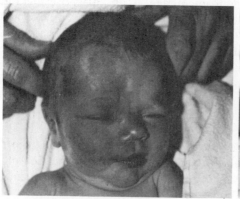

Figure 2–5  Sturge–Weber syndrome.

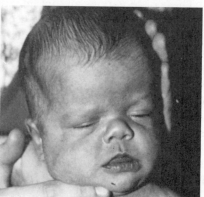

Figure 2–6  Achondroplasia.

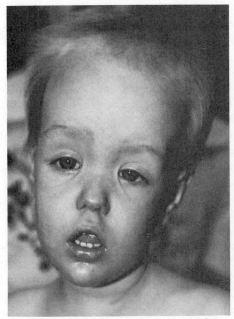

Figure 2–7 Sotos syndrome—cerebral gigantism.

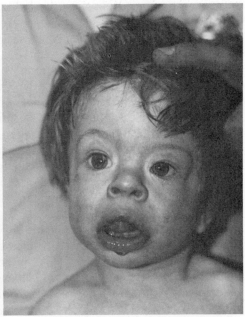

Figure 2–8 Williams syndrome.

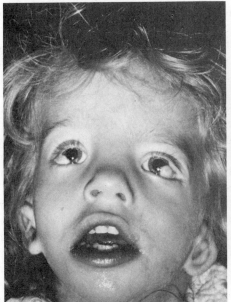

Figure 2–9 Goldenhar syndrome.

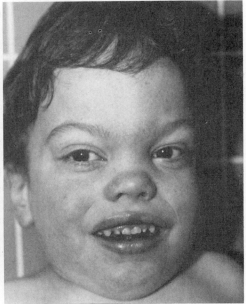

Figure 2–10 Hurler syndrome.

with cardiac failure is observed to be sitting up, not lying down; the child with peritonitis lies quietly and does not thrash about; the child with meningitis may lie on his side with the thighs flexed on the abdomen or in a position of opisthotonus; the patient with postencephalitis sequelae may demonstrate perseveration and hyperactivity. Clinical states apparent on general appraisal that warrant especial emphasis include dehydration, acidosis, sepsis and shock.

To an experienced clinician the following descriptive terms call forth definite mental images: vigorous, alert, cooperative, robust, weak, dull, exhausted, listless, lethargic, acutely ill, chronically ill, seriously ill, apprehensive, fearful, worried, complacent, writhing, comatose, delirious, malnourished, cachectic, moribund, confused, uncooperative, irritable, fretful, sad, prostrate, restless, toxic and unconcerned. One of the most difficult judgments for the student or young physician to make is the severity of a patient's illness. This comes with experience (e.g., the baby who is seriously ill cannot be made to smile).

The experienced clinician has learned to telescope his observations on the basis of experience. Once the physician has become adept and flexible in the procedures and findings of physical diagnosis, he is able to continue the interview while examining the patient, to observe meaningfully the behavior of both parents and child and to determine something about the interpersonal relations between parents and child and their interaction with himself.

The detailed examination of infants and children is no more difficult than that of adults. Their cooperation may be gained by learning and anticipating the reactions and responses of infants and children at various ages and by insight into their emotional development. The physician who is self-confident, enjoys infants and children and is patient will find physical examination in this age group productive and pleasant. The physician who is hurried, annoyed or baffled by these patients, who has many preconceived ideas of how to "handle" children or who has a rigid, disinterested, impersonal or patronizing approach without a capacity to adapt to the individual baby or child may find his experiences fruitless and frustrating.

A friendly, warm, seemingly unhurried and informal attitude should prevail. A few moments spent talking to the parents or becoming acquainted with the child, admiring a bracelet or cowboy boots before beginning the direct examination often prove to be time-saving. It may be helpful to let a child hold or play with a ball or some other small toy during the examination as a way of becoming acquainted. Children should be addressed by their names. If the child is reticent, appears frightened or is irritable, it may be best to proceed with the examination as rapidly as possible and with a more impersonal attitude. Sometimes whispering "secrets" into a child's ear and having the child whisper them back or saying, "You know, I like you," may place the child at ease. The adaptability of the physician to the individual situation will determine to a considerable extent his ability to establish a good relation. Children usually respond positively to those who they sense like them.

Patients should be completely undressed for each examination, with the exception of underpants for older children. The room should, of course, be at a comfortable temperature. Adolescents and some younger children often prefer to be treated with the same modesty as adults, if not more so. A nurse or the mother should be present during the examination of adolescent girls. Sometimes a young child will object to being undressed in the presence of the physician; hence, it is advisable to have this done before the physician enters the room. At times the child will not permit all his clothes to be taken off at once but will not object if the clothing is gradually removed, a piece at a time, as the examination proceeds and his anxiety lessens.

The physical examination should be conditioned by the age of the child. One specifically looks for physical findings that particularly characterize that period. The order of the examination also varies in different age groups. With older children, one may begin with the head, then proceed to the chest and so on. In infants and younger children, however, the order of the examination is adapted to the individual situation. The routine developmental examination of infants should be woven into the physical examination. Questions related to developmental achievements may be most naturally asked at this time.

The physical examination should not require much time since children tend to tire readily and become less cooperative. In making requests during the examination it is sometimes best to make positive statements such as, "Open your mouth, Johnny," rather than "Will you open your mouth for me?" The latter may be an open invitation to negativism.

In general, infants are not apprehensive until seven or eight months of age. Rarely, as early as the fourth month a baby seems to recognize that someone is a stranger and manifests resistance when approached. Actually, most infants enjoy the examination period and smile or babble in response to the physician. After this period, infants often show apprehension, poor cooperation and, occasionally, even terror. At this age, if the child appears timid or about to cry, it is well to begin the examination with the mother holding him. It may be necessary to complete the entire examination with the child held in the mother's arms or lying across her lap. Often the examination of the ears is most easily done with the child sitting on his mother's lap with the mother holding his head against her shoulder with one hand, and the other available to hold his free arm if necessary.

The child who appears friendly and not frightened may be placed on the examining table by the mother or nurse, and the examination begun. Most children, however, feel more secure sitting or standing in preference to lying supine, and as much of the examination as possible should be accomplished with the patient in these positions. Infants who have just learned to sit up often object to being placed supine. This may be avoided if the mother or the nurse, rather than the physician, puts the infant down. If two children in a family are to be examined, the one less likely to cry should be examined first. The physician should avoid looking directly into the face of an infant or young child who looks as if he is about to cry. In these instances the examination is best begun with auscultation of the back of the child's chest while he looks the other way.

Negativism and resistance to examination in young children are normal maturational events. Although such situations may not be frequent, they inevitably occur, no matter how the physician approaches the examination. The hyperactive child may be quiet if the pediatrician talks to him slowly and quietly and rubs his back.

If a child struggles when one begins to remove his clothes or examine him, and if it is not imperative that an examination be done at once, it is well to have the child return at a later date when cooperation may be more readily given. With anxious children, a number of brief "social" visits may be required before one can make much progress. At these times the child may be greeted in a gentle, friendly manner and given a balloon or tongue depressor. These are more unusual instances, of course, and there may be a need to determine why the child demonstrates excessive anxiety and unusual resistance. As they observe that the physician treats the child with understanding and kindness even though he is uncooperative and irritable, the parents may undertake to discuss their child-rearing difficulties constructively with the physician. Especially in the case of the baby who is retarded or who has congenital anomalies, the fact that the doctor holds and "talks" to the baby seems to make his acceptance of the baby and them very real and appears to be a powerful nonverbal communication.

The examiner's hands should always be warm and washed before the physical examination begins and after the examination is completed. Parents watch for this practice, and young children are sometimes intrigued by the soap dispenser. The stethoscope bell or diaphragm should also be warm and clean. It is sometimes well to allow children to become familiar with the diagnostic instruments before they are used. They may scrutinize the stethoscope carefully or try to listen with it.

Before using the otoscope, the physician may ask the child to try to blow out the light, flipping the switch off at the appropriate time. Younger children sometimes enjoy this very much. When it is necessary to darken the room for the ophthalmoscopic examination, the child should be told that the light will be turned out for a moment.

A pacifier may be used in small infants while examining the eyes or to quiet a crying infant so that the abdomen may be examined. Infants and young children who grab for the stethoscope or otoscope when these are being used can be distracted by giving them a tongue depressor for each hand.

One may also distract the child during the examination, especially palpation of the abdomen, by talking quietly with him about his pets, school, home or siblings. Some children cooperate well until the examination of the ears, nose and mouth; hence these often are best left until last. In order to allay apprehension it may be well to act as though this portion of the examination were a game. One may ask the child how many ears he has, pretend to be looking for potatoes in his ears, or jokingly say, "Let's get nosey," as one examines his nose. Of course these tactics depend upon the child; the sophisticated may resent this approach as juvenile. At best, however, examinations of the ears, nose and throat are not pleasant, and the doctor should perform them quickly and with minimal discomfort. Before examining the throat, one may ask to see the patient's teeth. A tongue depressor may then be introduced, and after the examination of the teeth one may say, "Let's look way back there. This will just take a second, then we'll be all through."

It is important to inform the child in a way understandable to him what to expect before any painful or unfamiliar procedure such as a throat swab, blood pressure determination, lumbar puncture, venipuncture or intradermal test, and to answer his questions truthfully. If the procedure is to be painful, he should be told that it will hurt somewhat. It is often helpful to liken a procedure such as an intradermal injection to some familiar sensation such as a mosquito bite. Manual restraint, when necessary, should be applied effectively and with dispatch and the procedure completed promptly and with as little anxiety as possible. The child should be told that the restraint is just to help him hold still until the procedure is completed and that he will be released at that time. Children often repeatedly ask, "All done?" as the physical examination or procedure nears completion. The physician may say, "Almost," or have the child count slowly with him until he is finished, at which time he can announce, "All done!" If a child cries because of anxiety or in response to pain, he should, of course, not be made to feel inadequate or that it is necessary to be the Spartan that the statement "Big boys don't cry" implies.

## GENERAL REFERENCES

Bergsma, D.: *Birth Defects Compendium.* 2nd ed. New York, Alan R. Liss, Inc., 1979.
Gellis, S. and Feingold, M.: *Atlas of Mental Retardation Syndromes – Visual Diagnosis of Facies and Physical Findings.* U.S. Dept. of HEW, Social and Rehabilitation Service, Rehabilitation Services Administration, Division of Mental Retardation, Washington, U.S. Government Printing Office, 1968.

Goodman, R.M. and Gorlin, R.J.: *Atlas of the Face in Genetic Disorders.* St. Louis, C.V. Mosby Co., 1977.
Gorlin, R.J., Pindborg, J.J. and Cohen, M.M., Jr.: *Syndromes of the Head and Neck.* 2nd ed. New York, McGraw-Hill Book Co., 1976.
Hatzilevich, B.: *Mental Retardation: An Atlas of Diseases with Associated Physical Abnormalities.* New York, The Macmillan Co., 1972.
McKusick, V.A.: *Heritable Disorders of Connective Tissue.* 4th ed. St. Louis, C.V. Mosby Co., 1972.
Schaffer, A.J. and Avery, M.E. (eds.): *Diseases of the Newborn.* 4th ed. Philadelphia, W.B. Saunders Co., 1977.
Smith, D.W.: *Recognizable Patterns of Human Malformation.* Philadelphia, W.B. Saunders Co., 1976.
Warkany, J.: *Congenital Malformations:* Chicago, Year Book Medical Publishers, Inc., 1971.

CHAPTER 3

# THE HEAD

## HEAD CONTROL

The head control of a young infant is an early indication of his motor development. When he is raised to a sitting position during the first month of life, the infant's head lags and remains overextended. In the sitting position, his head falls forward, with perhaps an occasional erect bob. In the supine position the infant lies with his head to one side, occasionally raising the side of his face. In the prone position, most newborn infants can transiently raise their heads slightly so that their chin just clears the surface. The head, however, cannot be maintained in the midline.

The *tonic neck attitude* describes the posture of the infant in which the head is turned to one side, the ipsilateral arm is extended and the contralateral arm is flexed. The tonic neck position is observed through the first three months of life but occurs only transiently in the fourth month as the infant begins to maintain his head in the midline.

By the end of the second month, the head can be maintained in the midline for a short time in the prone position and intermittently raised 2 or 3 inches. Toward the end of the third month, the infant begins to hold his head erect, though wobbly and unsteadily, when held in a sitting position. By four months of age, the head is held forward steadily in the sitting position; however, if the head is rotated much, control may disappear. During the fifth month, the position of the head is not disturbed by sudden rotation.

Failure to achieve head control by three months or persistence of the tonic neck attitude after four months is an indication of neuromotor retardation and may be the earliest clinical manifestation of cerebral palsy, other neurologic deficit or mental retardation. Loss of head control may occur in infant botulism.

## CIRCUMFERENCE

During infancy, the head circumference should be routinely measured at its maximum occipitofrontal circumference. In the term infant, the circumference of the head is usually about 2 cm. greater than that of the chest. In the premature infant the difference is even greater. Because of scalp edema or cranial molding, measurement of the circumference of the head may not be accurate until the third or fourth day of life.

## ENLARGEMENT OF THE HEAD (MACROCEPHALY)

The term *macrocephaly* is used when the occipitofrontal circumference exceeds 2.5 cm. above the mean. During the first six months of life, an increase in head circumference exceeding 2 cm./month is a cause of concern.

The differential diagnosis of an enlarged head or megalocephaly includes hydrocephalus, subdural hematoma or fluid, thickened skull and megalocephaly. Cerebral gigantism is characterized by a prominent forehead and a dolichocephalic head.

*Hydrocephalus* is the most frequent cause of macrocephaly. Because the ventricles are already markedly dilated by the time the head circumference is increased, determination of head circumference as a part of well-infant visits will, in itself, not permit early diagnosis of hydrocephalus. For this reason careful attention

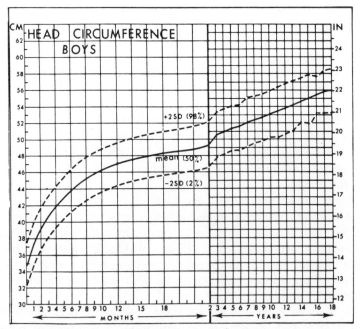

**Figure 3-1** Composite graph for males from birth through 18 years. From Nellhaus, G.: Head circumference from birth to 18 years: practical composite international and interracial graphs. *Pediatrics 41*:106, 1968.

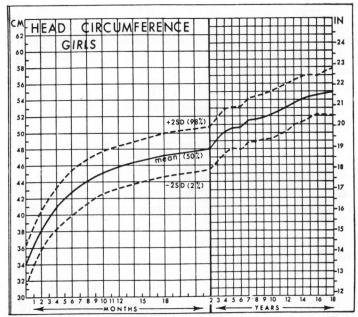

**Figure 3–2** Composite graph for females from birth through 18 years. From Nellhaus, G.: Head circumference from birth to eighteen years: practical composite international and interracial graphs. *Pediatrics 41*:106, 1968.

needs to be given routinely to the fontanels, sutures, skin texture and eye movement. Hydrocephalus may be caused by the following:

I. Noncommunicating hydrocephalus due to blockage within the ventricular system or at the foramina
   A. Congenital anomalies
      1. Atresia, stenosis or obstruction of the aqueduct of Sylvius or foramina of Luschka and Magendie
      2. Arnold-Chiari malformation
      3. Platybasia
      4. Achondroplasia
      5. Dandy-Walker syndrome
   B. Traumatic, due to organization of hemorrhage
      1. Wounds
      2. Hemorrhage associated with birth trauma
   C. Neoplasms – tumors and cysts
   D. Inflammatory
      1. Brain abscess
      2. Postmeningitis
II. Communicating hydrocephalus
   A. Increased production
      1. Hypertrophy or papilloma of the choroid plexus
   B. Decreased absorption
      1. Congenital failure of formation of the subarachnoid space
      2. Traumatic subdural hemorrhage and subarachnoid hemorrhage

    3. Neoplasm – gliomatosis, posterior fossa tumors
    4. Inflammatory
       Bacterial, including tuberculosis; toxoplasmosis; congenital syphilis
    5. Achondroplasia
    6. Intracranial arteriovenous fistula

Raimondi. A.J.: A critical analysis of the clinical diagnosis, management and prognosis of the hydrocephalic child. *Adv. Pediatr. 18*:265, 1971.

Patients with the Dandy-Walker syndrome have a *bulging or prominent occiput* along with hydrocephalus. A prominent occiput also occurs in trisomy 18. A sub-occipital dermal sinus may lead to an intracranial cyst that produces obstruction of the fourth ventricle and hydrocephalus.

*Hydranencephaly* is a rare cause of head enlargement in infants. The meninges and the skull are normal, but the cerebral hemispheres are not developed. The head transilluminates.

*Porencephaly* is a diagnostic consideration in infants with seizures, especially infantile spasms, focal motor deficits or delay in growth and development. Trans-illumination may be possible over the cystic area.

*Transillumination of the skull,* using a flashlight equipped with a narrow cuff of opaque sponge rubber placed around the glass end and firmly applied to the infant's scalp in a darkened room, should be a part of the physical examination of young infants under one year of age. Transillumination is an important screening procedure in infants with macrocephaly and in those suspected of having a sub-dural effusion, subdural hematoma, hydrocephalus, hydranencephaly, porence-phaly or increased intracranial pressure. Translucency that extends beyond 2 to 2.5 cm. in the frontal area or over 1 cm. in the occipital region may be abnormal. Subdural effusions may cause increased transillumination in the frontoparietal area. Suboccipital transillumination may suggest dilatation of the fourth ventricle as in the Dandy-Walker malformation. Transillumination is impaired by the presence of caput succedaneum, cephalohematomas, edema of the scalp, infiltration of scalp vein infusions, thick black hair and lack of dark adaptation by the examiner. Transillumination in hydrocephalus and porencephaly will not occur if the cortex is thicker than 1 cm.

Sjogren, I. and Engsner, G.: Transillumination of the skull in infants and children. *Acta Paediatr. Scand. 61*:426, 1972.

Swick, H.M.. Cunningham, M.D. and Shield, L.K.: Transillumination of the skull in premature infants. *Pediatrics 58*:658, 1976.

*Subdural hematoma* may cause enlargement of the head with or without hydro-cephalus. A posterior fossa subdural hematoma that may rarely occur in newborn infants causes enlargement of the head, respiratory difficulty and bloody cere-brospinal fluid.

*Subdural effusions* may complicate bacterial meningitis.

*Cerebral arachnoid cysts* in young infants produce signs that may suggest a subdural hematoma or hydrocephalus (i.e., excessive size or rate of growth of the head, tense fontanels, widening of sutures, localized bulging of the skull and transilluminability).

Anderson, F.M. and Landing, B.H.: Cerebral arachnoid cysts in infants. *J. Pediatr. 69*:88, 1966.

A rapid increase in head circumference may be the first clinical manifestation of an *intracranial tumor* in infants and young children.

*Premature infants* have heads that appear disproportionately large.

*Thickening of the skull* may be noted in osteopetrosis, osteogenesis imperfecta, orodigitofacial dysostosis, craniometaphyseal dysplasia, epiphyseal dysplasia, pycnodysostosis, leontiasis ossea and progressive diaphyseal dysplasia.

*Megalocephaly* may represent brain growth at the upper limits of normal, a familial pattern, cerebral gigantism or achondroplasia. Metabolic causes include the mucopolysaccharidoses and generalized gangliosidosis. Macrocranium also occurs with neurofibromatosis.

*Caravan's disease* (spongy degeneration of the central nervous system), an autosomal recessive disorder in Ashkenazi Jews, is characterized by megalocephaly in early infancy, developmental slowing and regression, hypotonia and opisthotonic response to auditory, visual and tactile stimuli. *Alexander's disease* is also characterized by enlargement of the head owing to obstruction of the aqueduct of Sylvius, mental retardation, spasticity and seizures.

DeMyer, W.: Megalencephaly in children. *Neurology* 22:634, 1972.

The *Russell dwarf* has a pseudohydrocephalus, that is, a normal-sized head with a dwarfed face and body.

Szalay, G.C.: Pseudohydrocephalus in dwarfs: the Russell dwarf. *J. Pediatr. 63*:622, 1963.

*Mulibrey nanism* is characterized by a pseudohydrocephalus, triangular facies, failure to thrive, prominent veins on the forehead and neck, muscle hypotonia, hepatomegaly, yellow dots on the fundi and constrictive pericarditis.

Perheentupa, J. et al.: Mulibrey nanism, an autosomal recessive syndrome with pericardial constriction. *Lancet 2*:351, 1973.

## MICROCEPHALY

*Microcephaly* is the term applied when the head circumference is two or three standard deviations below the mean for age, sex, height and weight. A small head circumference may reflect impaired brain growth, abnormalities of the skull or a generally small child.

*Cerebral dysgenesis* or *hypoplasia* is often accompanied by microcephaly since failure of brain growth provides a diminished stimulus for skull enlargement. At birth the brain has normally achieved about 25 per cent of its adult volume and at 1 year of age about 75 per cent. In *primary* or *familial microcephaly,* an autosomal recessive disorder, there is a low crown, a receding forehead and flattening of the occiput. Sex-linked microcephaly may be associated with spastic diplegia. *Secondary microcephaly* occurs as a result of trauma or central nervous system disorders. Microcephaly also occurs with these syndromes: incontinentia pigmenti, cri du chat, Cockayne's, Smith-Lemli-Opitz, Wolf-Hirschhorn, Rothmund-Thomson, fetal alcohol, fetal hydantoin and trisomy 13.

*Congenital viral infections* (e.g., cytomegalovirus, rubella and toxoplasmosis) may cause microcephaly.

Hanshaw, J.B.: Cytomegalovirus complement-fixing antibody in microcephaly. *N. Engl. J. Med. 275*:476, 1966.

*Premature synostosis of the sutures* or *craniosynostosis* may cause microcephaly or asymmetry of the head.

Infants with *Down's syndrome* usually have a small, brachycephalic head.

Avery, G.B., Meneses, L. and Lodge, A.: The clinical significance of "measurement microcephaly." *Am. J. Dis. Child. 123:*214, 1972.
Martin, H.P.: Microcephaly and mental retardation. *Am. J. Dis. Child, 119:*128, 1970.

## SKULL DEFECTS

*Craniotabes* refers to thin, parchment-like, soft, mushy areas in the skull that can be indented like a ping-pong ball. These are most common along suture lines and in the parietal bones at the vertex. Craniotabes may be physiologic up to three months of age. When caused by rickets, craniotabes usually does not occur before the third or fourth month of life. Hydrocephalus, syphilis, osteogenesis imperfecta or hypervitaminosis A may also be accompanied by craniotabes. A soft skull occurs in premature infants with hypophosphatasia.

*Lacunar skull* is characterized by thin areas in the skull due to defective formation of the diploë and the inner tables. On palpation these lesions resemble craniotabes. *Craniofenestria,* a defect due to a localized absence of membranous bone in the skull, is accompanied, at times, by herniation of cranial contents. Lacunar skull and craniofenestria usually occur in the parietal bones. Spina bifida is often an accompanying defect.

Enlarged *parietal foramina,* bilateral sharply demarcated, irregular depressions in the posterior portion of the parietal bones along the sagittal sutures, may be large enough to admit the tip of a finger.

*Meningoceles* or *encephaloceles* are rounded, compressible, usually midline tumors. They may also present through a suture line or bony defect elsewhere.

Delayed cranial ossification, large fontanels, widely open suture lines and frontal, parietal and occipital bossing may occur with *cleidocranial dysostosis.* Cranial findings may not be accompanied by abnormality of the clavicles.

## ASYMMETRY OF THE HEAD OR FACE

*Molding* of the skull with some overlapping of the bones during birth commonly causes temporary asymmetry. Normal shape of the head is largely regained by the end of the first week. Molding is not present in infants born by cesarean section or breech extraction.

Small, localized, rounded *depressions* sometimes seen in the frontal and parietal bones at birth are presumably due to abnormal intrauterine pressure associated with unusual fetal posture. These defects disappear during the neonatal period.

*Facial asymmetry* may also result from abnormal intrauterine pressure. A rounded depression may be present under the angle of the jaw on the involved side. Occasionally, this concavity may occur farther anteriorly, or it may extend posteriorly to the ear. When the lips are separated, the alveolar processes on the involved side are seen to touch while those on the other side do not. Usually the asymmetry is minimal and gradually disappears. Infants with breech or face presentations may demonstrate transient facial asymmetry owing to displacement of the mandible.

Cranial changes associated with *familial metaphyseal dysplasia* include diffuse symmetrical hyperostosis of the skull and mandible, hypertelorism and cranial nerve palsies.

Bumps on the head may also be noted with *myositis ossificans progressiva*.

*Fibrous dysplasia* of the facial bones is characterized by a firm painless swelling of bone with considerable asymmetry and deformity of facial structures. The bones most commonly involved include the maxilla, zygoma, mandible and calvarium. The orbits and teeth may be displaced.

Infants who lie predominantly in one position may have *flattening of the occiput*. Such flattening during the latter half of the first year suggests that the infant is not held often or that he is retarded. There is a high association between flattening of the head and maldevelopment of the brain. Infants with hydrocephalus are also prone to occipital flattening.

While an asymmetrical enlargement of the skull may suggest a cystic lesion on the enlarged side or an atrophic or malformed cerebral hemisphere on the smaller side, an etiologic diagnosis cannot be established by inspection. Such asymmetry may be especially evident when looking down on the top of the infant's head from above.

*Torticollis* that is permitted to exist over a period of years causes severe asymmetry of the head and face. Facial asymmetry may also occur in children with premature synostosis of the cranial sutures.


## FONTANELS

Since overriding of the sutures may be present immediately after delivery, the anterior fontanel may appear barely open. A few days later, after normal separation of the sutures has occurred, the anterior fontanel has a diameter of about 2.5 cm. on the average and in some infants as much as 4 to 5 cm. The anterior fontanel may normally enlarge somewhat in the first months of life. The posterior fontanel may remain palpable for four to eight weeks.

There is a wide range of normal variability in the shape, size and time of closure of the anterior fontanel. Closure ranges between 4 and 26 months of age. Ninety per cent close between the ages of 7 and 19 months, 2.7 per cent close by 6 months, 13.5 per cent by 9 months, and 41.6 per cent by the end of the first year. If head growth is proceeding normally and there is no ridging of the sutures, early closure of the fontanel should cause no concern. In prematures and other infants with delayed ossification of the membranous bones the anterior fontanel may be large, and the sagittal suture may extend almost to the base of the nose. The slight depression that may be present for a time after closure of the anterior fontanel is not to be confused with a sunken or open fontanel.

*Delayed closure* or a large open anterior fontanel is observed with rickets, hydrocephalus, syphilis, congenital hypothyroidism, osteogenesis imperfecta, Down's syndrome, cleidocranial dysostosis, mucopolysaccharidoses, achondroplasia, Apert's syndrome, hypophosphatasia, pycnodysostosis, Hallermann-Streiff syndrome, malnutrition, progeria, congenital rubella, Russell-Silver syndrome, trisomy 13 and trisomy 18.

Popich, G.A. and Smith, D.W.: Fontanels: range of normal size. *J. Pediatr.* 80:749, 1972.

An unusually *small fontanel* may occur in infants with slow brain growth and with craniosynostosis.

Though a slight depression of the fontanel is often present in normal infants, a *sunken fontanel* is an important sign of dehydration.

On palpation, the anterior fontanel is slightly depressed relative to the frontal and parietal bones. With crying the fontanel bulges but remains pulsatile. Such normal fullness is to be differentiated from true bulging, a sign of great clinical importance. Pulsation of the anterior fontanel occurs in normal infants held upright. In the hydrocephalic infant the anterior fontanel is usually not visibly pulsatile and almost always bulges.

On the first day of life, bulging may be due to extensive intracranial hemorrhage. Bulging that first appears on the third or fourth day is more likely due to meningitis than to intracranial hemorrhage. *A bulging fontanel in an infant should always suggest meningitis* and may be the only early physical indication of that infectious process. The meningeal signs present in older children are usually not present in infants.

Subdural hematoma, intracranial tumors and other space-occupying lesions may cause bulging of the fontanel. This physical finding is also noted with vitamin A poisoning, hypophosphatasia and pseudohypophosphatasia. A bulging fontanel and jaundice in a young infant should suggest galactosemia. Transient, unexplained, benign bulging of the fontanel may also occur in some normal infants. Rarely, this finding occurs with roseola infantum.

Huttenlocher, P.R., Hillman, R.E. and Hsia, Y.E.: Pseudotumor cerebri in galactosemia. *J. Pediatr. 76*:902, 1970.

## SUTURES

Sutures are fibrous septa between the cranial membranous bones. With the separation of these bones, which may overlap in the newborn infant, the sutures may be as much as one-fourth inch in width. Although suture lines are normally not palpable after the fifth or sixth month, final closure does not occur until early adult life except for the metopic suture that fuses in the early neonatal period.

During infancy, growth of the cranial bones occurs predominantly at their borders. Interference with such growth, as occurs with premature synostosis of the sutures, seriously hampers normal enlargement of the cranial vault. The most rapid growth of the brain occurs during the first two years of life. If closure of the sutures occurs during this time, compression of the brain and blindness will occur unless decompression is accomplished early. Craniostenosis may occur in some infants with the severe form of idiopathic hypercalcemia and with phenylketonuria, hypophosphatasia, rickets and thyrotoxicosis.

Johnsonbaugh, R.E., Bryan, R.N., Hierlwimmer, U.R. and Georges, L.P.: Premature craniosynostosis: a common complication of juvenile thyrotoxicosis. *J. Pediatr. 93*:188, 1978.

*Premature synostosis of the sutures or craniosynostosis* may lead to cranial distortions. A palpable ridge along a suture line occurs in all premature metopic closures, most sagittal closures and some unilateral or bilateral coronal closures. Such a ridge may also be present along the sagittal and metopic sutures in normal infants.

While craniosynostosis of the coronal suture compromises cranial growth in the anterior-posterior plane, it continues along the sagittal and, sometimes, the lambdoid sutures. The result is widening of the head, shortening of the anteroposterior diameter and, at times, a smaller than normal circumference. Other congenital anomalies, especially choanal atresia, are often present. With synostosis of the coronal, lambdoid and sagittal sutures, growth occurs only in the region of the anterior fontanel, resulting in a rounded pointing of the skull (oxycephaly, acrocephaly or tower skull). Unilateral synostosis of the coronal suture produces cranial asymmetry (plagiocephaly). With craniosynostosis of the sagittal suture, continued growth at the coronal and lambdoid sutures leads to an elongated, narrow head (scaphocephaly), which simulates an inverted boat. Premature or prenatal closure of the metopic suture between the frontal bones produces a prominent keel-shaped forehead (trigonocephaly). While such closure usually occurs alone, it may be associated with arhinencephaly. The anterior fontanel may be open even with premature closure of the metopic, sagittal or coronal sutures.

*Cranial dysostosis,* or *Crouzon's disease,* is characterized by oxycephaly, exophthalmos, exotropia, optic atrophy, a beak-shaped nose and protrusion of the mandible.

*Carpenter's syndrome* is characterized by acrocephaly, brachysyndactyly of the fingers, polydactyly and syndactyly of the toes and mental retardation.

Temtamy, S.A.: Carpenter's syndrome: acrocephalopolysyndactyly. An autosomal recessive syndrome. *J. Pediatr.* 69:111, 1966.

*Apert's syndrome* is characterized by flattening of the occiput and prominence of the forehead due to premature closure of the coronal sutures. Hypertelorism and ocular proptosis may also be noted. Marked syndactyly results in a "mitten" hand or "sock" foot.

Shillito, J., Jr. and Matson, D.D.: Craniosynostosis: a review of 519 surgical patients. *Pediatrics* 41:829, 1968.
Stewart, R.E.: Craniofacial malformations. Clinical and genetic considerations. *Pediatr. Clin. N. Am.* 25:485, 1978.

*Separation or widening of the sutures.* Because the sutures are not fused in infants and children, enlargement of the head due to hydrocephalus or space-occupying lesions may readily occur. Abnormal separation of the sutures can sometimes be detected by palpation. In infants with hydrocephalus, the sequence of splitting of the sutures is first the superior portion of the coronal sutures, then the sagittal suture from the anterior to the posterior fontanel and, finally, the lambdoid sutures. With such spontaneous decompression, other signs of increased intracranial pressure either disappear or are delayed. Separation of the sutures is frequent in patients with subtentorial tumors. In *cleidocranial dysostosis,* the sutures are wide and contain numerous wormian bones.

## ADDITIONAL CRANIAL FINDINGS

Cranial *bossing,* characterized by rounded prominences in the center of the parietal and frontal bones, occurs with rickets. Since the manifestations of rickets occur in actively growing bone and the head is the most rapidly growing part of the body in the first months of life, the earliest manifestations of rickets appear there. Bossing may also occur with congenital syphilis, cleidocranial dysostosis, pycnodysostosis, the fetal face syndrome, generalized gangliosidosis type I, Lowe's syndrome and hypohidrotic ectodermal dysplasia.

A *prominent forehead* occurs in patients with chondrodystrophy, mucopolysac-charidosis, craniofacial dysostosis, Laron's dwarfism, congenital ectodermal dys-plasia and Goldenhar's, Ehlers-Danlos, Williams elfin facies, nevoid basal cell car-cinoma, frontodigital, Pfeiffer's and Larsen's syndromes.

*Osteomas* may rarely arise in the membranous skull. Small cartilaginous exos-toses may appear at the base of the skull. Ectopic cartilage may also cause a parietal protuberance between the mastoid process and the occiput.

*Nodding of the head,* either up and down or side to side, once or twice a second, along with nystagmus occurs with *spasmus nutans.* Nodding may be greater in the sitting than in the supine position. In older children transient periods of head nodding or drooping may be a manifestation of petit mal epilepsy. Head nodding may also occur in infants with *ocular albinism.* Poor head control, nodding and cog-wheel nystagmus occurs in *Pelizaeus-Merzbacher disease.* Head banging, head nodding and other periodic movements may occur in emotionally deprived and retarded infants and in some normal children.

*Head bobbing* in infants may be a sign of respiratory distress. The infant's head, supported by his mother's forearm, bobs forward with each inspiration. *The bobble-head doll syndrome,* characterized by an unusual to-and-fro tremor of the head similar to the continuous bob seen in dolls with weighted heads set on a coiled spring, occurs in patients with hydrocephalus secondary to a cyst or other lesion in the region of the third ventricle. Rhythmic oscillation of the head and trunk occurs from side to side or up and down. The head bobbling does not occur during sleep and can be stopped voluntarily.

Russman, B.S., Tucker, S.H. and Schut, L.: Slow tremor and macrocephaly: expanded version of the bobble-head doll syndrome. *J. Pediatr. 87*:63, 1975.

Auscultation over the orbits and skull is indicated when an intracranial an-eurysm is suspected. An *intracranial bruit* occurs in 10 to 15 per cent of normal children, especially in the temporal area. Infants and young children with purulent meningitis have cranial bruits that may persist for one to four days after initiation of treatment. Recurrence of a bruit on the third to sixth day in a child with men-ingitis suggests a subdural effusion. Other conditions associated with bruits in-clude fever, increased intracranial pressure, anemia, thyrotoxicosis and loud car-diac murmurs.

Mace, J.W., Peters, E.R. and Mathies, A.W., Jr.: Cranial bruits in purulent meningitis in childhood. *N. Engl. J. Med. 278*:1420, 1968.

*Macewen's sign,* a "cracked-pot" sound on percussion of the skull, may be present with hydrocephalus, increased intracranial pressure or spreading of the sutures. It is also simulated in many normal infants.

*Osteomyelitis of the frontal bone* is characterized by local pain, increasing edema, especially of the upper eyelid on the involved side, and systemic toxicity.

## HEAD INJURIES

Head injuries are discussed on page 440.

The internal table of the infant's skull is largely absent at birth except frontally in the region of the sinuses. The remainder of the inner table is formed by about two years of age. Because of this, *skull fractures* in infants are usually linear, not comminuted, and do not produce depressions of the inner table as in older children. Depressed skull fractures involve only the external table in infants.

During cranial growth, osseous remolding takes place with bony resorption occurring in the center of the frontal, parietal and occipital bones. The dural attachments in these areas are relatively weak, and potential spaces exist for an *extradural hematoma*. If the ruptured vessel responsible for an extradural hematoma is not large and if the child's skull can expand to some extent, a latent period may occur before neurologic symptoms or signs of increased intracranial pressure appear. The child's condition may then rapidly deteriorate. Epidural hematomas, which may be caused by a fall from a highchair, are frequently associated with mildly depressed skull fractures; on the other hand, no fracture may be detected. Local swelling of the scalp is the most common finding, followed by hemiparesis and stupor. Persistent restlessness, irritability or pallor in a young child after a closed head injury is a source of concern.

*Cephalohematoma* is due to a subperiosteal collection of blood over one or more of the flat bones of the skull secondary to separation of the periosteum from the underlying bone. Since the periosteum is bound down at the edges of these bones, the swelling, unlike that of caput succedaneum, is limited by the edges of the affected bone and does not cross suture lines. At birth, a developing hematoma may be obscured by an overlying caput succedaneum and may not become apparent until the second day with maximal size usually reached by the third day. Involvement is usually unilateral but may be bilateral. The parietal bone is most commonly affected, but the occipital bone may also be involved. The swelling usually disappears by the third or sixth week. Since the elevated periosteum may produce new bone rapidly around the edge of the hematoma and occasionally over the clot, eggshell crepitation over the area may be noted after a few weeks. A peripheral ridge or parietal bossing may persist for months. An underlying skull fracture may be present, especially with bilateral cephalohematomas. Repeat skull roentgenograms should be obtained four to six weeks and three to four months after a skull fracture. If the fracture line has widened, a leptomeningeal cyst ("growing skull fracture") should be considered.

Rothman, L., Rose, J.S., Laster, D.W. and Tenner, M.: The spectrum of growing skull fracture in children. *Pediatrics* 57:26, 1976.

## SCALP

A *scalp abscess* at the site of electrode application may occur secondary to prolonged fetal heart rate monitoring.

*Caput succedaneum* is a diffuse, soft, boggy swelling of the scalp that usually disappears by the end of the first day or so. Ecchymoses and petechial hemorrhages may be noted over the involved area.

In infants with *hydrocephalus,* the skin of the scalp is thin and shiny, and the scalp veins are distended.

*Seborrheic dermatitis* or *cradle cap* may cause moist, greasy, dirty yellow scales and crusts in the scalp. Psoriasis, which may begin in the scalp, requires differentiation from seborrhea.

The occipital area may be bald in infants who lie chiefly in the supine position and in patients confined to bed for long periods of time. Localized loss of hair is also noted in young children with persistent head banging.

A localized, coin-sized congenital *absence of scalp* covered by a thin epithelial membrane or a serosanguineous exudate may occur, especially at the vertex. The defect heals with an atrophic, scarred area of alopecia. Pressure necrosis of the scalp over the parietal prominences may also occur in newborn infants. Scalp defects are present in trisomy 13 and in the Wolf-Hirschhorn and the focal dermal hypoplasia syndromes.

Absence of pigmentation of the skin over the forehead and of a triangular area of hair in the midfrontal portion of the scalp may be accompanied by white skin spotting. A *white forelock* may be noted in Waardenburg's syndrome.

## HAIR

The *hair of premature infants* is fine and wooly and occurs in bunches while that in term infants is silky, lies flat, occurs in single strands and is often long and dark. The hair present at birth is usually lost by four to six weeks of age and then gradually regrows.

In *congenital ectodermal dysplasia* the hair may be absent or scant and light brown and the underlying scalp shiny and smooth. Infants with hypothyroidism may have dry, thin, lusterless, brittle and coarse hair, which extends low on their forehead. In chronic idiopathic hypoparathyroidism, the hair of the scalp, eyebrows and eyelashes may be thin, patchy and coarse. Hyperthyroidism may rarely cause loss of scalp hair. In malnourished children the hair may be dry and gray.

*Progeria* is characterized by fine hair that later may be entirely lost. Abnormally fine, silky, sparse hair and short-limbed dwarfism occur in the *cartilage-hair hypoplasia syndrome*. The hair breaks off easily, and baldness may occur. Pigmentation of the hair does not occur in children with albinism. Thinning or loss of the hair, especially in the frontoparietal area, may occur in congenital syphilis. Vitamin A poisoning may also cause sparse hair.

*Fragility* and beading of the hair, the latter noted on microscopic examination, may occur in patients with *trichorrhexis nodosa* and with *monilethrix*. The former, which is the most common type of hair shaft anomaly and characterized by longitudinal splintering of the hair shaft (''paint-brush'' hair), has been attributed to unusual dryness of the hair caused by too frequent shampooing and excessive combing and brushing. With proximal trichorrhexis nodosa, which occurs only in black children, the hair is extremely fragile and will not grow more than a few centimeters in length. In monilethrix, usually a familial disease, the hair is a beaded, sparse and short stubble. *Keratosis pilaris,* with horny follicular papules, is present over the upper back and shoulders in these patients. *Pili torti* or *twisted hairs* also causes sparse scalp hair. Alopecia is evident, especially over the occiput, by two or three years of age. On microscopic examination, the hairs are noted to be twisted through 180 degrees at irregular intervals along the long axis. They are also short, broken, dull and sparse and shimmer in reflected light. Other ectodermal defects and sensorineural hearing loss may be present. *Bamboo hair* is associated with ichthyosiform skin changes and an atopic diathesis.

*Kinky hair disease,* which occurs in boys as the clinical expression of a sex-linked recessive trait, is characterized by stubby, white, kinky hair (pili torti) and seizures, especially myoclonic jerks. Hypothermia, susceptibility to infection, failure to thrive, drowsiness and lethargy may be presenting symptoms. In the newborn infant with this disorder the hair may appear normal.

Danks, D.M. et al.: Menkes's kinky hair syndrome. An inherited defect in copper absorption with widespread effects. *Pediatrics 50*:188, 1972.

*Unruly scalp hair,* which tends to stand up persistently over the top of the head, occurs in about 2 per cent of normal infants but more commonly with microcephaly.

Smith, D.W. and Greely, M.J.: Unruly scalp hair in infancy; its nature and relevance to problems of brain morphogenesis. *Pediatrics 61*:783, 1978.

*Pili annulati* ("spangled" hair), characterized by alternating dark and light bands, also shimmers in reflected light.

Argininosuccinicaciduria, an inborn error of metabolism, is characterized by brittle hair (trichorrhexis nodosa), seizures, ataxia and mental retardation.

The scalp hair in patients with *homocystinuria* is fine, fair, friable and easily removed by brushing.

*Alopecia* may follow a severe infectious disease or malnutrition. Congenital alopecia may be complete, patchy or characterized by diffuse hypotrichosis. Loss of hair occasionally occurs in hypothyroid infants after the initiation of thyroid therapy. *Trichotillomania,* in which the child pulls out and perhaps swallows his hair, may lead to partial alopecia. The eyebrows, eyelashes and the parts of the scalp, especially the crown and occipital areas, within ready reach of the dominant hand are most commonly involved. Twirling causes the hairs to be broken off close to the scalp so that the hair follicles appear as black dots. Occasionally, the involved areas appear circular and devoid of hair. When multiple areas are involved, trichotillomania may be confused with alopecia areata.

Muller, S.A. and Winkelmann, R.K.: Trichotillomania. *Arch. Dermatol. 105*:535, 1972.

*Alopecia areata* is characterized by a sudden loss of hair, perhaps overnight, leaving round, well-demarcated patches of smooth white scalp. "Exclamation point" hairs, colorless and thin at their roots, may occur at the border of these patches. With peripheral extension of these areas the entire scalp may become bald (alopecia totalis). Pitting and ridging of the nails may also occur.

Traction on the hair, usually from pony tails, braids or barrettes, may cause erythema, follicular pustules and alopecia.

Alopecia with loss of hair from the scalp, eyebrows and eyelashes occurs one to two weeks after ingestion of thallium. Ataxia or tremors may precede or accompany the hair loss.

In *hypohidrotic ectodermal dysplasia* the scalp hair is fine, stiff, short and blond.

Alopecia of the scalp, eyebrows and eyelashes occurs in *acrodermatitis enteropathica* along with vesicular and pustular dermatitis around the mucocutaneous orifices and on the extremities. Alopecia may accompany rickets.

Rosen, J.F., Fleischman, A.R., Finberg, L., Hamstra, B.S. and DeLuca, H.F.: Rickets with alopecia: an inborn error of vitamin D metabolism. *J. Pediatr. 94*:729, 1979.

Hypotrichosis involving the scalp (bald spots), eyelashes and eyebrows occurs in the Hallermann-Streiff syndrome.

*Tinea capitis, or ringworm of the scalp,* is characterized by bald, discrete, slightly inflamed, rounded, scaling patches of hair loss, ½ to 2 inches in diameter. Usually, several patches are present. Hairs are broken off close to the scalp. Involved areas may become erythematous, scaly, edematous, crusted and pruritic. Purulent folliculitis may develop. Examination with a Wood's light usually produces a green fluorescence over the lesions, but there are some types of tinea capitis that are unaccompanied by inflammatory changes and do not fluoresce with the Wood's light. Hair loss may also be patchy.

In patients with *pediculosis,* the patient complains of pruritis. A large number of ova or "nits," the size of a small grain of sand and firmly attached to the hair, occur especially near the scalp. Tiny lice may also be seen moving about. Suboccipital and postauricular adenopathy may develop.

*Hair casts,* which may be mistaken for the nits of pediculosis unless microscopic confirmation is used, are shiny, white, firm cylinders, 2 to 7 mm. in length, that encircle and can be moved along the scalp hairs.

In patients with an abnormally short neck caused by the Klippel-Feil syndrome or other anomaly, the scalp hair appears to extend far down on the neck posteriorly.

A tongue-shaped growth of hair may extend downward on the cheek in mandibulofacial dysostosis.

Orentreich, N.: Disorders of the hair and scalp. *Pediatr. Clin. N. Am. 18:*953, 1971.
Price, V.H.: Disorders of the hair in children. *Pediatr. Clin. N. Am. 25:*305, 1978.

*Subcutaneous nodules* may occur over the scalp, especially in the occipital area, with rheumatic fever or rheumatoid arthritis. The lesions of chickenpox, lymphosarcoma, eosinophilic granuloma and xanthomatosis may also occur in the scalp. The swelling associated with eosinophilic granuloma may be painful. Monilial infection of the scalp may cause keratinous horns.

*Dermoid tumors* of the scalp may occur over the bridge of the nose, along the midline of the head or in the occipital areas.

*Distention of the scalp veins* may occur secondary to hydrocephalus or other cause of increased intracranial pressure in infants. Distended scalp veins may also be noted with neonatal copper deficiency.

# CHAPTER 4

# THE EYES

In premature infants exposed to oxygen the possible occurrence of retinopathy of prematurity makes routine ophthalmologic examination mandatory.

As a screening procedure, the evaluation of the newborn infant should always include an examination for the *red reflex*. Using the "O" ophthalmoscopic lens from a distance of about 10 inches, the examiner focuses the light upon the infant's pupil. In white infants the pupillary area is seen as a bright orange-red circle. In black infants the reflex may be yellow-orange in color. The presence of a normal red reflex indicates that the lens is clear. If the reflex is not clearly seen, the pupils should be dilated and the eyes re-examined.

Newborn infants usually resist separation of their eyelids. Examination for a red reflex may therefore be delayed until the infant spontaneously opens his eyes.

## DEVELOPMENT OF VISION

In premature infants the eyes are closed most of the time. Occasionally one or both eyes may be transiently and partially or completely open. Newborn infants respond to the flashing of a bright light by frowning, blinking and by other withdrawal reactions. Their eyes may move about but do not fixate at this time. Larger premature infants are able to follow a dangling ring through an arc of 45 degrees.

The newborn term infant is able to differentiate between light and darkness. Pupillary contraction, blinking of the eyelids and contraction of the orbicularis muscle occur in response to the flashing of a bright light. A pupillary light reflex indicates that the peripheral visual apparatus is probably functional and that the infant has some vision unless cortical blindness is present. Thrusting one's hand toward the baby's eyes to elicit blinking is unreliable as a test of vision. A red ball or the examiner's face serves as a useful visual stimulus for newborn infants, especially if the baby is in an alert state and the room is not too brightly lighted.

A *fixation* reflex, in which a baby will instinctively look at a light, is present shortly after birth. During the early weeks of life the eyes move about with no particular fixation or evidence of perception. Occasional pauses do occur, however, during which the infant stares at a wall, a window or other source of light. He may transiently open one or both eyes but spends most of the time sleeping. In response to a visual stimulus the infant may demonstrate monocular fixation and generalized diminution of bodily activity as if giving almost total attention to the stimulus. Monocular fixation for near objects continues until about 16 weeks of age. The nonfixating eye may be kept closed, partially open or moving about. By the fourth week of life the infant is able to follow a dangling ring through a 90-degree arc.

It is not until the fifth or sixth week that an infant begins to be capable of binocular fixation. For the next three or four months the power of fusion is so weak that deviations from parallelism are frequent. By the fifth or sixth month a moderate degree of binocular fixation has developed. Convergence ability begins during the second month. At first, convergence is jerky and poorly coordinated. Similar incoordination of eye movements exists when moving objects are followed.

During the third and fourth months convergence and ocular following movements are comparatively well done. This increased coordination and visual acuity are due both to progression in neuromuscular control of the ocular muscles and to the more complete development of the macula during the third month. At three or four months of age the infant can perceive a small pellet. With attainment of improved head control at this time the infant is able to follow his mother as she moves about the room. Babies of this age also enjoy looking at their hands. At 12 weeks of age a dangling ring will be followed through an arc of 180 degrees. Some perception of colors may also begin by about four months. Between five and six months true coordination of eyes and hands begins to appear.

The eyeballs of most infants are relatively shorter in their anteroposterior diameter than is the case later. Thus, most infants have hyperopia, possibly of several diopters. Hyperopia in older children is usually due to an abnormally short longitudinal axis of the eye. The eye may attempt to compensate for this refractive error through accommodation. Overactivity of the internal rectus muscle may, however, occur with the development of a convergent strabismus. The normal lengthening of the anteroposterior diameter of the eye that occurs with growth accounts for the appearance or increase in myopia in some children. The eyes in infancy are relatively large compared with other facial features. As growth of the head proceeds, the eyes appear less prominent.

## VISUAL ACUITY

Visual acuity in the newborn is approximately 20/700. At four months of age it is about 20/200. Between 1 and 2 years it is 20/100 and at 3 years about 20/50. Since macular development is not complete until 6 or 7 years of age, a visual acuity of 20/30 or 20/40 as determined by the Snellen test charts may be considered normal at the age of 4 or 5 years. 20/20 vision is not usually developed until the age of 5 or 6.

Impairment of vision is usually due to a refractive error, most frequently myopia. In evaluating the vision of the young infant the examiner checks his pupillary light reaction, whether blinking occurs in response to a bright light, whether the infant fixes monocularly or binocularly and whether he follows a bright object or light.

In the infant suspected of blindness, the presence of vision may be demonstrated by a positive response (optokinetic nystagmus) to black and white stripes on a moving drum, that is, eye movement in the direction in which the stripes are moved followed by jerky movements back to the original fixation point.

Under the age of two to four years the determination of visual acuity in a child may be difficult without actual refraction unless the examiner determines the ability of the child to recognize standard objects such as white marbles of various sizes placed at standard distances in the examining room. At a distance of 18 to 20 feet recognition of a marble 1½ inches in diameter indicates a visual acuity of 20/200 and 1¾ inch in diameter corresponds to an acuity of 20/80. Recognition of a dime at a distance of 5 feet is consistent with at least 20/50 vision.

When the child has not learned to recognize the letters of the regular Snellen chart, the modified or illiterate Snellen chart, which has the letter "E" printed with the bars up or down and to the right or left, is used. The child is instructed to duplicate with his fingers the direction in which the bars of the "E" point. Testing of children with the illiterate Snellen "E" chart can usually be successfully accomplished by the age of three or four years and is an essential part of the general physical assessment at that time to detect myopia and amblyopia at an age when treatment may still be effective.

The use of the Snellen test charts alone, however, has limitations. Though myopia and amblyopia may be detected, hyperopia and strabismus, latent or manifest, may be overlooked. The first part of the Massachusetts screening test for visual testing in children uses a Snellen type of chart. Although the 20/20 line was originally recommended, the test may be more helpful in the 6- to 8-year-old child if inability to read correctly 4 of the 6 symbols on the 20/30 line is used as the basis for ophthalmologic referral. The following levels of visual acuity may be used as an indication for ophthalmologic referral: 20/50 or less in a 3 year old; 20/40 or less in 4 and 5 year olds; children who show one or more line difference in visual acuity between the 2 eyes; and 20/30 for children in the fourth grade and above. The second portion of the test screens for hyperopia. With a plus 1.50 lens placed before each eye, the ability to read the 20/20 or the 20/30 line with each eye is regarded as an indication for referral. Since some degree of hyperopia is normal in children, The National Society for the Prevention of Blindness recommends that a plus 2.25 sphere be used in children in the first 3 grades and a plus 1.75 for those in the fourth grade and above.

The Allen Picture Cards, the Sjögren Hand and the Titmus Screener are all reliable visual acuity tests. The Titmus stereo tester with Polaroid glasses may be used for determination of stereopsis. The Polaroid Fly Test may be used for binocular awareness at near vision.

In addition to referrals made on the basis of these screening tests, children with headache and ocular pain should receive an ophthalmologic examination with refraction unless the complaints are attributable to causes other than eyestrain.

Lin-Fu, J.S.: *Vision Screening of Children.* U.S. Dept. of HEW, Public Health Service Publication No. 2042, Washington, U.S. Government Printing Office, 1971.

Color vision may also be checked by simple charts. The incidence of benign red/green color blindness is 0.5 per cent in girls and 8 per cent in boys.

## IMPAIRED VISION

Developmental retardation and aberration may be caused by defective vision in infants. Motor development, especially for activities such as rolling over and sitting that require orientation in space, may be retarded in infants who are blind or severely myopic. Babies with impaired vision may demonstrate nystagmoid movements of the eyes and rub their eyes excessively.

*Hysterical amblyopia* may occur in children. In these children, the visual fields are constricted and tubular. *Acute cerebral blindness,* characterized by loss of vision, normal pupillary reflexes and absence of ophthalmologic disease, may be a complication of meningitis, head trauma, uremia, hypoxia, hydrocephalus, seizures and cardiac arrest. Recovery of vision occurs rapidly after head trauma but less rapidly with other disorders.

Barnet, A.B., Manson, J.I. and Wilner, E.: Acute cerebral blindness in children. *Neurology 20*:1147, 1970.
Griffith, J.F. and Dodge, P.R.: Transient blindness following head injury in children. *N. Engl. J. Med., 278*:648, 1968.
Tepperberg, J., Nussbaum, E. and Feldman, F.: Cortical blindness following meningitis due to Hemophilus influenzae type B. *J. Pediatr. 91*:434, 1977.

*Blindness* may be a sequela of cataracts, retrolental fibroplasia, optic atrophy, glaucoma, macular degeneration, retinoblastoma, chorioretinitis, trauma, ocular infections and a variety of cerebral degenerative diseases. The initial symptom in Spielmeyer-Vogt (Batten's) disease, for example, may be progressive loss of vision.

Parmelee, A.H., Jr. and Liverman, L.: Blindness in infants and children. *In* Green, M. and Haggerty, R.J. (eds.): *Ambulatory Pediatrics*. W. B. Saunders Co., 1968, p. 541.

Loss of vision or a change in the visual fields not accompanied by fundus changes suggests an *intracranial neoplasm*. Young children with brain tumors do not complain of diminished visual acuity until papilledema is advanced. Elevation of the disk may be present for many months without complaint of impaired vision. Loss of vision occurs with papillitis and with retrobulbar neuritis.

High-grade, progressive myopia may occur in infants. In the *Stickler syndrome* (hereditary arthro-ophthalmopathy), sudden, spontaneous retinal detachment may occur in the first decade of life.

Stickler, G.B.: Hereditary progressive arthro-ophthalmopathy. *Mayo Clin. Proc. 43*:433, 1965.

*Blurred vision* may be secondary to neuropathies caused by diphtheria or botulism, increased intracranial pressure, hypertension and migraine.

## EYELIDS

*Ptosis.* Newborn infants often have one eye widely open while the other eyelid droops a little or is closed. This pseudoptosis disappears with further maturation. *Congenital ptosis* is usually unilateral and sporadic. In the *Marcus Gunn phenomenon* (jaw-winking reflex), associated with congenital ptosis, protrusion or movement of the jaw to one side causes elevation of the paretic eyelid on the contralateral side. In infants, sucking may produce a similar response.

The triad of ptosis, blepharophimosis and epicanthus inversus is hereditary.

*Myotonic dystrophy* may cause congenital ptosis that precedes other signs by many years.

A pseudoptosis may occur with paralysis of the superior rectus muscle along with hypotropia of the involved eye and drooping of the upper lid. An epicanthal fold may also be present.

Ptosis may also be due to paralysis of the oculomotor nerve. Acquired ptosis may be due to encephalitis, thallitoxicosis, cervical neuroblastoma, botulism, myasthenia gravis (unilateral or bilateral), ocular myopathy, pineal tumors, Horner's syndrome, tuberculous meningitis and ocular rhabdomyosarcoma. Ptosis also occurs in the Aarskog, Noonan, Möbius, Leigh, multiple pterygium, whistling face, fetal alcohol and the Smith-Lemli-Opitz syndromes.

*Oculosympathetic paralysis* occurring during the course of acute otitis media in children is manifested by a slight droop of the upper eyelid. The affected lid can, however, be fully elevated.

Elevation or retraction of the upper lids in advanced hydrocephalus exposes the sclera above the cornea and produces an apparent exophthalmos or downward displacement of the eyes. Widening of the palpebral fissure due to exophthalmos and retraction of the lids may cause a staring expression in children with hyperthyroidism. The *lid lag sign*, the upper eyelid lagging behind the eyeball when the patient looks downward, may also be present.

An "eye-popping" appearance created by a sudden transient widening of the palpebral fissures may be noted in some infants when the examining light is removed after the pupillary reflexes are tested. A simultaneous downward deviation of the eyes may be noted.

Perez, R.B.: The eye-popping reflex of infants. *J. Pediatr. 81*:87, 1972.

Lower eyelid colobomas or notches are present in Treacher Collin syndrome; a unilateral upper eyelid coloboma may be present in Goldenhar's syndrome.

Excessive *blinking* of the eyes may indicate eyestrain or represent a habit spasm or tic.

*Squinting* or narrowing of the palpebral fissure is an indication for an ophthalmologic examination. Narrowing of the palpebral fissure also occurs secondary to puffy, edematous eyelids and with Duane's retraction syndrome.

*Palpebral fissure length* may be measured by sighting over a ruler that is held across the greatest horizontal axis of the eye from the medial to the lateral canthus. The mean length at 40 weeks' gestation is $1.85 \pm 0.13$ cm. Short palpebral fissures are found in the fetal alcohol, Williams elfin facies, whistling face and other syndromes as well as secondary to micro-ophthalmia.

Jones, K.L., Hanson, J.W. and Smith, D.W.: Palpebral fissure size in newborn infants. *J. Pediatr. 92*:787, 1978.
Jones, K.L. and Smith, D.W.: The Williams elfin facies syndrome. *J. Pediatr. 86*:718, 1975.

In *Duane's retraction syndrome,* sometimes confused with sixth nerve palsy, adduction of the eye is accompanied by narrowing of the palpebral fissure, retraction of the eyeball and superior or inferior deviation of the globe. There is also decreased or lost abduction with widening of the palpebral fissure on lateral gaze. Esotropia is present in the primary position.

*Staring* episodes may occur with petit mal epilepsy. A fixed stare may result from phenothiazine toxicity.

*Slanting of the palpebral fissures* from the lateral to the medial canthus occurs in children with Down's syndrome and occasionally in normal infants. Antimongoloid slanting occurs in Apert's, Pfeiffer's, cri du chat, Treacher Collins' and whistling face syndromes. There is also a droop at the outer canthus in patients with Treacher Collins' syndrome.

*Hordeolum,* or *stye,* a localized staphylococcal infection, is a painful, red and tender swelling, usually surmounted by a yellow punctum, at the edge of the eyelid.

*Chalazion,* or *meibomian cyst,* is a firm, discrete, nonpainful nodule on the bulbar aspect of the lid adjacent to the tarsal plate.

Swelling of the eyelid may be the first sign of an *orbital rhabdomyosarcoma.*

Embryonal rhabdomyosarcoma occurs most often at the upper inner angle of the orbit.

A *hemangioma* may cause bluish enlargement of an eyelid.

Thickening and eversion of the eyelid margins and pedunculated nodules on the palpebral conjunctiva may occur in the *multiple mucosal neuroma syndrome*.

Thickening and distortion of the upper eyelid may occur with *neurofibromatosis,* especially when associated with a glioma of the optic nerve. A *dermoid cyst* may present as a lump in the lateral part of the upper lid. The left eyebrow is the most common site for such cysts.

> Pollard, Z. F., Harley, R.D. and Calhoun, J.: Dermoid cysts in children. *Pediatrics 57*:379, 1976.

*Marginal blepharitis* is characterized by persistent erythema, scaling and crusting of the edges of the eyelids. *Staphylococcal blepharitis* produces tenacious scales, which on removal leave small ulcerated lesions. Pustules may develop around the base of the eyelashes, and the meibomian glands may contain pus. Some of the eyelashes may be lost. In seborrheic dermatitis the scales are greasy, waxy and easily removed.

*Orbital cellulitis* may be due to Staphylococcus aureus, Streptococcus pyogenes, Escherichia coli, Streptococcus pneumoniae and Hemophilus influenzae type B. In addition to redness and swelling of the lids (periorbital cellulitis), findings of orbital cellulitis may include conjunctival injection and edema, proptosis, tenderness, pain and restriction of eye movements. Hemophilus influenzae cellulitis often causes a blue-purple discoloration of the eyelids, but this is also seen in infections caused by Streptococcus pneumoniae.

> Barkin, R.M., Todd, J.K. and Amer, J.: Periorbital cellulitis in children. *Pediatrics 62*:390, 1978.
> Londer, L. and Nelson, D.L.: Orbital cellulitis due to Haemophilus influenzae. *Arch. Ophthalmol 91*:89, 1974.
> Thirumoorthi, M.C., Asmar, B.I. and Danani, A.S.: Violaceous discoloration in pneumococcal cellulitis. *Pediatrics 62*:492, 1978.

Children with *dermatomyositis* develop a lilac or heliotrope discoloration and scaling dermatitis of the eyelids that along with periorbital edema is virtually pathognomonic.

## EYELASHES AND EYEBROWS

Eyelashes and eyebrows are usually absent in premature infants.

Long, curved eyelashes may be hereditary. They are also common in chronically ill children and in de Lange's syndrome.

*Pediculosis* confined to the eyelashes may be detected only by careful examination. Frequent rubbing of the eyes or marginal blepharitis may be noted.

In patients with albinism the eyelashes are not pigmented. Poliosis or progressive whitening of the eyelashes is seen in the *uveomeningitis syndrome*.

*Distichiasis*, or *extra eyelashes*, may accompany familial lymphedema.

Eyelashes may be absent in the inner two-thirds of the lower eyelid in patients with Treacher Collins' syndrome. Patients with the Hallermann-Streiff and cartilage hair syndromes have hypotrichosis of the eyebrows and eyelashes.

Children with Hurler's syndrome have bushy eyebrows. The eyebrows meet in the midline with de Lange's and Waardenburg's syndromes.

The Coffin-Siris syndrome is characterized by hypertrichosis of the eyebrows and eyelashes and hypotrichosis of the scalp.

Carey, J.C. and Hall, B.D.: The Coffin-Siris syndrome. *Am. J. Dis. Child. 132*:667, 1978.

## SWELLING OF EYELIDS AND PERIORBITAL TISSUES

In the newborn, *chemical conjunctivitis* due to silver nitrate often results in edema of the eyelids. Prolonged crying may also cause mild edema. The eyelids in infants with hypothyroidism are characteristically puffy.

*Acute ethmoid sinusitis* may cause swelling of the periorbital region, especially medially. Initially, the swelling may be minimal and easily overlooked.

Slight puffiness of the eyelids and dark circles around the eyes may be seen in children with frequent respiratory infections or nasal allergy ("allergic shiners").

Other causes of edema of the lids include pollen allergy and conjunctivitis. Swelling of the eyelids may be noted in infants with pertussis after paroxysms of coughing. Measles and infectious mononucleosis may be accompanied by puffiness of the lids. In dermatomyositis the eyelids may have a heliotrope color as well as being edematous. The upper lids may also be swollen in trichinosis. Nephritis and nephrosis are classically characterized by puffy eyelids. Other causes of periorbital edema include angioneurotic edema, osteomyelitis of the frontal bone, cavernous sinus thrombosis and the superior vena caval syndrome.

*Blowout fracture* of the orbital floor following trauma to the orbit by fist- or baseball-sized objects may cause periorbital swelling, ecchymosis and conjunctival hemorrhage. If the inferior rectus or inferior oblique muscles herniate through the orbital floor into the maxillary sinus, mobility of the eyeball is reduced and enophthalmus occurs. The patient may complain of diplopia, especially on upward gaze.

Heller, R.M.: The clinical and radiological presentation of blowout fracture of the orbit in children. *Pediatrics 46*:796, 1970.

O'Neill, J.F.: Ocular trauma. *In* Green, M. and Haggerty, R.J. (eds.): *Ambulatory Pediatrics*. W. B. Saunders Co., 1968, p. 829.

## EPICANTHUS

A fold of skin extending down from the upper lid to cover the medial canthus of the eye may be noted in normal newborns. This fold usually disappears in one to three months.

In Down's syndrome the epicanthic fold is usually more prominent and extends farther down at the inner canthus. This fold may disappear as the child becomes older.

Patients with congenital ptosis of the eyelids may have an associated epicanthal fold as may patients with the cerebrohepatorenal, de Lange's, Smith-Lemli-Opitz, Ehlers-Danlos, Leopard, Möbius, Noonan's, Turner's, Williams elfin facies and fetal alcohol syndromes, and glycogenosis type II (Pompe's disease).

A pronounced semicircular epicanthic fold extends from the forehead downward onto the cheek in infants with bilateral renal agenesis (Potter's syndrome). These infants also have wide-spaced eyes.

*Ocular hypertelorism* refers to abnormally wide spacing of the eyes and a broadened bridge of the nose due to maldevelopment of the sphenoid bone. A number of physical findings, including epicanthal folds, flat nasal bridge or widely spaced eyebrows, may give a misleading impression of ocular hypertelorism. The interpupillary distance between the center of the eyes has diagnostic usefulness in craniofacial dysostosis and, with the exception of Waardenburg's syndrome, is the best indicator of ocular hypertelorism. Pryor has suggested the following formula: interpupillary distance is A–B/2 + B where A is the distance between the 2 outer angles of the palpebral fissures and B the distance between the 2 median angles. The determination of these distances is facilitated by having the patient look upward. Because there are racial differences in cranial configuration, appropriate normative values should be used.

Juberg, R.C., Sholte, F.G. and Touchstone, W.J.: Normal values for intercanthal distances of 5- to 11-year-old American blacks. *Pediatrics 55*:431, 1975.
Pryor, H.B.: Objective measurement of interpupillary distance. *Pediatrics 44*:973, 1969.

Ocular hypertelorism is also present in these syndromes: Aarskog, Noonan's, Apert's, craniofacial dysostosis, cerebral gigantism, craniometaphyseal dysostosis, multiple lentigenes, nevoid basal cell carcinoma, Rubinstein-Taybi, whistling face, orofaciodigital dysostosis, otopalatodigital, cri du chat and Ehlers-Danlos.

An unusually wide distance between the inner canthi of the eyes (dystopia canthorum), a broad nasal root, lateral displacement of the inferior lacrimal points, confluence of the eyebrows, heterochromia of the irises, white forelock and congenital deafness constitute *Waardenburg's syndrome.* The inner canthi are laterally displaced in the Carpenter's, orofaciodigital and multiple nevoid basal cell carcinoma syndromes.

The *orofaciodigital syndrome* is characterized by lateral displacement of the inner canthi, hypoplasia of the alar cartilages and broad nasal root.

*Orbital hypotelorism*, a decrease in the distance between the orbits, is found in the arhinencephaly group of malformations. These median faciocerebral defects include *cyclopia,* in which there is a single orbit in the nasal region, usually with a superior proboscis; *ethmocephaly,* with extreme hypotelorism, separate orbits and proboscis; *cebocephaly,* in which a flat, rudimentary nose similar to that of the platyrhine monkey is present; and *arhinencephaly,* with median or lateral cleft palate or with trigonocephaly.

DeMyer, W., Zeman, W. and Palmer, C.G.: The face predicts the brain: diagnostic significance of median facial anomalies for holoprosencephaly (arhinencephaly). *Pediatrics 34*:256, 1964.

Orbital hypotelorism also occurs in the Williams elfin facies syndrome.

Prominent *supraorbital ridges* are noted in congenital ectodermal dysplasia, Hurler's syndrome, Marfan's syndrome and frontometaphyseal dysplasia.

*Wrinkling of the skin* around the eyes is noted in ectodermal dysplasia, atopic eczema and older adolescents or adults with pituitary dwarfism.

## LACRIMAL GLAND AND NASOLACRIMAL DUCT

Most term or almost-term babies secrete tears.

Apt, L. and Cullen, B.F.: Newborns do secrete tears. *JAMA 189*:951, 1964.

In perhaps one third to two thirds of term infants, complete patency of the nasolacrimal duct has not been established at the time of birth. The lower end of the nasolacrimal duct is commonly separated from the inferior meatus by a thin membrane. Patency of the duct is usually present some weeks after birth. If not, watering of the eye is noted with the tears running over onto the cheek. Persistence of obstruction past the sixth month is an indication for ophthalmologic consultation. Failure of drainage may predispose to dacryocystitis with swelling and inflammation just below the inner canthus. A persistent conjunctivitis often develops, and the eyelids may stick together during sleep.

*Familial dysautonomia* is characterized by an absence or near absence of tears.

*Epiphora,* or *excessive tearing,* may occur with inflammatory disease, a corneal ulcer, foreign body plugging of the nasolacrimal duct or exophthalmos, or as an allergic reaction.

## EXOPHTHALMOS AND PROPTOSIS

While minimal exophthalmos cannot be measured directly, its progression or unilateral differences may be assessed by comparative readings.

*Neuroblastomas,* which frequently metastasize to the orbit, may cause ecchymosis, periorbital discoloration and unilateral or bilateral exophthalmos. Orbital sarcoma, retinoblastoma, glioma of the optic chiasm and retro-orbital tumors and abscesses may also be etiologic. Leukemic infiltration of the orbit is rare.

Progressive unilateral, nonpulsatile proptosis in association with diminishing visual acuity is usually the presenting finding in patients with a primarily *intraorbital glioma.* Such patients should be examined for café-au-lait spots. Neurofibromatosis may also cause a bony defect in the posterior orbit followed by proptosis that is more prominent when the patient is erect.

Other causes of exophthalmos or prominent eyes include:

Congenital cystic eye
Hyperthyroidism
Hand-Schüller–Christian syndrome
Ocular rhabdomyosarcoma — causes a rapidly progressive proptosis
Cavernous hemangioma
Cavernous sinus thrombosis
Arteriovenous aneurysm — pulsation may be present
Orbital and retro-orbital hemorrhage due to trauma or a bleeding disorder
Orbital cellulitis
Crouzon's disease
Apert's syndrome
Fibrous dysplasia of the facial bones
Basal skull fracture
Anterior meningocele or encephalocele — pulsation may be present
Acrocephalosyndactyly
Leopard syndrome
Pycnodysostosis

*Mucormycosis* may cause unilateral ophthalmoplegia, proptosis and extensive necrosis. A serosanguineous nasal discharge and necrotic nasal mucosa may occur. Leukemia and diabetes mellitus are predisposing diseases.

Landau, J.W. and Newcomer, V.D.: Acute cerebral phycomycosis (mucormycosis). *J. Pediatr.* 61:363, 1962.

Progressive unilateral proptosis may be an early sign of *cystic fibrosis.*

Strauss, R.G., West, P.J. and Silverman, F.N.: Unilateral proptosis in cycstic fibrosis. *Pediatrics 43*:297, 1969.

*Congenital glaucoma* is characterized by enlargement of the eyeball.

## OTHER ORBITAL FINDINGS

*Sunken, expressionless eyes* may be noted in malnourished infants, in infants who are severely dehydrated and in those who are critically ill.

*Microphthalmia* may occur in patients with persistent tunica vasculosa lentis, retinal dysplasia or encephalo-ophthalmic dysplasia, retrolental fibroplasia, toxoplasmosis, 13 and 18 trisomies and the focal dermal hypoplasia, Hallermann-Streiff and Lenz micro-ophthalmia syndromes.

*Anophthalmos,* or *congenital absence of the eye,* is a rare anomaly. The eye may be replaced by a large cyst, or an *ocular cyst* occurring below a congenitally small eye may cause protrusion of the lower eyelid.

A *meningocele* may rarely present as a cystic protrusion in the anteromedial aspect of the orbit.

"Allergic shiners" is the term given to the dark circles under the eyes in patients with nasal allergy.

## CONJUNCTIVA

*Subconjunctival hemorrhage,* common in newborn infants as a bright red, complete or incomplete band around the iris, generally has no clinical significance and disappears rapidly. Similar hemorrhage may occur after trauma and in patients with pertussis after paroxysms of severe coughing and in hemorrhagic disorders.

*Conjunctivitis.* Small vessels around the periphery of the bulbar conjunctiva that radiate toward the cornea become reddened and engorged. The palpebral conjunctiva also demonstrates inflammatory changes.

*Ophthalmia neonatorum,* or *conjunctivitis of the newborn,* has a number of etiologies. Shortly after birth about 90 per cent of infants demonstrate *chemical conjunctivitis* with edema of the eyelids as a reaction to silver nitrate instillation. This occurs in the first day, about the same time that gonorrheal infections become evident.

*Inclusion conjunctivitis,* the most common type of infectious neonatal conjunctivitis, occurs usually in the latter part of the first and in the second week. A thick yellow discharge, edema of the eyelids and diffuse conjunctival injection may be present or inflammatory changes may be minimal. *Chlamydia conjunctivitis* due to Chlamydia oculogenitalis cannot be differentiated from bacterial infection on clinical findings alone. Chlamydial and gonorrheal ophthalmia may occur concomitantly.

Rowe, D.S., Aicardi, E.Z., Dawson, C.R. and Schachter, J.: Purulent ocular discharge in neonates: significance of Chlamydia trachomatis. *Pediatrics 63*:628, 1979.

Bacteriologic studies are indicated with purulent conjunctivitis. Gonorrheal conjunctivitis is a special hazard during the immediate newborn period. Infections due to Hemophilus influenzae may also be serious.

Armstrong, J.H., Zacarias, F. and Rein, M.F.: Ophthalmia neonatorum: a chart review. *Pediatrics 57*:884, 1976.

Redness, watering of the eyes and swelling of the caruncle occur in patients with measles. Children with pertussis may demonstrate slight conjunctivitis. Chickenpox may also involve the conjunctiva. Acute mucopurulent or catarrhal conjunctivitis, caused by staphylococci, Diplococcus pneumoniae, Koch-Weeks bacillus, Hemophilus influenzae and Streptococcus viridans, is characterized by a mucopurulent discharge, swelling and redness of the conjunctiva and sticking of the lids on awakening ("Pink Eye").

Oculoglandular tularemia is characterized by conjunctivitis, usually unilateral, and by preauricular and cervical lymphadenopathy. Cat-scratch disease also causes preauricular adenopathy when the primary lesion is in the conjunctiva.

Carithers, H.A.: Oculoglandular disease of Parinaud. *Am. J. Dis. Child. 132*:1195, 1978.

Newcastle disease may cause conjunctivitis. Leptospirosis may cause a conjunctivitis as well as iritis and iridocyclitis. Conjunctivitis associated with nasopharyngitis and lymphadenopathy (pharyngoconjunctival fever) may be due to an adenovirus.

*Trachoma,* due to Chlamydia trachomatis, begins insidiously in children with few eye complaints. Positive signs include follicles on the upper tarsal conjunctiva and extension of limbal vessels.

Thygeson, P. and Dawson, C.R.: Trachoma and follicular conjunctivitis in children. *Arch. Ophthalmol. 75*:3, 1966.

Severe conjunctivitis occurs frequently with the *Stevens-Johnson syndrome.*

*Vernal conjunctivitis* has an allergic etiology, occurs most frequently during the spring and summer and is characterized by intense pruritus, photophobia and lacrimation. The palpebral conjunctiva has a bluish-white, cobblestone appearance, and plaques may be noted on the bulbar conjunctiva. A stringy, mucoid secretion is present.

*Epidemic keratoconjunctivitis,* caused by adenovirus type 8, is initially characterized by prominent follicles on the conjunctiva along with edema of the eyelids and ocular conjunctiva. Epiphora, pruritus, pain and photophobia are also present. A pseudomembrane may appear on the lids. Preauricular lymphadenopathy may be noted. Some days later punctate corneal opacities appear, and vision is temporarily impaired. Resolution occurs slowly.

Conjunctivitis may occur in preschool children after overexposure to sunlight.

*Pallor* of the conjunctiva may be a good clinical indication of anemia.

*Vitamin A deficiency* produces drying and injection of the bulbar conjunctiva. Yellowish patches (*Bitot's spots*) may occur on the bulbar conjunctiva.

The *ataxia-telangiectasia syndrome* is characterized by *conjunctival telangiectasis,* usually noted after five to six years of age. Other findings include progressive cerebellar ataxia; oculomotor apraxia; cutaneous telangiectasia of the face, pinnae, eyelids and arms; and susceptibility to pulmonary infections.

Careful examination of the conjunctiva is indicated when subacute bacterial endocarditis is suspected since petechiae in the conjunctiva may be an embolic phenomenon.

*Pinguecula* is a slightly elevated, yellowish, wedge-shaped benign lesion that extends from the outer canthus. Rare in infants and young children, this lesion is observed in Gaucher's disease.

*Pterygium* is a triangular membranous fold, the apex of which involves the cornea, while the base is continuous with the conjunctiva. This lesion is rare in childhood. Exposure to wind, dust and sun is thought to be etiologic.

*Epibulbar dermoids* and/or *lipodermoids* are noted in children with *Goldenhar's syndrome* (oculoauriculovertebral dysplasia) along with auricular appendices, preauricular fistulas and vertebral anomalies. The dermoid is a yellow or white flat or ellipsoidal lesion usually present at the corneal margin in the lower outer quadrant. The lipodermoid is usually noted in the upper outer quadrant.

Feingold, M. and Baum, J.: Goldenhar's syndrome. *Am. J. Dis. Child. 132*:136, 1978.

*Phlyctenular keratoconjunctivitis* is characterized by pinhead-sized, yellowish or grayish-white, conical, papular lesions accompanied by injection of the surrounding conjunctival vessels. Ciliary injection may also be present. These lesions may occur on the cornea, the bulbar conjunctiva or at the limbus. Photophobia, blepharospasm and epiphora may be notable, and ulceration may occur.

## SCLERA

The sclerae of infants and young children are usually bluish. Blue sclerae are also seen in patients with osteogenesis imperfecta or glaucoma and in the Russell-Silver, Ehlers-Danlos, Hallermann-Streiff and Marfan syndromes.

Melanin deposits in the form of nevi or freckles are frequently seen in the sclera.

Icterus may first become evident in the sclera. Pigmentation associated with carotenemia is manifested in the skin but not in the sclera.

## CORNEA

Congenital anomalies of the cornea include abnormalities in its size and curvature. A cone-shaped cornea is a rare anomaly. In *megalocornea*, the corneas are very large, but there is no increase in the intraocular pressure.

Hereditary abnormal enlargement of the eye (*megalocornea* or *macrophthalmia*) occurs almost exclusively in boys. The diameter of the cornea and the depth of the anterior chamber are increased. The pupil is contracted; the iris may be tremulous and the lens subluxated.

The cornea in newborn infants has a diameter of 9 to 10 mm. The adult size of about 12 mm. is reached between 6 and 12 months of age.

*Primary* or *congenital glaucoma* is usually present bilaterally at birth but may begin insidiously in the first year of life. The cornea is increased in diameter to greater than 10.5 to 11 mm. and may be cloudy. There is an increased depth of the anterior chamber between the cornea and the iris. Dilatation of the pupil occurs, and the sclerae appear thin and bluish-white. The cornea may appear clear, hazy or white. Photophobia, epiphora or excessive lacrimation and blepharospasm are usually the earliest symptoms and may be present for weeks before corneal hazing and enlargement are noted. *These findings should always arouse suspicion of congenital glaucoma.* Photophobia is the first sign of congenital glaucoma in 50 per cent of cases. The presence of this symptom in infants under 1 year of age should always suggest glaucoma. Because the eye often appears red and irritated, glaucoma has, at times, been confused with conjunctivitis. Some patients with unilateral glaucoma also have an ipsilateral capillary hemangioma (Sturge-Weber syndrome). Lowe's syndrome in males is characterized, in part, by glaucoma and cataracts along with mental retardation, hypotonia and aminoaciduria. Glaucoma also occurs in homocystinuria, retinoblastoma, congenital aniridia, neurofibromatosis, tuberous sclerosis and congenital rubella. It may occur in the Stickler and the cerebrohepatorenal syndromes and as a complication of retrolental fibroplasia.

Bettman, J.W. and Cleasby, G.W.: Congenital glaucoma. *Pediatrics 32*:420, 1963.

In the systemic mucopolysaccharidoses, corneal clouding occurs in these syndromes: Hurler's, Morquio's, Scheie's, Maroteaux-Lamy and beta-glucuronidase deficiency (MPS VII). The lysosomal storage diseases associated with corneal clouding include $GM_1$ gangliosidosis and mannosidosis. Corneal clouding also occurs in the mucolipidoses. Corneal opacities or haziness may occur in children with cystinosis caused by the deposition of cystine crystals in the cornea and visualized with the slit lamp. In the newborn, birth trauma with contusion of the eye, rupture of Descemet's membrane and edema of the cornea may cause corneal clouding, which lasts a few days. Unilateral corneal opacity always raises the possibility of congenital glaucoma.

*Interstitial keratitis* may occur during the latter half of the first decade with congenital syphilis. Initial involvement is usually unilateral. The cornea has a cloudy, ground-glass, reddish-gray appearance. Photophobia, blepharospasm and lacrimation may be intense. Injection of the ciliary vessels occurs around the limbus of the cornea. Uveitis may also develop.

*Corneal ulceration* due to the herpes viruses is characterized initially by a grayish or yellow infiltration of the cornea — at first localized but then more extensive — and by conjunctival and ciliary injection, intense pain, photophobia, lacrimation and blepharospasm.

*Corneal hypesthesia* is present in children with familial dysautonomia. The corneal reflex is absent.

After trauma to the eye or removal of a foreign body, careful examination of the cornea for abrasions is indicated.

## PUPILS

Pupillary contraction, blinking and closure of the eyelids occur in normal newborn infants in response to a bright light.

A *unilateral contracted pupil* indicates involvement of the cervical sympathetic chain. Such pupils still react to light, however, and dilate after the instillation of a cycloplegic drug. *Horner's syndrome* consists of constriction of the pupil, slight drooping of the upper lid and enophthalmos. At times, vasodilatation and anhidrosis occur on the involved side. Horner's syndrome may be caused by a cervical neuroblastoma.

*Oculosympathetic paralysis,* characterized by a slight ptosis of the upper eyelid and miosis of the ipsilateral pupil, may occur as a complication of acute otitis media. Inequality in size of the pupils is more evident in dim than in bright light, and the pupillary reaction to light is normal.

*Intracranial injury* may cause either dilatation or contraction of the pupils. Because of the importance of the comparative size and activity of the pupils in children who have sustained a head injury, mydriatics should not be used. Asymmetry of the pupils indicates unilateral brain damage. Dilatation of one pupil suggests ipsilateral, localized intracranial hemorrhage.

Dilatation of the pupil may occur late in *retinoblastoma* along with a yellow to gray-green, "cat's eye" pupillary reflex, visual impairment and squinting.

Glaucoma is characterized by dilatation of the pupil.

The pupils are widely dilated as a result of atropine, Jimson weed or barbiturate poisoning. Pinpoint pupils occur with morphine overdosage. Pupils respond poorly to light in botulism.

> McKee, K.T., Jr., Kilroy, A.W., Harrison, W.W. and Schaffer, W.: Botulism in infancy. *Am. J. Dis. Child. 131*:857, 1977.

*Adie's syndrome (tonic pupil)* is rare in childhood, and its significance is little understood. There is unilateral pupillary dilatation, and little or no reaction occurs to the direct or indirect light reflexes. In the dark, further dilatation may slowly occur. Conversely, the pupil will contract in bright light, often after a delay of minutes, and return to its original status when the light is removed. Pupillary contraction during accommodation-convergence for near vision occurs slowly but may be marked. Absence of tendon reflexes, especially the ankle jerks and segmental hypohidrosis, may be associated phenomena.

Pineal tumors may be accompanied by Argyll Robertson pupils. Dilatation and inequality of the pupils and impairment of their reaction to light may be noted in children with tumors of the brain stem.

Miosis in comatose patients may be due to ingestion of narcotics, barbiturates, phenothiazines and ethanol.

A dilated, poorly reactive pupil in an unresponsive child raises the possibility of *temporal lobe herniation* at the tentorium. Bilateral, *dilated and fixed pupils* unresponsive to light indicates damage to cranial nerve III due to transtentorial herniation, brain stem compression and death. Marked but transient anisocoria may occur during seizures.

> Pant, S.S., Benton, J.W. and Dodge, P.R.: Unilateral pupillary dilatation during and immediately following seizures. *Neurology 16*:837, 1966.

A *"white pupil,"* or *leukokoria,* may be caused, in order of their frequency, by cataracts, persistent hyperplastic primary vitreous, retrolental fibroplasia, retinal dysplasia, retinoblastoma and larval granulomatosis.

## LENS

*Cataracts* are circumscribed, central opacities of the lens and cause a white pupillary reflex. Ophthalmoscopically, the cataract appears as an opaque density surrounded, if the cataract is not complete, by a red fundal reflex. A positive ophthalmoscope lens (+ 8 to + 15) should be used with the examiner a few inches away from the child.

*Congenital cataracts* may be present at birth or first appear in early infancy. Some are bilateral and complete, others bilateral but incomplete and still others unilateral.

With small central cataracts the infant may have some vision when the pupils are dilated but not when they are constricted. Transient cataracts have been reported as an unusual finding in low birth weight infants.

Alden, E.R., Kalina, R.E. and Hodson, W.A.: Transient cataracts in low-birth-weight infants. *J. Pediatr. 82*:314, 1973.

Congenital rubella, toxoplasmosis, Herpes simplex infection and cytomegalic inclusion disease may cause cataracts. Hereditary congenital cataracts usually are an expression of an autosomal dominant trait. In 50 per cent of children with cataracts, the cause is unknown.

Galactosemia, galactokinase deficiency, hypoparathyroidism, aspartyl-glycosaminuria, Lowe's syndrome, osteopetrosis, diabetes, homocystinuria and mannosidosis are systemic processes that may be accompanied by cataract formation.

Other disorders associated with cataracts include these syndromes: pachyonychia congenita, Hallermann-Streiff, Rothmund-Thomson, chondrodysplasia punctata (Conradi's disease), incontinentia pigmenti, Marinesco-Sjögren, Stickler, mandibulo-dysostosis, Marfan's, cerebrohepatorenal and Smith-Lemli-Opitz. Cataracts are also seen in trisomy 13, 18, 21 and Turner's syndrome.

High-dose, long-term systemic corticosteroid therapy may produce translucent posterior subcapsular cataracts. Uveitis and trauma to the orbit as in perforating wounds may also lead to cataract formation.

*Congenital dislocation of the lens* leading to myopia may occur in Marfan's syndrome and with homocystinuria. Patients with *Marchesani's syndrome* have a small spherical lens with associated myopia and glaucoma. The lens may also be dislocated. Other clinical features of this disorder are short stature and short, stubby fingers.

Helveston, E.M.: Cataracts in children. *Ind. St. Med. Assoc. J. 69*:205, 1976.

Kohn, B.: The differential diagnosis of cataracts in infancy and childhood. *Am. J. Dis. Child. 130*:184, 1976.

## RETROLENTAL MEMBRANES

*Persistent tunica vasculosa lentis.* During fetal life the hyaloid artery and its supporting connective tissue, which constitutes the tunica vasculosa lentis, passes through the vitreous and supplies blood vessels to the posterior surface of the lens. Uncommonly, part of this tissue persists in full-term infants and produces a retrolental opacity that is most marked centrally and from which long ciliary processes extend peripherally. If part of the vitreous can be visualized, the persistent hyaloid artery may be seen. Involvement is usually unilateral, and some degree of microphthalmos may develop. Occasionally, a posterior cortical cataract is produced and results in complete opacity of the lens.

*Persistent hyperplastic primary vitreous* (PHPV) causes a white pupil as a result of a retrolental fibrovascular mass. Involvement commonly is present at birth, usually unilaterally, in full-term infants. Bilateral PHPV may be associated with trisomy 13.

*Persistent pupillary membrane* appears in premature infants as a brown or gray filamentous strand that projects across the pupil from the anterior surface of the iris to the lens or across the lens to the opposite side of the pupil.

*Retinal dysplasia* (Reese), or *encephalo-ophthalmic dysplasia* (Krause), occurs bilaterally in newborn infants and is characterized by a white pupil, retrolental membrane and, usually, microphthalmia.

*Retinopathy of prematurity* (retrolental fibroplasia) occurs almost exclusively in premature infants who have received supplemental oxygen. Rarely, it may develop in a term infant. Indirect ophthalmoscopy, especially of the temporal periphery, should be performed in all infants who receive continuing oxygen therapy, beginning two weeks after discontinuation of the oxygen and repeated at two-week intervals until discharge and then rechecked at six months. Early changes in infants with retinopathy of prematurity can be seen only with indirect ophthalmoscopy.

> Patz, A.: The continuing role of the ophthalmologist in the premature nursery. *Arch. Ophthalmol. 85*:129, 1971.

The earliest evidence of retinopathy of prematurity usually appears between the second and fifth weeks of life, uncommonly in the first week. If changes have not occurred by the age of three months, retinopathy of prematurity no longer remains a hazard. Peripheral retinal neovascularization is the earliest finding, followed by ingrowth into the vitreous. Dilatation of the retinal vessels, especially the veins, and tortuosity, especially of the arteries, then occur. Next, grayish-yellow elevations of the retina are evident at the extreme periphery. Fuzziness of the disk appears, and a grayish membrane due to folds of detached retina can be noted in the retrolental space. A number of vitreous bands then develop. The mild proliferative stage of retinopathy of prematurity spontaneously regresses in some infants.

The acute phase lasts through the third and fourth months and is followed by organization and cicatrization. In some cases continued fusion of the retinal folds produces a complete opaque retrolental membrane and loss of the red reflex. Other infants have only a partial membrane, a retinal fold extending peripherally from the disk or an opacity confined to the far periphery of the fundus. The anterior chamber may become shallow, and the iris and the lens may come into contact with the cornea, causing a corneal opacity. Microphthalmus, enophthalmos and dark circles around the eyes are late manifestations.

> McCormick, A.Q.: Retinopathy of prematurity. *Cur. Probl. Pediatr. 7*:3 (Sept.) 1977.

## UVEAL TRACT

In patients with *ciliary injection* the vessels radiate from the limbus toward the periphery and are not as brightly injected as in conjunctivitis.

The iris of newborn white infants is gray-blue, slate-colored or grayish-brown. In the black or brown races the iris is brown or grayish-brown. The permanent color of the iris appears in about 50 per cent of infants by the age of 6 months and in the others by the end of the first year.

In children with *albinism* the iris is pink, pale blue or dull gray. The iris trans-illuminates well when the sclera is illuminated by a light in contact with the orbit. In *ocular albinism* only the eye lacks pigmentation. The choroidal vessels are easily seen through the low-pigmented fundus. Visual acuity is low, especially in bright light. Pendular horizontal nystagmus and photophobia are noted.

"Salt and pepper" speckling of the iris (Brushfield's spots) is noted in infants with

Down's syndrome. This finding may be present with other types of mental retardation such as the cerebrohepatorenal syndrome, as well as in normal children.

Pigmented or nonpigmented iris nodules (Lisch spots) visible to the naked eye or on slit lamp examination occur bilaterally in many patients with neurofibromatosis.

A child may normally have one blue and one brown iris. Some instances of *heterochromia,* however, are associated with a chronic, low-grade iridocyclitis and secondary cataract formation in the eye with the lighter-colored iris (heterochromic iridocyclitis of Fuchs). Heterochromia may be noted in Waardenburg's syndrome.

Heterochromia may be associated with a Horner's syndrome present at birth, with the ipsilateral eye remaining blue. In cervical or mediastinal neuroblastoma, the iris on the involved side may be lighter in color.

Jaffe, N., et al.: Heterochromia and Horner syndrome associated with cervical and mediastinal neuroblastoma. *J. Pediatr. 87:*75, 1975.

*Iridodonesis,* a quivering movement of the iris, may be caused by dislocation of the lens in patients with Marfan's syndrome or homocystinuria.

*Coloboma* is a congenital notching or absence of part of the iris, lens, choroid or retina. A keyhole effect is produced in the iris. When the choroid and retina are involved, a depigmented area is noted on funduscopy. Colobomas occur in the focal dermal hypoplasia, trisomy 13 and Wolf-Hirschhorn syndromes.

The "cat's eye" syndrome, in which a lower vertical iridal and choroidal coloboma is present, may be accompanied by a number of congenital anomalies, including congenital heart disease.

Freedom, R.M. and Gerald, P.S.: Congenital cardiac disease and the "cat eye" syndrome. *Am. J. Dis. Child. 126:*16, 1973.

*Aniridia,* or absence of the iris, is inherited as an autosomal dominant trait. Nonfamilial aniridia may be associated with Wilms' tumor and neoplasms of the adrenal cortex and liver. Aniridia and hypoplastic iris also occur in Rieger's syndrome.

Haick, B.N. and Miller, D.R.: Simultaneous occurrence of congenital aniridia, hamartoma, and Wilms' tumor. *J. Pediatr. 78:*497, 1971.

The *Kayser-Fleischer ring,* a unilateral or bilateral complete or incomplete brown or grayish-green ring at the limbus of the cornea, may be seen in Wilson's disease at times with the naked eye or simple magnification but in some patients only with the slit lamp. The pigmentary deposits are most prominent at the 12 and 6 o'clock positions.

*Uveitis,* termed *anterior* when the iris and ciliary body are involved, *posterior* when the choroid and retina are affected and *pan* when all components are included, usually occurs secondary to systemic diseases such as sarcoidosis, rheumatoid arthritis, tuberculosis, syphilis, brucellosis or leptospirosis. Usually, however, the cause is unknown.

*Iritis* or *iridocyclitis* is characterized by a deep, perilimbal flush, dulling and discoloration of the iris; a contracted, sluggishly reacting, irregular pupil; ciliary injection; photophobia; epiphora; impairment of vision; and pain. The aqueous may be cloudy, and precipitates may appear on the posterior surface of the cornea. Exudates may be seen as opacities in the vitreous.

Iridocyclitis is a more frequent complication in pauciarticular than in polyarticular rheumatoid arthritis. Since early anterior uveitis may be asymptomatic, children with rheumatoid arthritis should have periodic slit lamp examinations and the parents should be urged to contact the physician promptly if photophobia, red eyes or decreased visual acuity occur. Iridocyclitis may precede or follow joint symptoms.

> Schaller, J., Kupfer, C. and Wedgwood, R.J.: Iridocyclitis in juvenile rheumatoid arthritis. *Pediatrics 44*:92, 1969.

The *uveomeningoencephalitic syndrome* (Vogt-Koyanagi-Harada) is characterized by uveitis, signs of meningeal irritation, other central or peripheral nervous system symptomatology, progressive whitening of hair and eyelashes (poliosis), vitiligo, alopecia, hearing impairment or tinnitus.

*Behçet's syndrome* is manifested by recurrent uveitis along with oral and genital ulcerations, meningoencephalitis, synovitis and cutaneous vasculitis.

*Choroiditis* and *chorioretinitis* produce chorioretinal atrophy characterized by irregular white patches and clumps of black pigment. Toxoplasmosis, cytomegalic inclusion disease, syphilis and tuberculosis may be etiologic. Though caused by a congenital infection, chorioretinitis may not be evident for some weeks after birth. In some instances the retinopathy is confined to the periphery, but involvement of the macular area is more common. Toxoplasmosis may cause solitary, yellow-white or gray cotton-like patches.

> O'Connor, G.R.: Manifestations and management of ocular toxoplasmosis. *Bull. N.Y. Acad. Med. 50*:192, 1974.

The "setting sun" sign, in which the irises appear to sink beneath the lower eyelids when the baby is quickly lowered from a sitting to supine position, may be normal in premature and some term infants. It may also be seen in kernicterus, hydrocephalus, lesions of the brain stem and Laron's dwarfism.

## RETINA

Funduscopic examination is usually readily performed in the older child, and mydriatics permit adequate visualization in infants. In infants, sedation may be required, but a pacifier or moistened sugar nipple may be effective. The examination may be facilitated if an assistant holds the infant's head steady and retracts one of the lids while the examiner retracts the other. Older children may be helped to hold their eyes reasonably fixed if the mother is asked to hold a colored object at an appropriate spot as a point of fixation. A brief respite is advisable if the examination is prolonged since funduscopy may rapidly fatigue the child. Supporting the back of the child's head in the upright position or performing the examination with the child lying down may facilitate cooperation. If a mydriatic is necessary, 2½ per cent phenylephrine (Neo-synephrine) or 1 per cent tropicamide (Mydriacyl) is a satisfactory agent.

As is true with other aspects of physical diagnosis, it is well to have some order in the examination of the retina. One may examine, in sequence, the disk, the vessels, the remainder of the fundus and the macular area. The macula appears as a dark, yellow-orange area lateral to and slightly below the optic disk. A bright light reflex is present around the fovea. The normal ratio of the caliber of the arterioles to that of the veins is 3:5.

Pulsation of the veins is present in most normal children. Disappearance of spontaneous venous pulsation is an early sign of papilledema. Venous pulsations in the retinal veins as they enter the optic nerve head indicate normal intracranial pressure. In infants the optic disks are pale, while in children they are light pink. The lateral portion of the disk is frequently pale, especially in children who are light-complexioned or anemic. This normal pallor is to be differentiated from that due to optic atrophy. A partial or complete brown or black pigmented ring is commonly present around the border of the disk. The medial edge of the disk may normally appear somewhat fuzzy.

A funduscopic examination to rule out increased intracranial pressure should be routine before lumbar puncture. Funduscopy is also important in children with impaired vision, convulsive disorders, retardation, microcephaly, headache, recurrent vomiting or with other findings that suggest neurologic disease. In most instances it is not difficult to differentiate between a normal and an abnormal fundus. There is considerable variation in the appearance of normal fundi, however, and at times such differentiation is difficult.

*Retinal hemorrhage* may be seen in the normal newborn infant as well as with subdural hematoma, scurvy or other generalized hemorrhagic states. Preretinal and retinal hemorrhages occur in most children with a subdural hematoma. Hemorrhagic retinopathy accompanied by retinal exudates may be seen in the abused child.

Tomasi, L.G. and Rosman, N.P.: Purtscher retinopathy in the battered child syndrome. *Am. J. Dis. Child. 129*:1335, 1975.

Retinal edema, hemorrhage and engorgement of the retinal veins may be due to cavernous sinus thrombosis. Increased intracranial pressure, especially when sudden, may lead to subhyaloid (preretinal) hemorrhages. Hemorrhage and exudation may occur in hypertension. Although fundus changes are uncommon in children with diabetes, capillary aneurysms and small round hemorrhages may appear. Retinal cytoid bodies resembling the cotton wool exudates seen in hypertensive disease and diabetic retinopathy may appear in lupus erythematosus and dermatomyositis.

Baum, J.D. and Bulpitt, C.J.: Retinal and conjunctival haemorrhage in the newborn. *Arch. Dis. Child. 45*:344, 1970.

Fruman, L.S., Sullivan, D.B. and Petty, R.E.: Retinopathy in juvenile dermatomyositis. *J. Pediatr. 88*:267, 1976.

Grover, W.D. and Harley, R.D.: Early recognition of tuberous sclerosis by funduscopic examination. *J. Pediatr. 75*:991, 1969.

The so-called *cherry red spot,* usually more of an orange-red colored area surrounded by a grayish-white areola, indicates involvement of the macula with $G_{M1}$ gangliosidosis, $G_{M2}$ gangliosidosis I (Tay-Sachs), $G_{M2}$ gangliosidosis II (Sandhoff's disease), infantile Gaucher's disease or Niemann-Pick disease. Macular cherry-red spots may also occur in patients with metachromatic leukodystrophy and mucoliposis I. The macular area should be carefully examined in all infants in whom degenerative disease is suspected. In late infantile amaurotic idiocy, fine brown pigment replaces the macular light reflex.

Menkes, J.H. Andrews, J.M. and Cancilla, P.A.: The cerebral retinal degenerations. *J. Pediatr. 79*:183, 11971.

*Lipemia retinalis,* characterized by a peculiar milky-white, pink, waxy appearance of the retinal vessels, rarely occurs in diabetic children and may be a finding in hyperlipoproteinemia.

Levy, R.I. and Rifkind, B.M.: Diagnosis and management of hyperlipoproteinemia in infants and children. *Am. J. Cardiol. 31*:547, 1973.

*Retinoblastoma* usually appears during the first three to five years of life as a unilateral, but often bilateral, gray or yellow-white glistening mass in the vitreous. If the macula is involved, strabismus (esotropia) may be the first sign. Tortuous vessels and hemorrhage may be present on the surface of the neoplasm. Unless the tumor is small, a whitish appearance or a grayish-yellow reflex through the pupil or unilateral dilatation of the pupil may be noted. *Nematode endophthalmitis* due to Toxocara canis may cause blindness, a white pupillary reflex and an intraocular tumor, findings suggestive of a retinoblastoma.

> Hogan, M.J., Kimura, S.J. and Spencer, W.H.: Visceral larva migrans and peripheral retinitis. *JAMA 194*:1345, 1965.

*Rubella retinitis* is characterized by unilateral or bilateral involvement of the posterior pole, especially the macula, with small black, irregular masses or fine to gross pigmentary speckling.

> Kresky, B. and Nauheim, J.S.: Rubella retinitis. *Am. J. Dis. Child. 113*:305, 1967.

*Tuberous sclerosis* causes a glistening, nodular, mulberry-like mass or oval, gray, flat areas in the retina. These lesions may be present in infancy. The retinal lesions of tuberculosis and neurofibromatosis may simulate those of tuberous sclerosis. Retinal angiomatosis (von Hippel's disease; the von Hippel-Lindau disease) is often associated with cerebellar as well as retinal involvement. One or more pairs of dilated and tortuous arterioles and veins may be followed from the disk into a peripherally placed white tumor mass.

In glycogenosis type I, multiple bilateral flat yellow lesions may be noted around the macula.

> Fine, R.N., Wilson, W.A. and Donnell, G.N.: Retinal changes in glycogen storage disease type I. *Am. J. Dis. Child. 115*:328, 1968.

*Retinitis pigmentosa* is characterized by degeneration, atrophy and pigmentation of the retina. Night blindness results from progressive constriction of the visual fields. The Laurence-Moon-Biedl syndrome consists of retinitis pigmentosa, obesity, mental retardation, hypogenitalism and polydactyly. Retinitis pigmentosa also appears in Refsum's syndrome with polyneuritis and ataxia, Cockayne's syndrome with dwarfism and deafness, Usher's syndrome with deafness, and Kearns-Sayre syndrome with progressive external ophthalmoplegia and heart block.

*Coats' disease* (exudative retinitis) occurs in boys between the ages of eight months and eight years. Strabismus and a detached retina may be present.

*Norrie's disease* is a sex-linked recessive disorder consisting of retinal detachment, deafness and mental retardation.

*Macular degeneration* produces a reddish or pigmented atrophic area in the macula.

## PAPILLEDEMA

Papilledema is caused by increased intracranial pressure and edema of the nerve fibers as they cross the disk. The optic disk becomes blurred and elevated. The amount of elevation of the disk is expressed in the number of diopters' difference in the ophthalmoscopic lenses used to see clearly a vessel or other area on the disk and a vessel or other area elsewhere on the retina. The continuity of the vessels becomes interrupted at the edge of the disk. Engorgement of the retinal veins, loss of venous pulsation and hemorrhages on or around the disk occur as the process advances. There is obliteration of the physiologic cup and an increase in the blind spot.

Papilledema is most commonly caused by space-occupying lesions such as tumor, tuberculoma, abscess or intracranial hematoma. Choking of the disk may also occur in patients with encephalitis, meningitis, chronic vitamin A intoxication or lead poisoning, occasionally in acute nephritis and rarely with hypoparathyroidism. Papilledema has also been reported in patients being treated with corticosteroids and in those with severe anemia. Premature synostosis of the cranial sutures may lead to papilledema.

Bilateral papilledema may also be associated with *pseudotumor cerebri*. This syndrome, which is more common in females, is characterized by the absence of neurologic signs and a normal electroencephalogram and computerized axial tomography.

Rothner, A. and Brujt, J.: Pseudotumor cerebri. *Arch. Neurol. 30*:110, 1974.

Secondary optic atrophy and impairment of visual acuity do not occur until papilledema has been present for a long time. With the onset of atrophy, swelling of the disk may recede.

Papilledema is present in 90 per cent of children with intracranial tumors. Elevation of the disk is an almost constant manifestation with cerebellar neoplasms but is much less frequent with a pontine glioma. Papilledema is usually bilateral, and unilateral differences are not of localizing value.

Papilledema, venous distention and tortuosity, retinal hemorrhages and cystic macular changes have been observed either separately or jointly in some patients with moderate to severe pulmonary disease due to cystic fibrosis and in cyanotic congenital heart disease.

Petersen, R.A. and Rosenthal, A.: Retinopathy and papilledema in cyanotic congenital heart disease. *Pediatrics 49*:243, 1972.

The differentiation of *true* and *pseudopapilledema* may be difficult early. In pseudopapilledema, which occurs in about 5 per cent of the population, especially whites, some blurring of the optic disk occurs. Elevation of the disk, if it occurs, is central rather than peripheral as with true papilledema. The vessels demonstrate preretinal branching, the disk does not obscure the origin of the vessels and venous pulsations are present. The blind spot is not enlarged. Since pseudopapilledema tends to be hereditary, ophthalmologic examination of relatives may reveal others with blurring or anomaly of the disk.

Conditions that may be confused with papilledema include medullated nerve fibers, drusen or hyaloid bodies and papillitis. When *myelination of the optic nerve* continues beyond the usual termination at the optic disk, whitish-yellow feather-edged areas may radiate from the disk into the retina. *Drusen* of the optic nerve, which are hyaline bodies in front of the lamina cribrosa and protruding through the disk, are the most common cause of pseudopapilledema.

Hoyt, W. and Pont, M.: Diagnoses of optic disk anomaly. *JAMA 181*:191, 1962.

## OPTIC NEURITIS

*Acute optic neuritis* causes edema of the disk or papillitis. The ophthalmoscopic findings of optic neuritis and papilledema may be similar and, at times, cannot be differentiated. In optic neuritis, visual acuity is reduced early. A similar loss of vision does not occur until papilledema is advanced. Loss of vision in patients with acute optic neuritis may be either largely central or complete. In the former, the retrobulbar pupillary reaction is present (i.e., pupillary contraction occurs in response to light), followed rapidly, with continued exposure to light, by dilatation. In the latter, the pupillary light reflex is absent. The visual acuity and visual fields should be evaluated in patients who have edema of the disks. In optic neuritis, there is moderate elevation and haziness of the disk, and the vessels, especially the veins, are widened and engorged. The disk is also hyperemic and may be covered by exudate and hemorrhages. Edema of the disk in optic neuritis may increase initially; however, the edema usually begins to disappear within two or three weeks, and pallor then becomes evident. In *retrobulbar neuritis* the disk may appear normal, but the patient has no vision in the affected eye. Secondary optic atrophy may occur.

Optic neuritis may occur as a complication of meningitis, chickenpox, measles, pertussis, mumps, influenza and, possibly, infectious mononucleosis. It has also been reported to follow diphtheria immunization and to be associated with lead poisoning. Multiple sclerosis in children may begin with optic neuritis.

*Neuromyelitis optica,* an uncommon condition in childhood, is characterized by gradual impairment of vision that may progress to total blindness. Neurologic findings, which may precede or follow ocular symptoms, may simulate transverse myelitis. The patient's difficulty in walking and talking may also suggest multiple sclerosis. Cerebrospinal fluid examination reveals elevation of protein, cells and pressure. Usually, normal vision returns after some weeks. The neurologic symptoms may, however, recur.

## OPTIC ATROPHY

With optic atrophy the disk is almost completely white, the margins well demarcated and the vessels and lamina cribrosa normal. Impairment of visual acuity and visual field defects also occur. Pallor of the disk, in itself, is not a reliable criterion for the diagnosis of optic atrophy in young children since the disks are normally pale then, and other factors may cause disk pallor. Distinction between primary and secondary optic atrophy may be impossible on ophthalmologic examination.

Optic atrophy may occur with tuberous sclerosis, Hurler's syndrome, toxoplasmosis, $G_{M1}$ gangliosidosis, Tay-Sachs disease, Schilder's disease, Krabbe's disease, Pelizaeus-Merzbacher disease, premature synostosis of the cranial sutures, osteopetrosis, craniometaphyseal dysostosis (leontiasis ossea), craniopharyngioma, optic glioma, Friedreich's ataxia, Conradi's disease, intracranial hemorrhage, hydrocephalus, lead poisoning, thallium intoxication, optic neuritis or retrobulbar neuritis. Optic atrophy, high frequency hearing loss and diabetes insipidus may occur in juvenile diabetes mellitus.

Gunn, T. et al.: Juvenile diabetes mellitus, optic atrophy, sensory nerve deafness, and diabetes inspidius — a syndrome. *J. Pediatr. 89:*565, 1976.

Central loss of vision may be the first clinical manifestation of degenerative disease of the central nervous system.

Schwartz, J.F., Chutorian, A.M., Evans, R.A. and Carter, S.: Optic atrophy in childhood. *Pediatries 34:*670, 1964.

## STRABISMUS

Strabismus represents nonparallelism of the visual axes in the various fields of gaze. Such ocular deviation is a common physiologic occurrence in infants three to six months of age before coordinated ocular movements develop. Occasionally, the deviation is so definite or constant that a true squint can be diagnosed at that time. Up to 18 months of age, transient unilateral deviation of an eye may normally occur for a few seconds. After this time, however, such deviation is not normal. The flat, relatively wide naso-orbital configuration of young infants may create the illusion of an internal strabismus. If constant or intermittent strabismus persists, an ophthalmologic consultation should be obtained.

Conditions that may predispose to strabismus include muscular defects, hyperopia, cerebral injury, differences in the refractive power of the two eyes, impairment of fusion ability and hereditary factors. An eye with impaired vision will tend to deviate: inward in young children and outward in older children. Infants with cerebral palsy may demonstrate strabismus. Strabismus may occur suddenly with intracranial hemorrhage, abscess or tumor, encephalitis, the Guillain-Barré syndrome, tuberculous meningitis, diphtheria, measles, lead poisoning and myasthenia gravis. Transient strabismus may occur with hypoglycemia. The sudden appearance of strabismus should suggest an intracranial, intraocular or intraorbital tumor. Unilateral or bilateral esotropia, often observed in children with intracranial tumors, may cause diplopia. Usually the increase in intracranial pressure is already well established before strabismus results from the effect of increased intracranial pressure on the abducens nerve.

External ophthalmoplegia, ataxia and absent or decreased deep tendon reflexes may be noted in Fisher's syndrome. Ophthalmoplegia with diplopia may occur in botulism. Extraocular palsies also occur in Leigh's syndrome.

*Ophthalmoplegic migraine* is characterized by episodes of severe pain involving the eye, forehead or hemicranium followed by ipsilateral ophthalmoplegia including third nerve palsy with mydriasis, ptosis and possibly paresis of cranial nerves IV and VI. The ophthalmoplegia may last several days.

Raymond, L.A., Tew, J. and Fogelson, M.H.: Ophthalmoplegic migraine of early onset. *J. Pediatr. 90*:1035, 1977.

External ophthalmoplegia may be caused by echo 9 viral infection and by ocular myopathy or neuropathy. The Kearns-Sayre syndrome consists of external ophthalmoplegia, retinitis pigmentosa and complete heart block.

Because of pressure on the corpora quadrigemina, patients who have a pineal tumor may be unable to elevate their eyes. This finding may also be seen with tumors of the cerebellum, the fourth ventricle, the pons and the diencephalon. Tumors of the pons may cause paralysis of conjugate movement of the eyes. Deviation of one eye upward and laterally and the other downward and medially (skew deviation) suggests a neoplasm in the posterior fossa. Paralysis of the ipsilateral third nerve may follow temporal lobe herniation. Rarely, a congenital aneurysm may cause ophthalmoplegia.

A phoria or tendency for strabismus may become converted to a tropia or manifest strabismus when a child is tired, emotionally disturbed or acutely ill.

## CLASSIFICATION OF STRABISMUS

*Esotropia*–convergent strabismus (eye turns medially)
*Exotropia*–divergent strabismus (eye turns laterally)
*Hypertropia*–upward deviation of the eye
*Hypotropia*–downward deviation of the eye
*Esophoria*–tendency to converge
*Exophoria*–tendency to diverge

*Concomitant (nonparalytic) strabismus* is characterized by a constant angle of deviation of the eyes in all fields. Frequently congenital, concomitant strabismus may be precipitated by febrile illnesses, head injury, fatigue or emotional upset. In *incomitant* or *paralytic strabismus* the angle of deviation of the visual axes is not constant in all directions but increases in the direction of movement normally produced by the paretic muscle. The paralysis may be congenital or acquired. *Constant (monocular) strabismus* is constantly present in the nonfixing eye. In *alternating strabismus* the eyes alternate in fixing and squinting. Esotropia is usually an alternating type of strabismus. Children with monocular strabismus, even though it is barely detectable, are at risk for amblyopia.

Since accommodation and convergence are closely associated movements, overactivity of the internal rectus muscle may lead to esotropia when the eye attempts to accommodate for a refractive error. Hyperopia is thus a common cause of convergent concomitant squint. This type of strabismus may become apparent during latter infancy or in early childhood. When first noted, the strabismus may be intermittent. Later, it is constantly present, either monocular or alternating. Impairment of fusion is an important factor in this development. Although myopia may be present in patients with convergent concomitant strabismus, this refractive error is usually associated with the less common divergent concomitant strabismus.

**Screening Tests for the Detection of Strabismus.** *Frank strabismus (tropia).* The child is asked to look at an otoscope light held about 13 to 15 inches in front of his eyes; meanwhile, the examiner seated in front of the child sights the position of the light reflex on the subject's pupil. The reflex should fall nearly in the center of each pupil. In children with strabismus the reflex falls somewhere between the center of the pupil and the limbus. If lateral displacement of the reflex occurs, the patient has a convergent squint. With medial displacement, a divergent strabismus exists. To evaluate the presence of strabismus when fixing on distant objects, the child is asked to look at a 75- or 100-watt light bulb 20 feet away. The examiner then determines the position of the light reflex. When one eye appears to be deviant, the other may be covered with a card. If the uncovered eye has been convergent, it will then move temporally. If divergent, it will move nasally. If no movement occurs, strabismus is not present.

*Tendency to strabismus (phoria).* The child is asked to focus on the light with both eyes uncovered. One eye is then covered with a card. When the card is removed, the examiner observes any movement of the eye. If a phoria is present, the eye will move from the convergent or divergent position assumed when covered to its original fixing position.

The oculomotor nerve also supplies the levator palpebrae superioris, the ciliary muscle and the sphincter of the pupil. The dilator of the pupil is supplied by sympathetic fibers. In older patients, diphtheritic neuritis may produce dysfunction of the ciliary muscle with resultant inability to read or do other work that requires

TABLE 4-1   ACTION AND INNERVATION OF OCULAR MUSCLES

| Muscle | Cranial Nerve | Action: Movement of Eye |
|---|---|---|
| Medial rectus | III | Medially |
| Lateral rectus | VI | Laterally |
| Superior rectus | III | Upward when eye is rotated laterally |
| Inferior rectus | III | Downward when eye is rotated laterally |
| Superior oblique | IV | Downward when eye is rotated medially |
| Inferior oblique | III | Upward when eye is rotated medially |

close accommodation. Patients receiving large doses of hydantoin may have difficulty with accommodation.

Head tilting or *ocular torticollis* may follow impaired function of the superior oblique. The head is tilted to the side opposite the involved muscle.

Infants with athetosis secondary to kernicterus are often unable to move their eyes upward and downward.

*Bell's phenomenon* is the automatic upward rotation of the eyes when the patient closes or, in the case of facial paralysis, attempts to close his eyes.

Third nerve palsies lead to ipsilateral ptosis, dilatation of the pupil and exotropia.

Ataxia-telangiectasia may be characterized by a pseudopalsy in which the child is unable to make rapid eye movements. The eyes tend to turn up on focusing.

## VISUAL FIELDS

Examination of the visual fields is indicated when edema of the optic disks is present or an intracranial space-occupying lesion is suspected. The confrontation test may be used as a screening examination. A more exact delineation of the visual fields requires the use of a perimeter. In the confrontation test the patient, seated about 3 feet from the examiner and with his back to the light, is asked to cover one eye and to look with his uncovered eye toward the opposite eye of the examiner. Using his finger or a small object, the examiner moves the test object from outside the patient's visual field toward his line of focus, keeping the object about 20 inches from the patient's eyes. This movement is performed in each of the principal meridians. Constriction of the visual fields may be noted in some patients with hysteria. Enlargement of the blind spot is an absolute criterion of papilledema. In children four to five years of age, finger counting may be used, the child being requested to hold up the same number of fingers as the examiner. Quantitative perimetry may be used after five to seven years of age.

## DIPLOPIA

Diplopia may occur in the Guillain-Barré syndrome, encephalitis, myasthenia gravis, pseudotumor cerebri, botulism, Sydenham's chorea and central nervous system leukemia. An intracranial tumor should always be considered when diplopia is precipitated by an acute paralytic strabismus. A child in whom double vision has suddenly developed may rub his eyes or squint as if photophobia were present, but he will not object to the ophthalmoscope light as will the patient with photophobia. The placing of a patch over one eye relieves the child of the disturbing double vision. Diplopia may occur in patients receiving hydantoin and with a blowout fracture of the orbit. Vertebrobasilar occlusive vascular disease is characterized by intermittent episodes of diplopia, vertigo, nausea, vomiting and mental confusion.

DeVivo, D.C. and Farrell, F.W.: Vertebrobasilar occlusive disease in children. *Arch. Neurol.* 26:278, 1972.

## PHOTOPHOBIA

Photophobia may be noted in the following conditions:

Measles
Vernal conjunctivitis
Foreign body
Iritis due to injury, bacterial infection or systemic illness
Corneal ulcer
Phlyctenular keratitis
Interstitial keratitis
Chronic idiopathic hypoparathyroidism
Xeroderma pigmentosa
Albinism
Cystinosis
Congenital glaucoma–*Photophobia may be the initial symptom*
Acrodermatitis enteropathica
Exposure to bright light
Botulism

Photophobia, partial albinism, atypical granules in the leukocytes and recurrent infections characterize the Chédiak-Higashi syndrome.

## NYSTAGMUS

Nystagmus is a rhythmic, usually rapid movement of the eyes that may be horizontal, vertical, rotary or mixed. The tremor may be about equal in rate in all directions *(pendular nystagmus)* or may demonstrate a quicker movement or component in one direction than in the other *(jerk nystagmus)*. The direction in which the fast component occurs is used to signify the direction of the nystagmus. The slight oscillating or nystagmoid movement *(end-point nystagmus)* with the fast component in the direction of gaze, which often occurs when normal children look out of the far corners of their eyes, is not true nystagmus.

The etiologic factors in nystagmus may broadly be regarded as neurologic, vestibular or ocular. In vestibular and neurologic disturbances, jerk nystagmus is usually present. Ocular defects are usually associated with the pendular type.

Ocular causes of nystagmus include cataracts, retrolental fibroplasia, astigmatism or other refractive errors, weakness of the extraocular muscles, and albinism. An unexplained congenital type of nystagmus may occur. In infancy pendular nystagmus and wandering of the eyes in an aimless searching manner suggest a visual defect. Ocular nystagmus may not be present, however, when total blindness has existed since birth or early infancy.

Vestibular causes of nystagmus are usually associated with labyrinthitis or other labyrinth disease. This type of nystagmus is discussed further on page 176.

Neurologic disorders associated with nystagmus include encephalitis, tuberculous meningitis, Friedreich's ataxia and Werdnig-Hoffmann disease. Nystagmus caused by an intracranial tumor suggests an infratentorial rather than supratentorial location. Nystagmus, usually on horizontal gaze, is present in most patients who have a posterior midline cerebellar tumor and is frequently present with tumors of the cerebellar hemispheres. This type of nystagmus is usually not spontaneous, as is common with vestibular disturbances, but develops when the patient focuses upon some point (*fixation nystagmus*). When the patient looks toward the side of the tumor, the nystagmus is slow and coarse. When the gaze is toward the opposite side, it is either not present or quick and minimal. In patients who have a tumor of the brain stem, nystagmus is often noted on horizontal and, occasionally, on upward gaze. Nystagmus may occur with cerebral palsy or organic brain damage. It may also be associated with systemic infections and drugs (e.g., children receiving large doses of hydantoin). Fixation nystagmus is seen in ataxia-telangiectasia. Cog-wheel rotary nystagmus, delayed head control and head nodding is seen in Pelizaeus-Merzbacher disease. Nystagmus also occurs in the craniofacial dysostosis and cerebrohepato-renal syndromes.

*Spasmus nutans,* or *nodding spasm,* is an uncommon disorder that occurs chiefly during the latter half or two-thirds of the first year in infants who have received relatively little stimulation. Often there is a history of inadequate lighting in the infant's environment. This syndrome is characterized by periodic, slight up-and-down or side-to-side nodding or rolling of the head. The movements occur once or twice a second for either brief or prolonged periods. There is also a unilateral or bilateral, intermittent and rapid nystagmus. Nodding of the head, which is especially prominent when the infant is sitting, may disappear when the infant lies down. Nystagmus may appear some weeks before the nodding.

Jayalakshmi, P., Scott, T. F. Mc., Tucker, S.H. and Schaffer, D.B.: Infantile nystagmus: a prospective study of spasmus nutans, congenital nystagmus, and unclassified nystagmus of infancy. *J. Pediatr. 77*:177, 1970.

*Opsoclonus ("dancing eyes"),* characterized by rapid, chaotic, irregular jerking of the eyes in all planes, but mainly horizontal, may be associated with occult neural crest tumors, especially neuroblastoma. In the Kinsbourne syndrome, opsoclonus is accompanied by myoclonic ataxia and extreme irritability in an infant or young child.

Dyken, P. and Kolar, O.: Dancing eyes, dancing feet: infantile polymyoclonia. *Brain 91*:305, 1968.

Moe, P.G. and Nellhaus, G.: Infantile polymyoclonia-opsoclonus syndrome and neural crest tumors. *Neurology 20*:756, 1970.

Solomon, G.E. and Chutorian, A.M.: Opsoclonus and occult neuroblastoma. *N. Engl. J. Med., 279*:475, 1968.

The *doll's eye phenomenon* is present in the first ten days of life and disappears in the second or third month. With the infant in the supine position, the baby's eyes lag behind when the head is turned gradually from side to side. The doll's eye maneuver may also be used in the evaluation of the older comatose child. Holding the patient's head first in a neutral position and with the eyelids held open, the examiner quickly rotates the head up and down and from side to side. In response to this maneuver, the eyes should move in a direction opposite to that of the head. Absence of doll's eye movements implies damage to the brain stem secondary to increased intracranial pressure and transtentorial herniation. Caution is advised if there is a possibility of a cervical fracture or if resistance is experienced to turning of the head.

## GENERAL REFERENCES

Costenbader, F.D.: Ocular affections and diseases. *In* Green, M. and Haggerty, R.J. (eds.): *Ambulatory Pediatrics.* 1st ed. Philadelphia, W. B. Saunders Co., 1968, p. 169.
Goldberg, M.E. (ed.): *Genetic and Metabolic Eye Disease.* Boston, Little, Brown and Company, 1974.
Harley, R.D.: *Pediatric Ophthalmology.* Philadelphia, W. B. Saunders Co., 1975.
Helveston, E.M.: Eye injuries, infections and screening. *In* Green, M. and Haggerty, R.J. (eds.): *Ambulatory Pediatrics II.* Philadelphia, W. B. Saunders Co., 1977, p. 242.
Liebman, S.D. and Gellis, S.S.: *The Pediatricians's Ophthalmology.* St. Louis, C. V. Mosby Co., 1966.

CHAPTER 5

# THE EARS

## HEARING

Normally, the newborn infant reacts to loud, sharp and sudden noises either by a startle response or by crying. In the second month he may demonstrate transient cessation of activity in response to sound. A month or two later the sound of his mother's voice brings anticipation. The five- or six-month-old child with well-developed head control often turns his head toward the source of sound.

Deaf infants may demonstrate a generalized indifference to sound in the presence of visual awareness and attentiveness. The five- to six-month-old infant experiences great pleasure in producing squealing and cooing sounds. A monotonal quality, a diminution or an absence of such sound experimentation suggests deafness. Such infants may also laugh less than normal babies.

When seeing infants during the first months of life, it is well to inquire about the infant's vocalizations and whether the mother believes that the infant can hear. In the older child, failure to develop or delayed development of adequate speech, difficulty in the enunciation of sibilants and a gradual loss of or a change in speech are indications for a hearing appraisal. When the cochlea is not functioning, speech disappears within a matter of weeks. The younger the child, the more rapid the disappearance.

Deafness or hearing impairment in a young child is often not obvious and may be difficult to determine. Deafness refers to hearing that is nonfunctional for ordinary purposes, even with a hearing aid. A *conductive* hearing loss is due to a problem in the external or middle ear whereas *sensorineural* or *nerve deafness* is due to a disorder medial to the stapes — in the inner ear, the auditory nerve or brain. A conductive hearing loss is seldom more severe than 60 decibels. A mixed hearing loss results from combined conductive and sensorineural impairments.

The fact that an infant can babble, perhaps say "Dada," or apparently notice the ringing of the telephone, the rumbling of a truck or similar noises does not mean that his hearing is adequate for speech perception. His response to the slamming of a door may be on a tactile or proprioceptive rather than an auditory basis. Young children with hearing impairment for the higher frequencies may in the home appear to understand many words and even begin to speak. A child with a loss of 30 to 45 decibels will be able to understand conversational speech from 3–5 feet but will have difficulty if the sound is faint or the speaker's face not visible.

Some mothers first suspect that something is wrong when they walk undetected into a room while their infant is looking in another direction. The baby appears startled when the mother finally comes into his line of vision. An infant with normal hearing and head control usually swings his head around almost instantly whenever someone enters the room.

Sometimes mothers are concerned about a possible hearing loss because the child turns up the sound of the radio or television until it is very loud. Usually this is a normal activity and does not indicate the presence of a hearing loss; however, such a possibility cannot always be immediately ruled out.

A child may be characterized as deaf if his hearing threshold across the speech frequencies is depressed 80 decibels in the better ear. Hearing impairment and deafness may be conductive or perceptive. Deafness may be genetic or acquired. Over 60 types of hereditary deafness exist, including autosomal recessive, autosomal dominant or sex-linked. Deafness may occur with diseases such as:

Retinitis pigmentosa (Usher's syndrome)
Recessive albinism
Pendred's syndrome of deafness and goiter
Leopard syndrome
Waardenburg's syndrome
Trisomies
Treacher Collins syndrome
Osteogenesis imperfecta
Osteopetrosis
Hurler's syndrome
Surdocardiac syndrome is characterized by deafness, electrocardiographic abnormalities (remarkably prolonged Q–T interval), syncopal attacks and sudden death.
Alport's syndrome–hereditary nephritis and deafness
Knuckle pads, leukonychia and hearing loss
Keratopachydermia, digital constriction and deafness
Congenital malformations of the ear.

Konigsmark, B.W.: Hereditary deafness in man. N. Engl. J. Med. 281:713, 774, 827, 1969.
Konigsmark, B.W.: Hereditary childhood hearing loss and integumentary system disease. J. Pediatr. 80:909, 1972.

Other children at risk of hearing loss include those affected by maternal rubella and those with neonatal hyperbilirubinemia, cleft palate, microtia, atresia of external auditory canal and recurrent otitis media.

Acquired deafness may be due to infections such as measles, meningitis and mumps, ototoxic drugs, anoxia and trauma. Deafness, usually severe and bilateral, is a complication of meningitis in about 3 per cent of patients, usually appearing on the first or second day. Serous otitis media is a common cause of a conductive hearing loss. Twenty-five per cent of children with cleft palates are estimated to have impaired hearing.

Infants and children with severe *mental retardation* may show little attentiveness or response to speech. The presence of retardation in other developmental areas may also suggest intellectual deficiency.

*Dysacusis* is characterized by an ability to hear but not discriminate sound. Discrimination impairment is an added handicap with neurosensory hearing losses.

*Psychogenic deafness,* characterized by an indifference to speech, is unusual in children. In this disorder, there is a discrepancy between the child's purported inability to hear ordinary conversation and his performance on repeated hearing tests. Because of their lack of response to speech, psychotic children may be referred for a supposed hearing problem.

**Hearing Tests.** It is often difficult to evaluate the status of hearing in infants and young children without careful observation over time and repeated hearing tests. Because of the complexity of the tests and the need for familiarity with their application, exact delineation of hearing loss in infants and children is usually a specialized procedure. Brain stem electrocochleography is a new noninvasive technique that may provide a quantitative assessment of the status of hearing in infants.

In the past the *aural palpebral* reflex was advised as a screening test to determine the presence of deafness with hearing supposedly present if the infant blinked his eyes in response to clapping of the hands or some other loud noise produced outside his field of vision. The test is not reliable and should be discarded.

The use of pure tones for testing may result in unreliable responses in infants and in many children under the age of three or four years. The use of tuning forks to test for air conduction is of little value. The same is true for bone conduction in the young child. A ticking watch is usually not satisfactory since ticking is a high frequency sound and does not necessarily mean that speech perception is adequate.

Turning of the head in response to a sound stimulus so that the eyes can see what the ears have heard is a fundamental and, probably, the best clinical reflex response for the testing of hearing. A number of noise-producing devices, including dog and police whistles, a squeaky toy mouse, cup and spoon, cowbells, cymbals, tom-toms, tambourines and ratchets, may be used out of sight of the child as qualitative office tests of hearing in young children. Cessation of activity or reflex turning of the head and eyes indicates ability to hear. Some quantitation can be obtained if the frequency and intensity of sound produced by these devices at various distances from the subject are known. Such quantitation may be difficult unless the examiner has had extensive experience and the circumstances of the test are carefully controlled. Infants and young children may normally respond to an auditory stimulus a few times, but they rapidly lose interest and fail to respond.

The *conditioned reflex* has been used as a hearing test in infants and children. A number of variations such as the peep show technique have been devised with the conditioned reflex as their basis. In some situations the child may be conditioned to react to various sounds by such responses as moving a block or pushing a button, or to pick up a ring and place it on a stand when the word "Go" is heard, the intensity of this word being gradually decreased. Similarly, the child who understands some language may be seated at a table with a few familiar objects or a picture book and asked to "Show me the cow," and the like, the intensity of the request being varied each time. Use of the audiometer without conditioned reflex responses is generally not possible before the age of four years. Even then, pure tone testing does not always permit a complete evaluation of a child's ability to perceive speech.

Downs, M.P.: Auditory screening. *Otolaryngol. Clin. N. Am. 11*:611, 1978.

The *Rinne test* compares loudness of the sound from a vibrating 512-cycle tuning fork that first is placed next to the external auditory canal and then is held in contact with the mastoid process. A normal or positive Rinne is obtained when the child hears the sound twice as long by air as by bone conduction. A child with conductive hearing loss will have difficulty hearing a 512-cycle tuning fork held near his ear but not when the handle is applied to the mastoid bone. With sensorineural hearing loss, both air and bone sound conduction are reduced, more so through the bone. In addition to hearing loss, children with severe deafness have problems with speech discrimination.

*Weber test.* When a vibrating 512-cycle tuning fork is placed on the center of the forehead in the presence of unilateral conductive loss, the sound will lateralize to the affected side. In unilateral sensorineural loss, the lateralization will be to the unimpaired ear.

Lesions of the vestibular branch of the auditory nerve may be detected by the use of the vestibular function tests described on page 26.

Bess, F.H.: *Childhood Deafness. Causation, Assessment, and Management.* New York, Grune & Stratton, 1978.
Fuller, C.W.: Hearing disorders in children: audiologic and educational management. *In* Green, M. and Haggerty, R.J. (eds.): *Ambulatory Pediatrics.* 1st ed. Philadelphia, W. B. Saunders Co., 1968, p. 550.

*Ringing* in the ears occurs with salicylism, the uveomeningoencephalitic syndrome and cerebellopontine tumors.

*Hyperacusia,* or hyperreactivity to sound, is frequent in Tay-Sachs and Sandhoff's diseases. Opisthotonus, flexion of the upper extremities and extension of the lower extremities occurs in response to a loud sound. Patients with tetanus or strychnine poisoning are also hyperreactive to sound.

## GESTATIONAL ASSESSMENT

In the premature infant, the ears lie flat against the scalp with only slight incurving of the superior part of the pinnae occurring at about 33 to 34 weeks' gestation. Since it contains no cartilage in preterm infants, the ear will remain folded when bent forward in early preterm infants. By 36 weeks of gestation, the pinna will spring back after folding. Incurving has occurred over two thirds of the ear by 38 to 40 weeks of gestation.

## CONGENITAL ANOMALIES

Anomalies of the pinna may be associated with deformities of the middle ear ossicles and a congenital hearing loss; therefore, deformity of the pinna is an indication for a hearing test. Anatomic landmarks of the pinna are illustrated in Figure 5–1.

> Jaffe, B.F.: Pinna anomalies associated with congenital conductive hearing loss. *Pediatrics 57*:332, 1976.

*Preauricular papillomas* or tubercles are not uncommon anomalies caused by maldevelopment of the first branchial arch. Single or multiple in number, they occur on the cheek, most commonly just anterior to the tragus and between the tragus and the corner of the mouth. Other anomalies of the external ear may be present as in Goldenhar's syndrome.

*Congenital aural fistulas* appear as unilateral or bilateral, pinpoint or slitlike openings from which a greasy, cheesy, white material can sometimes be expressed. The fistula is usually present immediately anterior and superior to the tragus or, more unusually, in the helix. Infection leads to inflammatory changes in the surrounding tissue.

A *darwinian tubercle* appears as a small nodule or thickening along the posterior segment of the helix near the tip of the auricle.

Abnormally protruding ears occur not infrequently. Patients with Marfan's syndrome may have prominent ears with pointing of the tips.

Infants with *Down's syndrome* have small low-set ears, measuring 3.4 cm. or less in their greatest vertical axis. The superior helix of the ear may be turned downward more than normally, and this border may be straight instead of curved.

Soft blister-like lesions or swellings occur in the first few days or weeks in newborn infants with *diastrophic dwarfism*. Spontaneous resolution of the lesions occurs after three to four weeks, leaving the ear hard owing to cartilaginous thick-

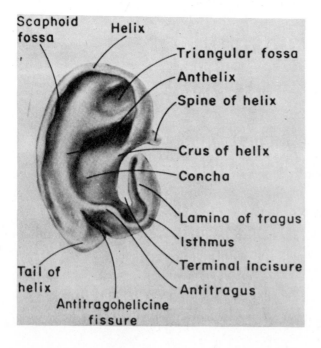

Figure 5–1 Anatomic landmarks of lateral aspect of right pinna. From Jaffe, B.F.: Pinna anomalies associated with congenital conductive hearing loss. *Pediatrics 57*:332, 1976.

ening and deformity. The lesions may later calcify. Infants with *bilateral renal agenesis* may have low-set, large and unusually floppy ears. Deformity of the pinna, microtia, atresia or stenosis of the external meatus and deafness may occur with *Treacher Collins* and *Goldenhar's syndromes*. In the latter, the maxillary, temporal and malar bones are unilaterally hypoplastic. Blind fistulas and extra skin tags may occur between the tragus and the angle of the mouth.

The ears may appear to be *low set* in children with a high cranial vault (e.g., with hydrocephalus and these syndromes: the Treacher Collins, Carpenter's, leopard, camptomelic, Smith-Lemli-Opitz, cri du chat, Turner's, Noonan's, Hallermann-Streiff, Williams elfin facies, Apert's, Pierre Robin, Potter's, trisomy 13, 18, 21, Wolf-Hirschhorn and fetal hydantoin).

Robinow, M. and Roche, A.F.: Low-set ears. *Am. J. Dis. Child. 125*:482, 1973.

Linear indentations of the ear lobes in the form of an inverted Y is a frequent finding in the *Beckwith-Wiedemann syndrome*.

*Tophi* may occur in the ears of patients with the Lesch-Nyhan syndrome.

## MASTOID

In infants with otitis media the mastoid area should be examined for swelling and tenderness. In patients with acute mastoiditis the pinna is displaced forward and the anteroposterior diameter of the meatus narrowed. Xanthomatosis is a rare cause of swelling in the mastoid region. Occasionally an enlarged lymph node is present over the mastoid area.

## EXTERNAL AUDITORY CANAL

*External otitis* may be due to bacteria or fungi and there is usually a history of water in the external auditory canal. Itching is the most common complaint, but exquisite pain may be present, especially if inflammatory edema occurs. Tenderness may be elicited with movement or pressure on the tragus. A wet, slimy aural discharge may be present.

A *foreign body* in the ear may cause a purulent or a serosanguineous discharge.

*Cerumen,* often in large amounts and sometimes impacted, may be softened by the instillation of hydrogen peroxide, warm sweet oil or light mineral oil once or twice. It may then be readily removed by washing gently with warm water if there is no perforation, or polyethylene tubes. Cerumen may also be removed with a Billeau earloop or spoon designed for the purpose. These procedures may be largely atraumatic in the older and cooperative child. In infants and young children, however, the procedure may cause traumatic bleeding unless the child is held tightly.

The *Ramsay Hunt syndrome* consists of herpes zoster of the auricle and external auditory canal with paralysis of the facial nerve, usually lasting only a few days to two weeks.

## TYMPANIC MEMBRANE

The manner of holding the otoscope depends upon the preference of the examiner. One method that permits flexibility of movement consists of grasping the upper end of the handle of the otoscope between the thumb and index finger so that the case rests on the metacarpophalangeal joint of the index finger perpendicular to the palm of the hand. Grasping the otoscope handle so that it is parallel to the palm does not permit the same range of motion.

In children, visualization of the tympanic membrane is facilitated if the auricle is pulled upward, outward and backward and if the speculum is directed anteriorly and superiorly. During infancy the auricle should be pulled slightly downward. The speculum may have to be rotated slightly to permit visualization of the entire tympanic membrane. A sketch of the normal tympanic membrane with landmarks is presented in Figure 5–2. These are easily seen in the older child but may be less distinct in the infant. The vertical and horizontal inclinations of the tympanic membrane observed in older children are greater in infants, the drum lying almost in a horizontal position with the posterosuperior portion of the membrane nearest the examiner.

On the first day of life, the tympanic membrane in the newborn is covered by vernix caseosa in the external canal. This may need to be irrigated away by a small-tipped medicine dropper and light mineral oil. A 2 or 3 mm. speculum should be used.

The tympanic membrane in infants is not as translucent as in older children. Once the examiner is well acquainted with the normal appearance of the tympanic membrane, pathologic findings may be recognized and interpreted quickly. The examination of the eardrums is of especial importance in children with respiratory infections, fever or pain. Slight injection along the manubrium and the periphery of the drum may be noted in normal infants and children. *Otitis media* occurs frequently in early life, especially between 4 and 12 months of age, but also in the newborn. Streptococcus pneumoniae is the most frequent cause of acute otitis media. Hemophilus influenzae, usually nontypable, is frequently the etiologic

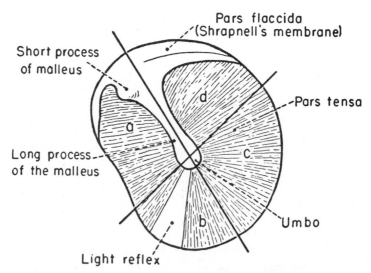

**Figure 5–2** Diagram of left tympanic membrane. *a,* Anterior-superior quadrant; *b,* anterior-inferior quadrant; *c,* posterior-inferior quadrant; *d,* posterior-superior quadrant.

agent in children under four years of age. Group A beta-hemolytic streptococcus and Staphylococcus aureus are uncommonly involved. Pseudomonas aeruginosa and other gram-negative enteric bacilli may be associated with chronic or recurrent middle ear diseases. Cultures of the nasopharynx or oropharynx are not helpful in determining bacterial etiology in otitis media. Needle aspiration is recommended if (1) the child is critically ill, (2) chronic otitis media is present, (3) there is no clinical response within 48 hours and (4) the patient is immunodeficient. Otitis media is to be looked for with symptoms of ear pain, fever, irritability or screaming. Acute and persistent crying or diarrhea and vomiting may be noted in infants with otitis media. Perforation of the drum and drainage may occasionally occur without pain. Some infants will pull at the involved ear while others will not. Pulling at an ear may also be a habit rather than a sign of otitis media.

Hyperemia or intense redness along the handle of the malleus, the periphery and pars flaccida of the drum occurs early in otitis media; however, this finding, in itself, does not support a diagnosis of otitis media. With continuation of the process, bulging appears, usually first in the posterosuperior quadrant, and then spreads forward. The light reflex and umbo are obliterated early.

The diagnosis of otitis media in the newborn is difficult since the symptoms of irritability, feeding problems, cough, diarrhea or rhinorrhea are nonspecific, and the tympanic membrane often looks dull, red and thickened. Since the short process of the malleus is almost always seen, its obliteration is diagnostic. Etiologic agents include Escherichia coli, Staphylococcus aureus and Klebsiella pneumoniae.

*Middle ear effusion.* The eardrum normally moves inward with positive pressure and outward with negative pressure obtained with the pneumatic otoscope. Fluid in the middle ear impedes drum mobility. A retracted drum usually does not move inward with positive pressure but somewhat outward with negative pressure. To evaluate tympanic mobility satisfactorily, a close fit must be obtained in the external ear canal. Rubber tubing slipped on the end of the speculum contributes to a tight seal.

In babies and young children, the diagnosis of otitis media is often difficult because of cerumen and because changes in retraction or fullness, color, translucency and mobility may be subtle. Tympanometry has been helpful in evaluating infants over six months of age in the office and in clarifying uncertain otoscopic diagnoses but is not recommended for mass screening on a routine basis for the detection of middle ear disease.

Bess, F.H. et al.: Use of acoustic impedance measurement in screening for middle ear disease in children. *Ann. Otol. Rhinol. Laryngol. 87*:288, 1978.
Paradise, J.L., Smith, G.G. and Bluestone, C.D.: Tympanometric detection of middle ear effusion in infants and young children. *Pediatrics 58*:198, 1976.

After an episode of acute otitis media, the tympanic membrane may appear retracted, dull and scarred.

*Blebs or bullae (bullous myringitis)* containing a serous or hemorrhagic fluid are occasionally noted on the tympanic membrane and, at first glance, may simulate a perforation. At other times hemorrhagic flecks may be noted on the drum. Severe otalgia and impairment of hearing may be associated symptoms. The cause is usually viral but may be bacterial.

*Serous otitis media* is a common cause of acute or chronic hearing loss. Although the older child may complain of a feeling of fullness or "water" in the ear, there are usually no complaints. Unsuspected hearing loss is usually detected on routine audiometric evaluation. The appearance of the tympanic membrane varies. Some retraction is usually present although, rarely, bulging may occur. A thickened tympanic membrane with obscured bony landmarks may be difficult to differentiate from a bulging drum. A fluid level or bubble may be seen. Frequently the tympanic membrane has an amber color, but this is variable and not diagnostic. The drum moves poorly when a pneumatic otoscope is used in either suppurative or serous otitis media.

Otitis media probably develops in all infants with *cleft palate* during the first months of life. A chronically draining ear may be observed with *histiocytosis*. *Rhabdomyosarcoma* arising in the ear may present with ear pain, chronic drainage, granulation tissue or polyp in the canal and facial paralysis.

*Chronic otitis media* may be relatively benign or serious. In the former the perforation is central whereas in the latter, usually associated with cholesteatomas, the perforation is marginal or in the pars flaccida. In the child with a central perforation the discharge is intermittent and usually associated with upper respiratory tract infections whereas with a cholesteatoma, white greasy flakes may be visualized in the attic perforation, and there is an intermittent foul-smelling discharge.

Bluestone, C.D. and Shurin, P.A.: Middle ear disease in children. Pathogenesis, diagnosis and management. *Pediatr. Clin. N. Am. 21*:379, 1974.
Howie, V.M., Ploussard, J.H. and Lester, R.L., Jr.: Otitis media: a clinical and bacteriological correlation. *Pediatrics 45*:29, 1970.
Klein, J.O.: Middle ear disease in children. *Hosp. Pract. 11*:45 (July) 1976.
Rowe, D.S.: Acute suppurative otitis media. *Pediatrics 56*:285, 1975.
Tetzlaff, T.R., Ashworth, C. and Nelson, J.D.: Otitis media in children less than 12 weeks of age. *Pediatrics 59*:827, 1977.

### GENERAL REFERENCE

Bluestone, C.D. and Stool, S.E.: *Disorders of the Ear, Nose and Throat in Children.* Philadelphia, W. B. Saunders Co., 1978.

CHAPTER 6

# THE NOSE

The nose is frequently misshapen and somewhat flattened after birth. Usually the normal shape is regained within a short time, either spontaneously or with gentle manipulation. Deformity of the nose and a short columella are frequent in the infant with a cleft lip.

Sneezing, a common occurrence in newborn infants, is generally interpreted as the infant's only method of effectively clearing his upper respiratory tract.

## OBSTRUCTION AND CONGESTION

Obstruction of the nasal airway may be due to unilateral or bilateral *congenital closure of the posterior choanae.* A wisp of cotton held below the involved side does not move with respiration. Obstruction may be confirmed by attempting to pass a No. 8 French rubber catheter through the nose. Skull roentgenograms after instillation of a liquid contrast medium may confirm the clinical impression. Since infants are obligate nose breathers, sleeping with their mouth closed and breathing through their nose, patent nasal airways are important for normal respiration. Bilateral choanal atresia precipitates respiratory distress immediately after birth. Unilateral choanal atresia causes few symptoms. Nasal obstruction may lead to irritability, cyanosis, dyspnea and feeding difficulty. A persistent nasal discharge may be present. A large amount of glairy, translucent, mucoid secretion may be removed from the involved nostril.

Nasal congestion may occur and persist for several days in newborn infants whose mothers have received reserpine. Hypothyroidism has also been reported as a cause of difficulty in nasal breathing in infants. Allergic rhinitis may be a rare cause of nasal obstruction in the young infant.

Ingall, M., Glaser, J., Meltzer, R.S. and Dreyfuss, E.M.: Allergic rhinitis in early infancy. *Pediatrics 35*:108, 1965.

Fibrous dysplasia of the facial bones is an unusual cause of bony nasal obstruction in childhood.

## CONGENITAL ANOMALIES

A flat, *depressed nasal bridge,* or *saddle nose,* may be noted with syphilis, Down's syndrome, congenital ectodermal dysplasia, craniometaphyseal dysostosis, congenital hypothyroidism, Conradi's syndrome, chondrodystrophy, Larsen's syndrome, osteopetrosis, cleidocranial dysostosis and Hurler's syndrome.

The nose in chondrodystrophy and Hurler's syndrome may be somewhat large and *turned up* at the end with relatively large nostrils. The Smith-Lemli-Opitz syndrome is also characterized by a broad nose with upturned nares. The fetal alcohol syndrome includes a low nasal bridge with a short or upturned nose. A small nose and anteverted nares occurs in the Aarskog syndrome.

A thin, *beak-like nose* occurs in patients with progeria and craniofacial dysostosis including Apert's syndrome and pycnodysostosis. In the Hallermann-Streif syndrome, the nose is thin, curved and pointed, giving a parrot-like facial profile. A beak nose is also seen in patients with craniofacial dysostosis and the Rubinstein-Taybi syndrome.

*Holoprosencephaly* (arhinencephaly) may be characterized by a proboscis-like structure instead of a nose or a rudimentary nose that resembles that of the platyrhine monkey (cebocephaly).

## OTHER FINDINGS

Flaring or movement of the alae nasi with respiration may occur in patients with pneumonia, peritonitis, hyperpyrexia, acidosis, paralysis of the respiratory musculature and other conditions characterized by hyperpnea, tachypnea and dyspnea. It may accompany the short inspiratory movements caused by chest pain.

A *dermoid* may appear, usually in adolescence, as a persistent small nodule, cystic swelling or dimple in the midline of the nose.

*Wegener's granulomatosis* or *idiopathic lethal granuloma* of the nose and face is a progressively destructive process characterized by persistent nasal discharge, crusted and pustular lesions, swelling, induration and finally ulceration of midline structures of the face such as the nasal septum, inferior choanae, lip and hard palate.

## SINUSES

Although the sphenoid sinuses are present at birth, the ethmoid and maxillary sinuses are the ones that become infected during early life. The frontal sinuses do not appear until four to six years of age. During infancy, the ostia of the sinuses are relatively larger than later in life, and the sinuses usually become infected during an acute rhinitis. Such involvement usually clears spontaneously.

*Chronic sinusitis,* unusual in children unless there is some other problem, may occur secondary to diving into water feet first, nasal allergy, cystic fibrosis, cleft palate, Kartagener's syndrome, choanal atresia, immunologic disorders and Hurler's syndrome.

> Jaffe, B.F.: Chronic sinusitis in children. *Clin. Pediatr. 13*:944, 1974.

Chronic sinusitis is associated with a chronic nasal discharge and obstruction. A yellow, mucopurulent, purulent or clear mucoid discharge may be seen draining from above or below the middle turbinate. The inferior turbinates may be so engorged that the middle turbinates cannot be visualized. During an acute infection, tenderness and swelling may be present over the affected sinus. Digital pressure does not produce pain in chronic infections. Acute ethmoid sinusitis may cause swelling of the periorbital region, especially medially. This swelling may initially be minimal and easily overlooked. Slight puffiness of the eyelids and dark circles around the eyes may be noted in children with chronic sinusitis. On gagging, a postnasal drip may be seen coming from the nasopharynx. Sinusitis may also be present without evidence of a nasal discharge. Frontal sinusitis may occasionally be complicated by osteomyelitis of the frontal bone producing localized pitting edema.

Transillumination of the sinuses in children is not of value.

## EPISTAXIS

Epistaxis most commonly arises from Kiesselbach's area, the anastomotic site for a number of terminal arterioles, on the nasal septum about 0.5 cm. within the nose and above the nasal floor. Varicosities that develop under the thin mucous membrane here are easily traumatized by nose picking, the most common cause of epistaxis in children, and excessive drying of the mucous membrane.

Other causes of epistaxis include rheumatic fever, infectious mononucleosis, sickle cell anemia and systemic hemorrhagic disorders. Hemangiomas and hereditary telangiectasis are unusual causes of epistaxis. A chronic bloody nasal discharge may be caused by nasal diphtheria or a foreign body in the nose.

*Juvenile angiofibroma of the nasopharynx,* which develops after the age of ten years almost exclusively in boys, is manifested by progressive unilateral or bilateral nasal obstruction, mucoid or mucopurulent discharge and recurrent, severe epistaxis. The tumor may protrude into the nasal passages anteriorly or hang down below the soft palate. Olfactory neuroepithelial tumors may also cause nasal obstruction and recurrent epistaxis.

Pimpinella, R.J.: The nasopharyngeal angiofibroma in the adolescent male. *J. Pediatr.* *64*:260, 1964.

*Lymphoepithelioma,* an uncommon malignant nasopharyngeal tumor, is characterized by unilateral, tender, cervical lymphadenopathy, and epistaxis, trismus and painful torticollis. These findings are indications for a skilled examination of the nasopharynx.

Pick, T., Mauer, H.M. and McWilliams, N.B.: Lymphoepithelioma in childhood. *J. Pediatr.* *84*:96, 1974.

## NASAL DISCHARGE

A unilateral, persistent nasal discharge accompanied by obstruction of the airway may be caused by a foreign body or an imperforate choana. Snuffles is the term applied to the persistent and profuse mucopurulent or bloody nasal discharge in infants with congenital syphilis.

## TURBINATES

The turbinates may be pale and boggy in children with allergic rhinitis. Similar findings may be caused by chronic use of nose drops and by vasomotor rhinitis. *Nasal polyps* are soft, glistening, smooth, pinkish-gray and movable. While these may occur in children with sinusitis, allergic rhinitis and Kartagener's syndrome, *cystic fibrosis of the pancreas* should be ruled out since multiple and recurrent polyps frequently obstruct the nasal airways in children with this disorder.

Baker, D.C. and Smith, J.T.: Nasal symptoms of mucoviscidosis. *Otolaryngol. Clin. N. Am.* *3*:257, 1970.

*Septal deviation* may result from trauma to the nose.

CHAPTER 7

# THE MOUTH

## EXAMINATION

Inspection of the oral cavity and pharynx is usually the most disturbing part of the physical examination for young children and generally best done last. It should be performed quickly, yet completely, and with minimal discomfort to the child. Before examining the throat one may ask to see the patient's teeth. A tongue depressor may then be introduced, and after the examination of the teeth one may say, "Let's look way back there," and then proceed to examine the throat. Many cooperative children are able to open their mouths so widely and protrude their tongues so actively that a tongue depressor is unnecessary. The procedure need not gag the patient, although gagging, at times, may be necessary to allow satisfactory visualization. Gagging may be avoided in the older child if he breathes actively through his mouth during the examination. Some children have extremely active gag reflexes and tend to gag and sometimes even vomit when a tongue blade is placed on the back of their tongues. At times the examination of the pharynx may be facilitated by first depressing one side of the base of the tongue and then the other. Examination of an infant's pharynx may be difficult because the mouth is often kept tightly closed. In such event one should wait until the infant relaxes his clenched jaws or until he cries. Actually, one may obtain a fair view of the mouth and part of the pharynx during crying. The posterior pharynx is not easily seen in young infants. Forcing the mouth open or holding the infant's nose shut is unnecessary and undesirable. During the examination of the pharynx, infants and young children may have to be held by a parent or nurse. The child's arms may be extended above and held tightly against his head. This may be accomplished best if the mother cups her fingers around the child's elbows and uses her thumbs to rest on and control the infant's head. In this position the child cannot move his head. After examination of the pharynx, the head may be turned to either side for the examination of the ears.

Good intraoral lighting is essential. A pocket flashlight or a large flashlight with a condensing or spotlight lens is satisfactory. Usually the otoscope light is not bright enough to permit good visualization. A small-sized tongue blade may be used to facilitate inspection of various areas of the mouth. Compact, combined spotlight and tongue blade holders may be substituted for the otoscope head during the examination of the mouth. This attachment is helpful in that one hand is free to hold the child or to take a throat culture under direct vision.

## ORAL DEVELOPMENT

Developmentally, the *sucking and swallowing* reflexes should be present in the term newborn infant. These reflexes are poorly developed or absent in some premature infants. Failure to suck well and difficulty in swallowing may suggest cerebral injury. Infants with such neuromuscular impairment feed slowly, gag easily and choke. Increased sucking behavior is noted in infants of drug-addicted mothers. In infant botulism, which occurs usually between the ages of three and six months, sucking and swallowing may be impaired with resultant pooling of secretions.

During early infancy, semisolid food introduced into the anterior part of the mouth is often pushed out by the tongue. By two and one-half to three months, and sometimes even earlier, neuromuscular maturation has proceeded to the point at which pureed foods can be carried back from the anterior part of the mouth to the pharynx and swallowed. At eight or nine months of age or later, licking and chewing motions are noted, and the infant enjoys chewing on toast, a crust of bread or a piece of bacon.

Infants normally sleep with their mouths closed. Nasal obstruction due to an upper respiratory tract infection or atresia of the posterior choanae may lead to dyspnea, difficulty in sucking and cyanosis.

Little salivation occurs in the newborn infant, being minimal until two to four months of age, at which time drooling may occur. Babies often drool excessively when teething. Drooling may also be excessive and abnormally persistent in children with cerebral palsy because of pharyngeal incoordination and in those with mental retardation and with familial dysautonomia, especially when the child is excited.

## CLINICAL FINDINGS

*Excessive saliva and mucus coming from the mouth of a newborn infant should always suggest esophageal atresia.* When one suspects that an esophageal atresia is present, a No. 8 or 10 French soft rubber catheter should be passed into the esophagus. If the catheter passes into the stomach as verified by fluoroscopy, esophageal atresia is ruled out.

Yawning, frequent swallowing movements and facial grimacing may be signs of nausea in infants.

Hiccups in young infants possibly are a reflection of neuromuscular immaturity and the gastric distention that frequently follows feeding.

*Sucking pads,* which produce a fullness of the cheeks anterior to the masseter muscle, become prominent in malnourished infants.

The loss of subcutaneous fat that occurs gradually from the upper half of the body in patients with *progressive lipodystrophy* is especially noticeable in the cheeks.

*Mouth breathing* in older children may be due to sinusitis, hypertrophy of adenoid tissue or other nasopharyngeal obstruction. Snoring and cogwheel breathing may occur when the child sleeps on his back. Chronic mouth breathing may lead to an "adenoid facies" with an open mouth, narrow pinched nose, short upper lip, a high palate and a dull facial expression. The upper incisors may be spaced and protrude beneath the lip. Mouth breathing may also occur with a retropharyngeal abscess, pneumonia or weakness of the respiratory musculature.

*Risus sardonicus* occurs in some patients with tetanus. The corners of the mouth are pulled outward and downward, and the lip is stretched across the upper incisors to produce a sardonic grin. The eyebrows may also be drawn upward and the palpebral fissures narrowed.

A large, fish-like mouth occurs in these syndromes: Treacher Collins, Williams elfin facies, oculoauriculovertebral dysplasia, congenital myotonic dystrophy and idiopathic hypercalcemia. Microstomia is characteristic of the whistling face syndrome.

Weinstein, S. and Gorlin, R.J.: Cranio-carpo-tarsal dysplasia or the whistling face syndrome. *Am. J. Dis. Child. 117*:427, 1969.

Children with the athetoid form of cerebral palsy often "tuck in" their chin when they walk. The mouth may also remain open because of the depression of the lower jaw.

Failure of one corner of the mouth to move downward and outward, especially noticeable when the child cries, may be due to *congenital absence or hypoplasia of the depressor anguli oris muscle,* a disorder that must be differentiated from congenital facial palsy. The lateral part of the lower lip may feel thinner on the involved side.

Nelson, K.B. and Eng, G.C.: Congenital hypoplasia of the depressor anguli oris muscle; differentiation from congenital facial palsy. *J. Pediatr. 81*:16, 1972.

"Bad breath," or halitosis, may be attributable to the following causes:

Poor oral hygiene
Vomiting
Dry mouth due to dehydration
Tonsillitis
Blood in the mouth
Sinusitis
Hypertrophy and infection of adenoid tissue
Herpetic and Vincent's stomatitis
Typhoid fever and other enteric infections
Ingestion of strong-smelling, volatile foods that produce odors because of pulmonary excretion

*Acetone odor* to the breath occurs with ketoacidosis.

## LIPS

In *cleft lip* the unilateral or bilateral defect may range from a simple notching to a complete separation of the maxillary and premaxillary processes and an extension of the cleft into the nostril. Cleft of the palate is often an associated defect.

*Congenital lip pits or fistulas* are bilateral blind sinuses, usually on the vermilion border of the lower lip, which may occur with or without an associated cleft lip and/or palate, popliteal pterygia and genital anomalies.

Fusion of the upper lip to the underlying gum occurs in some patients with *chondroectodermal dysplasia* (Ellis-van Creveld syndrome).

The *labial or sucking tubercle* in the middle of the upper lip in young infants disappears after weaning. Sucking plaques are also frequently noted along the edges of the upper and lower lips, particularly in infants whose sucking movements are vigorous.

The distance between the columella of the nose and the upper lip is greater than normal with Hurler's syndrome.

The lesions of *herpes simplex* may appear on the lips either singly or grouped. Beginning as a small erythematous macule, the lesion rapidly progresses to the papular stage followed by a minute, painful vesicle. Rupture of the vesicle, crusting and secondary infection then occur.

*Cheilitis* with drying, wrinkling, cracking and scaling of the lips may occur during acute febrile illnesses or with contact sensitivity or chapping.

*Acrodermatitis enteropathica* is characterized by an erythematous, moist skin eruption and fissuring around the mouth and other orifices; vesiculobullous or crusted lesions on the buttocks, elbows, knees, hands and feet; alopecia and stomatitis.

*Perleche,* characterized by fissuring, scaling, maceration and crusting of the angles of the mouth, is usually due to a monilial or, at times, streptococcal infection. *Cheilosis* is a form of fissuring caused by a nutritional deficiency. *Rhagades* are moist, radiating lesions around the corners of the mouth due to congenital syphilis. Fissuring may also be noted in children who drool excessively.

In the *Peutz-Jeghers syndrome* discrete bluish black and brown pigmented spots may occur around the eyes, nose and mouth, lips and oral mucosa.

*Angioneurotic edema* may cause an acute, nonpitting, perhaps pruritic, massive swelling of the lip or face.

The *mucosal neuroma syndrome* may present early with neuromas of the lips, anterior part of the tongue and the conjunctiva. The lips are protuberant with a "blubbery" appearance. Medullary carcinoma of the thyroid and pheochromocytoma may appear later. The patient has a Marfan-like habitus.

> Schimke, R.N.: Phenotype of malignancy: the mucosal neuroma syndrome. *Pediatrics* 52:283, 1973.

The *fetal alcohol* syndrome is characterized by a thinned upper vermilion border of the lip.

*Electrical burns of the mouth,* usually caused by the child chewing on an electrical cord, initially cause a painless, white, parchment-like lesion of the skin followed in a few hours by considerable edema. Since the burn is always more extensive than initially appears to be the case, serious bleeding may occur one day to three weeks later from erosion of the labial artery.

> Gifford, G.H., Jr., Marty, A.T. and MacCollum, D.W.: The management of electrical mouth burns in children. *Pediatrics* 47:113, 1971.

*Self-mutilative behavior* with a section of the lip or part of a finger bitten away occurs in the Lesch-Nyhan syndrome.


## BUCCAL MUCOSA

*Thrush,* caused by Monilia albicans, is characterized by white, raised membranous patches, which resemble milk curds, on the buccal surfaces, lips, tongue and pharynx. The patches are removed with some difficulty and leave mucosal lesions slightly oozing with blood.

*Acute necrotizing ulcerative gingivitis* or *Vincent's stomatitis* (trench mouth) is characterized by crater-like ulcerated lesions on the marginal gingiva covered by a white pseudomembrane and surrounded by a zone of erythema. The gums are severely tender, painful and bleed easily. The breath has a fetid odor. Submaxillary lymphadenopathy may be present.

In *pachyonychia congenita* the buccal mucosa and the dorsum of the tongue are thick and white or gray-white.

*Herpetic gingivostomatitis,* due to the herpes simplex virus, is characterized by fever, irritability and small vesicles that rupture to leave shallow ulcers on the gums, tongue and buccal mucous membrane. The lesions are irregular, 0.3 to 1.0 cm. in diameter, and have a gray center and a red, elevated edge.

*Canker sores* appear as pinhead-sized vesicles that rupture quickly to leave small grayish or yellowish ulcers, which may be encircled by a reddish areola and covered by a greenish or yellowish-gray membrane. Removal of the membrane leaves a raw area. Canker sores are often seen in children with inflammatory bowel disease.

Recurrent stomatitis may occur in patients with *cyclic neutropenia*.

*Behçet's syndrome* consists of recurrent oral and genital ulcerations, uveitis, meningoencephalitis, arthritis or arthralgia and erythema nodosum. The oral lesions, which may be single or multiple, are usually under 1 cm. in diameter with a yellow center surrounded by erythema.

Mundy, T.M. and Miller, J.J., III: Behçet's disease presenting as chronic aphthous stomatitis in a child. *Pediatrics 62*:205, 1978.

*Herpangina* is a manifestation of an acute, epidemic, febrile disease due to an enterovirus. Occurring in the summer, this syndrome is characterized by dysphagia, a mildly sore throat and papulovesicular lesions that range in size from 1 to 4 mm. The vesicles are surrounded by a zone of intense erythema. Their rupture leads to grayish-yellow or white ulcers. The lesions, usually few in number but at times numerous, appear chiefly on the anterior tonsillar pillars, occasionally on the tonsils and soft palate, and more unusually on the tongue. The pharynx may be diffusely injected. In contrast to herpetic gingivostomatitis, the buccal mucosa and gingivae are uninvolved.

*Hand-foot-and-mouth disease* is characterized by vesiculoulcerative lesions of the oropharynx accompanied by a maculopapular exanthema on the palms, soles, heels and, at times, the knees and legs.

One or a few small white or yellow follicles on an erythematous base may be seen on the anterior tonsillar pillars on the second or third day of life. These benign lesions disappear in two to four days.

*Leukemia* may cause ulcers on the buccal mucosa.

*Koplik's spots* occur during the prodromal phase of measles as grayish-white, opalescent specks surrounded by a light red, blotchy areola. Best seen in natural light, they appear first on the buccal mucosa opposite the lower molars. Occasionally, they may be extensively distributed in the mouth.

*Chickenpox* lesions may occur on the palate as well as elsewhere in the mouth and pharynx.

*Epidermolysis bullosa* lesions may involve the buccal mucosa.

Brown or blue-black pigmented areas may occur on the buccal mucous membrane in *Addison's disease*. Similar pigmentation may also be observed in the *Peutz-Jeghers syndrome*.

Small submucosal hemorrhages or grayish-white plaques in the region of the molars may be of traumatic origin due to malocclusion or jagged teeth. A bluish, translucent retention cyst of a labial or buccal mucous gland may develop on the lower lip secondary to trauma.

*Popsicle panniculitis* caused by exposure to cold is characterized by a deep, movable, firm, slightly elevated, red nodule on the cheek.

Epstein, E.H., Jr. and Oren, M.E.: Popsicle panniculitis. *N. Engl. J. Med. 282*:966, 1970.

*Papillomas* may arise from the buccal epithelium as pedunculated, smooth or verrucous tumors with a whitish surface.

Bulging cheeks occur in the *whistling face syndrome*.

## GINGIVAE; ALVEOLAR PROCESSES

*Epulis* is a nonspecific term for any of the benign neoplasms or hyperplasias of the gingiva. Congenital epulis of the newborn is a benign, pedunculated, smooth soft tissue growth from the maxillary or mandibular gingival edge.

Bhaskar, S.N.: Oral tumors of infancy and childhood. *J. Pediatr. 63*:195, 1963.

Occasionally the midline membranous labial frenum from the upper lip to the labial surface of the upper alveolar process may continue on between the central incisors to the lingual side of the arch as an *alveolar frenum* and cause spacing between the central incisors.

In the *orofaciodigital syndrome,* a median notching of the upper lip extends through the vermilion border. Multiple fibrous bands course from the lower lip and cheeks onto the mandibular alveolar process and cause clefting there.

The gingival mucosa in the region of the unerupted molars is often pale or nearly colorless. Occasionally a pearly white retention cyst persists for months on the gingival margin in infants.

*Histiocytosis X* may cause gingivitis, swelling of the palate and loss of teeth.

Hydantoin therapy may cause extensive, painless, firm and lobulated *gingival hypertrophy.* Hypertrophy and injection of the gingivae may occur in persistent mouth-breathers. Poor dental hygiene may be contributory.

*Periapical abscesses* or "gum boils" occasionally occur at the base of a tooth, either lingually or labially. Localized areas of swelling and redness usually indicate a periapical infection. Pus may be noted to escape around the tooth, which is usually nonvital and loose.

The gingivae of black children are brownish-red while the marginal aspects of the gingivae and the interdental papillae are bluish-gray.

*Gingivitis* may be noted in adolescents. The margin of the gum is red and edematous and bleeds easily. Gingivitis also occurs in patients with neutropenia or myelomonocytic leukemia when the absolute granulocyte count is less than 1000/mm$^3$.

Polson, A.M.: Gingival and peridontal problems in children. *Pediatrics 54*:190, 1974.


## PALATE

There are four chief types of cleft palate:
1. Involvement is limited to the soft palate.
2. The cleft extends through both the soft and hard palates up to the alveolar process.
3. The soft and hard palates are both involved, and there is a unilateral cleft of the alveolar process.
4. The soft and hard palates are both involved, and there is a bilateral cleft of the alveolar process.

Patients with a *submucous cleft* have no overt cleft, but the midline of the palate on palpation seems to be very thin. The palate may also be foreshortened and velopharyngeal closure incomplete. The uvula is bifid, and a notch in the posterior border of the hard palate is palpable. The speech has a prominent nasal quality due to excessive nasal resonance. A bifid uvula is not pathognomonic for a submucous cleft. A submucous cleft of the primary and secondary palate occurs in the orofaciodigital syndrome.

Cooper, H.K. et al.: *Cleft Palate and Cleft Lip: A Team Approach to Clinical Management and Rehabilitation of the Patient.* Philadelphia, W. B. Saunders Co., 1978.


Cleft palate may occur as an isolated defect but is often part of a syndrome (e.g., with congenital lip fistulas, diastrophic dysplasia, mandibulofacial dysostosis, and the Larsen, orofaciodigital, popliteal pterygium, trisomy 13, trisomy 18 and Wolf-Hirschhorn syndromes).

Lis, E.F.: Management of children with cleft lip and cleft palate. *In* Green, M. and Haggerty, R.J. (eds.): *Ambulatory Pediatrics*. 1st ed. Philadelphia, W. B. Saunders Co., 1968, p. 581.

The *Pierre Robin syndrome* is characterized by a posterior cleft of the palate, micrognathia and glossoptosis. These findings may be seen in the Stickler, Beckwith-Wiedemann, diastrophic dysplasia and fetal hydantoin syndromes.

Schreiner, R.L., McAlister, W.H., Marshall, R.E. and Shearer, W.T.: Stickler syndrome in a pedigree of Pierre Robin syndrome. *Am. J. Dis. Child. 126*:86, 1973.

*Palatopharyngeal incompetence* occurs when the soft palate and related pharyngeal musculature do not effectively separate the nasopharynx from the oropharynx. Associated symptoms include hypernasal speech, escape of fluid through the nose when swallowing, and inability to hiss, whistle, gargle, blow out a candle or inflate a balloon.

The palate should elevate when a tongue blade is gently applied to each pillar of the palatal arch. This *gag reflex,* which tests for function of cranial nerves IX (afferent) and X (efferent), is clinically significant only if one side persistently does not respond. It is absent in *botulism*. Patients with diphtheria may have paralysis of the palate.

*Epstein's pearls* or *Bohn's nodules* are small, localized accumulations of epithelial cells or cysts on each side of the median raphe of the hard palate or along the alveolar ridge in newborn infants. The lesions, which are white, firm and raised, vary from pinhead to 3 mm. in size.

*Petechial spots* are occasionally observed on the soft palate with pharyngitis or other respiratory diseases.

A *high, arched palate* may occur with Marfan's, Treacher Collins, Ehlers-Danlos, cerebral gigantism and Rubinstein-Taybi syndromes and in mouth breathers.

Two reddened or yellow-gray, slightly eroded lesions sometimes called *Bednar's aphthae* may occur far back on the hard palate in young infants, one on each side of the midline. These lesions are usually due to trauma from the nipple or to overvigorous cleansing of the mouth at the time of birth.


CHAPTER 8

# THE TONGUE


## NORMAL FINDINGS

Since it follows the neural growth curve, the tongue may appear relatively large at birth and during early infancy. Occasionally, slight protrusion of the normally large tongue may suggest macroglossia.

Functional or neurologic impairment of tongue movements may interfere with feeding and speech. The movements of the tongue necessary for normal feeding and speech include the ability to extend the tongue forward between the lips and the teeth, retract it back into the mouth, move the tongue laterally and elevate the base or tip of the tongue.

## CLINICAL FINDINGS

The dorsal surface of the tongue is covered with conical, filiform, fungiform and vallate papillae. The fungiform papillae, which appear as red, pinhead-sized elevations clustered near the tip of the tongue among the gray-white filiform papillae, are absent in *familial dysautonomia*.

> Smith, A.A., Farbman, A. and Dancis, J.: Tongue in familial dysautonomia. A diagnostic sign. *Am. J. Dis. Child. 110*:152, 1965.

Enlargement of the tongue, or *macroglossia,* may be due to congenital hypothyroidism, Down's syndrome, rhabdomyoma, lymphangioma, cystic hygroma, hemangioma, Hurler's syndrome, mannosidosis, glycogenosis type II (Pompe's disease or acid maltase deficiency) and neurofibromatosis. Enlargement of the tongue may also occur in amyloidosis type I, generalized gangliosidosis, Sandhoff's disease and the syndrome of congenital muscular hypertrophy. At times, the cause of the hypertrophy is unknown.

> Engel. A.G. et al.: The spectrum and the diagnosis of acid maltase deficiency. *Neurology 23*:95, 1973.

The *Beckwith-Wiedemann syndrome* consists of macroglossia, omphalocele, increased birth weight, hepatomegaly, ear lobe anomalies and, at times, hypoglycemia and hemihypertrophy.

> Filippi, G. and McKusick, V.A.: The Beckwith-Wiedemann syndrome. *Medicine 49*:279, 1970.

Lobulations, bifurcation or multifurcation of the tongue and a shortened frenulum occurs in the *orofaciodigital syndrome*.

> Ruess, A.L., Pruzansky, S., Lis, E.F. and Patau, K.: The oral-facial-digital syndrome: A multiple congenital condition of females with associated chromosomal abnormalities. *Pediatrics 29*:985, 1962.

A *thyroglossal duct cyst* at the base of the tongue may lead to enlargement and protrusion of the tongue and to respiratory obstruction. The base of the tongue should be palpated in infants with otherwise unexplained stridor or dysphagia.

*Glossoptosis,* or posterior positioning of the tongue, is usually associated with hypoplasia of the mandible. Because of the resultant small airway and the tendency to hypoxia, infants with glossoptosis have great difficulty in feeding; they fail to thrive and may have episodes of dyspnea and cyanosis. The respiratory difficulty may be greatest when the infant is supine. Glossoptosis occurs along with cleft palate in the Pierre Robin syndrome.

Although the frenulum of the tongue may occasionally be short and cause a notch at the tip of the tongue, true *tongue-tie* or congenital ankyloglossia is extremely rare.

*Ranula* is a translucent, bluish retention cyst of the sublingual glands, usually on one side of the frenulum underneath the tongue.

Frequent *protrusion of the tongue* occurs in infants with mental retardation, Down's syndrome, congenital hypothyroidism and Niemann-Pick disease. Foote's sign, rhythmic protrusion of the tongue, suggests intracranial hemorrhage or cerebral edema in the newborn. A kind of tongue thrusting may occur in children with familial dysautonomia.

In *Sydenham's chorea,* the tongue is often undulating and cannot be held still on protrusion. When the child is asked to smile, his response lasts only a fleeting moment. Tremor of the protruded tongue is also noted in hyperthyroidism. *Werdnig-Hoffmann disease* is characterized by fibrillation and atrophy of the tongue.

Dryness of the tongue may be due to dehydration or mouth breathing.

White, grayish or brownish-white *coating of the tongue* occurs commonly in febrile illnesses and in the early stages of scarlet fever, measles and other exanthemata. The coating consists of desquamated cells, food debris and bacteria.

The *white strawberry tongue* is characterized by red, congested and edematous fungiform papillae present against a white-coated background produced by the smaller filiform papillae. Such coating may occur between the second and fifth days in patients with scarlet fever, occasionally in patients with measles and, at times, in patients who have other febrile illnesses.

In patients with a *red strawberry or raspberry tongue* desquamation of the white coating and filiform papillae has occurred, leaving the red, swollen fungiform papillae against a raw, beefy-red background. This occurs on or about the sixth or seventh day in scarlet fever. It may also accompany other severe febrile illnesses, including Kawasaki disease.

In *ariboflavinosis* the tongue is purplish-red and has a smooth to pebbly surface. In pellagra, redness and induration of the edges occur early. With more advanced deficiency, a beefy-red color and swelling of the papillae occur, followed by their atrophy and matting.

*Pernicious anemia* is a rare cause of glossitis in childhood.

*Fissured tongue* is characterized by irregular fissures or grooves in a leaflike, cerebriform or scrotal pattern.

In *geographic tongue,* annular, smooth, red patches with slightly raised gray margins begin posteriorly on the dorsum and spread anteriorly and laterally. Somewhat similar but more transient patches may be noted in acute febrile illnesses.

Furrowed tongue occurs with recurrent facial nerve palsy in the *Melkersson-Rosenthal syndrome.*

*Venous congestion* occurs under the tongue in congestive cardiac failure, constrictive pericarditis and the superior vena caval syndrome.

CHAPTER 9

# SPEECH

## SPEECH DEVELOPMENT

Crying is largely an undifferentiated noise in the neonatal period, but in a few weeks many mothers are able to differentiate the type of cry depending upon its cause. During the second month of life, the baby may begin to make cooing sounds, and in the third month the mother may report that her baby "talks" to her. This is the "babbling" stage of vocalization. At first, most of the sounds produced are vowels, with consonants appearing later.

In the latter half of the first year the infant enters the period of vocal verbal play. He enjoys squealing and making other sounds of varying frequency and intensity, listening, and then repeating the sounds. Infants with severe hearing impairment do not spontaneously progress beyond the babbling stage. Blind children may also demonstrate a prolonged babbling period.

Toward the end of the first year the infant begins to repeat the speech of his parents. During the eighth month most infants can say "Dada," and at the end of the first year their vocabulary may consist of one to three words in addition to "Mama" and "Dada." About the age of one year or at times somewhat before, a definite meaning begins to be attached to words. By 18 months the infant's vocabulary includes 6 to 50 words. Children between the ages of 21 and 24 months may begin to use 2-word phrases. Between 2 and 3 years they may begin to speak in sentences. There is, of course, great variation in the time at which these stages of language development normally occur. Referral to a speech and language consultant is indicated if a child has no words by 20 months of age, no 2-word phrases by 30 months of age or fails to use sentences by 36 months of age. Other indications for referral are obvious echolalia or speech unintelligible to parents after 2 years of age, failure to understand appropriately for his age the speech of others and speech unintelligible to strangers after 3 years of age.

Instruments that may be used for the office evaluation of language development include the Denver Developmental Screening Test, the Peabody Picture Vocabulary Test, the Utah Test of Language Development and the Mecham Verbal Language Development Scale.

## DELAYED SPEECH

Mental retardation is the major cause of language delay. Emotional disturbance and family turmoil is another common cause. Speech retardation also occurs in the child with a hearing loss and other sensory defects secondary to prolonged illness and lack of appropriate environmental stimulation. The overdependent

83

child may also be slow in talking. Immaturity and unusual negativism may be present. Twins and the children of deaf and mute parents may show delayed speech as may the neurologically injured child. Autistic children are frequently first seen because of failure to speak. Speech retardation occurs with histidinemia.

Fuller, C.W.: The child who does not talk. *In* Green, M. and Haggerty, R.J. (eds.): *Ambulatory Pediatrics.* 1st ed. Philadelphia, W. B. Saunders Co., 1968, p. 564.

*Dysphasia* is characterized by motor or expressive difficulties in using speech and/or defective perception with an inability to understand the meaning of words. Speech may be completely lacking or primitive and unintelligible.

*Elective mutism* is the clinical situation in which the child will speak to members of his family or close friends but not with strangers or at school.

Elson, A., Pearson, C., Jones, C.D. and Schumacher, E.: Follow-up study of childhood elective mutism. *Arch. Gen. Psychiatry 13*:182, 1965.

## STUTTERING

*Repetitive or mildly dysfluent speech* occurs as a transient finding in almost all children during the preschool period. Some hesitation or unevenness in speech may be noted and repetitiveness may occur with syllables, words or combinations of words. This normal developmental process should not be termed stuttering.

*Stuttering,* much more common in boys than in girls, is a kind of speech dysfluency accompanied by secondary manifestations such as blocking, apprehension about speaking, mannerisms, tic-like movements of the face and changes in breathing when the child tries to speak fluently and avoidance of troublesome sounds and words.

*Cluttering* is an unusual type of speech characterized by repetition of words or phrases, repeated false starts, changes in context in the middle of the sentence and general verbal confusion.

## HEARING IMPAIRMENT AND SPEECH

The child who has a hearing impairment may also have retarded speech, an articulatory speech defect or an abnormality in pitch, loudness or other vocal quality.

Cooing, crying and babbling are stages of speech development that occur in children with impaired hearing as well as in those who are normal. That an infant can babble and perhaps say "Dada" does not necessarily mean that his hearing is adequate for speech perception. The infant with serious hearing impairment is handicapped in progressing to the next stage of speech development since this depends upon verbal vocal play and the imitation of sounds made by himself and others.

## ARTICULATORY SPEECH DISORDERS

The time at which distinct speech is achieved is variable. Though some children demonstrate correct articulation relatively early in life, more frequently this is not perfected until the late preschool or early elementary school period. Some articulatory speech defects are minor and, in time, disappear. In extreme instances, speech is largely or completely unintelligible.

Four types of articulatory speech defects are usually considered: *substitution,* in which one sound is substituted for the correct sound, as w for r (*run* becomes *wun*); *omission,* in which a sound is omitted; *insertion,* in which an extra sound is added to a word; and *distortion,* in which the sound is not made correctly and therefore is indistinct. *Lisping* is characterized by the use of the "th" sound for the "s" sound.

As already noted, some articulatory defects are within the limits of normal development. Persistence of infantile speech in an otherwise normal child may reflect social and emotional immaturity or overdependence. Some functional difficulty in the use of the structures involved in speech must also be considered. Office assessment of articulation may be based on the Denver Articulation Screening Examination.

*Dysarthria* is the term applied to difficulty in articulating the individual sounds of speech secondary to an organic motor defect in the speech mechanism. *Dysphasia* is a language disturbance due to damage or dysfunction of those areas in the brain involved in symbolic formulation. *Dyslalia* is the term applied to an articulatory disorder in which no organic basis can be found. Children with cerebral palsy or central neurologic damage may have articulatory difficulty due to a poorly functioning tongue, paralysis of the palate or incoordination of the pharyngeal muscles. A cleft palate, submucous cleft, severe malocclusion, malalignment of the teeth or other oral deformity may be etiologic. Intellectual retardation and a hearing loss are other important considerations. Slurred speech may occur in patients with Wilson's disease.

*Hyponasal speech,* which sounds about the same whether the nostrils are open or pinched shut, may be due to nasal allergy or enlarged adenoids. *Hypernasality* may be due to complete or submucous cleft palate with velopharyngeal insufficiency or neurogenic dysfunction of the palate.

Normal speech depends upon normal respiratory movements since a relatively long and sustained expiratory phase is needed. In the child with *cerebral palsy* the respiratory excursions may be rapid, irregular, spasmodic or nonsynchronized. Consequently his speech may be halting, strained and dysrhythmic, with short, irregular spurts. The pitch of the speech may also be abnormal. Patients with Friedreich's ataxia or chorea may have similar speech.

Shanks, J.C.: The child who speaks defectively. *In* Green, M. and Haggerty, R.J. (eds.): *Ambulatory Pediatrics.* 1st ed. Philadelphia, W. B. Saunders Co., 1968, p. 572.

Speech consultation is desirable for an articulatory speech defect if a four-year-old child talks in a jargon unintelligible to strangers. If speech is intelligible, the decision as to speech therapy may be delayed until school entrance.

## QUALITY OF SPEECH

Children with paralysis of the palatal and pharyngeal muscles have a nasal twang to their voice. Sinusitis and adenoid hypertrophy cause the so-called adenoid voice that results from impairment of nasal resonance.

Differential diagnosis of *hoarseness* includes vocal abuse through excessive shouting, screaming or singing. When the pitch is extreme in the child between five and ten years of age, abuse may lead to vocal cord nodules with hoarseness or a husky quality. *Papilloma of the larynx,* the commonest cause of persistent hoarseness in children, occurs most frequently between the ages of one and four years. Progressive airway obstruction may develop. Direct laryngoscopy is required. Other causes of hoarseness include:

Chronic or acute sinusitis, especially upon arising
Laryngitis or croup
Laryngeal foreign body
Unilateral paralysis of the recurrent laryngeal nerve
Ectodermal dysplasia
Measles

Infants with hypothyroidism may have a weak, low-pitched, hoarse cry.

Lipoid proteinosis may cause hoarseness.

Some infants with congenital heart disease may have a weak or hoarse cry due to pressure of enlarged pulmonary vessels on the left recurrent laryngeal nerve.

Hoarseness may be noted at birth in infants with disseminated lipogranulomatosis.

In the *cri du chat* syndrome, the cry during the first year of life is high-pitched and plaintive, similar to that of a distressed kitten.

Deepening of the voice occurs in boys during adolescence. Premature deepening and coarsening of the voice appears with precocious sexual development or masculinization.

A patient's speech may give an impression of his affect (e.g., the slow, monotonal and, at times, almost inaudible speech of the chronically ill or depressed child or the whisper of the child with hysteria).

### GENERAL REFERENCES

Fuller, C.W.: Speech and hearing problems. *In* Green, M. and Haggerty, R.J. (eds.): *Ambulatory Pediatrics II.* Philadelphia, W. B. Saunders Co., 1977, p. 321.

CHAPTER 10

# THE THROAT, PHARYNX, TONSILS AND LARYNX

The tonsils are normally large in childhood, an expression of the luxuriant lymphoid growth characteristic of this age period. When tonsillar enlargement occurs during an infection, normal size is usually regained two or three weeks later.

*Tonsillitis and pharyngitis* are discussed on page 497. During the first few days of life the infant's pharynx may normally appear red.

The patient who has a *peritonsillar abscess* is not able to open his mouth wide and may hold his head toward the involved side. Frequent swallowing movements may be noted. Because of the severe pain on swallowing, drooling may occur. The limited pharyngeal examination that is possible reveals anterior and superior displacement of the involved tonsil, bulging of the soft palate and movement of the uvula toward the opposite side.

*Retropharyngeal abscess* occurs largely in infants. Patients with a retropharyngeal abscess tend to lie with their head either tilted to one side or retracted. Cervical adenopathy is usually present on the affected side. Stiffness of the neck, mouth breathing and stridor may also occur. Extreme caution is indicated in the examination of the pharynx in these patients since forceful depression of the tongue with a blade may precipitate respiratory arrest. Lateral soft tissue x-rays of the neck should be obtained. Palpation of the retropharyngeal abscess is to be performed quickly, gently and without pressure. Standing at the head of the patient, the examiner may insert his finger dorsally along the roof of the mouth and posterior pharyngeal wall until the abscess is palpated, or the tongue may be gently depressed with a tongue blade and the examining finger introduced at the corner of the mouth and passed over the base of the tongue to the posterior pharyngeal wall. On palpation the abscess is felt as a smooth, tense and perhaps fluctuant swelling, sometimes more prominent on the side than in the center of the pharynx.

*Lymphosarcoma* may rarely involve a tonsil. Unilateral enlargement of a tonsil is an indication for a tonsillectomy-biopsy.

*Rhabdomyosarcoma* in the nasopharynx may cause denasalized speech, a persistent nasal discharge, enlargement of the cervical lymph nodes in the upper third of the neck and cranial nerve palsies.

Ulceration of the pharynx may occur in patients with leukemia or agranulocytosis.

*Infectious mononucleosis* may cause a thick, dull-white pseudomembrane over the tonsils and lymphoid tissue on the posterior pharyngeal wall. The membrane does not extend beyond the lymphoid tissue.

*Tangier disease* is characterized by huge, lobulated or honeycombed yellowish-gray tonsils, hepatosplenomegaly, lymphadenopathy and transient neuropathy. Hypocholesterolemia, moderate hypertriglyceridemia and very low levels of plasma high-density lipoproteins are laboratory findings.

*Hyperplasia of lymphoid follicles* on the posterior pharyngeal wall may occur in children who have chronic sinusitis or recurrent pharyngitis. The mucosa of the posterior pharynx becomes granular and pebbled with small glistening islands of lymphoid tissue.

In children with sinusitis or chronic nasopharyngitis a yellowish, glairy, mucopurulent curtain may hang down or drain from the nasopharynx.

The *gag reflex* should be checked in patients thought to have cranial nerve palsies. Pharyngeal pooling of saliva may occur in patients with bulbar palsy or botulism.

Indirect *visualization of the larynx* by the use of a laryngeal mirror may be possible in older children and adolescents. Direct laryngoscopy is necessary in young children.

# CHAPTER 11

# THE JAW

The mandible, which appears relatively small in newborn infants, grows forward and downward during early life and by the latter half of the first year is more proportionate to the rest of the face. *Micrognathia* or hypoplasia of the mandible may be accompanied by glossoptosis. The *Pierre Robin syndrome* consists of a cleft palate, micrognathia and glossoptosis.

A small mandible with the typical *Vogelgesicht* (bird facies) may occur in juvenile rheumatoid arthritis owing to interference with growth at the temporomandibular joint. Ankylosis of the temporomandibular joint may also be due to birth injury, postnasal trauma or infection. The involved side of the mandible fails to grow normally, and the midpoint of the jaw is displaced toward the injured side.

Micrognathia may be noted in *Treacher Collins syndrome* along with hypoplasia of the facial bones. The malar bones, the zygomatic arch and the infraorbital ridges are either absent or defective. In hemifacial microsomia, the mandibular ramus and condyle do not develop on the involved side.

The *Hallermann-Streiff syndrome* is characterized by a hypoplastic mandible, bird facies, scaphocephaly, brachycephaly, beaked nose, hypotrichosis, atrophy of the skin, dental anomalies, congenital cataracts and understature.

Micrognathia also occurs in these syndromes: Smith-Lemli-Opitz, cri du chat, fetal alcohol, pycnodysostosis, trisomy 13, trisomy 18, Rubinstein-Taybi and Russell-Silver.

Prominence of the mandible, or *prognathism,* may be noted in chondrodystrophy and in Crouzon's disease. Soft tissue prognation may be seen in the mucosal neuroma sydrome. The mandible is prominent in acromegaly.

Mandibular involvement occurs in *infantile cortical hyperostosis* as a soft tissue swelling that may simulate mumps.

*Grooves* in the chin occur in the whistling face syndrome.

*Cherubism* is a hereditary, hard, painless, symmetrical swelling of the jaw beginning in early childhood. This disorder is accompanied by abnormal dentition in the mandible and by regional lymphadenopathy. Fibrous dysplasia may also cause a prominent mandible.

A draining fistula in the submandibular area may arise from a periapical dental abscess.

Disorders to be considered in the differential diagnosis of *tumors of the jaw* in childhood include osteomyelitis, eosinophilic granuloma, giant cell tumor, Ewing's tumor, fibrosarcoma, osteogenic sarcoma and odotogenic tumors. Tender, localized swelling of the jaw, fever and inability to open the mouth may occur in association with mandibular cyst formation in patients with the nevoid basal cell carcinoma syndrome.

*Burkitt's lymphoma* may present as a soft tissue tumor or swelling in the mandible or maxilla.

*Trismus,* an inability to open the mouth, most commonly occurs in patients with tetanus but may be noted with phenothiazine toxicity, encephalitis, brain tumors, primary hypoparathyroidism, the infantile form of Gaucher's disease and tumors of the jaw such as rhabdomyosarcoma.

Dislocation or subluxation of the temporomandibular joint may be caused by the intermittent extensor thrust of the jaw in patients with athetosis.

Familial, perpendicular, rhythmic *trembling of the chin* may be seen especially during periods of emotional stress.

Newborn and young infants demonstrate some trembling of the chin during periods of crying.

CHAPTER 12

# THE SALIVARY GLANDS

*Mumps* causes a tender, somewhat painful, unilateral or bilateral swelling of the parotid and, rarely, the submaxillary glands. The swelling is below and anterior to the lobe of the ear and extends onto the face, below the mandible and to the mastoid region. The ear lobe may be pushed out from the face, and the angle of the mandible may not be palpable. Swelling, greatest during the second and third days of the illness, persists for a week to ten days. A brawny, gelatinous edema surrounds the swelling, and the overlying skin may be slightly erythematous and shiny. Presternal edema may occur. The orifice of Stensen's duct opposite the upper second molar tooth may be injected and puffy. Submaxillary or sublingular mumps may occur without parotid involvement.

Lymphadenopathy in the parotid area may require differentiation from mumps. With lymphadenopathy, the swelling is usually more discrete, the angle of the mandible can be palpated and, except for preauricular adenopathy, most of the swelling is submandibular. Preauricular lymphadenopathy may occur with conjunctivitis or other ocular infection.

*Purulent parotitis* may occur in newborn infants or in older children. The submaxillary glands may be similarly involved. The gland is enlarged, tender and the overlying skin red and warm. With fluctuation, pus may be expressed from Stensen's duct.

David, R.B. and O'Connell, E.J.: Suppurative parotitis in children. *Am. J. Dis. Child.* *119*:332, 1970.
Leake, D. and Leake, R.: Neonatal suppurative parotitis. *Pediatrics 46*:203, 1970.

*Recurrent swelling of the parotid gland* usually begins after the age of two years and continues throughout childhood. Tenseness and erythema of the skin over the parotid area are noted. A sense of fullness and pain may be present, but there are no systemic symptoms. Attacks usually last two or three weeks. Spontaneous remission is the rule, but suppuration occasionally occurs. Salivary gland involvement, including recurrent parotitis, has been reported with *mixed connective tissue disease.*

Chronic or recurrent enlargement of the salivary glands, usually the parotid but at times the submaxillary, occurs in *Sjögren's syndrome* along with keratoconjunctivitis sicca, xerostomia and often an associated connective tissue disease. Chronic enlargement of the parotid glands causes a chipmunk appearance.

Athreya, B.H., Norman, M.E., Myers, A.R. and South, M.A.: Sjögren's syndrome in children. *Pediatrics 59*:931, 1977.

Parotid enlargement may rarely be caused by a calculus in Stensen's duct.

*Hemangioma,* probably the most common of parotid tumors and frequently present at birth, enlarges rapidly in the first few weeks and months of life. Discoloration of the overlying skin may be present. The tumor feels compressible, elastic and lobulated. *Lymphangiomas* may also be present at birth or appear during the first year. *Mixed tumor,* a common benign tumor of the parotid gland, usually presents as a round, firm, painless mass beneath and just in front of the ear. Burkitt's lymphoma may involve the salivary glands.

*Mikulicz's syndrome* is characterized by bilateral, firm, painless enlargement of the parotid, lacrimal and, at times, submaxillary glands with resultant dryness of the mouth and an absence of tears. The syndrome may be due to tuberculosis, lymphoma or leukemia.

The *auriculotemporal syndrome,* which follows injury to the auriculotemporal nerve near the parotid gland, is characterized by a sense of warmth, sweating, erythema and, occasionally, pain involving the cheek when the patient eats.

*Uveoparotid syndrome.* In addition to uveitis, indurated, painless enlargement of the parotid glands occurs, perhaps unilaterally at first, but later bilaterally. The patient may complain of dryness of the mouth. Unilateral or bilateral facial nerve paralysis may be an associated finding.

*Hypertrophy of the masseter and/or temporalis muscles* due to excessive chewing or malocclusion may be confused with swelling of the parotid glands. Swelling of the masseter muscle occurs anterior to the ramus of the mandible while that of the temporalis muscle is anterior to and above the tragus.

Kalish, G.H. and Gellis, S.S.: Hypertrophy of the masseter or temporalis muscles or both. *Am. J. Dis. Child. 121*:346, 1971.

# CHAPTER 13

# THE TEETH

## DECIDUOUS TEETH

**Eruption.** Although the eruption of teeth follows a pattern, there is much individual variation. Deciduous teeth tend to erupt in three groupings with an interval of one and one-half to three months between each group:

| | |
|---|---|
| 2 lower central incisors | 5–10 months |
| 2 upper central incisors | 8–12 months |
| 2 upper lateral incisors | 9–13 months |
| 2 lower lateral incisors | 10–14 months |
| 2 lower anterior molars | 13–16 months |
| 2 upper anterior molars | 13–17 months |
| 4 canines | 12–22 months |
| 4 posterior molars | 24–30 months |

Rarely, one or two teeth are prematurely present at birth. These supernumerary teeth usually are loosely held and easily removed. The tooth buds of the deciduous teeth are readily evident in the gums of the young infant. Eruption of the deciduous teeth may be delayed normally until the end of the first year. Further delay may occur in infants with hypothyroidism and hypopituitarism. All 20 deciduous teeth should be present before the end of the third year. The lower central incisors are usually the first deciduous teeth to be lost, with the last deciduous tooth shed by about 12 years of age. During the preschool period, spacing of the anterior deciduous teeth is normal. Similarly, the deciduous teeth may be irregularly aligned when they erupt. Realignment then occurs under the influence of muscular forces exerted by the lips, cheeks and tongue.

Prolonged retention of deciduous teeth may be noted in pycnodysostosis and cleidocranial dysostosis.

## PERMANENT DENTITION

The permanent teeth usually erupt in the following order:

| | |
|---|---|
| First molars | 6–7 years |
| Incisors | 7–9 years |
| Premolars | 9–11 years |
| Canines | 10–12 years |
| Second molars | 12–16 years |
| Third molars | 17–25 years |

During the first years after their eruption the permanent teeth appear relatively large and may be irregularly spaced and aligned. With further growth of the face, however, the teeth no longer appear disproportionately large. The malalignment usually does not persist, and the spacing between the upper permanent incisors usually disappears after eruption of the canine teeth.

The incisal margin of the newly erupted anterior permanent teeth have three saw-toothed projections, or mamelons, which are remnants of the developmental lobes of the teeth. These projections are worn down after a time.

The first (sixth-year) molar of the permanent dentition erupts behind the deciduous molars. This tooth, which has an extremely important role in the positioning of other teeth, has been termed the keystone of the dental arch.

Davis, W.B.: Dental health in children. *In* Green, M. and Haggerty, R.J. (eds.): *Ambulatory Pediatrics.* 1st ed. Philadelphia, W. B. Saunders Co., 1968.

## MALOCCLUSION

Malocclusion may be categorized as malpositioning of the teeth with normal relation of the jaws, as retrusion of the mandible with accompanying protrusion or retrusion of the upper incisors and as protrusion of the mandible. Vigorous and persistent thumb sucking may lead to malpositioning, especially if it continues after the age of five or six years.

Normally, alignment of the teeth is maintained by the muscular forces of the lip, cheeks and tongue. The upper lip in mouth breathers becomes shortened and slack and does not exert its normal molding action on the upper dental arch. The lower lip may also become flaccid and everted and with retrusion of the mandible may be held behind the upper incisors. Spacing and protrusion of the upper incisors result.

Protrusion and spacing of the teeth may occur in children with *thalassemia major.*

## DISTURBANCES OF THE TEETH

Total or partial *anodontia,* or absence of teeth, may occur with hypohidrotic ectodermal dysplasia, Marfan's syndrome and cleidocranial dysostosis. In congenital ectodermal dysplasia the upper lateral incisors, and occasionally other teeth, are cone- or peg-shaped. Deformity of the teeth may also occur in children with chondroectodermal dysplasia.

*Premature loss of teeth,* or "floating teeth," may occur in patients with histiocytosis, vitamin D–resistant rickets, cyclic neutropenia, hypophosphatasia and neoplasms such as reticulum cell sarcoma or Ewing's sarcoma. In histiocytosis the gingivae are friable, swollen and ulcerated, especially on the lingual or palatal side of the erupting molars. With juvenile periodontitis in adolescents, extensive bone loss occurs around the permanent first molars and lower incisors with resultant increased tooth mobility. Premature loss of the deciduous teeth may occur with palmar-plantar hyperkeratosis.

Gorlin, R.J., Sedano, H. and Anderson, V.E.: The syndrome of palmar-plantar hyperkeratosis and premature periodontal destruction of the teeth. *J. Pediatr. 65*:895, 1964.

*Enamel hypoplasia,* characterized by pitting or grooving of the enamel surface, may be due to tetracycline administration, rickets, oculodentoosseous dysplasia, congenital syphilis, malnutrition, diarrhea or other severe systemic disease in early life. Enamel hypoplasia, hypodontia and other dental malformations occur in *Rieger's syndrome* along with aniridia and glaucoma.

Feingold, M., Shiere, F., Fogels, H.R. and Donaldson, D.: Rieger's syndrome. *Pediatrics 44*:564, 1969.

During the period of tooth development from the latter half of gestation to eight years of age, *tetracycline* causes yellow-gray-brown permanent discoloration of the teeth, occasionally accompanied by enamel hypoplasia.

*Brown teeth,* or *amelogenesis imperfecta,* results from malfunctioning of the ameloblasts or enamel-forming cells. The brown dentin is not covered by an adequate coating of enamel.

Grooving and pitting of the enamel may occur in chronic idiopathic hypoparathyroidism.

*Opalescent dentin,* or *dentinogenesis imperfecta,* may occur with osteogenesis imperfecta. The deciduous and permanent dentition may be characterized by a brownish opalescence and rapid attrition.

In *congenital syphilis* the upper central permanent incisors may be peg-shaped and notched on their distal border. These so-called *Hutchinson teeth* are shaped like the tip of a screw driver. "Mulberry" molars, which have irregularly formed, crowded cusps on a dwarfed occlusal surface, are also a stigma of congenital syphilis.

*Infection of a tooth bud,* usually that of the first molar, may occur in newborn infants, causing inflammatory changes in the lip, cheek, orbital region and the underlying alveolar process. A purulent nasal discharge may also develop.

*Grinding of the teeth,* or *bruxism,* occurs chiefly during sleep, but may be diurnal as well. A grating, rasping sound is produced, and the teeth may be worn down rapidly.

Greenish-black discoloration near the gingival margin of the teeth in children is due to *tartar* and *calculus deposits.*

*Nursing bottle caries* with rampant decay, especially on the labial aspect of the primary canine and incisor teeth, may occur in infants over one year of age with prolonged bottle feeding during sleep.

Shelton, P.G., Berkowitz, R.J. and Forrester, D.J.: Nursing bottle caries. *Pediatrics 59*:777, 1977.

Neonatal jaundice may cause a permanent greenish color (the *green neonatal ring*) in the enamel being formed at birth. As a result, the portion of the deciduous teeth formed prenatally is completely green.

*Erythrodentition* with pink or reddish-brown coloration of the teeth may occur with chronic porphyria.

# CHAPTER 14

# THE NECK

The neck is normally short in infants. Patients with Morquio's, Hunter's, Hurler's, Klippel-Feil, Noonan's, Turner's and Goldenhar's syndromes, platybasia, spondyloepiphyseal dysplasia congenita, cretinism, pterygium colli, bilateral Sprengel's deformity and chondrodystrophia calcificans congenita have abnormally short necks.

## CERVICAL MASSES

*Cervical adenopathy* is a common cause of enlargement of the neck.

A *thyroglossal duct cyst* appears as a round, smooth, firm swelling, ¼ to 1½ inches in diameter, in or near the midline of the neck between the foramen cecum of the tongue and the suprasternal notch, usually at or about the level of the thyroid cartilage. The cyst moves upward in the neck when the patient protrudes his tongue or swallows. It may first become apparent during a respiratory infection as a painful, tender and rapidly increasing mass. Differentiation between a thyroglossal cyst above the hyoid bone and enlargement of a submandibular lymph node may be difficult. Inflammatory changes may be intermittently present in both.

A *thyroglossal duct sinus,* which may present anywhere along the midline from the level of the hyoid bone to the suprasternal notch, retracts on protrusion of the tongue. Occasionally, a few drops of a clear, mucoid or purulent discharge may drain from the sinus and produce a local inflammatory reaction. Rarely, an ectopic thyroid gland in the midline may simulate a thyroglossal duct cyst.

Kaplan, M., Kauli, R., Lubin, E., Grunebaum, M. and Laron, Z.: Ectopic thyroid gland. *J. Pediatr. 92*:205, 1978.

*Dermoid or sebaceous cysts* in the midline of the neck are attached to the overlying skin whereas thyroglossal duct cysts, unless infected, are attached to underlying structures.

A *first branchial cleft anomaly* may present as a sinus or cyst at or above the level of the hyoid bone about halfway between the midline of the neck and the anterior border of the sternocleidomastoid muscle. A fistulous tract opening into the external auditory canal may cause chronic drainage of the ear.

*Branchial cleft cysts* are slightly movable, smooth, tense, nontranslucent, unilocular subcutaneous swellings from 1 to 5 cm. in diameter that appear in late childhood along the anterior border of the sternocleidomastoid muscle. The overlying skin is freely movable. A sticky, clear mucoid secretion may occasionally drain from an opening along the anterior border of the sternocleidomastoid muscle between the hyoid bone and the suprasternal notch.

An enlarging, firm, usually painless mass in the neck in a child with Horner's syndrome suggests a *neuroblastoma* of the cervical sympathetic chain.

A *cystic hygroma* may occur just above the clavicle or elsewhere in the neck as a

94

soft, diffuse, poorly demarcated cystic mass that is moderately movable, translucent and multilocular. In some instances, the tumor does not seem lobulated. The overlying skin may be thin and bluish.

*Lipomas* rarely appear as lobulated masses in the neck.

*Edema* of the neck may occur in diphtheria, infections of the deep cervical spaces, herpetic stomatitis and anasarca.

Rapidly enlarging lumps or swellings in the neck, neck pain or trismus raise the possibility of a rhabdomyosarcoma or neuroblastoma.

Jaffe, B.F. and Jaffe, N.: Head and neck tumors in children. *Pediatrics 51*:732, 1973.

Pratt, C.B. et al.: Factors leading to delay and affecting survival of children with head and neck rhabdomyosarcoma. *Pediatrics 61*:30, 1978.

## MOVEMENT OF THE NECK

The *Klippel-Feil syndrome,* due to a fusion of two or more cervical vertebrae, is characterized by limitation of movement, shortening of the neck and a low posterior hairline.

*Congenital torticollis* occurs in the first several weeks of life. Tilting of the head toward the affected side is usually the presenting complaint. In the first month a circumscribed, firm or hard, fusiform mass, ¾ to 1½ inches in diameter, is palpable in the sternocleidomastoid muscle. The tumor, which may be most readily demonstrated when the infant's shoulders are elevated so that his head falls backward, is usually not present at birth. The mass may enlarge for two to four weeks and then regress with complete disappearance between four and eight months of age. Unresolved torticollis leads to asymmetry of the face and skull. Growth on the involved side is diminished.

Infants and children with *strabismus* may tilt their heads to one side to avoid a double visual image (ocular torticollis).

Patients with an *astrocytoma* or other *tumor of the cerebellar hemispheres* may rotate or tilt the occiput toward the shoulder on the involved side. Tumors of the cervical spine and syringomyelia may cause torticollis.

*Paroxysmal torticollis* of infancy, the infantile form of benign paroxysmal vertigo, is characterized by episodes of head tilting that recur two or three times a month and last from ten minutes to three days. Other symptoms may include vomiting, pallor and restlessness.

Snyder, C.H.: Paroxysmal torticollis in infancy. A possible form of labyrinthitis. *Am. J. Dis. Child. 117*:458, 1969.

Torticollis may occur in the *Klippel-Feil syndrome*.

Torticollis due to muscle spasm may accompany *acute cervical adenitis*. Cervical Pott's disease and retropharyngeal space abscesses also cause torticollis.

*Eosinophilic granuloma* is a possibility in a child with neck pain, torticollis and a cervical vertebral lesion.

Davidson, R.I. and Shillito, J., Jr.: Eosinophilic granuloma of the cervical spine in children. *Pediatrics 45*:746, 1970.

An *osteoid osteoma* in the cervical spine may cause torticollis.

*Acquired torticollis* may be due to a nontraumatic *subluxation of the atlantoaxial joint* associated with inflammatory processes around the neck such as pharyngitis and cervical adenitis. Clinical manifestations include pain and tenderness at the base of the skull and limitation of rotation of the head. Three types of subluxation are possible: anterior bilateral, anterior unilateral and posterior unilateral. With bilateral anterior subluxation the patient holds his head rigidly in the midline and tilted forward with the chin depressed. With an anterior unilateral subluxation, the head is tilted foward and toward the involved side, and the neck is rotated away from the affected side. In a unilateral posterior subluxation, tilting of the head and rotation of the neck occur toward the involved side. Careful roentgenographic examination, including stereoscopic views, is indicated with an acquired torticollis.

*Occipitalization,* in which the bony ring of the atlas is partially or completely fused to the base of the occiput, is manifested by torticollis, a low posterior hairline, a short neck and limitation of motion.

Congenital *anomalies of the odontoid* may cause torticollis or subtle neurologic symptoms. Patients with mucopolysaccharidoses and spondyloepiphyseal dysplasia often have odontoid anomalies. Laxity of the transverse ligament may occur in children with rheumatoid arthritis or Down's syndrome.

> Hensinger, R.H.: Orthopedic problems of the shoulder and neck. *Pediatr. Clin. N. Am.* 24:889, 1977.

*Sandifer's syndrome* is characterized by bizarre movements of the head and neck, usually during or immediately after eating, in some children with a hiatus hernia. Usually the neck is extended and the head rotated to one side.

> Kinsbourne, M.: Hiatus hernia with contortions of neck. *Lancet 1*:1058, 1964.

## NUCHAL RIGIDITY

*Meningitis* and other central nervous system disorders characterized by nuchal rigidity are listed on page 180.

*Tetanus* is characterized by progressive stiffness of the neck muscles.

*Cervical and posterior auricular adenopathy* associated with rubella, infectious mononucleosis or acute cervical lymphadenitis may cause slight stiffness of the neck. Nuchal rigidity may also occur with a retropharyngeal abscess.

Neck pain, stiffness and limitation of motion may be early symptoms of *rheumatoid arthritis*.

*Calcification of the cervical intervertebral disc* may cause localized pain, limitation of motion, muscle spasm, tenderness and torticollis.

> Melnick, J.C. and Silverman, F.N.: Intervertebral disc calcification in childhood. *Radiology 80*:399, 1963.

## OTHER LESIONS AND ANOMALIES

A hernia of the lung may present in the midline above the sternum as a soft, spongy, lemon-shaped mass. The apices of the lungs above the clavicles may rarely appear to puff out in infants during crying.

> Jones, J.G.: Cervical hernia of the lungs. *J. Pediatr. 76*:122, 1970.

*Venous engorgement in the neck,* best seen with the patient sitting, is observed in:

Congestive cardiac failure
Constrictive pericarditis

Enlarged mediastinal nodes

Pneumomediastinum

Superior vena cava syndrome along with edema and cyanosis of the head and neck, stridor and dyspnea.

A *cervical aortic arch* presents as a pulsating mass, best seen with the patient sitting and the head retracted, in the suprasternal region or above the clavicle. A systolic murmur and thrill may be present. Symptoms due to compression of the trachea and esophagus may be reported.

Mullins, C.E., Gillette, P.C. and McNamara, D.G.: The complex of cervical aortic arch. *Pediatrics 51*:210, 1973.

*Unusual pulsation of the carotid arteries* may occur with aortic insufficiency. Pulsation of the neck vessels also occurs with a large patent ductus arteriosus.

*Takayasu's disease* may be characterized by a bruit in the neck.

*The hepatojugular reflex* is present with congestive heart failure. With the patient recumbent, venous distention in the neck becomes accentuated when pressure is applied over the liver.

*Pterygium colli,* webbed neck or "sphinx neck," is characterized by a thick web of skin that extends from behind the ears to the distal portion of the clavicle and to the acromial process. Pterygium colli is sometimes seen in *Turner's and Noonan's syndromes.* Redundant, loose longitudinal folds of skin may also occur over the neck.

Nora, J.J. et al.: The Ullrich-Noonan syndrome. (Turner phenotype.) *Am J. Dis. Child. 127*:48, 1974.

Redundancy and laxity of the skin around the neck occurs in *Down's syndrome.*

Small, subcutaneous *cartilaginous tags* or remnants rarely occur in the neck, most commonly anterior to the sternocleidomastoid muscle. The tags may be pedunculated or extend into the tissues of the neck.

## TRACHEA

Deviation of the trachea may be evident on inspection or palpation.

An "auditory slap," a "palpatory thud" and an "asthmatoid wheeze" may occur in patients with a tracheal foreign body.

## THYROID

The size and other characteristics of the isthmus and lobes of the thyroid may be determined by standing behind the patient, hyperextending his head, and palpating the gland with the fingers of both hands as it moves upward during swallowing. Another method is to face the patient, place one's thumbs along the upper border of the isthmus and the fingers along the posterior border of the sternocleidomastoid muscle and ask the patient to swallow. Moderate enlargement of the thyroid is, of course, readily evident on inspection. Normally, the right lobe may be larger than the left.

*Neonatal goiters,* characterized by either a slightly nodular or a soft, diffuse enlargement, usually disappear in a short time. A large goiter may cause tracheal compression, respiratory difficulty and hoarseness. Babies whose mothers received propylthiouracil during pregnancy may be born with a goiter. An enlarged thyroid may also appear a few days after birth in babies whose mothers received iodides prenatally. Maternal iodine deficiency may be associated with neonatal goiter. The cause for some neonatal goiters is unknown.

Senior, B. and Chernoff, H.L.: Iodide goiter in the newborn. *Pediatrics 47*:510, 1971.

*Simple or endemic goiter* due to iodine deficiency is characterized by a diffuse, smooth, compressible enlargement of the thyroid gland. A bruit and thrill may be present. Enlargement of the thyroid may also be due to excessive iodine intake.

Doland, T.F., Jr. and Gibson, L.E.: Complications of iodide therapy in patients with cystic fibrosis. *J. Pediatr. 79*:684, 1971.

Patients with *hyperthyroidism* have a diffuse, smooth and firm enlargement of the thyroid. A bruit and a palpable thrill are often present. The thyroid is usually very prominent but occasionally may be only slightly enlarged.

Vaidya, V.A., Bongiovanni, A.M., Parks, J.S., Tenore, A. and Kirkland, R.T.: Twenty-two years' experience in the medical management of juvenile thyrotoxicosis. *Pediatrics 54*:565, 1974.

A soft, diffuse and usually transitory increase in size of the thyroid may occur physiologically during or immediately after adolescence, especially in rapidly growing girls. The gland is smooth and its edges indistinct.

Since irregular *nodular enlargements* of the thyroid may be neoplastic, immediate surgical removal appears indicated. Enlargement of the Delphian and other cervical lymph nodes may occur with thyroid neoplasms and may be the presenting complaint.

*Medullary carcinoma* of the thyroid gland may be associated in the *mucosal neuroma* syndrome with a Marfan-like body habitus and multiple nodularities of the tongue and lips. Pheochromocytoma and ganglioneuroma may also be present.

Levin, D.L., Perlia, C. and Tashjian, A.H., Jr.: Medullary carcinoma of the thyroid gland: the complete syndrome in a child. *Pediatrics 52*:192, 1972.

*Hashimoto's thyroiditis* or *chronic lymphocytic thyroiditis* is a common cause of goiter in children and adolescents, especially girls. The patient may complain of local pressure, difficulty in swallowing and hoarseness. Coarsely granular or firm in consistency, the gland is nontender. Similar firmness may be noted in simple goiters. The Delphian node may be palpable above the isthmus.

*Subacute thyroiditis,* likely a viral disease, is characterized by fever, exquisite tenderness on palpation and pain, which is at times referred to the angle of the jaws. Spontaneous resolution occurs in a few weeks.

*Goiters* may be a manifestation of a defect in thyroid hormone synthesis. Hypothyroidism appears in infancy or early childhood with the soft, diffuse goiter noted late in the first decade of life or in adolescence.

## GENERAL REFERENCES

Ferguson, C.F. and Kendig, E.L.: *Pediatric Otolaryngology* Vol II. *Disorders of the Respiratory Tract in Children.* Philadelphia, W. B. Saunders Co., 1972.
Strome, M.: *Differential Diagnosis in Pediatric Otolaryngology.* Boston, Little, Brown and Company, 1975.

# CHAPTER 15

# THE CHEST

In early infancy the chest is circular or barrel-shaped with some flattening in the axillae. In older children, the chest has an elliptical shape. A barrel-shaped chest in the older child usually indicates chronic obstructive pulmonary disease.

The circumference of the chest at birth (about 33 cm. or 12 inches for the fiftieth percentile) is usually equal to or slightly larger than that of the head.

Subcutaneous fat in well-nourished infants makes the ribs, clavicles, scapulae and the interspaces less prominent on physical inspection than is the case with premature infants or malnourished children.

## RESPIRATIONS

During early infancy, and especially in prematures, respiratory movements may be irregular, intermittent and variable in rate and depth — deep for a while and then shallow. Apneic episodes may occur. During sleep, breathing may be almost imperceptible. At times the respiratory rate may be rapid. Variable pauses may occur between inspiration and expiration. *Periodic breathing* with brief apneic periods interrupting the breathing cycle is common in premature infants and may be normal for six weeks. Periodic breathing during sleep is present in excessive amounts in infants with a history of near-miss sudden infant death syndrome.

Kelly, D.H. and Shannon, D.C.: Periodic breathing in infants with near-miss sudden infant death syndrome. *Pediatrics 63*:355, 1979.

Breathing during infancy is characteristically abdominal or diaphragmatic. A thoracic respiratory component in young infants suggests pulmonary disease unless abdominal distention or another abdominal problem is present. The thoracic type of respiration, more prominent as the child grows older, becomes predominant at about seven or eight years of age.

In full-term newborn infants the respiratory rate averages about 45 per minute when awake and 35 per minute when asleep with a considerable normal range on either side of these averages. An increase to a rate of 70 or 80 may occur with very little excitation. Because of this, accurate respiratory rates are best obtained while the infant is asleep. The rate also tends to be higher in the premature infant. At 1 year of age the rate is around 30 per minute. During the preschool period it averages from 20 to 25 per minute. At the age of 10 years the rate is about 20 per minute. Table 15–1 lists the respiratory rates for children of various ages.

A *rapid respiratory rate* may occur with pneumonia, paroxysmal atrial tachycardia, interstitial myocarditis, congestive heart failure, meningitis, fever, pain, severe anemia, metabolic acidosis, hyperammonemia, shock and acute anxiety. Tachypnea ranging from 50 to 100 per minute during sleep may be the first sign of left heart failure. In infants, abdominal distention may be an important cause of respiratory

TABLE 15–1   RESPIRATORY RATES PER MINUTE OF NORMAL CHILDREN, BOTH SEXES, SLEEPING AND AWAKE*

| Age | Sleeping | | | Awake | | | Mean Difference Between Sleeping and Awake |
| --- | --- | --- | --- | --- | --- | --- | --- |
| | No. | Mean | Range | No. | Mean | Range | |
| 6–12 months | 6 | 27 | 22–31 | 3 | 64 | 58–75 | 37 |
| 1– 2 years | 6 | 19 | 17–23 | 4 | 35 | 30–40 | 16 |
| 2– 4 years | 16 | 19 | 16–25 | 15 | 31 | 23–42 | 12 |
| 4– 6 years | 23 | 18 | 14–23 | 22 | 26 | 19–36 | 8 |
| 6– 8 years | 27 | 17 | 13–23 | 28 | 23 | 15–30 | 6 |
| 8–10 years | 19 | 18 | 14–23 | 19 | 21 | 15–31 | 3 |
| 10–12 years | 11 | 16 | 13–19 | 17 | 21 | 15–28 | 5 |
| 12–14 years | 6 | 16 | 15–18 | 7 | 22 | 18–26 | 6 |

*From Waring, W. W. *In* Kendig, E. L., Jr. and Chernick, V. (eds.): *Disorders of the Respiratory Tract in Children*. 3rd ed. Philadelphia, W. B. Saunders Co., 1977, p. 84.

difficulty, producing dyspnea, rapid respiratory rate and even cyanosis, especially in the presence of patchy atelectasis or pneumonitis. Because of the pain associated with abdominal breathing, respiratory movements in patients with peritonitis are chiefly thoracic, rapid and accompanied by grunting. Expiratory grunting may also be noted with pneumonia, heart failure, pulmonary edema and the respiratory distress syndrome.

Since salicylate poisoning may cause an increase in the respiratory rate, a blood salicylate level should be obtained in all young children with hyperpnea even if aspirin ingestion is denied.

Intermittent hyperventilation and irregular respiration occurs with *subacute necrotizing encephalomyelopathy* (Leigh's syndrome). There may be irregular, sighing respirations.

*Kussmaul breathing*, due to metabolic acidosis and characterized by deep respiratory movements and use of the accessory respiratory musculature, may occur in diabetes, renal failure, salicylism, inborn errors of metabolism and lactic acidosis.

Hypoxic states in infants and children are usually accompanied by apprehension, anxiety, restlessness and by an increase in the respiratory rate.

*Orthopnea* occurs with asthma, pulmonary edema, croup and cystic fibrosis.

*Bulbar or central involvement of the respiratory center* may lead to irregular and shallow respiratory movements characterized by spasmodic or jerky, hiccup-like inspirations and intervals of apnea. The early diagnosis of *intercostal or diaphragmatic paralysis* permits prompt use of assisted ventilation to prevent fatigue and hypoxia. Early signs of respiratory insufficiency include irregular, shallow respiration with perhaps an increase in respiratory rate, use of the accessory muscles of respiration, dilatation of the alae nasi, slight grunting, unwillingness to talk or frequent interruptions in speech, monosyllabic speech, restlessness, anxiety, fear of falling asleep, mental confusion, headache and, occasionally, euphoria. Decreased vital capacity can be demonstrated by asking the patient to count rapidly to ten. Patients with respiratory difficulty cannot do this. Cyanosis and unresponsiveness are *late* signs, as is forced use of the accessory muscles of respiration with gasping and opening of the mouth for each breath.

Intercostal and diaphragmatic paralysis may occur simultaneously or independently. In young children it may be possible to localize paralysis of the intercostals or diaphragm by splinting the chest and then the abdomen while observing the action of the alternate group of muscles. With paralysis of the intercostals the patient cannot inhale but is able to exhale. The converse is true with diaphragmatic involvement. When the intercostal muscles are paralyzed, abnormal expansion of the abdomen occurs on inspiration unaccompanied by enlargement of the chest or by pulling in of the chest wall unilaterally or bilaterally. When the diaphragm is paralyzed, the chest expands on inspiration and the upper part of the abdomen retracts. With unilateral paralysis of the diaphragm, wide flaring of the ribs on the ipsilateral side occurs if the intercostals are intact.

Respiratory difficulty may occur in patients with the Guillain-Barré syndrome. Diaphragmatic paralysis may be a manifestation of diphtheritic neuritis. Patients with chorea may have paradoxical respiration with retraction instead of expansion of the abdomen occurring at the beginning of a deep inspiration *(Czerny's sign)*.

Because of incoordination of the respiratory musculature, respiratory difficulty and irregularity in both duration and amplitude may occur in children with spastic cerebral palsy. The respiratory excursions may be jerky and halting.

## RETRACTIONS AND BULGING

When expansion of the lungs lags behind the forced expansion of the thoracic cage during labored breathing, increased negative intrathoracic pressure results, and retractions occur. While the sternum and ribs are lifted during inspiration, the soft tissues in the suprasternal, infrasternal, intercostal, subcostal and supraclavicular spaces are drawn inward.

Slight retractions are normal. More marked retractions occur with atelectasis, pneumonia, bronchiolitis, cystic fibrosis and asthma. They are an important physical finding with respiratory tract obstruction, especially laryngeal obstruction. Mild retractions may occur in young infants when the nasal airway is blocked by a purulent discharge or in infants with congenital choanal atresia. With congenital hypoplasia of the mandible and glossoptosis, the airway may be compromised, causing retractions to occur.

Because of the poorly developed and yielding thoracic skeleton in prematures and in some term infants, retraction of the thoracic cage, especially the anterior chest wall and along its line of attachment, may occur when the diaphragm contracts during inspiration. During infancy the sternum may demonstrate paradoxical motion on respiration, moving inward rather than outward on inspiration. Retraction of the sternum during inspiration does not always imply insufficient pulmonary aeration, particularly in small premature infants. Inspiratory collapse of the thoracic wall in such infants is also not necessarily the cause or result of atelectasis.

*Unequal expansion and respiration lag* suggest
Atelectasis. Flattening of the involved side of the chest and narrowing of the intercostal spaces may occur with massive atelectasis.
Pneumonia
Pleurisy
Pneumothorax, empyema, hydrothorax
Diaphragmatic hernia
*Intercostal bulging* may occasionally be noted when there is a large amount of fluid or exudate in the pleural spaces or marked expiratory effort.

*Precordial bulging* may occur in patients with pneumomediastinum and with right ventricular hypertrophy.

## STRUCTURAL ANOMALIES

*Funnel chest,* or *pectus excavatum,* is characterized by a depression of the sternum and costal cartilages, most prominent during inspiration. The defect usually begins at about the second interspace and becomes more prominent as the xiphoid is approached. The apex of the depression may be in the midline, over or slightly lateral to the xiphoid. Lateral funnel chest may be associated with absence of the pectoralis major and minor. Pectus excavatum occurs with Marfan's and Noonan's syndromes.

*Pigeon breast,* or *pectus carinatum,* is characterized by a prominent, protruding sternum with vertical depressions along the costochondral junctions lateral to the sternum. Patients with Morquio's disease, spondyloepiphyseal dysplasia congenita and Noonan's syndrome have notable pigeon breast deformities.

*Harrison's groove* is a horizontal depression of the rib cage along the line of attachment of the diaphragm from the lower end of the sternum to the midaxillary line. Some flaring of the costal margins is present below this groove. The deformity may be congenital or due to rickets.

A *barrel-shaped chest,* in which the sternum appears to be pushed out and the ribs are more horizontal than normal, may develop as a result of chronic obstructive pulmonary diseases such as asthma and cystic fibrosis.

*Asphyxiating thoracic dystrophy,* a generalized skeletal abnormality, causes a narrow, fixed thorax. The circumference of the chest at the nipple line is decreased. Respiratory distress and cyanosis occur when the dystrophy is severe.

Oberklaid, F., Danks, D.M., Mayne, V. and Campbell, P.: Asphyxiating thoracic dysplasia: clinical, radiological and pathological information on 10 patients. *Arch. Dis. Child.* 52:758, 1977.

In *Morquio's syndrome* the vertical length of the chest is decreased, and the anterior-posterior diameter and width increased. Protrusion of the sternum develops during early childhood.

The costochondral junctions are palpable in many normal infants, but not to the extent they are with rickets or scurvy. The *rachitic rosary* consists of rounded, knob-like prominences or beading at the costochondral junctions.

*Scorbutic beading* is characterized by sharp, angular deformities of the costochondral junctions. The sternum and the adjacent cartilage may be displaced inward or dorsally at the costochondral junction, producing the so-called bayonet deformity. Enlargement of the costochondral junctions may also be noted in chondrodystrophy and hypophosphatasia.

*Agenesis or hypoplasia of the pectoralis major and minor muscles* is accompanied by hypoplasia or absence of the breast and nipple. Lack of a well-developed anterior axillary fold is evident on inspection. In Poland's syndrome, ipsilateral hypoplasia of the upper extremities and syndactyly occurs in some instances along with defects of the ribs and costal cartilages.

Brooksaler, R.S. and Graivier, L.: Poland's syndrome. *Am. J. Dis. Child. 121:*263, 1971.

*Tietze's syndrome* is characterized by a firm, tender and painful fusiform swelling of one or more of the upper four costal cartilages. Although usually localized to the involved cartilage, the pain may radiate.

## PERCUSSION

Percussion is performed in infants and children much as in adults, either indirectly by striking the middle phalanx of the left middle finger with the tip of the right middle finger or by percussing the chest wall directly with the finger tips. Because of the thinness of their chest wall the percussion findings in infants differ from those in older children. Tactile sensations, such as a feeling of resistance or fullness, may be more informative than the percussion note.

In the examination of the lung fields in infants and children, the examiner may use light percussion over the interspaces, beginning in the supraclavicular spaces and proceeding downward, comparing the percussion notes obtained on both sides of the chest. Physical findings related to the upper lobes will be represented over the upper half of the chest anteriorly, the upper axillae laterally and over the upper third of the back posteriorly. The lower lobes largely account for pulmonary findings over the rest of the thorax except in the nipple and midaxillary areas on the right.

Liver dullness in infants usually extends up to the lower border of the sixth rib anteriorly. The dullness shades off above this point to about the region of the fourth rib. An impaired percussion note may be present over the left lower hemithorax anteriorly when the stomach of an infant is distended with fluid. Usually, however, a tympanitic percussion note is elicited on the left side below the sixth rib owing to the gastric air bubble.

In infants or in children who are too ill to sit up or who do not wish to, the patient should lie as straight as possible so that flexion of the trunk and uneven contact with the bedclothing do not produce misleading percussion notes. It is preferable, of course, for the child to sit or to stand erect during percussion of the chest.

*Impairment of the percussion note* with dullness or flatness may be noted in the following diseases:

Lobar pneumonia during consolidation.

Patchy atelectasis may be characterized by areas of impaired resonance, but usually the percussion note is modified by the compensatory emphysema. Dullness or flatness is present over areas of massive atelectasis.

In the presence of pleural effusion or empyema the percussion note is flat over the involved area, duller than over areas of pneumonic consolidation. The interspaces may feel full and resistant. If the effusion is only moderate in amount, a tympanitic percussion note may be found above the area of dullness. Except in the presence of massive effusion, shifting dullness may be noted when the patient changes from a sitting to a recumbent position.

Wolfe, W.G., Spock, A. and Bradford, W.D.: Pleural fluid in infants and children. *Am. Rev. Resp. Dis.* 98:1027, 1968.

Pleural thickening
Intrathoracic neoplasms
Diaphragmatic hernia

*Hyperresonance* may be noted in the following:

Pneumothorax

Lobar emphysema

Asthma, bronchiolitis and cystic fibrosis in infants when associated with generalized expiratory obstruction

Tympany on percussion may be obtained in some infants with a diaphragmatic hernia.

## AUSCULTATION

With patience and experience one may perform auscultation of the chest with confidence and dispatch. For auscultation of the chest of older children the examiner may have the child breathe deeply through his mouth ("pant like a dog") after demonstrating what is desired and then following the respirations by saying "In" and "Out" as auscultation proceeds. Since this forced respiration may be tiring, the child should be given a brief respite during the examination.

The choice of a bell or a diaphragm type of stethoscope is a matter of individual preference and experience. The bell or diaphragm should be small, however, so as to fit closely over the interspaces.

In prenasal and preoral auscultation, one listens to the breath sounds with the bowl of the stethoscope held ½ to 1 inch in front of the nose or mouth of the infant. This permits an evaluation of the infant's respiration without awakening him or causing him to cry.

In infancy the breath sounds are relatively louder and harsher than in adults. This relative increase in the intensity of breath sounds is present up to the age of five or six years. The breath sounds over the medial and upper portions of the chest are characterized by a relatively prolonged expiratory phase as compared to the same areas in adults. These sounds, which resemble the bronchovesicular breathing of the adult, have been called puerile breathing. In young infants there may be no noticeable pause between expiration and the next inspiration; on the other hand, expiration may be quiet, and a brief pause may be noted before the inspiratory phase.

Breath sounds may be classified as vesicular, tracheal (bronchial, tubular) and bronchovesicular.

In older children *vesicular breath sounds* are heard over most of the chest except for those limited areas characterized by tracheal or bronchovesicular breathing. Inspiration is louder, higher-pitched and longer in duration than expiration. Expiration may be so brief and faint as to be almost imperceptible in the older child. Vesicular breath sounds are most intense over the upper part of the chest and axillae. As in percussion, one begins with the examination of the supraclavicular fossae and proceeds downward an interspace at a time, comparing findings on both sides of the chest. Slight variations in the sounds on the two sides of the chest may be present, but with experience one learns the normal limits of this variation. As noted earlier, the breath sounds are more intense and harsh in early life, and puerile or bronchovesicular sounds with relative prolongation of the expiratory phase are present medially and over the upper portion of the chest.

Diminished or suppressed vesicular breathing, characterized by a decrease in intensity, may occur early in pneumonia. Early pneumonia is present in the area with diminished breath sounds rather than in the region in which the breath sounds are intensified. In infants and young children the transmission of breath sounds through an area of pleural effusion may be only slightly diminished though the percussion note is dull. Tubular breathing may be present over areas of pulmonary consolidation. Diminished vesicular breathing may also be noted with hydrothorax, pneumothorax, lobar emphysema, pleurisy, patchy atelectasis, massive atelectasis if the associated bronchus is closed, pulmonary edema, bronchitis and paralysis of the respiratory musculature.

*Tracheal breath sounds* are normally heard over the trachea, larynx and the upper part of the sternum, and along the vertebral column above the first thoracic vertebra. These breath sounds are louder and more tubular and have a much higher pitch than the vesicular breath sounds. The expiratory phase is also longer and louder. A brief pause may occur between inspiration and expiration. *Tubular breathing* may be heard in pneumonia during consolidation, tuberculosis, atelectasis if the bronchus to the atelectatic area remains open, massive pericardial effusion and in some instances of pleurisy with effusion.

In infants and young children, *bronchovesicular breath sounds* are heard parasternally and over the upper part of the chest. In older children these findings are limited to the area over the larger bronchi: the manubrium, along the sternal angle of Louis and posteriorly in the upper interscapular area. These sounds vary, being either chiefly bronchial or vesicular. Usually, the expiratory phase is longer, louder and higher-pitched than the inspiratory phase.

In patients with a *congenital diaphragmatic hernia,* breath sounds may be distant or absent on the involved side. Bowel sounds may be heard in the chest. Occasionally bowel sounds can be heard in the left lower hemithorax anteriorly in normal infants.

*Rhonchi* are musical, continuous sounds, wheezes and vibrations.

*Rales* are crackling or bubbling discontinuous sounds or vibrations. Rales of the medium or fine variety may be heard in a number of disease states, such as bronchitis, pneumonia, atelectasis, pulmonary edema, heart failure, bronchiectasis and tuberculosis.

Expiratory wheezing is discussed on page 494.

A *pleural friction rub* causes a grating, jerky, leathery, creaking, rubbing sound that seems close to the examiner's ear. It can be intensified by slight pressure with the stethoscope on the chest wall. The rub is usually most distinct at the end of inspiration but may be present in both phases and disappears when the patient holds his breath. A pleuropericardial rub has clinical features of both pleural and pericardial rubs.

## GENERAL REFERENCES

Pulmonary Terms and Symbols: A Report of the American College of Chest Physicians–American Thoracic Society Joint Committee on Pulmonary Nomenclature. *Chest* 67:583, 1975.

Waring, W.W.: The history and physical examination. *In* Kendig, E.L., Jr. and Chernick, V. (eds.): *Disorders of the Respiratory Tract in Children.* 3rd ed. Philadelphia, W. B. Saunders Co., 1977, Chapter 3, p. 71.

CHAPTER 16

# THE BREASTS

Examination of the breasts is helpful in assessment of gestational age in the newborn. In the premature the areola and nipple are barely visible, and there is no palpable breast tissue. The areola becomes evident at about 34 weeks. The term infant has 5 to 6 mm. of palpable breast tissue, and the areola is raised. In the postmature infant, there is 10 to 12 mm. of palpable breast tissue.

Unilateral or bilateral *engorgement of the breasts* may occur in both male and female newborn infants. This enlargement appears on the second to fourth day, gradually increases for a time and may persist for several weeks. A colostrum-like secretion from the breasts may be noted. Such engorgement occurs in most term infants but not in prematures. *Mastitis,* or infection of the breast in the newborn infant, characterized by local redness, heat and swelling, is usually due to Staphylococcus aureus but may rarely be caused by gram-negative organisms.

Supernumerary nipples may occasionally be seen in the axillary line or below and medial to the nipple. Increased inter-nipple distance may be associated with Noonan's or Turner's syndromes, but is not a constant finding.

Collins, E.: The illusion of widely spaced nipples in the Noonan and the Turner syndromes.
J. Pediatr. 83:557, 1973.

*Breast development,* one of the earliest of the secondary sexual characteristics to appear, begins in adolescent girls between the ages of 10 and 14 years. There is a considerable difference in the status of such development and in breast size and contour among girls of the same chronologic age. In the individual girl there may be some difference in the development of each breast, one developing perhaps somewhat in advance of the other. The Tanner stages of breast development are as follows:

Stage 1.  Preadolescent, in which only the papilla is elevated.
Stage 2.  The breast bud stage, in which the breast and the papilla are both elevated as a small mound, and the diameter of the areola is enlarged.
Stage 3.  Further enlargement and elevation of the breast and areola with no distinct separation of their contours.
Stage 4.  Projection of the areola and the papilla to form a secondary mound above the level of the breasts.
Stage 5.  The mature stage, in which only the papilla projects because of the recession of the areola to the general contour of the breast.

Examination of the breasts should be a part of the routine examination of adolescent girls. An explanation as to the necessity of the examination helps the child to accept it without embarrassment.

Occasionally, *precocious breast development (premature thelarche)* may be noted during infancy or childhood in the absence of other signs of sexual maturation. This unilateral or bilateral breast enlargement usually does not proceed beyond the bud stage. Continued observation for other signs of precocious development is indicated.

Children who proceed to complete sexual precocity usually have advanced height and bone age.

Precocious breast development has also been reported in young children owing to accidental ingestion of diethylstilbestrol. Intense, dark brown areolar pigmentation in a girl with pseudoprecocious puberty suggests exogenous estrogen as a cause for the precocity.

During the prepubertal period a unilateral or bilateral, transient, indurated, *discoid swelling,* 1 or 2 inches in diameter, may occur behind the areola in both boys and girls. This swelling may be painful and secretion of a colostrum-like substance may occur.

Enlargement of the breast and nipple and an underlying disc-like mass occurs in patients with *leprechaunism.*

Some degree of unilateral or bilateral breast enlargement or simple *adolescent gynecomastia* is common in adolescent boys. In some instances the enlargement may be moderate. Spontaneous regression should occur within a few months to two or three years. Obese children may appear to have enlarged breasts, but this appearance is usually due to adipose and not to glandular tissue. Most instances of gynecomastia in adolescent males are nonendocrine.

> August, G.P., Chandra, R. and Hung, W.: Pubertal male gynecomastia. *J. Pediatr. 80*:259, 1972.
> Latorre, H. and Kenny, F.M.: Idiopathic gynecomastia in seven preadolescent boys. *Am. J. Dis. Child. 126*:771, 1973.

*Klinefelter's syndrome* is characterized by bilateral gynecomastia that appears some time after the onset of puberty. The breast enlargement may be notable. Other secondary sexual characteristics are normal. The testes are small, and spermatogenesis does not occur.

Rare pathologic causes for gynecomastia in adolescent boys include severe liver disease, congenital virilizing adrenal hyperplasia, feminizing tumors of the adrenal, interstitial cell tumors of the testis, mixed gonadal dysgenesis, Reifenstein's and Rosewater's syndromes, chorionepitheliomas and exogenous estrogens. Gynecomastia may be a result of Leydig-cell dysfunction in adolescent boys secondary to chemotherapy for malignant disease.

> Sherins, R.J., Olweny, C.L.M. and Ziegler, J.L.: Gynecomastia and gonadal dysfunction in adolescent boys treated with combination chemotherapy for Hodgkin's disease. *N. Engl. J. Med. 299*:12, 1978.

Breast development does not occur in girls with Turner's syndrome unless cyclic estrogen treatment is used.

Occasionally, unilateral or bilateral massive *virginal breast hypertrophy* may occur in otherwise normal girls.

The most common tumor of the adolescent female breast is the benign *fibroadenoma.* This tumor is palpable as a rubbery, firm, mobile, 2.5 by 3.0 cm. mass with a smooth or slightly irregular surface.

> Daniel, W.A., Jr. and Mathews, M.D.: Tumors of the breast in adolescent females. *Pediatrics 41*:743, 1968.
> Turbey, W.J., Buntain, W.L. and Dudgeon, D.L.: The surgical management of pediatric breast masses. *Pediatrics 56*:736, 1975.

*Galactorrhea,* a rare occurrence in adolescent males, may be idiopathic or may be due to hyperprolactinemia, a pineal tumor or a chromophobe adenoma. In girls, galactorrhea may occur with pituitary tumors or the use of tranquilizers, oral contraceptives and steroids.

# CHAPTER 17

# THE HEART

## APEX BEAT

The apex beat is usually not apparent in infants and young children unless the heart is enlarged or there is minimal subcutaneous fat over the chest. It may be palpable although not as well localized as in older children. Because of the relatively horizontal position of the heart, the apex beat is usually present in the fourth interspace outside the mammary line up to three years of age. From the fourth to seventh years it is usually in the fifth to sixth interspace within the mammary line. The right border of the heart normally extends to the right sternal margin, and the left border is usually within the mammary line. The apex beat is best palpated with the child sitting and leaning forward.

The apical impulse may be diffuse and almost inapparent in patients with pneumomediastinum, pericarditis with effusion and pleurisy with effusion. With hyperthyroidism, excitement or anxiety the apex beat may be prominent.

When the heart is enlarged, the apex beat is displaced to the left. Location of the apex beat more than 1 cm. lateral to the midclavicular line in the fourth interspace in young children and outside this line in the fifth interspace in older children suggests cardiomegaly. In the presence of pleurisy with effusion, pneumothorax or lobar emphysema, the apex beat shifts toward the uninvolved side. With atelectasis, the apex beat shifts toward the involved side.

The apex beat is present on the right in dextrocardia.

## THRILLS

The palm or finger tips may be used in palpating for a thrill. Light palpation is usually best although at times a thrill is more readily detected by firm palpation. Differentiation between an active but normal cardiac thrust and a thrill may be difficult, especially in the patient with a thin chest wall. Other than reflecting the loudness of a murmur (at least Grade IV), a thrill has no significance.

**Systolic Thrill.** Aortic stenosis is almost always accompanied by a thrill over the base of the heart to the right of the sternum, over the right side of the neck and at the suprasternal notch. A systolic thrill may be present in the second and third left interspaces and atrial septal defects, especially if another anomaly such as pulmonary stenosis or interventricular septal defect is also present, and over the third and fourth left interspaces in interventricular septal defects. Pulmonary stenosis, either isolated or in the tetralogy of Fallot, may be accompanied by a thrill in the second and third left interspaces.

**Continuous Thrill.** About half of the patients with a patent ductus arteriosus have a systolic or continuous thrill at the base of the heart, parasternally along the first and second left interspaces and below the left clavicle.

## PULSE

Since it is unaffected by exercise, anxiety or excitement, the sleeping pulse permits a baseline heart rate in infants and children. This is important in relation to rheumatic fever and hyperthyroidism, since tachycardia during sleep is of diagnostic interest. It is difficult to determine the pulse rate in infants by radial palpation, and auscultation of the heart must be used. The approximate rate at various ages is given in Table 17-1. An increase in rate occurs in patients with fever, severe anemia, hypoxia, hyperthyroidism, active rheumatic heart disease and myocarditis.

*Tachycardia,* with a rate of 150 to 200 in infants and 100 to 150 in older children, is a constant finding in children in congestive cardiac failure. In sinus tachycardia, the rate will vary some 10 to 15 beats a minute in contrast to paroxysmal atrial tachycardia, in which the rate remains constant during an episode.

*Myocarditis* accompanies many viral diseases. The initial symptoms of interstitial myocarditis in children may simulate those of a severe pneumonitis or a mild gastroenteritis. These patients soon, however, exhibit tachycardia, a change in the quality of the heart sounds, gallop rhythm, cardiac enlargement, dyspnea, hepatomegaly, edema and possibly cyanosis. T-wave changes appear on the electrocardiogram.

*Bradycardia* in the presence of fever suggests a salmonella infection. Rheumatic fever patients treated with cortisone may also have bradycardia.

The heart rate is an important diagnostic and prognostic sign in neonatal asphyxia. Rates under 100 warrant special concern.

Patients with aortic insufficiency have a bounding pulse with a quick rise and fall. Capillary pulsations may be noted in the fingernails.

*Palpation of the femoral pulse* should be performed routinely in infants and children too young for routine blood pressure determinations and in infants with cardiac enlargement. An absent or weak femoral pulse suggests coarctation of the aorta and is an indication for determination of the blood pressure. The presence of a palpable femoral pulse does not, however, exclude coarctation of the aorta. Simulta-

### TABLE 17-1  AVERAGE PULSE RATES AT REST*

| Age | Lower Limits of Normal | | Average | | Upper Limits of Normal | |
|---|---|---|---|---|---|---|
| Newborn | 70 | | 120 | | 170 | |
| 1-11 months | 80 | | 120 | | 160 | |
| 2 years | 80 | | 110 | | 130 | |
| 4 years | 80 | | 100 | | 120 | |
| 6 years | 75 | | 100 | | 115 | |
| 8 years | 70 | | 90 | | 110 | |
| 10 years | 70 | | 90 | | 110 | |
| | *Girls* | *Boys* | *Girls* | *Boys* | *Girls* | *Boys* |
| 12 years | 70 | 65 | 90 | 85 | 110 | 105 |
| 14 years | 65 | 60 | 85 | 80 | 105 | 100 |
| 16 years | 60 | 55 | 80 | 75 | 100 | 95 |
| 18 years | 55 | 50 | 75 | 70 | 95 | 90 |

*From Vaughan, V. C., III and McKay, R. J. (eds.): *The Nelson Textbook of Pediatrics.* Philadelphia, W. B. Saunders Co., 1979, p. 1252.

neous palpation of both the radial and femoral pulses may be helpful. Normally, both impulses are felt at the same time. In coarctation of the aorta the femoral pulse wave may be slightly delayed.

In *Takayasu's disease,* the carotid, brachial and radial pulses may be absent or diminished.

> Warshaw, J.B. and Spach, M.S.: Takayasu's disease (primary aortitis) in childhood. *Pediatrics 35*:620, 1965.

Although an *arrhythmia* may be noted clinically, a specific diagnosis depends on an electrocardiogram.

In *sinus arrhythmia* the pulse rate increases during inspiration and slows during expiration. A normal finding in most children above the age of three years, this arrhythmia is especially prominent during later childhood and puberty and infrequent during infancy. In older children sinus arrhythmia may occasionally superficially suggest dropped beats or premature contractions.

*Pulsus paradoxus,* characterized by a diminution or disappearance of the pulse during inspiration, may occur in patients with cardiac tamponade due to pericardial effusion, bleeding, purulent pericarditis, constrictive pericarditis, severe asthma, pleural effusion and pneumothorax. This phenomenon is more clearly demonstrated by use of the sphygmomanometer. A significant drop in the systolic pressure is noted at the end of a full inspiration compared with expiration. A difference of over 20 mm. is highly suggestive of cardiac tamponade whereas values between 10 mm. and 20 mm. are suspicious.

*Extrasystoles,* premature cardiac contractions not followed by a compensatory pulse, occur in normal children and are of no significance unless associated with rheumatic carditis or congenital heart disease. Extrasystoles occurring in normal children usually disappear after exercise, while those associated with cardiac lesions may become more pronounced.

*Premature contractions* followed by a compensatory diastolic pause may cause cardiac irregularity. The compensatory pause that follows the premature contraction may suggest dropped beats.

> Jacobsen, J.R., Garson, A., Jr., Gilette, P.C. and McNamara, D.G.: Premature ventricular contractions in normal children. *J. Pediatr. 92*:36, 1978.

*Dropped beats* occurring with a partial heart block also cause irregularity of the cardiac rhythm. Cardiac arrhythmias and bradycardia may be caused by digitalis toxicity.

Patients with acute carditis may demonstrate a *"tic-tac" rhythm,* in which the interval between the first and second sounds is equal to or even longer than diastole. Instead of the normal 1:2 relation between the systolic and diastolic intervals, the ratio becomes more nearly 1:1.

During episodes of *paroxysmal tachycardia* the heart rate may be too rapid to count. In infancy these attacks are characterized by restlessness, irritability, cyanosis or pallor, rapid respiratory rate, anorexia, vomiting, fever and, in some patients, hepatomegaly and other signs of congestive heart failure. These episodes may last for minutes, hours or days. Paroxysmal episodes of tachycardia may occur in infants with endocardial fibroelastosis or underlying congenital heart disease such as coarctation.

# PERCUSSION

Light indirect or direct percussion along the interspaces from the periphery toward the midline may be used for an estimation of heart size. Although moderate or marked enlargement may be detected by this technique, the determination of heart size by percussion is of limited accuracy, especially in infants. The position of the apex beat may be a better reflection of heart size.

In patients with massive atelectasis the area of cardiac dullness shifts toward the involved side. In the presence of pleurisy with effusion or pneumothorax, this area shifts to the uninvolved side.

*Pericarditis with effusion* may cause an increased area of dullness over the precordium.

*Enlargement of the heart* in infants may be due to, among other causes, congestive heart failure, endocardial fibroelastosis, glycogenosis type II (Pompe's disease), idiopathic hypertrophy of cardiac muscle, rhabdomyoma, coarctation of the aorta, anomalous origin of the coronary arteries, aortic stenosis, septal defects and a large patent ductus. Cardiomegaly is also present in some infants of diabetic mothers. Cardiac enlargement in older children may be due to rheumatic fever, severe anemia and hypertension.

With *pneumomediastinum* the area of cardiac dullness may be reduced. Hyperresonance may be present over the precordium, especially when the patient is supine. This finding may not be present when the patient leans forward in the sitting position.

# AUSCULTATION

The preferred stethoscope for cardiac auscultation in children is one with a combined bell (for murmurs of low frequency) and diaphragm (for murmurs of high frequency) with the smallest diameter available. The room should be quiet and the child cooperative.

Attention may be given to the rate, rhythm, regularity, intensity and quality of the heart sounds. Patients should be examined in the supine, upright and left lateral positions and leaning forward. Because of the thinness of the chest wall in infants, cardiac murmurs are widely transmitted and heard over a wider area than in older children and adults. The location and transmission of murmurs, therefore, is not always as significant in infants as in older children.

In childhood, except in young infants, the intensity of the first apical heart sound is greater than that of the second. The converse is true in the pulmonic area. This difference in loudness facilitates timing of the cardiac cycle. *Splitting of the pulmonary second sound,* heard best in the second left intercostal space using the diaphragm of the stethoscope, is a common normal finding. The sounds are widely split during inspiration but almost synchronous during expiration. Accentuation of the aortic second sound may accompany hypertension, and diminution may be noted in congenital aortic stenosis. A quiet or absent unsplit pulmonary second sound is characteristic of valvular pulmonary stenosis whereas pulmonary hypertension is suggested by a loud, high-pitched, booming pulmonic second sound. An incomplete bundle branch block accompanying an atrial septal defect may be suspected when the second pulmonic sound is widely split and remains fixed during both inspiration and expiration. In the newborn infant, the pulmonary second sound is either single or minimally split.

In patients with pericardial effusion the intensity of the heart sounds may be so diminished that they become difficult to hear. The pulse, however, usually remains full and strong.

Myocarditis should be considered when the heart sounds are of poor quality and difficult to hear.

Pneumothorax may also cause the heart sounds to be distant and weak.

With pneumomediastinum, subcutaneous emphysema may appear, and a concomitant pneumothorax, usually on the left, is often present. *Hamman's sign*, the occurrence of crackling, bubbling, crunching and churning sounds, may occasionally be heard on auscultation over the precordium with pneumomediastinum. Though these sounds may be present through the entire cardiac cycle, they are usually most apparent during systole, in the left lateral recumbent position and during the expiratory phase of respiration.

A *pericardial friction rub* is a rough and grating or soft and scratchy, superficial, to-and-fro or inconstant sound usually heard best in the third and fourth left interspaces parasternally and over the sternum. The sound, similar to the rustling of hair, is transient and easily missed. The rub may occur synchronously with the heart beat and may be intensified by firm pressure of the stethoscope on the chest. Except for the time relation with the respiratory movements, pleural friction rubs may simulate the pericardial rub. With the development of a purulent or serous effusion, the rub usually disappears except, perhaps, at the base of the heart. Echocardiography is a useful diagnostic tool when pericardial effusion is suspected.

*Purulent pericarditis,* often secondary to a primary infection elsewhere, is a pediatric and surgical emergency. Diagnostic pericardiocentesis should be done promptly and the purulent effusion drained.

Gersony, W.M. and McCracken, G.H., Jr.: Purulent pericarditis in infancy. *Pediatrics 40*: 224, 1967.
Vanreken, D., Strauss, A., Hernandez, A. and Feigin, R.D.: Infectious pericarditis in children. *J. Pediatr. 85*:165, 1974.

Pericarditis with effusion may be associated with rheumatic fever, viral infections, rheumatoid arthritis, uremia and metastatic malignancy.

Bernstein, B., Takahashi, M. and Hanson, V.: Cardiac involvement in juvenile rheumatoid arthritis. *J. Pediatr. 85*:313, 1974.
Cayler, G.C., Taybi, H., Riley, H.D., Jr. and Simon, J.L.: Pericarditis with effusion in infancy and children. *J. Pediatr. 63*:264, 1963.

In the *postpericardiotomy syndrome,* which may occasionally occur after cardiac surgery, pericardial and pleural reactions and effusion accompanied by the abrupt onset of fever and chest pain appear in the second postoperative week or later. The pain frequently radiates from the precordial region to the neck and shoulder unilaterally or bilaterally and may be accentuated by a deep breath. A pericardial friction rub may be heard, especially with the patient supine.

A continuous, loud *venous hum* may frequently be heard over the upper sternum, clavicle and vessels of the neck, especially on the right, but occasionally also along the left parasternal border in normal children. The intensity of this hum varies greatly with changes in position of the head and neck, being loudest during diastole with the patient in the upright position and diminishing or disappearing in the recumbent position or with compression over the neck vessels. A prominent systolic hum may be heard over the pulmonic area in hyperthyroidism.

A *third heart sound* is often heard during diastole in normal children. This low-pitched, short sound, best heard at the apex, is thought to occur at the end of rapid filling of the left ventricles. There are a number of differences between a split second sound and a third heart sound. The interval between the split second sound is less than that between the beginning of the second and third heart sound. This difference may be detected clinically. The duplicated second sounds have identical quality and pitch whereas the third heart sound has a quiet, dull, lumplike or thudlike quality. Split second sounds are most frequent at the base of the heart and parasternally on the left. The third heart sound is usually heard best at the apex or just medial to and above the apex with the child in the left recumbent position. This sound may also be optimally heard with the patient in the left lateral decubitus position and with the bell of the stethoscope lightly applied after exercise or with the slowing of the heart rate that occurs during the expiratory phase of respiration. In active rheumatic fever it may be difficult to differentiate a third heart sound from an early diastolic murmur, especially when the heart rate is rapid.

Differentiation is required, at times, between a third heart sound and a *gallop rhythm*. As a general rule, if other evidences of carditis are present, the three sounds usually represent a gallop rhythm; on the other hand, if there is no evidence of cardiac disease, the diastolic sound may be considered a third heart sound. Gallop rhythm may be a manifestation of carditis, severe anemia, thyrotoxicosis, mitral and aortic insufficiency, patent ductus and septal defects causing ventricular diastolic overloading and a protodiastolic gallop. Presystolic gallops may be associated with systolic overloading caused by such lesions as aortic stenosis, coarctation of the aorta and pulmonary stenosis when they are of a moderately severe grade. *Protodiastolic gallop* is generally best heard in the apical region or between that region and the lower portion of the sternum. *Presystolic gallop* is heard best along the left sternal border and the base of the heart. Gallop sounds are faint and heard best in a quiet room with the stethoscope bell lightly applied.

## MURMURS

*Ejection murmurs* begin after a short pause following the first sound. They are crescendo-decrescendo (diamond-shaped) and usually innocent in type.

It is sometimes difficult to be sure about the presence of a murmur, and whether it is *innocent* or *organic*. Whereas the characteristics of some murmurs are diagnostic, others require correlation with additional clinical findings, including the history. Their significance may not be evident until the child has been observed over time.

Each murmur may be described according to the following characteristics:

Position in the cardiac cycle (i.e., systolic [early, middle or late] or diastolic [early, middle, late or presystolic]). Location of the murmur and the point of maximal intensity is of diagnostic interest, but murmurs of specific lesions may be variable.

Ejection or regurgitant. *Ejection murmurs* occur during the ejection phase of ventricular systole. A short interval occurs between the first heart sound and the onset of the murmur. Many have a crescendo-decrescendo quality and end before the second heart sound. They may occur in normal patients as well as those with lesions such as aortic stenosis. *Regurgitant systolic murmurs* have an organic etiology and are due to an abnormal flow of blood from a ventricle, as in mitral insufficiency or ventricular septal defect. The regurgitant murmur is holosystolic. Regurgitant diastolic murmurs may also occur in aortic or pulmonic insufficiency.

Transmission
Duration (e.g., holosystolic murmurs are caused by an organic lesion)
Quality–blowing, rasping, rumbling
Pitch
Intensity
Response to exercise and change of position.

The intensity of murmurs may be graded from I to VI. A grade I murmur is just barely audible after careful auscultation for a time. In the absence of other findings, a grade I murmur is of no clinical significance. Grade II is also faint but heard immediately; grade III, a moderate murmur; grade IV, a loud murmur; and grade V a very loud murmur. Grade VI can be heard without a stethoscope. Although this classification may be helpful in describing what is heard, the intensity of a murmur, in itself, is not diagnostic.

Murmurs may be produced or intensified by an increase in cardiac output due to hypermetabolic states such as fever, exercise, hyperthyroidism, anemia (hemic murmur) or anxiety. Crying may cause murmurs to diminish or disappear because of changes in blood flow.

During the neonatal period, *transient* systolic ejection *murmurs* may be heard, especially in the third and fourth interspaces parasternally. Usually these murmurs disappear after a few days. If the murmur persists, a congenital defect is probably present; on the other hand, the murmur of a congenital defect may be initially almost inaudible but may become moderately loud in a few days or weeks (e.g., the murmur of a patent ductus arteriosus or a ventricular septal defect). Harsh murmurs heard on the first day of life are often caused by pulmonic or aortic stenosis.

*Innocent murmurs* occur in a large number of normal children at the base of the heart or along the left parasternal or pulmonic areas. They are more commonly heard during a febrile illness. Though these murmurs can often be readily recognized as nonorganic, differentiation from organic murmurs is occasionally difficult and may require a period of observation and further studies. Innocent murmurs are systolic and of short duration. Almost all systolic murmurs in otherwise asymptomatic children are either innocent or due to a ventricular septal defect. Usually soft and blowing, they occasionally may be loud and harsh. The intensity of the murmur does not permit categorization as either innocent or organic. Innocent murmurs may diminish in intensity or disappear after exercise, but they may also become more prominent. They may also be heard in the back. The nature of the murmur may vary, depending upon the phase of the respiratory cycle. Innocent murmurs usually have a lower pitch than the blowing murmur of mitral insufficiency, which is heard maximally at the apex and transmitted to the axilla.

The *vibratory murmur* is the most commonly encountered innocent murmur in children, especially between the ages of three and seven years. About grade II or III in intensity, brief in duration, early to midsystolic in time, maximal at the third or fourth left interspace or medial to the apex, the murmur transmits to the apex. Vibratory murmurs are usually heard best with the bell of the stethoscope and with the patient recumbent. They decrease or disappear when the patient is erect. Their vibratory, buzzing, low-pitched "twanging-string" or groaning quality is usually diagnostic. The location of maximal intensity of the innocent murmur medial to the apex is helpful in differentiation from the murmur of mitral insufficiency. At times, it is difficult to differentiate the murmur from that due to a ventricular septal defect or cardiomyopathy. An electrocardiogram and chest x-ray may be indicated, especially with grade IV or louder murmurs.

Bloomfield, D.K. and Liebman, J.: Idiopathic cardiomyopathy in children. *Circulation* 27:1071, 1963.

The *pulmonic ejection murmur,* another common innocent murmur, especially in young adolescents, is well localized parasternally in the second and third left interspaces. Grade I to III, short, early to midsystolic and blowing in quality, it is transmitted along the sternum and toward the apex. The murmur may be caused by an increase in pulmonary blood flow associated with fever, anxiety, exercise or anemia. A similar murmur may be due to mild pulmonic stenosis or an atrial septal defect. The latter may be suggested by a pulmonary second sound that remains widely split in both inspiration and expiration.

The pulmonic ejection murmur in the *straight back syndrome* is an innocent murmur heard in children who do not have the normal thoracic kyphosis. This syndrome has its highest incidence in infants up to two years of age. Although not readily apparent clinically, it is easily recognized roentgenographically when the ratio of the anteroposterior diameter to the transverse diameter of the thorax is determined. Functional murmurs may also occur in patients with scoliosis, kyphoscoliosis and pectus excavatum.

The *cardiorespiratory murmur,* a benign finding occasionally encountered in children, may be heard over the precordium, the apex or the cardiopulmonary borders. Characteristically mid- or late systolic in time and sharply localized, the murmur begins and ends suddenly, diminishes during inspiration and sounds like a high-pitched, short squeal close to the examiner's ear. Sometimes called the *"systolic whoop,"* it may begin with a systolic click. This murmur may be heard in patients with deformities of the chest.

Isolated *systolic clicks* may be heard infrequently in normal children.

*Mitral valve prolapse,* which is usually asymptomatic in children, may cause a midsystolic click, a high frequency sound with a scratchy quality, a mid-late grade II–III/VI systolic murmur heard best between the mitral area and the apex in the left lateral decubitus or standing positions, and whoops or whistles heard even without a stethoscope. The prevalence of mitral valve prolapse is high in children with Duchenne's progressive muscular dystrophy.

Brown, L.M.: Mitral valve prolapse in children. *Adv. Pediatr.* 25:327, 1978.

A *carotid bruit* may be heard as a well-localized early or midsystolic grade II to III murmur over the neck vessels supraclavicularly on the right but not in the aortic area.

In *rheumatic carditis* the murmurs and heart sounds are inconstant and vary in quality from one examination to the next. The sounds may appear muffled and dull. Impairment of the quality of the first heart sound and shortening of diastole produce a "tic-tac" rhythm characteristic of acute carditis. A gallop rhythm may also be present. Occasionally, a high-pitched, vibrant, somewhat raucous "seagull" murmur is heard at the apex in addition to the murmur of mitral insufficiency. A transient, low frequency, protodiastolic murmur may also be heard at the apex.

Markowitz, M. and Kuttner, A.G.: *Rheumatic Fever.* Philadelphia, W. B. Saunders Co., 1965.

## SYSTOLIC MURMURS

*Mitral insufficiency* is characterized by a soft to moderately loud, high-pitched, blowing apical murmur, generally holosystolic. The murmur is maximal at the apex and transmitted toward the left axilla, the base of the heart and, at times, to the back. The murmur may, in time, become louder and harsher and replace or muffle the first sound. It is best heard with the diaphragm during expiration with the patient in the left lateral recumbent position.

*Aortic stenosis* is characterized by a harsh, very loud, systolic ejection, crescendo-descrescendo murmur that is maximal in the second right interspace and widely transmitted to the right shoulder, the clavicle, up the vessels of the neck and toward the apex. Occasionally, in infants and young children the murmur may be loudest at the apex. Diastolic murmurs may also be heard in some patients. Aortic ejection clicks are common. A systolic thrill is present along the base of the heart and over the neck vessels.

*Pulmonic stenosis* of mild degree may produce a murmur identical to that of the innocent pulmonary ejection murmur or an atrial septal defect. The pulmonic second sound is decreased with severe but not mild stenosis.

A *ventricular septal defect* causes a grade III or IV, harsh, widely transmitted holosystolic murmur along the left parasternal area at the third and fourth interspaces and over the xiphoid process. The murmur may not be noted until days or weeks after birth. A systolic thrill is also often present. With a very large defect, a low-pitched, early diastolic murmur may be heard in the mitral area. With very small defects the murmur may be grade II and blowing. If the septal defect closes, the murmur gradually decreases, becomes confined to early systole and then disappears. The murmur may also diminish in intensity and duration if pulmonary hypertension develops. In the latter event the murmur may be accompanied by a loud single pulmonary second sound. The murmur of an arteriovenous canal simulates that of a ventricular septal defect.

An *atrial septum defect,* more commonly the secundum type, is usually characterized by a relatively soft, less than grade III, blowing systolic ejection murmur maximal in the second and third left interspaces and well transmitted. A systolic thrill may be present. The pulmonic second sound demonstrates a wide splitting with the second component louder than the first. A low-pitched, early diastolic murmur may be heard over the end of the sternum. The murmur of an atrial septal defect may not be noted for several months or years after birth. In defects of the ostium primum type with a split mitral valve, the murmur may be lower and accompanied by a prominent holosystolic apical murmur. The murmur accompanying an ostium primum defect is harsh, loud and well transmitted. An atrial septal defect murmur is often indistinguishable from an innocent functional pulmonic ejection murmur.

Patients with *isolated pulmonary stenosis* may have a loud, harsh and widely transmitted or a soft, scratchy and localized systolic murmur in the second or third left interspace parasternally. The murmur may be transmitted toward the left clavicle and posteriorly to the interscapular area. A systolic thrill may be present. The pulmonary second sound may be normal but is usually diminished in intensity or absent. Increased splitting of the second sound occurs in mild to moderate pulmonic stenosis. In the tetralogy of Fallot the pulmonic murmur is maximal in the third left interspace along the sternum. Duplication of the second sound heard best in the third and fourth interspaces does not occur in patients with tetralogy. With mild stenosis of the pulmonic valve, an ejection click may be heard just before the murmur. A pulmonic murmur may be absent in some infants who have severe, isolated pulmonic stenosis.

When a murmur occurs with *coarctation of the aorta,* it is usually a soft or moderately loud systolic or, rarely, continuous murmur, especially prominent at the base in the left infraclavicular area and transmitted to the left interscapular area. In a few patients, it is more prominent posteriorly than precordially.

Moss, A.J.: The "incidental" systolic murmur. *Pediatrics* 45:687, 1970.

## DIASTOLIC MURMURS

*Mitral stenosis* is characterized by a soft to loud, harsh, rumbling, though occasionally blowing, low-pitched mid-diastolic or crescendo presystolic murmur. The latter may terminate in an accentuated and snapping first sound. Not widely transmitted, the murmur is heard best with the bell type of stethoscope in a limited area just medial to and above the apex, after exercise and with the patient in the left lateral recumbent position. The patient should be asked to hold his breath in moderate expiration. The murmur of mitral stenosis usually does not appear for a number of years. During active rheumatic carditis a brief, blowing apical murmur may be audible in proto- or mid-diastole. This murmur, which is probably related to myocardial disease and cardiac dilatation, disappears as the rheumatic process becomes quiescent.

*Aortic insufficiency* is characterized by a soft to loud, high-pitched, blowing, decrescendo diastolic murmur, usually maximal along the left sternal border in the second and third interspaces and heard best with the diaphragm of the stethoscope firmly applied. This murmur, which is usually not transmitted to the apex, becomes most prominent when the patient leans slightly forward and holds his breath in expiration. The Austin Flint murmur, a presystolic or protodiastolic apical murmur, may accompany that of aortic insufficiency.

Diastolic murmurs may also be heard in some patients with atrial or ventricular septal defects, Eisenmenger's syndrome, patent ductus arteriosus, pulmonary hypertension and cardiomegaly.

## CONTINUOUS MURMUR

Diagnosis of a *patent ductus arteriosus* can be made on the basis of the physical examination alone in almost every instance. The murmur of a patent ductus is present in the second and third left interspaces and transmitted to the precordium, the vessels of the neck, the left axilla and the interscapular area, especially on the left. Since the systolic component is more widely transmitted than the diastolic, the double murmur is not heard in all areas. Characteristically harsh, rumbling, rasping, humming or sounding like machinery in type, the murmur is usually continuous throughout the heart cycle, loudest during systole and softest in mid- or late diastole. A systolic thrill is usually palpable. A continuous murmur may be present in new-born infants in association with prematurity and the respiratory distress syndrome. In other infants, no murmur or only the systolic component is noted at this time. Before one year of age, absence of the diastolic component does not rule out a patent ductus. An apical systolic murmur may also occur. Rarely, there may be no murmur. In a small number of patients with a patent ductus only a systolic component is present, even after the age of three or four years. This has been noted in patients with either an extremely small shunt or an extremely large ductus with a high pulmonary artery pressure. Patients with extremely large shunts sometimes have a diastolic murmur in the mitral area and a systolic murmur in the aortic area in addition to the classic continuous murmur. The sudden onset of a continuous precordial murmur, maximal on the right, is observed with a ruptured congenital aneurysm of the sinuses of Valsalva. Chest pain, dyspnea and a widened pulse pressure are accompanying features. High interventricular septal defects may be difficult to differentiate from a patent ductus. Some of these patients also have an atrioventricular conduction defect and a low diastolic pressure. Patent ductus arteriosus may occur as an isolated defect or be accompanied by other congenital lesions such as ventricular septal defect or coarctation of the aorta.

A continuous murmur may be heard over a *pulmonary arteriovenous fistula*.

## GENERAL REFERENCES

Castle, R.F. and Craige, E.: Auscultation of the heart in infants and children. *Pediatrics 26*:511, 1960.
Moss, A.J., Adams, F.H. and Emmanouilides, G.C. (eds.): *Heart Disease in Infants and Adolescents.* 2nd ed. Baltimore, The Williams and Wilkins Co., 1977.
Nadas, A.S. and Fyler, D.C.: *Pediatric Cardiology.* 3rd ed. Philadelphia, W. B. Saunders Co., 1972.

CHAPTER 18

# BLOOD PRESSURE

All children three years of age and above should have an annual determination of blood pressure. The room should be quiet for this procedure and, except for infants, the blood pressure should be taken with the child sitting and the manometer at the examiner's eye level.

Figures 18–1 and 18–2 give the percentiles of blood pressure measurements for children over the age of two years.

## DETERMINATION

The use of a proper-sized cuff is important in the determination of the blood pressure in children, especially in the obese child. The greater the length of the arm, the wider the blood pressure cuff should be. An appropriately sized cuff usually

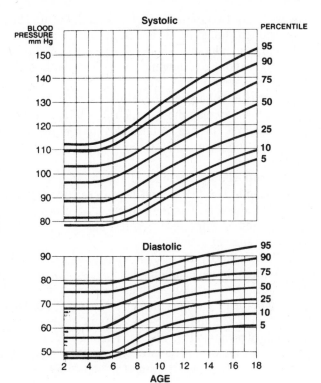

**Figure 18–1** Percentiles of blood pressure measurements in boys (right arm, seated). From the Report of the Task Force on Blood Pressure Control in Children. Prepared by the National Heart, Lung and Blood Institute's Task Force. *Pediatrics 59*: 797, 1977.

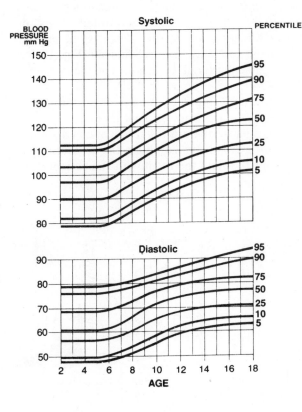

**Figure 18–2** Percentile of blood pressure measurements in girls (right arm, seated). From the Report of the Task Force on Blood Pressure Control in Children. Prepared by the National Heart, Lung and Blood Institute's Task Force. *Pediatrics 59*: 797, 1977.

covers about two thirds of a child's upper arm. The largest size cuff that will fit the arm or thigh should be used without overlying the antecubital or popliteal fossae. In addition, the inflatable bladder within the cuff should completely and snugly encircle the arm without overlapping itself. The stethoscope diaphragm should be applied lightly over the brachial artery. While a 2.5-cm. cuff is available for newborn infants and infants under 1 year of age, the 5-cm. cuff is often to be preferred. For children under 8 years of age, the 9-cm. cuff for children may be used and a 12.5-cm. cuff for children above this age. A false elevation of the blood pressure reading is obtained if the cuff is too narrow. With too wide a cuff, the blood pressure reading obtained is too low.

The cuff should be inflated rapidly but deflated slowly at the rate of 2 to 3 mm./second. The first sound heard (Korotkoff Phase I) signifies the systolic pressure. The diastolic reading represents the point at which the sounds become low-pitched and muffled (Korotkoff Phase IV). The fifth phase is characterized by disappearance of sound.

The auscultatory method of determining the blood pressure is used in older infants and children. In small infants the palpatory, flush or Doppler method must usually be used since the Korotkoff sounds are almost inaudible on auscultation. If the baby is given a bottle or pacifier, one may, however, be able to use the auscultatory method. In the flush method a 2.5-cm. cuff is wrapped around the ankle or wrist in the customary manner (Fig. 18–3A). The infant may be given a bottle or a pacifier so that he does not cry during the procedure. Before the cuff is inflated, rubber sheeting or a rubber glove is wrapped around the foot or hand, beginning at the distal portion of the extremity and proceeding proximally toward the cuff (Fig. 18–3B). The cuff is then inflated above the expected systolic pressure, and the rubber wrapping is removed (Fig. 18–3C). The pressure within the cuff is permitted to fall slowly, not faster than 6 to 7 mm. per second. Good lighting is necessary. The systolic pressure is that at which the blanched foot or hand suddenly becomes flushed (Fig. 18–3D). This value usually approximates the mean arterial pressure. The flush method usually requires two examiners.

The Doppler ultrasound method, now widely employed, permits the determination of both systolic and diastolic pressures in the newborn or older infant.

Whenever the blood pressure is elevated in one arm, determinations should be made in the other arm and in the lower extremities. To obtain the pressure in the lower extremities, a large cuff is wrapped around the thigh with the patient in the

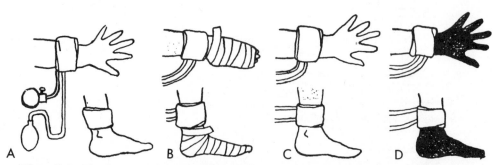

A    B    C    D

**Figure 18–3**   Blood pressure determination by the flush method. From Moss, A.J. et al.: An evaluation of the flush method for determining blood pressures in infants. *Pediatrics 20*:54, 1957.

prone position, and the sounds are noted over the popliteal artery. The diastolic pressure is about the same in both the upper and the lower extremities; however, the intra-arterial pressure in the lower extremities ranges from 10 to 40 mm. of mercury higher than that in the upper extremities.

Moss, A.J.: Indirect methods of blood pressure measurement. *Pediatr. Clin. N. Am. 25*:3, 1978.

In the term newborn, hypertension may be defined as systolic pressure over 90 mm. Hg and diastolic pressure over 60 mm. Hg. Similar values for the premature infant are 80 mm. and 45 mm. respectively.

When the blood pressure is unexpectedly elevated in older children and no related complaints or findings are present, the patient and the parents should be informed that the adolescent has a high normal blood pressure and asked to return for additional examinations to determine whether the elevation is transient, perhaps owing to anxiety, or is true and persistent. Borderline hypertension is frequent.

Julius, S.: Clinical and physiologic significance of borderline hypertension at youth. *Pediatr. Clin. N. Am. 25*:35, 1978.
Rames, L.K. et al.: Normal blood pressures and the evaluation of sustained blood pressure elevation in childhood: the Muscatine study. *Pediatrics 61*:245, 1978.

Elevation of the blood pressure above the 95th percentile on three separate occasions is abnormal. Once an elevation of the blood pressure is established, the following etiologic possibilities may be considered:

## ETIOLOGIC CLASSIFICATION OF HYPERTENSION

I. Renal
   A. Acute glomerulonephritis. Sudden elevation of the pressure over a few hours in these patients may cause hypertensive encephalopathy. Restlessness, irritability, vomiting, nausea, headache or visual disturbances are danger signs in the presence of a rising blood pressure. Acute poststreptococcal glomerulonephritis may present with hypertensive encephalopathy as its only clinical manifestation.

Hoyer, J.R., Michael, A.F., Fish, A.J. and Good, R.A.: Acute poststreptococcal glomerulonephritis presenting as hypertensive encephalopathy with minimal urinary abnormalities. *Pediatrics 39*:412, 1967.

   B. Congenital dysplastic kidney
   C. Hydronephrosis and obstructive uropathy
   D. Wilms' tumor may infrequently be associated with hypertension.
   E. Polycystic kidney
   F. Chronic pyelonephritis; chronic glomerulonephritis
   G. Henoch-Schönlein purpura with nephritis
   H. Acute renal failure
   I. Hemolytic-uremic syndrome
   J. Unilateral or bilateral stenosis of renal arteries; anomalous renal artery. Renal artery stenosis may be a cause of hypertension in patients with neurofibromatosis. Takayasu's arteritis may also cause hypertension.

Mena, E., Bookstein, J.J., Holt, J.F. and Fry, W.J.: Neurofibromatosis and renovascular hypertension in children. *Am. J. Roentgenol. Rad. Ther. Nuclear Med. 188*:39, 1973.
Wiggelinkhuizen, J. and Cremin, B.J.: Takayasu arteritis and renovascular hypertension in childhood. *Pediatrics 62*:209, 1978.

    K. Renal tubular acidosis with nephrocalcinosis
    L. Idiopathic hypercalcemia
    M. After renal transplantation
    N. Fabry's disease
    O. Familial nephritis
    P. Cystinosis

Leumann, E.P., Bauer, R.P., Slaton, P.E., Biglieri, E.G. and Holliday, M.A.: Renovascular hypertension in children. *Pediatrics 46*:362, 1970.

Robson, A.M.: Special diagnostic studies for the detection of renal and renovascular forms of hypertension. *Pediatr. Clin. N. Am. 25*:83, 1978.

II. Cerebral
    A. Increased intracranial pressure may cause an increase in blood pressure, bradycardia and abnormal respiration.
    B. Diencephalic disorders, hypothalamic tumors
    C. Pontine tumors
    D. Encephalitis
    E. Guillain-Barré syndrome

Stapleton, F.B., Skoglund, R.R. and Daggett, R.B.: Hypertension associated with the Guillain Barré syndrome. *Pediatrics 62*:588, 1978.

    F. Anxiety

Eden, O.B., Sills, J.A. and Brown, J.K.: Hypertension in acute neurological diseases of childhood. *Dev. Med. Child Neurol. 19*:437, 1977.

III. Cardiovascular
    A. Coarctation of the aorta. If the systolic pressure determined in the upper extremities is high and that in the lower extremities is low, coarctation of the aorta probably exists. When the coarctation is proximal to the point of origin of the left subclavian artery or when an atresia of the proximal portion of the left subclavian artery is present, a difference of 30 or 40 mm. of pressure may be found in the blood pressure readings between the two upper extremities, that in the left arm being lower than the right. The blood pressure values in the upper extremities are the converse if there is stenosis of the right subclavian artery or an anomalous right subclavian artery that originates from a left aortic arch distal to the coarctation. Differences in pressure in the two arms may also be present when the coarctation is distal to the origin of the left subclavian artery. In those instances in which the coarctation is not severe or there is an accompanying subaortic or aortic stenosis, the blood pressure in the upper extremities may be only slightly elevated while that in the lower extremities is relatively decreased. The *mesenteric arteritis syndrome* occurs in an occasional patient, predominantly males, on the third postoperative day following surgical repair of a coarctation of the aorta. Symptoms and signs include hypertension, abdominal pain, abdominal tenderness, vomiting, intestinal hemorrhage, fever and leukocytosis.

Ho, E.C.K. and Moss, A.J.: The syndrome of "mesenteric arteritis" following surgical repair of aortic coarctation. *Pediatrics 49*:40, 1972.

    B. Periarteritis nodosa
    C. Lupus erythematosus
    D. Takayasu's arteritis

IV. Hormonal
  A. Pheochromocytoma
  B. Cushing's syndrome
  C. Neuroblastoma
  D. Primary aldosteronism
  E. Adrenal virilizing tumors
  F. Occasionally, children with 11–beta–hydroxylase or 17–hydroxylase deficiency associated with congenital adrenal hyperplasia have hypertension.
  G. Turner's syndrome when accompanied by coarctation of the aorta
  H. Hyperthyroidism (systolic only)
  I. Corticosteroid administration
V. Miscellaneous
  A. Psychologic factors may produce transient elevation of the blood pressure.
  B. Familial dysautonomia may be characterized by a transient elevation of the blood pressure. Postural hypotension is also a frequent finding. A fall in systolic and diastolic pressures of 10 to 60 mm. of mercury may occur over several minutes with a change from the supine to the erect position.
  C. Vitamin D poisoning
  D. Burns. About 30 per cent of children with burns are hypertensive and some of them have convulsions.
  E. Lead poisoning
  F. Porphyria during acute attacks
  G. Oral contraceptives
  H. Idiopathic, primary or essential hypertension

A *diminution of the blood pressure* may occur in patients with pericardial effusion, Addison's disease and hypothyroidism. The systolic pressure may be decreased to between 60 and 80 mm. of mercury with severe cardiac failure. The onset of a narrow pulse pressure is a serious sign in pericarditis with effusion. The pulse pressure may be low in chronic constrictive pericarditis, shock or severe aortic stenosis. An increase in the pulse pressure may occur with a patent ductus arteriosus, aortic insufficiency, hyperthyroidism, ruptured congenital aneurysm of the sinuses of Valsalva, complete heart block, peripheral arteriovenous fistula, anemia and fever. With a small patent ductus, the diastolic pressure may not be decreased; however, if the fistula is large, the diastolic pressure may fall to 50 or 40 mm. of mercury.

## GENERAL REFERENCES

Adelman, R.D.: Neonatal hypertension. *Pediatr. Clin. N. Am. 25*:99, 1978.
Gill, D.G., Medes de Costa, B. and Cameron, J.S.: Analysis of 100 children with severe and persistent hypertension. *Arch. Dis. Child. 51*:951, 1976.
Loggie, J.M.H.: Hypertension in children and adolescents. *Hosp. Pract. 10*:81(June) 1975.
Loggie, J.M.H., New, M.I. and Robson, A.M.: Hypertension in the pediatric patient: a reappraisal, *J. Pediatr. 94*:685, 1979.
Londe, S.: Causes of hypertension in the young. *Pediatr. Clin. N. Am. 25*:55, 1978.
Report of the Task Force on Blood Pressure Control in Children. Prepared by the National Heart, Lung, and Blood Institute's Task Force on Blood Pressure Control in Children. *Pediatrics 59*:797, 1977.

# CHAPTER 19

# THE ABDOMEN

## EXAMINATION

Abdominal examination in infants and children requires patience. The tendency of the infant and young child to be apprehensive or to cry may make an adequate examination difficult or impossible. The approach to the child with an acute abdominal problem must be especially well considered, since accurate diagnostic appraisal is possible only with the child's cooperation. It is often well to have the child undressed by his mother so that the physician need not chance resistance in uncovering the child. Also, the examination may begin with the child on his mother's lap. With the child who is especially apprehensive it is usually well to leave the otoscope and other diagnostic instruments out of sight until the abdominal examination has been completed. Time may also be allowed for mutual inspection, perhaps at some distance. The amount required varies considerably with different children. Once the physician has been accepted, however, valid physical findings can be elicited within a relatively short time.

When an immediate and exacting examination is essential for diagnosis and therapy and cooperation cannot be obtained, the rectal administration of a rapidly acting barbiturate provides sufficient relaxation for examination. The rectal dose of Seconal is 6.4 mg. or 0.1 grain per pound of body weight up to a maximum of 200 mg. or 3 grains. This is mixed with 8 ml. of water and administered rectally through a catheter with an attached funnel. After administration of the sedative, the buttocks are taped together with a strip of 1-inch tape to prevent escape of the medication. In the presence of an upper respiratory tract infection or anemia this dose should be reduced by one half.

## INSPECTION

Inspection is of great value in the clinical assessment of the child with an acute abdominal complaint. In the presence of peritoneal irritation the child lies almost immobile on his back, and movement of the abdominal wall on inspiration is greatly restricted. Localized fullness in the right lower quadrant due to an appendiceal abscess may sometimes be noted on inspection.

Visible *peristaltic waves* usually indicate obstruction in the gastrointestinal tract, more commonly at the pylorus or in the duodenum. Gastric peristaltic waves, passing across the abdomen from left to right, are classically present with pyloric stenosis. Peristaltic waves and projectile vomiting may also occur with malrotation of the bowel, duodenal stenosis or atresia, duodenal ulcer, gastrointestinal allergy, urinary tract infection and adrenal insufficiency.

The *superficial abdominal veins,* normally prominent in infancy, become increasingly conspicuous with abdominal distention. Normally the venous flow is downward in the veins below the umbilicus. With obstruction of the inferior vena

124

cava, dilatation of the abdominal veins and reversal of venous flow may occur. The direction of venous flow may be determined by stripping the vein: first placing one's index fingers together and then pushing in opposite directions along the vein. Filling of the vein from below should not occur when the pressure exerted by the lowermost finger is released. Pushing one's index finger upward along the course of the vein does not empty the vessel if the venous flow is reversed since the vein continues to fill from below.

The abdomen normally bulges at the beginning of inspiration. In patients with chorea, retraction of the abdomen may occur at this time *(Czerny's sign)*.

A *scaphoid abdomen* in the newborn infant may imply a diaphragmatic hernia.

*Diaphragmatic flutter* may occur in clinical tetany.

## ABDOMINAL ENLARGEMENT

A prominent, "potbelly" contour is normal in infants and young children. Pathologic enlargement of the abdomen may be due to ascites, tympanites, enlargement of an organ, the presence of a neoplasm or cyst or an abnormality of the abdominal wall. Since the respiratory pattern of infants is chiefly abdominal, enlargement may be a serious problem in infants with pneumonia or atelectasis.

*Ascites* is accompanied by a tense abdominal wall, shifting dullness (unless the amount of fluid present is large) and a fluid wave. The mechanisms involved in ascites formation and the differential diagnosis are discussed on page 541. Chylous ascites is characterized by the collection of lymph within the peritoneal cavity. Paracentesis may be diagnostically helpful, especially if it reveals bile, blood, chyle or evidence of infection.

INTESTINAL OBSTRUCTION. High intestinal obstruction may lead to epigastric or right upper quadrant distention while that of the jejunum or ileum causes generalized distention.

*Intestinal patterning* may occur with intestinal obstruction or distention. Because of their thin abdominal wall, intestinal patterning is occasionally observed in normal premature and in some term infants. The rectus muscles may also be clearly outlined in these infants.

Other causes for *tympanites* include:

Peritonitis

Paralytic ileus

Chronic idiopathic intestinal *pseudo-obstruction syndrome* consists of symptoms of intermittent intestinal obstruction and abdominal distention due to a disturbance in intestinal motility.

Byrne, W.J. et al.: Chronic idiopathic intestinal pseudo-obstruction syndrome in children — clinical characteristics and prognosis. *J. Pediatr.* 90:585, 1977.

Pneumonia and other acute infectious diseases may be accompanied by paralytic ileus, especially in infants.

Celiac syndrome

Meconium ileus

Megacolon may be accompanied by gaseous distention.

Fecal impaction

Aerophagia may accompany crying, faulty feeding techniques and comatose states. Air swallowing is a habit in some children.

A tracheoesophageal fistula is frequently accompanied by abdominal distention due to forcing of air into the stomach and alimentary tract.

Pneumoperitoneum

Gastric perforation in the newborn

Interposition of the colon between the liver and the diaphragm (Chilaiditi's syndrome)

Hypopotassemia may cause abdominal distention, usually accompanied by hypotonia of the abdominal musculature.

Viral diarrhea in the newborn

Acute enteritis

Chronic ulcerative colitis, especially with toxic megacolon

Intestinal perforation

Hardy, J.D., Savage, T.R. and Shirodaria, C.: Intestinal perforation following exchange transfusion. *Am. J. Dis. Child. 124*:136, 1972.

Necrotizing enterocolitis in premature infants

Santulli, T.V. et al.: Acute necrotizing enterocolitis in infancy: a review of 64 cases. *Pediatrics 55*:376, 1975.

ENLARGEMENT OF AN ORGAN.    Occasionally a distended urinary bladder is mistaken for an abdominal tumor. With high intestinal obstruction, abdominal distention is chiefly present over the upper abdomen. Distention is more generalized with obstruction of the lower intestinal tract. Other causes of organ enlargement are:

Malrotation with or without midgut volvulus

Volvulus without rotation

Congenital peritoneal bands

Gastric dilatation

Hirschsprung's disease

Intussusception

Renal enlargement (e.g., hydronephrosis or congenital multicystic kidney with or without atresia of the ureteropelvic juncture accounts for one half of the abdominal masses in the newborn)

Hepatomegaly

Splenomegaly

Duplication of the bowel

Hydrops of the gallbladder may be associated with right-sided abdominal pain and tenderness. Vomiting and a right upper quadrant mass may be noted.

Chamberlain, J.W. and Hight, D.W.: Acute hydrops of the gallbladder in childhood. *Surgery 68*:899, 1970.

Hydrocolpos may cause a large mass in the lower abdomen.

Pregnancy

Adrenal hemorrhage in the newborn infant may cause a palpable mass in the region of the kidney.

Torsion of a fallopian tube and ovary may cause a freely movable, midabdominal mass in the newborn infant.

NEOPLASMS AND CYSTS.    Transillumination of the abdomen with a bright light in a dark room is a valuable technique in differentiation of solid and cystic masses. The transillumination that occurs in normal infants with abdominal distention is easily differentiated from that due to a large cyst.

Wilms' tumor

Neuroblastoma

Embryonal rhabdomyosarcoma

Lymphomas, including Hodgkin's disease

Ovarian cyst or tumor

Mesenteric cyst or tumor

Omental cyst

Choledochal cyst

Duplication of the bowel

Urachal cyst

Vitelline duct cyst

Retroperitoneal sarcoma

Retroperitoneal teratoma

Pancreatic pseudocyst should be considered as a diagnostic possibility in children with chronic abdominal pain, epigastric tenderness or fullness appearing after even minimal abdominal trauma.

Hepatic cyst or tumor

Dermoid cyst

Teratoma

Polycystic kidneys

A large hydronephrotic kidney may appear cystic and transilluminate well. Hydronephrosis is the most common abdominal tumor in patients under one year of age.

## THE ABDOMINAL WALL

The atonic musculature in patients with anemia, rickets, hypothyroidism or Down's syndrome may predispose to abdominal distention.

Umbilical hernia

Omphalocele, a defect of the umbilical ring covered by both peritoneum and amnion, is more likely to occur in premature infants, in the Beckwith-Wiedemann syndrome, in trisomy disorders and in association with other congenital gastrointestinal, genitourinary and cardiac anomalies.

Gastroschisis occurs as a defect lateral to the umbilicus with evisceration of the bowel and chemical peritonitis. Intestinal atresia occurs in 10 to 15 per cent of these patients.

Abscess of the abdominal wall.

Neoplasms of the abdominal wall — hemangioma, lipoma, teratoma, fibroma, desmoid tumors

Obesity

Edema and discoloration of the abdominal wall may occur with perforation of the stomach or peritonitis in the newborn.

With complete or partial *absence of the abdominal muscles* (prune belly syndrome) the abdominal wall is flabby, balloons out in the flanks and does not contract during crying. Skin creases may radiate laterally and downward from the umbilicus. Genitourinary tract anomalies, undescended testes, enlargement of the bladder, hydroureter and hydronephrosis are common associated findings.

Pagon, R.A., Smith, D.W. and Shepard, T.H.: Urethral obstruction malformation complex: a cause of abdominal muscle deficiency and the "prune belly". *J. Pediatr. 94*:900, 1979.

Williams, D.I. and Burkholder, G.V.: The prune belly syndrome. *J. Urol. 98*:244, 1967.

## HERNIAS AND HYDROCELES

UMBILICAL HERNIA. An umbilical hernia appears as a soft, bulging but easily reducible mass that becomes especially prominent during crying. A hernial ring is palpable around the abdominal defect. Umbilical hernias are most common in black infants, and in those with Down's syndrome, hypothyroidism, chondrodystrophy or Hurler's syndrome. Most umbilical hernias gradually close over a period of months. An abdominal neoplasm or organomegaly may cause an acquired umbilical hernia as a result of increased intra-abdominal pressure. Flattening or a slight protrusion of the umbilicus occurs with abdominal distention.

LINEA ALBA HERNIA may be characterized by abdominal pain and the finding, on light palpation with the finger tips along the linea alba in the region of the umbilicus, of a small, tender, fixed, subcutaneous nodule.

Bugenstein, R.H. and Phibbs, C.M., Jr.: Abdominal pain in children caused by linea alba hernias. *Pediatrics 56*:1073, 1975.

INGUINAL HERNIA. Congenital inguinal hernias may not be evident until the second or third month of life. The parent may first notice a bulge at the internal ring, along the inguinal canal or in the scrotum when the infant is crying, coughing or straining. This history is diagnostically important since the hernia may not be evident at the time of consultation and demonstration of a hernia sac may be difficult. Inspection for a hernia should be made with the patient in both the supine and erect positions. Hernias are usually readily reducible and slip back into the abdominal cavity rapidly with a swishing or gurgling sensation. In general, hernias do not transilluminate well unless the herniated loop is empty and distended. An expansible impulse on coughing or straining may be noted in older children. In children one does not invaginate the scrotum and palpate the external inguinal ring as in adults.

At times, an ovary along with a fallopian tube may be palpated in an inguinal hernia sac as a bean-sized movable nodule. Femoral or direct inguinal hernias may rarely be the cause of an inguinal mass. In the *testicular feminization syndrome* the external genitalia appear unambiguously female, but the uterus and fallopian tubes are absent. These children are often seen because of an inguinal hernia or a labial lump.

Children initially presenting with a left inguinal hernia have about a 50 per cent chance of developing a hernia on the right. Those with a right inguinal hernia usually do not develop one on the left. Bilateral hernias occur frequently in patients with exstrophy of the bladder. Unrecognized inguinal hernias may account, at times, for irritability in infancy. With incarceration, the mother is unable to reduce the hernia. The infant is fretful and in pain. Rapid breathing, abdominal distention and vomiting may occur. The herniated loop in the inguinal canal or scrotum may become firm and tender.

Fonkalsrud, E.W., deLorimier, A.A. and Clatworthy, H.W., Jr.: Femoral and direct inguinal hernias in infants and children. *JAMA 192*:597, 1965.

Kaplan, S.A., Snyder, W.A., Jr. and Little, S.: Inguinal hernias in females and the testicular feminization syndrome. *Am. J. Dis. Child. 117*:243, 1969.

SPIGELIAN HERNIAS may rarely occur in the anterior abdominal wall along the spigelian semilunar line, which extends from the eighth or ninth costal cartilage to the pubic tubercle. The usual finding is a mass in the lower abdominal wall that disappears on external pressure or reclining.

Graivier, L. and Alfieri, A.L.: Bilateral spigelian hernias in infancy. *Am. J. Surg. 120*:817, 1970.

HYDROCELES, which represent an accumulation of fluid in the tunica vaginalis, may be congenital or acquired, acute or chronic, unilateral or bilateral. Swelling may be limited to the cord or be present around both the cord and testis. The former represents a hydrocele of the cord while the latter is a hydrocele of the tunica vaginalis testis. Depending upon the presence or absence of a communication with the peritoneal cavity through an incompletely closed processus funicularis, the hydrocele may be communicating or noncommunicating or encysted.

A *hydrocele of the tunica vaginalis testis* appears as an elastic, fluctuating, smooth, occasionally tense and usually translucent scrotal swelling. The testis is displaced posteriorly and somewhat upward, and fluid in the hydrocele sac may make palpation of the testis difficult. The swelling in the communicating type can sometimes be reduced by pressure and may be less evident after sleep. This type of hydrocele, which occurs frequently at birth, usually resolves in a few weeks or months.

A *hydrocele of the cord* causes a small, elastic, translucent, usually irreducible, sausage-shaped swelling above the testis or within the inguinal canal. The testis is in its normal position and not displaced upward.

Acquired hydroceles are usually due to trauma or infection and epididymitis. The cause of the chronic hydrocele that may occur in older boys usually cannot be determined.

Differentiation between hydrocele and hernia may be difficult, and they may coexist. Unless the tunica vaginalis is considerably thickened, hydroceles usually transilluminate well. Although hernias may not, they may be translucent, especially in infants. Hernias are usually readily reducible with a swish, but hydroceles commonly are irreducible or reduce slowly. Except in the communicating type, the top of the scrotal swelling caused by a hydrocele can be palpated in contrast to that of a hernia.

Occasionally a *hydrocele of the canal of Nuck* may occur in a girl as a firm, cystic, nonmovable and nontranslucent swelling, 1 to 2 cm. in diameter, along the inguinal canal.

The finding of firm masses in the inguinal regions of patients with normal female genitalia should raise the possibility of *testicular feminization*. This disorder may require differentiation from the prolapse of normal ovaries into an inguinal hernia. The nuclear chromatin pattern may be diagnostically helpful.

## UMBILICUS

The umbilical cord normally is pearly white. Green or yellow staining suggests pathology. Mummification occurs during the first week, and the cord usually separates in the latter part of the first or early part of the second week. A moist, pink to bright red, small nubbin of friable granulation tissue with a grayish mucoid or mucopurulent discharge may then appear. This usually heals within a few days with scab formation and epithelization.

Normally the umbilical cord contains one large vein, usually centrally placed, and two smaller umbilical arteries. A number of anomalies have been associated with a *single umbilical artery*.

In infants with an *amniotic navel,* the thin, transparent amniotic membrane that covers the umbilical cord extends over the surrounding abdominal wall. If the defect is small, umbilical healing occurs without event, and a flat scar may remain.

*Omphalocele* is a rare anomaly in which the anterior abdominal wall around the umbilicus consists of amniotic membrane and peritoneum. This defect, 3 to 4 inches in diameter, may permit protrusion of the abdominal viscera covered only by the translucent or opaque amniotic membrane and peritoneum.

Ravitch, M.M.: Omphalocele. *Pediatr. Clin. N. Am. 51*:1383, 1971.

The *Beckwith-Wiedemann syndrome* consists of omphalocele or umbilical hernia, macroglossia, enlargement of the kidneys and liver, nevus flammeus over the forehead, ear lobe grooves and, at times, symptomatic hypoglycemia. Complications may include hemihypertrophy and intra-abdominal malignancies (e.g., adrenal cortical carcinoma, Wilms' tumor, hepatoblastoma and gonadoblastoma).

Cohen, M.M., Jr., Gorlin, R.J., Feingold, M. and ten Bensel, R.W.: The Beckwith–Wiedemann syndrome. *Am. J. Dis. Child. 122*:515, 1971.

In infants with a *cutis or skin navel* the skin of the abdominal wall extends up the cord for an inch or more, and a long, protruding stump remains after separation of the cord.

*Gastroschisis* is a paraumbilical full-thickness abdominal wall defect, usually a few centimeters in diameter and commonly to the right of the umbilicus, through which the herniated abdominal viscera, usually the small and large bowel, present as an adherent, dark purple mass covered by a thick, gelatinous or fibrinous material. A normal umbilicus and umbilical cord are present, and there is no covering membrane.

Children with *exstrophy of the bladder* have a flattened umbilicus without the usual depression.

*Diastasis recti,* or separation of the abdominal rectus muscles, occurs frequently in infants and small children, especially above the umbilicus. A bulge may occur in this area when the intra-abdominal pressure is raised by crying or defecation. Diastasis recti commonly accompanies exstrophy of the bladder.

A *patent omphalomesenteric duct* may open into the center of a moist and glistening, red umbilical polyp. Serous, mucoid or fecal discharge from the duct may excoriate the surrounding skin. Prolapse of the duct may occur when the infant strains or cries. Peristaltic movements in the walls of the duct have also been reported. A *vitelline cyst* in the intermediate part of the omphalomesenteric duct may present as an umbilical mass.

In infants with a *patent urachus,* urine may leak from the umbilicus, especially with pressure on the bladder. A *urachal cyst* may occur as a deep swelling in the midline between the umbilicus and the bladder. A *urachal rest* may be palpated as a cordlike structure that extends from the umbilicus to the bladder.

*Omphalitis* is characterized by a red, warm, moist, periumbilical inflammation and a foul, purulent discharge.

The *Cruveilhier-Baumgarten syndrome* is characterized by prominent collateral circulation around the umbilicus, a localized venous hum and thrill, portal hypertension and splenomegaly.

## AUSCULTATION

In patients with peritonitis the bowel sounds, which at first may be increased, later diminish and disappear. Bowel sounds are increased in the presence of hyperperistalsis, and tumultuous bowel sounds may be heard with diarrhea. With obstruction of the intestine the sounds at first are high-pitched and tinkling, but later they disappear. Bowel sounds are diminished or absent with paralytic ileus.

## PALPATION

Light palpation should generally be used in the abdominal examination of infants and children. The examiner's hand should be warm. With the hand flat on the abdominal wall, palpation is performed with the finger cushions rather than the tips. The examiner's fingernails should be trimmed. Flexion of the patient's knees and the placing of a pillow beneath his head may promote abdominal relaxation. Palpation is greatly facilitated if the child is distracted by conversation. It is usually best to perform the examination of the abdomen seated at the bedside rather than standing over the child. If the child is lying quietly on his parent's lap, it is often wise to begin the abdominal examination there rather than chance upsetting him.

In the presence of abdominal tenderness the nontender areas are palpated first, and the area of tenderness is approached *slowly* and *gently*. The child's facial expression is a sensitive indicator of tenderness and should be watched for wincing or other signs of distress. It is not necessary to ask the child whether it hurts; the examiner can tell by watching his face. With superficial and gentle palpation, voluntary muscle tenseness may gradually be overcome. The physician may also have the child palpate his own abdomen under the examiner's hand when there is a question of tenderness. The child will often palpate it much more vigorously than the physician!

*Tissue turgor,* or resiliency of the tissues, an important index of hydration and nutrition, may be determined by grasping and then releasing a fold of skin and subcutaneous tissue. The turgor may be rated as good, fair or poor.

**Palpation of Masses.** Position, size, surface configuration, consistency, tenderness and mobility may be noted in the palpation of abdominal masses. If an abdominal mass is suspected to be neoplastic, palpation should be performed only by the persons immediately concerned with management. Unnecessary palpation may cause dissemination of neoplastic cells. Palpation for intra-abdominal masses is always difficult in the presence of ascites. Ballottement of the mass may be attempted by quickly dipping one's finger tips into the abdomen in the hope that enough fluid is displaced to permit palpation.

In addition to palpation, other aids to the diagnosis of an abdominal mass include anteroposterior and lateral films of the abdomen with the patient supine and upright, an intravenous pyelogram through an ankle vein, an arteriogram, ultrasonography or CAT scan.

*Wilms' tumor* is a firm, smooth, but occasionally irregular abdominal mass. It is usually unilateral and, unless large, does not extend across the midline.

The abdominal *neuroblastoma* is firm but not as hard as a Wilms' tumor. The surface is finely nodular and irregular. Neuroblastomas frequently extend across the midline.

*Embryonal rhabdomyosarcoma,* the third most common malignant abdominal tumor in childhood, usually arises in the genitourinary tract and presents as a hard, immobile mass in the pelvis, bladder or vagina. It may also occur retroperitoneally or elsewhere in the abdomen.

The *choledochal cyst* (cystic dilatation of the common bile duct) may be palpable as an easily outlined or ill-defined mass in the right upper quadrant immediately below the liver. Since its cystic nature is often not apparent on palpation, differentiation from a localized enlargement of the liver may be difficult or impossible. Colicky, right upper quadrant abdominal pain, vomiting and intermittent obstructive jaundice may also occur, but the triad of pain, mass and jaundice is infrequent. In the young infant, obstructive jaundice may be the presenting symptom, with the patient often thought to have biliary atresia. Abdominal distention and hepatomegaly may be other presenting signs. Ultrasonography may be useful diagnostically.

Barlow, B. et al.: Choledochal cyst: a review of 19 cases. *J. Pediatr. 89:*934, 1976.

Localized abdominal tenderness and a mass in the right upper quadrant may occur with *cholecystitis. Hydrops of the gallbladder* causes a palpable right upper quadrant mass. Gallbladder hydrops may occur in Kawasaki disease.

Andrassy, R.J., Treadwell, T.A., Ratner, I.A. and Buckley, C.J.: Gallbladder disease in children and adolescents. *Am. J. Surg. 132:*19, 1976.

Magilavy, D.B., Speert, D.P., Silver, T.M. and Sullivan, D.B.: Mucocutaneous lymph node syndrome: report of two cases complicated by gallbladder hydrops and diagnosed by ultrasound. *Pediatrics 61:*699, 1978.

A *pseudocyst of the pancreas* may present as a tender, firm, globular, upper abdominal mass. Abdominal pain, anorexia and vomiting may be reported. Ascites may be present.

Stone, H.H. and Whitehurst, J.O.: Pseudocysts of the pancreas in children. *Am. J. Surg. 114:*448, 1967.

Large, hard *fecal masses* can often be palpated along the large bowel with chronic constipation. The masses may be large enough to suggest an intraabdominal neoplasm. Fecal retention in children with cystic fibrosis may cause a right lower quadrant abdominal mass and intestinal obstruction.

Snyder, W.H., Jr., Gwinn, J.L., Landing, B.H. and Asay, L.D.: Fecal retention in children with cystic fibrosis. Report with three cases. *Pediatrics 34:*72, 1964.

The *abdominal aorta* is palpable in many normal children.

An *anterior meningomyelocele* can sometimes be palpated through the abdominal wall.

A *duplication of the bowel* may occasionally be palpable as a movable, smooth, round, nontender mass.

In *superior mesenteric artery thrombosis,* the gangrenous proximal bowel may cause a palpable mass.

In *chronic ulcerative colitis* the ascending and sometimes the descending and sigmoid colons may be palpable as tender tubes.

The intestinal loops of newborn infants with *meconium ileus* are rubbery or hard and easily outlined on palpation. Palpable, hard fecal masses, 3 to 5 cm. in diameter, in the right lower quadrant may cause obstructive symptoms and abdominal pain *(meconium ileus equivalent).*

Mullins, F., Talamo, R. and Di Sant' Agnese, P.: Late intestinal complications of cystic fibrosis. *JAMA 192*:841, 1965.

A sausage-shaped tumor can be palpated, characteristically in the right or left upper quadrant, in about 85 per cent of infants and children who have an *intussusception.* At times, only an unusual fullness is noted, and a mass cannot be definitely outlined.

Palpation of a *pyloric tumor* is possible in 95 to 98 per cent of infants with *hypertrophic pyloric stenosis.* This finding is diagnostic. The tumor can best be felt immediately after the infant has vomited because of the relaxation of the abdominal wall occurring at that time. The examiner stands or sits on the infant's left side, places his hand on the infant's abdomen and palpates with his middle finger flexed at nearly a right angle. Usually the tumor is found, at times somewhat deep within the abdomen, between the edge of the rectus muscle and the costal margin on the right. Occasionally, it is present below this and, rarely, even underneath the costal margin. The pyloric tumor is usually moderately firm and olive-shaped and sized, although at times smaller and harder. Though usually readily palpable, the tumor may be elusive, so persistent or repeated examinations may be necessary.

A palpable pyloric mass may occur in some infants with duodenal obstruction due to malrotation of the intestine or to other causes. Such a mass appears and disappears, depending upon the pressure within the distended first portion of the duodenum.

Koop, C.E.: Abdominal mass in the newborn infant. *N. Engl. J. Med. 289*:569, 1973.

**Peritonitis.** Abdominal pain, tenderness and constant involuntary, boardlike rigidity or spasm of the abdominal wall and rebound tenderness is characteristic of peritonitis, at least in older children. Young infants may not demonstrate such rigidity. Abdominal distention, a doughy feeling, and tenderness occur in this age group, as may edema and a reddish-blue discoloration of the abdominal wall, flanks and genital region. Patients with peritoneal irritation do not thrash around but lie very still. The abdominal wall may have a doughy, inelastic feel in some patients with tuberculous peritonitis, but this finding is also present in dehydrated or malnourished patients. In fibrinous tuberculous peritonitis, irregular masses may be palpable. Localized erythema of the abdomen may occur with neonatal necrotizing enterocolitis.

*Bile ascites,* in its acute form referred to as *bile peritonitis,* may present as an acute surgical abdomen in young infants, with pain, distention and toxicity.

Hansen, R.C., Wasnich, R.D., DeVries, P.A. and Sunshine, P.: Bile ascites in infancy: diagnosis with $I^{131}$-rose bengal. *J. Pediatr. 84*:79, 1974.
McDougal, W.S., Izant, R.J. and Zollinger, R.M., Jr.: Primary peritonitis in infancy and childhood. *Ann. Surg. 181*:310, 1975.

**Appendicitis.** Abdominal tenderness, especially *localized or point tenderness,* is the finding of greatest diagnostic significance in children with acute appendicitis and almost always present. Before palpation the child may be asked to point to the "spot where it hurts the most." Young children, of course, cannot localize this very well, and they almost invariably point to the umbilicus. Since the appendix is relatively long and mobile, the point of maximal tenderness is often not localized at McBurney's point, even by an older child. Rather, it may be in the right upper quadrant, in the flank, near the inguinal canal or, rarely, even on the left side. Tenderness in the right flank may indicate an inflamed retrocecal appendix. Instead of localization to one point, the abdominal tenderness may be diffuse.

Abdominal rigidity, usually in the right lower quadrant, indicates that extension of the inflammatory process to the parietal peritoneum has occurred. Although often present when the patient is first seen, rigidity is not necessary for diagnosis, which optimally is made before much peritoneal involvement has occurred. Absence of abdominal rigidity or spasm may occur if the inflamed appendix is pelvic, retrocecal or surrounded by the omentum so that it does not contact the peritoneum. Infants often demonstrate no abdominal resistance.

Differentiation between voluntary and involuntary muscle spasm is important since many extra-abdominal disease processes are accompanied by the former. Such differentiation may, however, be difficult. The examiner's hand is gently placed on the abdominal wall and permitted to rest there for a time before gradually increasing the pressure. The patient should be distracted during this time. Spasm of the abdominal muscles due to extra-abdominal causes may diminish or disappear with this gentle but continued pressure while that due to peritonitis persists. The child may wince, shift position or try to push the examiner's hand away. Occasionally a young child is too irritable to permit an adequate abdominal examination. Rectal administration of a rapidly acting barbiturate may permit such appraisal without masking tenderness and involuntary muscle spasm.

*Rebound tenderness,* elicited by the sudden release of manual pressure on the abdominal wall, denotes peritoneal involvement. Besides being painful, this sign has limited reliability in the young child. Testing for it is best omitted.

When firm pressure is exerted along the descending colon, the patient with appendicitis may experience pain in the right lower quadrant *(Rovsing's sign).* This sign is of limited reliability in young children.

The child with appendicitis may walk with a limp and may lie with his right thigh flexed. When the psoas muscle is involved in the inflammatory process, hyperextension of the right leg, e.g., having the child drop his right leg off the bed, may be very painful *(psoas sign).* This finding may also be present with a perinephritic abscess. Flexion and internal rotation of the right thigh may also cause abdominal pain *(obturator sign).*

With rupture of the appendix, the abdomen may become soft and nontender, and the child may complain less of pain for an hour or two. The pulse rate, however, usually increases during this time, and extreme abdominal tenderness and boardlike rigidity soon appear. Localization and abscess formation may lead to a palpable abdominal mass.

Rowe, M.I.: Appendicitis in childhood. *Pediatrics 38*:1057, 1966.

Savrin, R.A. and Clatworthy, W., Jr.: Appendiceal rupture: a continuing diagnostic problem. *Pediatrics 63*:37, 1979.

Other disease processes characterized by abdominal pain, tenderness and muscle spasm include pleurisy, right lower lobe pneumonia, acute pyelonephritis, rheumatic fever, diabetic acidosis, torsion of an ovarian cyst, enteritis, ulcerative colitis, Crohn's disease, primary peritonitis, Meckel's diverticulitis and sickle cell anemia. Boardlike abdominal rigidity is also seen in tetanus and may be present with primary hypoparathyroidism and black widow spider poisoning.

The diagnosis of appendicitis is often difficult and may require repeated examinations over a few hours, especially when abdominal tenderness is minimal and rigidity absent.

Patients with Addison's disease or acute adrenal insufficiency may demonstrate pain and tenderness in the costovertebral angles. These complaints decrease as the patient improves.

Upper abdominal tenderness may occur in patients with *pancreatitis*. Gastroenteritis may be characterized by mild, generalized abdominal tenderness.

*Ileac adenitis* may cause constant lower abdominal pain. Physical findings include deep lower abdominal tenderness, a positive psoas sign and limp. Localized edema, induration and a palpable mass below and medial to the anterior superior spine may develop later.

*Acute salpingitis* is characterized by sudden bilateral lower abdominal pain accompanying menstruation and associated with a vaginal discharge, fever and chills. Palpation reveals bilateral lower abdominal tenderness. Right upper quadrant tenderness may also be noted if perihepatitis is also present.

## PERCUSSION

The abdomen is usually tympanitic on percussion, especially in patients with intestinal obstruction, aerophagia and ileus. Occasionally, a distended bladder may be detected by percussion. Shifting dullness may be noted in patients with ascites unless the presence of a large amount of fluid causes generalized dullness.

CHAPTER 20

# THE SPLEEN

## EXAMINATION

Palpation of the spleen may be performed from the patient's right by placing the examining hand flat on the abdomen and feeling for the edge of the spleen with the finger tips. By placing the left hand under the child's left flank and pressing up, the edge of the spleen may be felt to slip under the examiner's fingers on the abdomen as the patient breathes normally or inspires deeply. Another method is to stand on the patient's left, place the right hand flat on the lower left hemithorax and slip the fingers under the costal margin from above as the patient breathes deeply. In infants and children with apparent enlargement of the abdomen the edge of the spleen should first be sought below the level of the umbilicus; otherwise, one may palpate on top of the spleen and miss the edge. Palpation of the spleen may be facilitated by placing the patient on his right side. The tip may be just palpable on deep inspiration. An enlarged spleen seems to lie superficially, immediately under the abdominal wall. The splenic edge is firm, notched and usually sharp. Rarely, ptosis of the spleen ("floating" spleen) may need to be differentiated from splenomegaly. Scanning may be diagnostically helpful in patients with splenomegaly and hepatomegaly.

Rosenfield, N. and Treves, S.: Liver-spleen scanning in pediatrics. *Pediatrics 53*:692, 1974.

Congenital absence of the spleen may be accompanied by congenital heart disease and Howell-Jolly bodies in the peripheral blood.

Careful examination of the left upper quadrant is important after blunt trauma. In addition to the signs of shock, traumatic *rupture of the spleen* may be accompanied by tenderness and muscle spasm in the left upper quadrant. Pain may be reported in the left shoulder with pressure over the left upper quadrant. Palpation of the spleen in patients with infectious mononucleosis should be gentle since spontaneous rupture sometimes occurs. The finding of a ruptured spleen in a child under the age of three years suggests child abuse.

Upadhyaya, P. and Simpson, J.S.: Splenic trauma in children. *Surg. Gynecol. Obstet. 126*: 781, 1968.

**Splenomegaly.** Enlargement of the spleen is usually but one manifestation of a systemic disease. Hepatomegaly and other symptoms and signs are often also present. On the other hand, splenomegaly may be the only finding. The following is a partial list of diseases in which enlargement of the spleen may occur.

## ETIOLOGIC CLASSIFICATION OF SPLENOMEGALY

I. Infectious diseases
   A. Bacteremia
   B. Subacute bacterial endocarditis
   C. Salmonella infections, typhoid fever
   D. Abscess of the spleen
   E. Brucellosis
   F. Tuberculosis
   G. Syphilis
   H. Toxoplasmosis
   I. Histoplasmosis
   J. Malaria
   K. Infectious mononucleosis
   L. Q fever
   M. Leptospirosis
   N. Other severe infectious diseases
II. Blood diseases
   A. Hemolytic disease of the newborn
   B. Congenital hemolytic anemia

C. Acute acquired hemolytic anemia. Splenomegaly is not a constant finding.

D. Thalassemia

E. Sickle cell anemia. Fibrosis of the spleen gradually occurs in these patients, and the spleen becomes nonpalpable after about the age of six years. Acute enlargement may occur owing to splenic sequestration of erythrocytes accompanied by severe anemia and shock.

F. Other hemoglobinopathies, such as sickle cell–hemoglobin C disease or hemoglobin C disease

G. The spleen may be enlarged in children with iron deficiency anemia.

H. Thrombocytopenic purpura may be accompanied by splenomegaly.

III. Congestive splenomegaly–portal hypertension

A. Splenic vein thrombosis

B. Cavernous transformation of the portal vein

C. Hepatic cirrhosis

D. Hepatic fibrosis

E. Galactosemia

F. Chiari's disease — thrombosis of the hepatic vein

G. Congestive heart failure

H. Constrictive pericarditis

I. Cystic fibrosis

Voorhees, A.B., Jr. et al.: Portal hypertension in children: 98 cases. *Surgery* 58:540, 1965.

IV. Metabolic diseases

A. Gaucher's disease

B. Niemann-Pick disease

C. Sandhoff's disease

D. Histiocytosis X

E. Hyperlipoproteinemia

F. Letterer-Siwe disease

G. Familial hemophagocytic reticulosis

McClure, P.D., Strachan, P. and Saunders, E.F.: Hypofibrogenemia and thrombocytopenia in familial hemophagocytic reticulosis. *J. Pediatr.* 85:67, 1974.

H. Hemosiderosis

I. Hurler's syndrome

J. Amyloidosis

Strauss, R.G., Schubert, W.K. and McAdams, A.J.: Amyloidosis in childhood. *J. Pediatr.* 74:272, 1969.

K. Cystinosis

L. Porphyria

M. Wolman's disease is characterized by failure to thrive, vomiting, diarrhea, anemia and punctate calcification of the adrenals.

Crocker, A.C., Vawter, G.F., Neuhauser, E.B.D. and Rosowsky, A.: Wolman's disease: three new patients with a recently described lipidosis. *Pediatrics* 35:627, 1965.

N. Fucosidosis

O. Mannosidosis

P. Mucolipidoses

Q. $G_{M1}$ gangliosidosis type I (generalized gangliosidosis)

V. Neoplastic diseases
   A. Leukemia
   B. Lymphosarcoma
   C. Hodgkin's disease
VI. Cysts
VII. Miscellaneous
   A. Serum sickness
   B. Sarcoidosis
   C. Rheumatoid arthritis
   D. Lupus erythematosus
   E. Osteopetrosis
   F. Infant of a diabetic mother
   G. Porphyria erythropoietica
   H. Chronic active hepatitis

CHAPTER 21

# THE LIVER

## EXAMINATION

The methods described for palpation of the spleen may also be used on the right side in palpation of the liver. The liver edge is usually palpable in premature infants and may be found 1 to 3 cm. below the costal margin in term infants and young children. Riedel's lobe, a congenital hepatic anomaly, may be felt extending downward on the right. Except for its more medial location, an enlarged left lobe of the liver may be mistaken for an enlarged spleen. In patients with situs inversus the liver edge is palpable on the left. Absolute liver dullness is usually present on percussion below the sixth rib on the right anteriorly and about the level of the ninth rib posteriorly. Relative dullness is present for one or two interspaces above this. Apparent enlargement of the liver as detected by abdominal palpation should be confirmed by percussion of the upper and lower borders of hepatic dullness.

Table 21–1 lists the expected liver span of infants and children determined by percussion of the upper and lower borders in the midclavicular line with the child supine. Determination of liver size by abdominal palpation alone is unreliable. Younoszai and Mueller, who based their measurements on palpation rather than percussion of the lower border, found the mean liver span to increase from around 7 cm. at 5 years to about 9 cm. at 12 years, with a standard deviation of 1.0 to 1.3.

Lawson, E.E., Grand, R.J., Neff, R.K. and Cohen, L.F.: Clinical estimation of liver span in infants and children. *Am. J. Dis. Child. 132*:474, 1978.
Younoszai, M.K. and Mueller, S.: Clinical assessment of liver size in normal children. *Clin. Pediatr. 14*:378, 1975.

TABLE 21-1  EXPECTED LIVER SPAN OF INFANTS AND CHILDREN*

| Males | | | Females | | |
|---|---|---|---|---|---|
| Age, yr | Mean Estimated Liver Span | SEM | Age, yr | Mean Estimated Liver Span | SEM |
| 6 mo | 2.4 | 2.5 | 6 mo | 2.8 | 2.6 |
| 1 | 2.8 | 2.0 | 1 | 3.1 | 2.1 |
| 2 | 3.5 | 1.6 | 2 | 3.6 | 1.7 |
| 3 | 4.0 | 1.6 | 3 | 4.0 | 1.7 |
| 4 | 4.4 | 1.6 | 4 | 4.3 | 1.6 |
| 5 | 4.8 | 1.5 | 5 | 4.5 | 1.6 |
| 6 | 5.1 | 1.5 | 6 | 4.8 | 1.6 |
| 8 | 5.6 | 1.5 | 8 | 5.1 | 1.6 |
| 10 | 6.1 | 1.6 | 10 | 5.4 | 1.7 |
| 12 | 6.5 | 1.8 | 12 | 5.6 | 1.8 |
| 14 | 6.8 | 2.0 | 14 | 5.8 | 2.1 |
| 16 | 7.1 | 2.2 | 16 | 6.0 | 2.3 |
| 18 | 7.4 | 2.5 | 18 | 6.1 | 2.6 |
| 20 | 7.7 | 2.8 | 20 | 6.3 | 2.9 |

*From Lawson, E. E., Grand, R. J., Neff, R. K. and Cohen, L. F.: *Am. J. Dis. Child. 132*:475, 1978.

Systolic *pulsation* of the liver may occur with tricuspid insufficiency or with congestive failure. Presystolic hepatic pulsation may be caused by tricuspid stenosis, constrictive pericarditis and pulmonary stenosis.

*Hepatic tenderness* may occur with infectious hepatitis, infectious mononucleosis, leptospirosis, passive congestion secondary to cardiac failure, and liver abscess. Gonococcal perihepatitis, characterized by right upper quadrant tenderness, hepatomegaly and elevated SGPT, may be accompanied by gonococcal salpingitis.

Litt, I.F. and Cohen, M.I.: Perihepatitis associated with salpingitis in adolescents. *JAMA 240*:1253, 1978.

**Hepatomegaly** may be but one manifestation of a generalized disease process, often accompanied by splenomegaly. Rarely, apparent but not true hepatomegaly may be due to downward displacement of the liver secondary to thoracic deformity or pulmonary hyperinflation.

## ETIOLOGIC CLASSIFICATION OF HEPATOMEGALY

I. Infections
  A. Bacteremia
  B. Infectious hepatitis
  C. Infectious mononucleosis
  D. Syphilis
  E. Leptospirosis
  F. Histoplasmosis
  G. Brucellosis
  H. Toxoplasmosis
  I. Tuberculosis
  J. Ascariasis

K. Amebiasis or amebic abscess

L. Pyogenic abscess of the liver may cause fever, abdominal pain and hepatomegaly. Scintillation scanning is diagnostically useful with lesions larger than 2 cm.

Chusid, M.J.: Pyogenic hepatic abscess in infancy and childhood. *Pediatrics* 62:554, 1978.

M. Visceral larva migrans

N. Cytomegalic inclusion disease

O. Q fever

P. Reye's syndrome

Q. Gonococcal perihepatitis

II. Hemolytic anemias

A. Hemolytic disease of the newborn

B. Other hemolytic anemias

C. Sickle cell anemia

III. Passive congestion

A. Congestive cardiac failure. In the first year of life, liver size is important in assessing cardiac failure. Liver tenderness is uncommon.

B. Constrictive pericarditis. Hepatomegaly and ascites may be caused by constrictive pericarditis.

Idriss, F.S., Nikaidoh, H. and Muster, A.J.: Constrictive pericarditis simulating liver disease in children. *Arch. Surg.* 109:223, 1974.

C. Chiari's disease—thrombosis of the hepatic vein

D. Mulibrey nanism, secondary to constrictive pericarditis

IV. Metabolic diseases

A. Glycogenosis type I (glucose–6–phosphate deficiency). Hepatomegaly may be present at birth or appear soon thereafter. Other symptoms in early infancy include hypoglycemia, ketosis and lactic acidosis. Glycogenosis type III (debrancher enzyme deficiency) and glycogenosis type VI (phosphorylase deficiency) are also characterized by hepatomegaly.

B. Glycogenosis type IV is characterized by an enlarged, nodular liver, splenomegaly and cirrhosis.

C. Glycogenosis types IX, XI and XII present with hepatomegaly.

D. Galactosemia. Enlargement of the liver is usually present early in infancy.

E. Cystinosis. Hepatomegaly is a late manifestation.

F. $GM_1$ gangliosidosis type I (generalized gangliosidosis)

G. I cell disease

H. Niemann-Pick disease

I. Sandhoff's disease

J. Gaucher's disease

K. Lipogranulomatosis

L. Wolman's disease

M. Hyperlipoproteinemia

N. Hereditary tyrosinemia is characterized by failure to thrive, vomiting, diarrhea, rickets and cirrhosis.

O. Tangier disease is a familial disorder characterized by hepatosplenomegaly, tonsillar hypertrophy, lymphadenopathy, hypocholesterolemia and absence or almost complete absence of plasma alpha-lipoproteins.

P. Wilson's disease

Silverberg, M. and Gellis, S.S.: The liver in juvenile Wilson's disease. *Pediatrics 30*:402, 1962.

Q. Congenital porphyria
R. Hurler's and Hunter's syndromes; beta-glucuronidase deficiency
S. Hereditary fructose intolerance; fructose–1,6–diphosphatase deficiency
T. Methylmalonic acidemia
U. Lysosomal acid phosphatase deficiency
V. Ornithine transcarbamoylase deficiency
W. Argininosuccinicaciduria
X. Fucosidosis
Y. Mannosidosis
Z. Mucolipidoses
V. Obstruction to the biliary tract
VI. Neoplastic disease
    A. Hepatoma
    B. Hepatic cell carcinoma
    C. Infantile choriocarcinoma is characterized in young infants by hepatomegaly, anemia and hemorrhage in the form of hemoptysis, hematemesis, hematuria or melena. Chorionic gonadotropin concentration in the urine is elevated.

Witzleben, C.L. and Bruninga, G.: Infantile choriocarcinoma: a characteristic syndrome. *J. Pediatr. 73*:374, 1968.

    D. Hepatoblastoma or embryonal cell carcinoma
    E. Hemangioma, hemangioendothelioma. Multiple cutaneous hemangiomas, hepatomegaly and high-output cardiac failure due to arteriovenous shunts may occur. An epigastric systolic bruit may be present.

Gates, G.F., Miller, J.H. and Stanley, P.: Scintiangiography of hepatic masses in childhood. *JAMA 239*:2667, 1978.
Rocchini, A.P., Rosenthal, A., Issenberg, H.S. and Nadas, A.S.: Hepatic hemangioendothelioma: hemodynamic observations and treatment. *Pediatrics 57*:131, 1976.

    F. Leukemia
    G. Hodgkin's disease
    H. Metastatic neuroblastoma
VII. Cysts
    A. Congenital cysts
    B. Echinococcus cyst
    C. Traumatic cyst
    D. Inflammatory cyst

Johnston, P.W.: Congenital cysts of the liver in infancy and childhood. *Am. J. Surg. 116*: 184, 1968.

VIII. Miscellaneous diseases
    A. Congenital hepatic fibrosis. In addition to hepatosplenomegaly and polycystic kidneys, portal hypertension may develop.

McCarthy, L.J., Baggenstoss, A.H. and Logan, G.B.: Congenital hepatic fibrosis. *Gastroenterology 9*:27, 1965.

B. Fatty infiltration of the liver may occur in patients receiving cortisone therapy.
C. Fatty infiltration may occur secondary to malnutrition or poorly controlled diabetes.
D. Hepatic cirrhosis
E. Alpha–1–antitrypsin deficiency
F. Juvenile rheumatoid arthritis

Schaller, J., Beckwith, B. and Wedgwood, R.J.: Hepatic involvement in juvenile rheumatoid arthritis. *J. Pediatr.* 77:203, 1970.

G. Sarcoidosis
H. Subcapsular hematoma due to trauma may occur in the newborn or older child.
I. Lupus erythematosus
J. Infants born to diabetic mothers
K. Cerebrohepatorenal syndrome

Patton, R.G., Christie, D.L., Smith, D.W. and Beckwith, J.B.: Cerebro-hepato-renal syndrome of Zellweger. *Am. J. Dis. Child. 124:*840, 1972.

L. Chronic active hepatitis
M. Histiocytosis X; Letterer-Siwe disease, xanthomatosis
N. Familial hemophagocytic reticulosis
O. Cystic fibrosis of the pancreas
P. Vitamin A poisoning
Q. Poisons and toxins
R. Hemosiderosis
S. Amyloidosis
T. Osteopetrosis

CHAPTER 22

# THE KIDNEYS AND BLADDER

## EXAMINATION

Because of their relatively low position, the kidneys in premature and term infants may be felt on deep palpation. They are usually not palpable in older infants and children although occasionally a lower pole may be felt, especially on the right. To palpate for the left kidney, the examiner stands on the patient's left and presses anteriorly with his right hand in the posterior flank. The left hand, placed laterally to the rectus muscle and immediately below the thoracic cage, is used for abdominal palpation. When the patient takes a deep breath, an enlarged kidney may be felt to move between the examiner's hands. Ballottement may also be helpful in determining renal size. At the end of a deep inspiration the kidney is quickly pushed upward against the upper hand, which has been pressed deeply into the abdomen.

In newborn infants, abdominal muscular relaxation may be obtained by flexing the baby's knees on the abdomen, supporting the infant in a 45-degree upright posture with one hand under the occiput and cervical region and flexing the infant's head. The fingers of the examining hand support the flank posteriorly while the thumb palpates the abdomen.

Mims, L.C.: Palpation of the kidneys in the newborn. Letter to the editor. *Pediatrics* 47: 1097, 1971.

Museles, M., Gaudry, C.L., Jr. and Bason, W.M.: Renal anomalies in the newborn found by deep palpation. *Pediatrics* 47:97, 1971.

Perlman, M. and Williams, J.: Detection of renal anomalies by abdominal palpation in newborn infants. *Br. Med. J.* 2:347, 1976.

## RENAL ENLARGEMENT

*Hydronephrosis,* which causes an intermittent or constant cystic enlargement in the flanks, may be confused with a Wilms' tumor or other abdominal neoplasm. A large hydronephrotic kidney often transilluminates well, especially in infants and young children.

*Congenital polycystic disease of the kidneys* may occasionally account for renal enlargement in young infants. The lobulated and cystic nature of these organs may be apparent on careful palpation.

Gwinn, J.L. and Landing, B.H.: Cystic diseases of the kidneys in infants and children. *Radiol. Clin. N. Am.* 6:191, 1968.

*Wilms' tumor* is a primary consideration in the differential diagnosis of an intra-abdominal mass. When a Wilms' tumor is suspected, the work-up should be accomplished within a few hours. Usually unilateral, the Wilms' tumor has a hard consistency and a smooth or gently lobulated surface. It may range in diameter from a few inches to a mass that fills over half of the abdomen. Unless very large, it does not extend across the midline as frequently as an abdominal neuroblastoma. Differentiation from an enlarged liver or spleen should not be difficult since these organs do not extend far back into the flank.

A *perinephritic abscess* is characterized by tenderness and spasm in the costovertebral area and by systemic symptoms such as fever and chills. The patient splints his back when walking and lies with the thigh on the involved side flexed. Diffuse swelling, cutaneous inflammatory changes and fluctuation may occur in the flank.

Costovertebral tenderness after blunt abdominal trauma suggests renal damage.

Unilateral or bilateral *thrombosis of the renal vein* may occur in severely dehydrated infants with diarrhea or septicemia. Symptoms include sudden renal enlargement, shock, hematuria and oliguria or anuria.

Rarely, a *pelvic kidney* may be palpated as a pelvic mass.

*Megaloureters* can sometimes be palpated through the abdominal wall.

## BLADDER

*Distention* of the urinary bladder may be evident on inspection, percussion or palpation, especially during infancy and early childhood when the bladder is largely an intra-abdominal organ. A distended bladder may reach the umbilicus. Although a distended bladder may occasionally be confused with some other suprapubic mass, spontaneous voiding or catheterization quickly permits differentiation. A distended bladder is to be looked for in patients with meningitis, the Guillain-Barré syndrome and transverse myelitis; in patients who are comatose or stuporous; and postoperatively. Children with chronic bladder distention may dribble constantly or intermittently. *Investigation for posterior urethral valves or other partial urethral obstruction is indicated in these children.* When urethral obstruction is suspected, it may be well to observe the patient as he urinates for abnormality of the urinary stream.

*Neurogenic bladder dysfunction* may occur in myelodysplasia and the caudal regression syndrome. In addition to distention of the bladder, dribbling may occur either spontaneously or with external bladder compression.

Colodny, A.H.: Evaluation and management of infants and children with neurogenic bladders. *Radiol. Clin. N. Am. 15*:71, 1977.

*Exstrophy of the bladder* is characterized by absence of the anterior abdominal wall over the bladder area with complete or partial exposure of the bladder mucosa. The mucosa, which is bright red, moist and raised in irregular folds, may be hypersensitive to touch. The trigone is usually apparent, and urine may drip intermittently from the elevated ureteral orifices. Usually the testes are undescended, the penis is short and there is a complete epispadias. In girls, the clitoris and vulvar area are cleft and the uterine cervix exposed. Bilateral inguinal hernias are commonly present. The child has a waddling gait due to separation of the symphysis pubis.

*Exstrophy of the cloaca,* accompanied by an omphalocele, is characterized by a stoma or prolapsed terminal ileum over the opening of the colon.

Franken, E.A., Jr.: Anomalies of the anterior abdominal wall: classification and roentgenology. *Am. J. Roentgenol. Rad. Ther. Nucl. Med. 112*:58, 1971.

CHAPTER 23

# ANUS, RECTUM AND SACROCOCCYGEAL AREA

## CONGENITAL ANOMALIES

A careful inspection of the anus after birth is usually sufficient to determine its patency. Digital examination is not necessary if meconium stools are passed and signs of intestinal obstruction are absent.

The various types of *imperforate anus* are discussed in Chapter 31. Since anomalies of the urinary tract and vertebral column frequently occur in association with an imperforate anus or another anorectal anomaly, an intravenous pyelogram is indicated early. Rectovesical, rectourethral, rectoperineal or rectovaginal fistulas occur in over 50 per cent of these patients. Meconium or flatus may be passed from the urethra or vagina in the presence of rectal fistulas. The urine may contain meconium. A rectoperineal fistula in a baby with an imperforate anus has, at times, been confused with a normal anus.

The *VATER association* of anomalies consists of *V*ertebral defects, *A*nal atresia, *T–E* fistula with esophageal atresia, *R*adial and *R*enal dysplasia. Ventricular septal defects and single umbilical artery are other associated anomalies.

Quan, L. and Smith, D.W.: The VATER association. *J. Pediatr. 82*:104, 1973.

*Anorectal stenosis* may be palpable on rectal examination as a fibrous ring or diaphragm about ¾ to 1 inch above the anus. High-grade rectal stenosis that fails to respond to conservative dilatation therapy raises the question of a presacral teratoma, anterior sacral meningocele or bony anomaly as the underlying extrinsic cause.

Malangoni, M.A., Grosfeld, J.L., Ballantine, T.V.N. and Kleiman, M.: Congenital rectal stenosis: a sign of a presacral pathologic condition. *Pediatrics 62*:584, 1978.

*Anomalous anal papillae* may appear as small, smooth and rounded anal tags. Fissures at their base may cause severe pain on defecation and bright red blood in the stools.

## ACQUIRED LESIONS

*Rectal prolapse* appears as a bright red, tube-like protrusion of the rectum. There may be a history of bright red blood on the stools. Prolapse may occur in patients with constipation, chronic diarrhea, chronic ulcerative colitis, infravesicular urinary tract obstruction, pertussis, malnutrition, cord lesions, polyps and hypothyroidism. Prolapse of the rectum may be the initial complaint in some patients with cystic fibrosis.

*Acquired anorectal fistulas,* which usually open on the perineum near the anus, may develop from a recurring, exquisitely painful and deep perianal abscess. Perianal abscesses may occur in children with chronic ulcerative colitis and in infants with severe and prolonged diarrhea. Perirectal and perianal fistulas and abscesses occur frequently in regional enteritis and may precede, by months, the occurrence of diarrhea and abdominal pain. Perirectal abscesses may also occur in children with leukemia or immunodeficiency.

Ament, M.E. and Ochs, H.D., Gastrointestinal manifestations of chronic granulomatous disease. *N. Engl. J. Med. 288*:382, 1973.
Enberg, R.N., Cox, R.H. and Burry, V.F.: Perirectal abscess in children. *Am. J. Dis. Child. 128*:360, 1974.

*Anal fissures* or excoriations are an important cause for otherwise unexplained crying in infants. A careful examination for these lesions is indicated in infants who cry excessively. Bright red blood may also be present in the stools. A fissure near the mucocutaneous junction may not be seen unless the infant is in the knee-chest position, the buttocks are spread widely apart and a bright light is used. A well-lubricated anoscope or otoscope speculum may be used to visualize lesions not evident on external inspection. Constipation in the early months of life is a common cause of fissures and excoriations that may persist for months.

Occasionally, the external anal sphincter may not function well after surgical repair of an imperforate anus, resulting in *fecal incontinence*. Similar findings may occur in the caudal regression syndrome and myelodysplasia. Fecal incontinence occurs only when the somatic innervation of the external striated muscle anal sphincter is impaired.

> Gryboski, J.D., Spiro, H.M. and Gelfand, M.: Anal sphincter in fecal incontinence. *Pediatrics 41*:750, 1968.
> White, J.J. et al.: A physiologic rationale for the management of neurologic rectal incontinence in children. *Pediatrics 49*:888, 1972.

*Hemorrhoids* are extremely rare in children.

*Pruritus ani* may be due to poor perianal hygiene or to pinworms.

*Perianal cellulitis* due to group A streptococci is characterized by a marked erythema of the perianal tissues and a history of painful defecation.

> Amren, D.P., Anderson, A.S. and Wannamaker, L.W.: Perianal cellulitis association with group A streptococci. *Am. J. Dis. Child. 112*:546, 1966.

An *ischiorectal abscess* is characterized by local pain, swelling and warmth.

Ulcerating anorectal lesions may be seen with *leukemia*.

## DIGITAL EXAMINATION OF THE RECTUM

Digital examination of the rectum is not routine in the physical examination of infants and children but should be performed when it may provide necessary diagnostic information. When indicated, a rectal examination may often be substituted for a vaginal examination. If a child is old enough to understand, he should be told briefly and in words intelligible to him what the physician is going to do in this examination and why it is necessary. He should also be informed that he will experience some discomfort and perhaps pain. Unless the child remains cooperative, one cannot be certain about the finding of tenderness.

The child is placed or lies on his side, in the knee-chest position or on his back. The little finger may be used in infants and the index finger in older children. Using a well-lubricated finger cot or glove, the examining finger is introduced slowly and gently so that spasm of the sphincter may be overcome. If the child cries or complains of pain, one may have to pause a moment before attempting to palpate adjacent structures. At times a combined abdominal-rectal palpation may be informative.

In the absence of anorectal stenosis the little finger can be easily inserted into the rectum of newborn infants. In newborn female infants a relatively large uterus may be palpated. In young boys the flat and small prostate, about 1 cm. in diameter, is usually not palpable unless inflammatory changes have occurred.

Rectal examination in infants with Hirschsprung's disease reveals a normal sphincter, a well-formed anal canal and a small, empty or nearly empty rectal ampulla. In megacolon secondary to chronic constipation, rectal examination reveals a patulous anal sphincter, a short anal canal and a large amount of feces in the rectal ampulla.

In infants and children with a cord tumor, meningomyelocele or other cord anomaly, anal sphincter tone may be lacking, and the anus gapes or pouts open during crying. Fecal incontinence may be present. Perineal sensation may be absent.

A mass resembling the uterine cervix may be palpable on rectal examination in some patients who have an *intussusception*. Rarely, the mass may advance so as to protrude from the anus. Such protrusion can be differentiated from a rectal prolapse by inserting the examining finger between the presenting mass and the anal ring.

A *duplication of the rectum* may be palpable on digital examination. Occasionally a rectal polyp may also be detected in this manner.

Though *appendicitis* can often be diagnosed on the basis of abdominal findings and history alone, the finding of tenderness on the right on rectal examination may be helpful if the other signs are equivocal or the appendix is pelvic in position. An appendiceal abscess is often not evident on abdominal examination but may be palpable as a bogginess or as a tender mass anterior to and pressing on the rectum. A diffuse, boggy tenderness may be noted if generalized pelvic peritonitis has developed.

In girls with right-sided or left-sided pain due to torsion of an ovarian pedicle, rectal examination may reveal a small, firm mass on the right or left side. An ovarian tumor may also be palpated by rectal or a combined abdominal-rectal examination.

## SACROCOCCYGEAL AREA

A *postanal dimple* is not infrequently present in the sacrococcygeal area. Nevi, hemangiomas, cystic lymphangiomas, lipomas and tufts of hair are other cutaneous lesions in the sacrococcygeal area that may be accompanied by neurologic disorders and spinal cord defects.

A *pilonidal sinus* may also open in this area. Infection of an associated pilonidal cyst may be accompanied by inflammatory skin changes, perhaps with fluctuation and purulent drainage from the sinus tract.

Any mass that involves the sacrococcygeal area, the buttocks or the perineum in newborn infants is to be considered a *sacrococcygeal teratoma* until proved otherwise. The mass can be palpated rectally. It may range from a few centimeters in diameter to a mass almost half the size of the baby and may be hard or largely cystic in consistency. Dermoid cysts, anterior myelomeningoceles, lipomas, sarcomas and hemangiomas are other tumors that may occur in this region.

If the mass is completely cystic, differentiation from a meningocele may be difficult. A meningocele may be accompanied by neurologic abnormalities in the lower extremities and by roentgenographic evidence of a spina bifida. The meningocele may also become tense when the infant cries or strains with a bowel movement. Pressure applied to a meningocele may be transmitted to the fontanel. Similar transmission of pressure may occur when an anterior meningocele is palpated through the rectum.

Donnellan, W.A. and Swenson, O.: Benign and malignant sacrococcygeal teratomas. *Surgery 64*:834, 1968.
Lemire, R.J., Graham, C.B. and Beckwith, J.B.: Skin-covered sacrococcygeal masses in infants and children. *J. Pediatr. 79*:948, 1971.

# CHAPTER 24

# GENITALIA

Inspection of the genitalia is an important aspect of the examination of infants and children. In the newborn infant, such examination permits early detection of the genital anomalies that characterize patients with pseudohermaphroditism, congenital adrenocortical hyperplasia and other developmental defects. Additional discussion of normal and abnormal genital development is presented in Chapter 42.

## FEMALE GENITALIA

The examination of the female external genitalia is best conducted with the patient in the supine position and with the thighs flexed. In older girls, a rectal examination may give considerable information about the presence of a vaginal foreign body or other vaginal or pelvic pathology; however, because of the small size of the pelvic organs in children, it is often difficult to be sure about the normality of such structures when they are palpated through the rectum. In the young child, the adnexa are not palpable unless there is an abnormality. In the bimanual abdominal-rectal examination of the adolescent girl, one can palpate the cervix and uterus but not normal ovaries or tubes. The cervix may be palpated on rectal examination. In the sexually immature child, the small mass palpable in the midline is usually the uterine cervix rather than the fundus. The ratio of fundus to cervix increases from 1:3 in the infant to 1:1 at puberty to 3:1 in the mature female. A combined rectovaginal examination may be indicated when a foreign body is suspected. In this approach a blunt-nosed probe is inserted into the vagina as a sound for the foreign body while the little finger of the right hand is simultaneously introduced into the rectum as a guide for the instrument.

Since digital examination of the prepubertal vagina is not possible, a vaginoscopic examination is necessary for direct visualization and perhaps biopsy. A number of instruments may be used for inspection of the vagina and uterine cervix (e.g., the Huffman-Graves vaginoscope with a 1 × 11 cm. blade or a straight urethroscope [diameters of 24, 30 and 33 F and lengths of 8 and 12 cm.] with an obturator). Because it is painful, stretching of the hymenal ring should be avoided when the speculum is opened. The vulva is also sensitive so it is a good practice for the examiner to touch the thigh or lower abdomen before separating the labia majora. Because a cotton-tipped applicator causes discomfort, vaginal secretions for smear and culture should be obtained with a bacteriologic loop.

Gynecologic examination in girls should be performed by a physician who is especially skilled in this procedure. Children who are old enough to understand should be told the reasons for the examination and the nature of the procedure before its performance. Depending upon the child's preference, either her mother or a nurse should be present if the examination is done by a male physician. The examination should proceed slowly and gently.

Emans, S.J.H. and Goldstein, D.P.: *Pediatric and Adolescent Gynecology.* Boston, Little, Brown and Co., 1977.

The external genitalia are not fully developed in premature and in some term infant girls. The labia minora are relatively prominent and protrude between the labia majora as a red, taglike cuff around the hymen and vaginal orifice. The greater the immaturity of the infant, the more prominent is this protrusion. Normally the edges of the labia minora in premature and full-term newborn girls are darkly pigmented. Turgescence and swelling of the external genitalia may be present during the early neonatal period. The clitoris may also appear relatively prominent in the newborn girl and in leprechaunism. If it is abnormally large, the possibility of virilization is to be considered. Occasionally, an isolated congenital hypertrophy of the clitoris occurs. In girls with *congenital adrenocortical hyperplasia* varying degrees of masculinization of the external genitalia are noted (p. 388). Virilizing adrenal hyperplasia should be considered a diagnostic possibility in seriously ill infants with anomalies of the external genitalia.

*Adhesion of the labia minora* with occlusion of the vaginal orifice may occur in infant girls. The thin, semitransparent membrane between the labia is easily broken by a blunt probe or may rupture spontaneously.

During the first week or two of life, and especially on the second and third days, a *vaginal discharge* may be present between the labia in term infants. This discharge may be tenacious or thin, mucoid or glairy and grayish or milky. Occasionally it is blood-tinged.

*Nonspecific vaginitis* is not uncommon in young girls. The mother may report that a slight discharge stains the girl's underpants. There may also be some pruritus, frequency and dysuria. Predisposing factors include poor local hygiene and tight clothing. Often no particular cause is evident. Culture reveals mixed bacterial flora.

In patients with *bacterial vulvovaginitis* the discharge is profuse and causes secondary inflammatory changes involving the vulva. The etiologic agent may be the pneumococcus or streptococcus. Gonococcal or Shigella flexneri vaginitis is characterized by reddening of the vulva and genital mucosa along with a thick, yellow, creamy discharge. Cultures should be obtained of all purulent vaginal discharges. While gonorrhea may cause dysuria or a vaginal discharge in girls, it is frequently asymptomatic and diagnosable only by culture.

In *acute salpingitis,* a purulent vaginal discharge is present and genital movement of the cervix causes pain.

Primary *herpetic vulvovaginitis* due to herpes type II is characterized by vesicular lesions on the vulva, in the vagina and around the anus, which go on to ulceration. Vesicles may also be present on the surrounding skin. The lesions may be very painful. *Cytomegalovirus* may cause urethritis.

Vulvovaginitis may also be associated with pinworm, ascaris or whipworm infestation. Trichomonas may also cause vaginitis in infants and children. Monilial vaginitis may also occur in childhood.

Al-Salihi, F.L., Curran, J.P. and Wang, J-S.: Neonatal trichomonas vaginalis. *Pediatrics* 53:196, 1974.

Davis, T.C.: Chronic vulvovaginitis in children due to Shigella flexneri. *Pediatrics 56*:41, 1975.
Litt, I.F., Edberg, S.C. and Finberg, L.: Gonorrhea in children and adolescents: a current review. *J. Pediatr. 85*:595, 1974.
Nahmias, A. et al.: Genital infection with Herpesvirus hominis types 1 and 2 in children. *Pediatrics 42*:659, 1968.

A vaginal *foreign body* may account for an otherwise unexplained vaginal discharge, especially one that is sanguineous in character.

*Hydrocolpos,* caused by the retention of vaginal secretions in newborn girls due to an imperforate hymen, may present as a midline, lower abdominal mass or as a small, cystic and somewhat displaceable swelling between the labia. Spontaneous release of the retained secretions may occur or surgical drainage may be necessary.

*Hydrometrocolpos* may appear in newborn or young infants, causing a lower abdominal mass that may extend above the umbilicus and may lead to retention of urine. Often, hydrometrocolpos is caused by an atresia of the vagina or a transverse vaginal septum that may not be immediately obvious. *Hematocolpos,* due to retention of menstrual discharge in adolescent girls with an imperforate hymen, is characterized by lower abdominal pain and a suprapubic mass. The hymen may appear bluish and bulge. In the infant, a mass may protrude between the labia.

*Verrucae acuminatae* (condylomata acuminata) are filiform, papular and, at times, coalescing lesions in the perineal and genital areas, usually associated with poor hygiene. Moist, flat plaques (condyloma latum) occurring in the genital area may be due to syphilis.

*Sarcoma botryoides* arise from beneath the vaginal epithelium and appear at the vulva as moist, grape-like, fleshy masses. There may be a history of bleeding or hematuria. *Clear cell adenocarcinoma of the genital tract* has shown a sharply increased incidence in recent years in adolescent girls, partly as a result of prenatal intrauterine exposure to diethylstilbesterol. Presenting symptoms have been abnormal vaginal bleeding or discharge; however, in many instances, the patient had been asymptomatic, and the tumor is found in the pelvic examinations that such patients at risk should routinely receive.

Soyka, L.F.: Prenatal exposure to stilbestrol and adenocarcinoma of the female genital tract: the pediatrician's responsibility. *Pediatrics 55*:456, 1975.

Chickenpox lesions may occasionally occur on the genital mucous membranes. Genital ulcers on the vulva and vagina may be due to *Behçet's disease.*

Edema of the vulva may occur in Schönlein-Henoch purpura.

*Lichen sclerosis et atrophicus* is a rare disorder of the external genitalia in premenarchal girls in which the skin of the perineum and vulva appears atrophied, thin, white, wrinkled and excoriated. Moderate pruritus may be present.

*Prolapse of the urethra* in young girls is characterized by an abnormal protrusion around the urethra, pain on urination, hematuria and vaginal bleeding.

Klaus, H. and Stein, R.T.: Urethral prolapse in young girls. *Pediatrics 52*:645, 1973.

*Epispadias* in girls is characterized by a midline division of the mons and clitoris and a dorsal opening of the urethra.

## MALE GENITALIA

During early infancy, adhesions are usually present between the prepuce and glans of the penis. In many instances these adhesions prevent retraction of the prepuce so that the urethral meatus and glans cannot be uncovered. To help identify possible posterior urethral obstructions, well-baby appraisals should include a question about the force of the urinary stream in boys.

*Paraphimosis* occurs when the foreskin has been retracted behind the corona of the glans and cannot be slipped forward again. Swelling and discoloration of the glans develop rapidly.

Small, white epithelial pearls or inclusion cysts may be transiently present on the distal portion of the prepuce in the newborn boy.

*Balanitis* refers to an inflammation of the glans. *Posthitis* refers to an inflammation of the prepuce.

In boys with *epispadias* the urethral opening is on the dorsal surface of the penis. The types of epispadias depend upon the position of the urinary meatus: the balanitic type, which involves the glans; the penile form, in which a groove is present along the shaft and glans of the penis; and the penopubic type, in which the epispadias is complete and the urinary opening is present beneath the symphysis. The penis is variously malformed in these children. Urinary incontinence and separation of the pubic rami may also be present.

The urethral meatus opens on the ventral surface of the penis in *hypospadias*. Although the meatus in these patients usually occurs near the glans, it may be anywhere along the shaft of the penis or, rarely, in the perineum in association with a bifid scrotum. The various types include glandular or balanitic, penile, and penoscrotal, perineal or pseudovaginal. A hooded prepuce that covers the dorsal but not the ventral surface of the glans may occur, and the penis may be otherwise malformed or rudimentary. Cryptorchidism is a frequent finding. Pseudohermaphroditism is to be considered in infants with a small penis and a hypospadias. Hypospadias occurs in the Smith-Lemli-Opitz syndrome.

Congenital *stenosis of the urethral meatus* is occasionally noted.

Urethral meatal stenosis in males: Statement of the Urology Section of The American Academy of Pediatrics. *Pediatrics 61*:778, 1978.

Superficial *ulceration of the urethral meatus* occurs frequently in infant boys, especially those who have been circumcised. The meatus is reddened and inflamed. There is excoriation and ulceration of the surrounding glans. Frequently a serous crust may interfere with the passage of urine. Micturition is painful, and urinary retention results. Irritant diaper dermatitis is often contributory.

Ulcers of the penis and scrotum may be due to Behçet's disease.

*Torsion of the spermatic cord,* which may occur during the neonatal period or in later infancy and childhood, is a surgical emergency. Characteristically, there is swelling of the involved side of the scrotum and testis with severe testicular pain, tenderness and ipsilateral bluish or erythematous discoloration of the scrotum. Pain may be referred to the lower abdomen. The epididymis usually cannot be palpated. A shock-like state may be present.

In patients with *orchitis* the scrotum is swollen, painful and tender. The skin overlying the involved testicle may be reddened and shiny. Coxsackievirus or echovirus may be etiologic.

*Leukemic* infiltration of the testes may occur during complete bone marrow remission with recurrence of the disease restricted to this site. While there may be swelling or discomfort of the testes, the child may be asymptomatic.

Finklestein, J.Z., Dyment, P.G. and Hammond, G.D.: Leukemic infiltration of the testes during bone marrow remission. *Pediatrics 43*:1042, 1969.

*Epididymitis* is characterized by swelling of the scrotum and enlargement and tenderness of the epididymis. Dysuria and frequency may be present. The testes are usually not involved. In young boys, epididymitis may be the outward manifestation of a major urologic anomaly or disorder.

Amar, A.D. and Chabra, K.: Epididymitis in prepubertal boys. Presenting manifestation of vesicoureteral reflux. *JAMA 207*:2397, 1969.

*Torsion of the appendix testis* is characterized by the sudden onset of severe pain followed within hours by edema of the involved side of the scrotum. A small, extremely tender mass may be palpated between the testis and globus major of the epididymis.

Scrotal edema and acute, severe testicular pain and/or swelling may occur in boys with Schönlein-Henoch purpura.

Sahn, D.J. and Schwartz, A.D.: Schönlein-Henoch syndrome: observations on some atypical clinical presentations. *Pediatrics 49*:614, 1972.

During infancy the proximal portion of the scrotum is usually wider than the distal portion. After adolescence, the converse is true. The scrotum in some newborn infants is small and firm while in others it may be loose and pendulous.

In the premature infant the testes are in the inguinal canal, and few scrotal rugae are present. Normally the testes are in the scrotum at birth in term infants although frequently one or both testes are in the inguinal canal. This may occur in infants who have an active cremasteric reflex or in response to chilling or crying. Repeated, gentle examinations are indicated in determining the presence of undescended testes. Placing the child in a warm bath for a time may cause descent of the testes into the scrotum. The majority of *undescended testes* are of this migratory or retractile type in which spontaneous descent may be expected before or during adolescence.

Another method of differentiating pseudocryptorchidism and true cryptorchidism is to have the child sit on a straight-backed chair and flex his knees tightly against his chest so that his feet rest on the seat of the chair. The pressure thus exerted on the inguinal canal may cause a migratory testis to appear in the upper part of the scrotum. The examiner may also have the boy sit in the cross-legged tailor or catcher position so that an active cremasteric reflex is prevented from causing upward retraction of the testis.

Testes that cannot be palpated along the inguinal canal or in the scrotum may be either intra-abdominal or absent. Rarely, a testis may lie ectopically above and superficial to the external inguinal ring, in the femoral area, at the base of the penis or in the perineum. In children with cryptorchidism these areas should be palpated for a testis. An extrascrotal migratory testis can sometimes be brought down into the scrotum by gentle traction. If not, the testis may be considered anatomically fixed, perhaps by adhesions or bands. Unusual shortness of the spermatic cord, which may prevent full descent, usually undergoes spontaneous correction with adolescent growth of the cord. Extrascrotal testes that have been present in the scrotum at some time may be expected to redescend spontaneously.

Lattimer, J.K. Smith, A.M., Dougherty, L.J. and Beck, L.: The optimum time to operate for cryptorchidism. *Pediatrics 53*:96, 1974.

Buccal smears for nuclear chromatin pattern should be obtained in all patients with true cryptorchidism, since a phallic urethra and a normal-appearing scrotum and penis may occasionally occur in female pseudohermaphrodites.

Weldon, V.V., Blizzard, R.M. and Migeon, C.J.: Newborn girls misdiagnosed as bilaterally
    cryptorchid males. *N. Engl. J. Med. 274*:829, 1966.

An inguinal hernia is frequently present in patients with an incompletely descended testis.

Before the age of 11 years the testis is between 1.5 and 2.0 cm. in length. Little growth of the testis occurs before this time. Rapid growth of the testis begins at about 11 years and is accentuated between 12 and 16 years of age. By the end of the eighteenth year the length has increased to between 3.5 and 5.0 cm. This enlargement is almost entirely attributable to growth of the spermatic tubules.

The testes in boys with neurogenic or idiopathic isosexual precocity are abnormally enlarged for their chronologic age. This enlargement does not usually occur, however, in patients whose sexual precocity is due to adrenal cortical carcinoma or hyperplasia. The rare occurrence of aberrant cortical tissue in the testes is an exception to the latter generalization. These patients evidence stimulation of the Leydig cells, which add little to the growth in size of the testes, but no spermatogenesis. When sexual precocity is caused by a testicular tumor, the involved testis is abnormally enlarged, but the other testis remains normal for chronologic age. During adolescence the testes in boys with adrenocortical hyperplasia develop normally; however, testicular tumors have been reported in some of these adolescents. Precocious testicular enlargement may occur with hypothyroidism.

Laron, Z., Karp, M. and Dolberg, L.: Juvenile hypothyroidism with testicular enlargement.
    *Acta Paediatr. Scand. 59*:317, 1970.

The testes are small in *Klinefelter's syndrome*. They are also relatively small in patients with hypopituitarism, the size attained depending upon the level of gonadotropins.

*Testicular tumors* are rare in childhood; nevertheless, the possibility of a testicular malignancy must be considered when a generalized, firm, nonpainful enlargement of a testis is noted or a hard or cystic nodule is palpated within a testis. Careful examination for a testicular teratoma or an interstitial cell tumor is indicated in boys with isosexual precocity.

Infants who are *male pseudohermaphrodites* may have external genitalia that resemble those of a female. Anatomic features vary widely. In some instances these children resemble those with female pseudohermaphroditism due to congenital virilizing adrenal hyperplasia except that testes are present in the male pseudohermaphrodite. The scrotum may be cleft and resemble labia. Examination of infants with pseudohermaphroditism should include careful palpation of the inguinal region and labia or scrotum for testes.

Grumbach, M.M. and Van Wyk, J.J.: Disorders of sex differentiation. *In* Williams, R.H.
    (ed.): *Textbook of Endocrinology.* 5th ed. Philadelphia, W. B. Saunders, 1974, pp.
    423–501.

The size and state of development of the penis, scrotum and the prostate provide good clinical indications of the adequacy of androgen production. Growth of these structures commensurate with the patient's age is a reflection of normal androgenic activity. During adolescence the penis doubles in length and diameter. The prostate, which usually cannot be palpated during early life, may become palpable at puberty.

In *Tanner maturational stages* for genital development, *stage 1* is preadolescence. In *stage 2* the scrotum and testes enlarge, and the skin of the scrotum becomes reddened and altered in texture. With *stage 3* the penis enlarges, initially in length, and there is further growth of the testes and scrotum. *Stage 4* is characterized by further growth of the penis in width, increased darkening of the scrotum and continued growth of the scrotum and testes. Progress from stage 2 to stage 4 requires about 2 years as does development from stage 4 to 5. The adult genital size is referred to as *stage 5*. The maturation of pubic hair is described on page 383.

Early enlargement of the penis, prostate and scrotum occurs in boys with *congenital virilizing adrenocortical hyperplasia*. This may be noted at birth or may not appear until months or years later. The scrotum is darkly pigmented in infants with virilizing adrenal hyperplasia.

*Micropenis* refers to an obviously small penis that is more than two standard deviations below the mean length for the child's age. This finding may occur in patients with pituitary dwarfism.

> Guthrie, R.D., Smith, D.W. and Graham, C.B.: Testosterone treatment for micropenis during early childhood. *J. Pediatr. 83*:247, 1973.

Transitory erection of the penis occurs commonly during infancy. Priapism or persistent erection may be associated with local irritation, urethritis, urethral or bladder calculi, spinal cord lesions, leukemia, sickle cell anemia, thrombosis of the corpora cavernosa and Fabry's disease.

> Jaffe, N. and Kim, B.S.: Priapism in acute granulocytic leukemia. *Am. J. Dis. Child. 118*:619, 1969.


CHAPTER **25**

# NEUROMOTOR, SPEECH AND PSYCHOSOCIAL DEVELOPMENT IN THE FIRST THREE YEARS

Assessment and interpretation of behavior that reflects the neurologic, social, intellectual and emotional aspects of development is an important part of the history and physical examination and a necessary prelude to anticipatory guidance. Although the organization of such information, which comes from neurology, psychiatry, general pediatrics and the social sciences, into a clinically useful pattern or developmental map is no easy task, the description of *typical* or *expected behaviors* in a sequence that has at least an approximate time frame provides reliable guidelines for pediatric diagnosis.

---

This chapter was written by Dr. Sally Provence, Professor of Pediatrics, Child Study Center, Yale University.

In assessing the development of a young child it is useful to focus on two major kinds of questions: (1) What has the child achieved in the various sectors of development that can be observed, described or measured and how does his behavior compare with what is usually expected? and (2) How does he make use of the skills and functions available to him? The answer to this second question is useful in permitting inferences about the child's coping behavior and other adaptive functions.

This chapter presents an overview of the three-year-old child. Next, the developmental assessment of the newborn infant and the child from two months to three years is reviewed, including a discussion of motor, speech and psychosocial development.

## THE THREE-YEAR-OLD

The normally developing child of three is an experienced, competent and interesting person. He walks, runs and climbs with skill and pleasure. He speaks in complete sentences, using pronouns without confusion and generates new sentences that express his ideas, interests and feelings. He is strongly attached to his parents and a few other people, misses them when separated and usually wishes to please them. He is capable of playing alone briefly and able to show concern, empathy and cooperation as well as jealousy, anger and competitiveness with another child of his age. He feels shame and to some degree guilt, though he continues to need his parents (external controls) as the major regulators of his social behavior. He will usually have established sphincter control and in other ways will have made discernible progress in the long process of self-regulation of body functions and the assumption of responsibility for his own behavior. He has a developing sense of his personal and gender identities and some awareness of himself as a family member. Some of the ambivalence of attitudes and reactions to others and the contradictory behavior of the classical toddler have given way to behavior that conveys the impression of a more reasoning and reasonable person, more comfortable with himself and with others. But he is by no means bland. Rather he is venturesome, curious, energetic and self-motivated in much of his play. His capacity for symbolic thinking is demonstrated in his verbal performance and in his ability to play imaginatively.

## THE NEWBORN

The newborn comes into the world with a certain endowment, with potentials for development that are shared with other newborn infants but are also unique to him. Development proceeds as the maturational process unfolds and is in constant interaction with environmental forces. The determination of neurologic normality in the newborn is based upon observation of spontaneous behavior and response to certain stimuli. The clinical neurologic examinations described by Prechtl in 1977 and Beintema in 1964, and by Andre-Thomas and colleagues in 1960 are well standardized. Versions of them are incorporated into the pediatrician's examination of the newborn and older infant. An approach to neonatal assessment that promises to be more useful than the neurologic examination alone is systematically presented in Brazelton's Neonatal Behavior Assessment Scale, which includes a neurologic assessment. Brazelton's assessment takes into account the relevance of the infant's state for the findings and the importance of the examiner's technique in their interpretation. This examination includes observations of behavior and administration of specific stimuli through six states from deep sleep to fully awake crying.

Andre-Thomas, Chesni, C.Y. and Saint Anne Dargassies, S.: *Neurologic Examination of the Infant,* Little Club Clinics in Developmental Medicine, No. 1. London, National Spastics Society, with Heinemann Medical Books, Ltd., 1960.

Beintema, D.J.: A Neurologic Study of Newborn Infants. *Clinics in Developmental Medicine* Vol. 28. London, Spastics International Medical Publications, 1968.

Brazelton, T.B., Parker, W.B. and Zuckerman, B.: Importance of behavioral assessment of the neonate. *Curr. Probl. Pediatr. 7:*4 (Dec.), 1976.

Brazelton, T.B.: *Neonatal Behavioral Assessment Scale. Clinics in Developmental Medicine.* No. 50. London, Spastics International Medical Publications. Philadelphia, J. B. Lippincott Co.. 1973.

Prechtl, H. and Beintema, D.: *The Neurological Examination of the Full Term Newborn Infant.* Little Club Clinics in Developmental Medicine, No. 12. London, Heinemann Medical Books, Ltd., 1964.

Prechtl, H.: *The Neurological Examination of the Full Term Newborn, 2nd ed. Clinics in Developmental Medicine.* No. 63. London, Spastics International Medical Publications. Philadelphia, J. B. Lippincott Co., 1977.

Several other investigators in recent years (Escalona, Wolff, Anders) have pointed out that reactions to stimuli may vary markedly as the infant passes from one state to another; that is, variable states influence the behavioral response repertoire. This means that pediatric diagnosis regarding the nervous system of the infant, as well as other aspects of behavior, will have the greatest validity when the findings are interpreted in the context of state. Among the observations on the Brazelton Scale are the standard neonatal reflexes such as hand and plantar grasp, Babinski, automatic walking, Moro, placing, rooting and sucking responses and others. There are also scales for tonus, motor maturity and alertness. Other responses rate excitement, defensiveness, lability of states and self-quieting activities. Criteria for determining states and the motor activity and other responses usually associated with them are outlined. Although the general pediatric clinician may not wish to master the Brazelton Scale, which requires special training, it is important to recognize that an interpretation of the relevance of behavioral findings in the neonate, including their relevance for neurologic development, must take into account considerations such as these.

Anders, T.F.: State and rhythmic process. *J. Am. Acad. Child Psychiatry 17:*401, 1978.

Escalona, S.K.: The study of individual differences and the problem of state. *J. Acad. Child Psychiatry 1:*11, 1962.

Wolf, K.M.: Observations of individual tendencies in the first year of life. *Sixth Conference on Problems of Infancy and Childhood.* New York, Josiah Macy, Jr. Foundation. 1953.

## THE CHILD FROM TWO MONTHS TO THREE YEARS

*Motor* and *speech development* are the two areas most commonly noticed and described by parents. Both are relevant areas for pediatric diagnosis and are not difficult to check against established norms. These developmental landmarks are described in condensed form below and in Table 25–1.

TABLE 25-1 DEVELOPMENTAL CHARACTERISTICS AND LANDMARKS (0 to 36 MONTHS)

| Age (Months) | Body Mastery | Manipulative Skills and Eye-Hand Coordination | Play and Response to Objects | Language | Relation to Others and Emotions | Self-Awareness and Self-Help |
|---|---|---|---|---|---|---|
| 0 | Movements are mostly undirected | | | | | |
| 1 | Raises head slightly when lying on belly and looks around briefly | Hands partially open or fisted | Looks at object and follows with eyes | Makes small throaty noises | Looks at face of adult / Follows moving person with eyes / Smiles responsively to people (social smile) | |
| 2 | Holds head erect when held upright | Grasps voluntarily when toy is placed in hand | Holds toy (rattle) briefly | | Distinguishes "mother" from others; responds more to her | |
| 3 | | Clasps hands together | Shows interest in playthings; looks and begins to reach | Vocalizes in response to others (musical cooing) | | Gazes at own hand |
| 4 | Raises head high when lying on stomach / Rolls from front to back | Grasps object held near hand | Looks briefly for toy that disappears | Vocalizes spontaneously to self, to people and to toys | Makes social contact by smiling or vocalizing (i.e., actively initiates contact) | Plays with hands and clasps them together / Comforts self by sucking thumb or finding pacifier |
| 5 | Rolls from back to front / Holds trunk erect when supported in sitting position | Reaches out and grasps toy | Shows displeasure at loss of toy | | | Plays with own foot |
| 6 | Sits alone when placed | Transfers toy from one hand to the other | | | | |
| 7 | Holds two toys at once | | Uncovers toy hidden by cloth | Vocalizes da, ma, ba | Pushes away someone he does not want / Reacts to strangers with soberness or anxiety; / actively clings to or seeks familiar person when distressed | Discovers genitals |
| 8 | Pulls self into standing position | | | Understands meaning of no / Vocalizes dada, mama (nonspecific) | | Feeds self cookie or cracker |
| 9 | Creeps on hands and knees | Bangs two toys together | Explores toy with eyes and fingers (examines and pokes) | Says dada, mama, as names / Recognizes (looks or moves toward) familiar object when named | Plays social games with adult (peek-a-boo; pat-a-cake; so-big; bye-bye) | Can take bottle without help |

TABLE 25–1 DEVELOPMENTAL CHARACTERISTICS AND LANDMARKS (0 to 36 MONTHS) (Continued)

| Age (Months) | Body Mastery | Manipulative Skills and Eye-Hand Coordination | Play and Response to Objects | Language | Relation to Others and Emotions | Self-Awareness and Self-Help |
|---|---|---|---|---|---|---|
| 10 | Walks forward with two hands held | Grasps small object with index finger and thumb (pincer grasp) | Shows preference for one toy over another | Has at least one word besides mama and dada | Expresses several clearly recognizable emotions; (e.g., anger, anxiety, sadness, pleasure, affection, excitement) May object to separation from parent | |
| 11 | Walks holding to crib or furniture | Takes covers from boxes, etc. | | | Plays simple ball game (rolls ball to another) | |
| 12 | Walks a few steps alone | | Puts one object inside another | | | Cooperates in dressing (pushes arm into shirt, foot into shoe, etc.) |
| 13 | Climbs stairs on hands and knees | | Finds toy hidden by screen, furniture or door | Says three to six words besides mama and dada | | |
| 14 | Walks well alone; starts and stops with good control | Imitates scribbling with crayon | | | | |
| 15 | | | Likes to play with possessions of parents (pots and pans, hats, shoes, tools, cosmetics) | Vocalizes with elaborate jargon Indicates wants by pointing | Hugs parent | Partially feeds self with fingers and spoon |
| 18 | Throws ball Climbs into adult chair or on couch; seats self in small chair | Makes single imitative stroke with crayon on paper | Carries or hugs doll or teddy bear Explores cabinets and drawers | Has vocabulary of about ten words Identifies 1 or more parts of own body (eye, nose, etc.) Follows simple directions Names or identifies 1 or more pictures of common objects | Is often negativistic but is also loving; seeks affection Kisses with pucker | Identifies 1 or more parts of own body (eye, nose, mouth, etc.) |

## TABLE 25-1 DEVELOPMENTAL CHARACTERISTICS AND LANDMARKS (0 to 36 MONTHS) (Continued)

| | | | | | | |
|---|---|---|---|---|---|---|
| 21 | Squats in play and returns to standing position | Uses spoon well | | Combines two or three words spontaneously Uses words to make wants known | | Tries to put on clothing Handles cup well Uses spoon well |
| 24 | Runs with good co-ordination Walks up and down stairs; may hold rail | Executes circular stroke with crayon | Shows interest in play of others but has little ability to join Begins fantasy play; Takes care of doll or teddy, "goes to store," etc. | Has vocabulary of 20–50 words Uses three-word sentences Begins to use pronouns I, you, me | Imitates adult activities, (housekeeping, use of tools, etc.) Likes to please parents | Refers to self by name |
| 30 | Jumps from step or low chair to ground | Holds crayon with fingers, simulating adult grasp Imitates vertical, horizontal and circular strokes with crayon | Signs of pretending in play are clearly evident, especially with adult participation. Plays briefly with other children | Names or identifies 5–7 objects or pictures Speaks full sentences and uses pronouns correctly Identifies 6 or more body parts | "Helps" mother with housework and putting away Knows own family members very well and relates selectively to them | Takes pride in what he can do Refers to self by pronoun (me or I) Has partial or complete control of bladder and bowel movements Identifies 6 or more body parts |
| 36 | Rides tricycle using pedals | Handles small toys skillfully (blocks, beads, pegs, etc.) Copies circle from picture Imitates cross after demonstration(+) | Pretend play becomes more elaborate; uses miniature objects as well as life-size Understands taking turns | Tells use of objects (e.g., ball, key, pencil, etc.) | Gradually becomes less negativistic Begins to play with other children Has interest in sex differences | Puts on simple garment: cap, slippers Tells full name Knows own sex and that of others Feeds self well with little spilling |

Yale Child Study Center, New Haven, 1977.

## MOTOR DEVELOPMENT

The infant's *neuromotor development* proceeds so that he first gains control over the muscles that support his head and move his arms. By the age of two months his head is held erect and steady; by four to five months he rolls from supine to prone and back again; by five to six months he can hold his trunk erect when supported in the sitting position and sit alone briefly when placed. In regard to fine motor skills, by two months he has progressed from the reflex grasping of the first weeks to voluntary grasping when a toy is placed in his hand. Clasping hands together in the midline occurs by four months, and the ability to reach out to grasp a toy, first in a corralling movement with two hands and then with each hand independently, is achieved by five to six months. By this time he can easily get his thumb to his mouth and can touch all of the parts of his body at will. Between six and seven months his mastery of the large muscles results in his being able to get himself into a sitting position without help. Between eight and nine months he first crawls on his abdomen and then creeps on all fours with reciprocal, coordinated movements of the upper and lower extremities. By nine months of age most infants are able to pull to stand and soon thereafter begin to cruise around the furniture or the crib rail with a sidestepping gait. Walking forward with two hands held and walking without assistance are accomplished by many infants by 15 months and by others a month or so later.

In respect to manipulative skills and eye-hand coordination, there is an impressive increase in precision between six months and one year. The grasp matures from whole hand to finger grasping and from the ulnar to the radial side of the hand. At about eight to nine months the child uses a radial-digital grasp for picking up objects; by 11 to 12 months he can grasp even tiny objects between index finger and thumb in a pincer grasp of impressive precision. The coordination and integration of motor skills are evident in the child's ability to manipulate toys in the midline, to transfer them from one hand to another, to manipulate two at a time and combine them in a variety of ways.

Motor skills are also coordinated with development in the other areas. They are dependent not only on the integrity of the motor apparatus but also on the quantity and quality of the infant's experiences with his environment, especially with nurturing persons. Both deprivation and overstimulation can disrupt motor functioning. It is useful for the clinician to look both at the progressive acquisition of motor skills and at the use to which these are put by the child. Motility both expresses and serves the rapidly expanding mental life of the infant. Fluctuations in motor activity are often reliable indicators of feeling states (e.g., some infants become still and inactive when feeling upset or fearful while others become agitated and overactive).

Early in the second year the toddler walks well alone with a heel-toe gait, starting and stopping with good control. Between 15 and 18 months he is able to walk fast and to run a little. He has also become interested in climbing onto couches or large chairs and going up stairs on hands and knees. By the middle of the second year he will climb stairs in an upright position if someone holds his hand; by the end of the second year he can negotiate stairs without assistance. By the middle of the second year, too, he will have learned to throw a ball overhand from a standing position with fair accuracy. The one- to two-year-old child is noteworthy for his enormous pleasure in motor activity. When he first masters walking, the pure pleasure in mastery seems reason enough to stand upright and walk. Very soon, however, the mastery of walking becomes coordinated with other aspects of his development: he walks or runs in order to get to some attractive object, to go to his mother or father or to avoid something about which he is apprehensive or that he does not like. In the second year also he demonstrates his interest and versatility in the many ways he uses his manipulative skills. For example, he is able to remove the covers from boxes or bottles, to pile cubes or other objects, to play at filling and emptying games or losing and finding. He may be able to manage a spoon well enough by 20 to 21 months to feed himself partially. With a crayon early in the second year he does little more than imitate scribbling but by the end of the year his control increases, and he also reveals his progressive cognitive development in his ability to discern and imitate specific forms such as vertical, horizontal and circular strokes.

Between two and three years of age he further consolidates and extends his mastery of his body through such accomplishments as walking backward or on tiptoes and jumping from a step or chair. Before the age of three, children who have had an opportunity to do so have usually mastered tricycle riding using the pedals and steering competently. During this period, too, they are impressive in their ability to handle small toys such as blocks, beads or pegs and to hold a crayon with their fingers, simulating an adult type of grasping. The young child's motor skills, utilization and style of activity tell much about him: the integrity and the maturation of his neuromotor apparatus as well as many aspects of his experiences. In situations in which a neurologic problem is suspected, the behavioral observations described are an important supplement to the standard pediatric neurologic examination.

## SPEECH DEVELOPMENT

*Speech* is one of the more highly valued and conspicuous aspects of the child's development. It is also a sensitive indicator of normality and of adversity, whether organic or psychosocial. Though speech production is one of the more variable functions in normally developing children, it is nevertheless important to check it against the norms. The child's vocabulary, the length and structure of sentences, the presence or absence of pronouns, the ability to generate new sentences and the clarity of speech are all significant pediatric observations. The following are average findings.

The small throaty noises of the one-month-old and the musical cooing and responsive vocal socialization of the two- to three-month-old are followed by spontaneous vocalization in the four-month-old, who babbles to himself when alone, to other people and to his toys. His responsive and spontaneous vocalization is one of the major indicators of his interest in others. The differentiation of speech is such that by seven months he is able to vocalize vowel and consonant combinations such as da, ma, and ba and by eight months dada, mama, baba, though these verbalizations are not yet names. By 9 to 10 months he will use these sounds as names for the important persons and about a month later he will have at least one other word for some familiar object, person or action. At this time also he shows his understanding of the speech of others by recognizing the names of familiar persons or objects when named for him. At 13 to 14 months he will usually have three to six words besides the names of his parents and a little later he will be vocalizing with elaborate jargon. By 18 months his vocabulary will have increased to about 10 words, by 2 years to 20 to 50 and by 3 years more than one can easily count. The child's ability to speak becomes very serviceable during the second year, when he can say the names of things he wants. Two- to three-word phrases appear in the middle of the second year.

By age two he will speak in short sentences, perhaps three words or so, and will have begun to use pronouns such as I, you and me. By age two and one-half to three he can name many objects and answer questions about what they are for as well as commenting on many aspects of his immediate experience. By age three he speaks in complete sentences, using pronouns without confusion and generating new sentences that express his ideas, interests and feelings. The child's speech is also one of the important functions through which his intellectual development can be examined. As with other functions, it is relevant not only to take note of the child's ability to speak but also of how he utilizes speech in adapting to his daily life. Can he express his wants and protests? Can he ask and answer questions?

## PSYCHOSOCIAL DEVELOPMENT

The information to follow on psychosocial development is organized around the development and characteristics of the child's relationship with others. This choice is made not only because of the importance of these relationships for many aspects of the child's development but also because the pediatric diagnostician operates in a social context and most of the relevant findings are interactional: pediatrician and child, pediatrician and parent, parent and child.

From the moment of birth an infant interacts with people. He is born with a readiness for social contact. In the beginning, many of the contacts that meet his psychosocial needs take place at the same time his bodily needs are being met. One has only to observe to be impressed with the frequency and variety of interactions between an infant and those who take care of him. Since the infant's ability to express his needs is poorly differentiated in the earliest months the person who cares for the baby "reads" his changes in behavior and decides what to do for him. There is wide variation in the ability of parents to take cues from their babies and in styles of infant care within the norm. Eye contact between parent and infant occurs from the newborn period onward. The beginning of what some have called *reciprocity* and others have called *mutuality* is easily discernible during the first weeks of the baby's life (e.g., the infant moves or makes sounds to which the mother responds). Compared with later development, however, the baby's facial expression at first is vague and his eyes focus on the adult only briefly. If restless or crying, he may become quiet when spoken to or lifted. More specific reactions develop gradually. Some time during the second month the baby develops an unmistakable social smile; he adjusts his body when picked up and held; he visually follows a person across the room; and he vocalizes when spoken to. By the third or fourth month he responds with much smiling, musical cooing and increased body activity when someone smiles at, speaks to or touches him. He is likely to respond happily to everyone at this age, but usually most strongly to the primary caregiver. It appears that these stronger reactions are the first clear sign of his recognition of that person. By about the fourth month he is capable of a strong, definite show of displeasure when social contact is broken, and he may cry in protest when the adult moves out of sight or sound. While the human face is by far the most appealing stimulus, he gradually becomes attentive to and interested in other things as well. He recognizes and anticipates situations, especially those in which the adult does something with and for him. For example, he recognizes the breast or bottle and shows some eagerness when the feeding situation is being readied. At about the same age (around four months) he is usually able to wait a short time for feeding if he is watching the preparation. It appears that this is one of the first indicators of an important event in mental development, namely, an interaction of perception and memory that brings about an anticipation of the future: the infant is able to wait, for a short while, because he remembers from past experience that he is going to be fed and he looks forward to the forthcoming satisfaction. It is believed, too, that this behavior means that the baby is developing a sense of confidence that he is going to be cared for. This confidence (Benedek, 1959) or trust (Erikson, 1959) is built upon such experiences as being fed when hungry, being warmed when cold and being comforted by the adult in other ways. At first, the infant probably responds only to the total experience that is responsible for the comfort, but later, around four months, he shows signs of recognizing and responding specifically to the particular person who provides the comfort and pleasure. One can now propose that he shows signs of entering into the first love relationship with another person.

Benedek, T.: Parenthood as a developmental phase. *J. Am. Psychoanal. Assoc.* 7:389, 1959.
Erikson, E.: Identity and the life cycle. *In Psychological Issues.* 1:1, New York, International Universities Press, 1959.

At about four to six months one sees a reaction in most infants that has been called *stranger anxiety*. The infant who, though discriminating, has previously accepted everyone quite amiably now shows signs of psychological distress when an unfamiliar person appears. This is likely to happen for the first time with someone whose hair color or tone of voice differs markedly from the adults to whom he is accustomed, or when a familiar person appears different to him in some way (e.g., new glasses, hat, etc.). At this time, too, he may cry when taken to an unfamiliar place. This behavior appears to herald both another dimension of the infant's growing perception and his ability to express clearly recognizable psychologic distress in contrast with physical discomfort. This awareness, which reflects the increased distinction between the familiar and unfamiliar, probably operates also to strengthen existing attachments to people. The child's visual attentiveness and response to all aspects of his visual environment are very vivid at this time.

In the second half of the first year the baby's contacts with people rapidly become more varied and complicated as does his repertoire of feelings. He actively initiates social contact through reaching, smiling and vocalizing. He expresses pleasure, excitement, anger, eagerness, delight and protest, especially through voice, facial expression and motility. He signals with his voice when he wants attention. The infant who has had good care not only signals but behaves precisely as if he expects a response. For example, an infant of nine or ten months whose mother is out of sight in another room will call her with a sharp "ah" sound and look expectantly toward the door for her to appear. Among other things the behavior illustrates the further development of his ability to develop mental images of the important persons in his world who now exist in his mind, at least briefly, even when out of sight and sound. At some time during the six- to nine-month period, on the average, the baby begins to show reactions of distress when strangers appear and/or his mother leaves him. This behavior signals another step in psychologic growth: the infant's feelings of love for the mother have grown more intense. Advances in cognition permit increasingly acute perceptions of her and his need for her. This person who is so important çan, he perceives, also be lost. Anxiety specifically in regard to loss enters his psychic life.

The child of 9 to 12 months also has many facial expressions that make it easier for others to recognize his more differentiated emotions. In addition to the pleasure and displeasure reactions one now recognizes behaviors that reveal anxiety, confusion, curiosity or puzzlement. He appears, at times, joyful, tender, angry, gleeful or sad. Furthermore, he shifts rapidly from one mood to another. He is able to be more active both in making contact with a person and avoiding or rejecting such interaction. In so doing, he uses the various skills he has developed: he may make a contact with another person by smiling, by using his voice or by looking; he may hold out a toy, sometimes giving it to the other person, sometimes pulling it back playfully. If held, he may gently pat the face of the adult or not so gently pull her hair or push against her. He expresses his wish for contact as well as his ability to turn away or refuse it. One sees at this time, too, a rapid development of the interest and ability to imitate the actions of others that continues and becomes more complicated over time. Some examples are the games played with babies, such as peek-a-boo, pat-a-cake, bye-bye and so-big. The peek-a-boo play usually begins to be seen at around eight months; the other games about a month later. At first the baby imitates an adult; later he starts these games on his own and expects the adult to respond. The infant who is not playful in this way should arouse concern. If he has not had adequate nurturing he is often apathetic and does not enter vigorously into or initiate playful interchanges with others. Age-appropriate social play is both a healthy sign and a stimulus to further learning.

The relationship to persons also influences the child's interests in toys and other aspects of the material world. It is believed that the infant's development of a concept of the consistency and constancy of a world of things is dependent upon the consistency and constancy of those who provide care for him. To put it another way, object permanence as defined by Piaget as one aspect of sensorimotor intelligence is crucially influenced for better or worse by the nature of the child's relationship with parent figures. The linkages between social and cognitive development are demonstrated in such observations. It has also been established that while play with toys, interest in the environment and playful activity in general develop a momentum of their own after a time, they are closely entwined with and reflective of the child's relations with other people. Diminished interest in toys and play or their utilization at a delayed level may be due, of course, to a mental handicap, but it also occurs frequently in response to adverse experiential factors.

Another facet of normal development apparent in the latter part of the first year reflects that along with the attachment to and fear of loss of the primary caregiver the baby develops meaningful attachments to other persons and can accept and trust them as substitutes for the mother. In a family this attachment is most often formed with the father, but it may be made with another adult or, at times, with an older child. Thus, the infant can accept another person who cares for him without having his main attachment disturbed. The world in which he is comfortable and secure is thus expanded.

Another kind of substitute for the parent that is also accepted gradually is the *transitional object*. This is usually an object with sensuous qualities associated with experiences of pleasure — conventionally a stuffed toy or blanket — with which the child may comfort himself in his mother's absence. A prominent characteristic of the transitional object is that while the child's attachment appears to be associated with feelings of safety, comfort and need satisfaction similar to those provided by the ministrations of the mother, it is somewhat apart from her and under the child's control.

Another sign of healthy emotional growth during the last part of the first year and beyond is that the child can use the various skills he has developed to defend or assert himself. He can pull hard on a toy, insisting on his right to have it; he creeps toward something he wants; he can push away the hand of the adult, try to wriggle out of her arms or go away from something he fears or dislikes. When being seen by the doctor at this age he may push away from the physician's hand or instrument. These defensive flight and fight patterns will remain as aspects of the child's ability to cope with stress. The infant of this age as well as the older child who cannot be active both in seeking positive contact and in avoiding threatening or unpleasant situations should immediately raise questions in the clinician's mind.

In the second year, the child's relationship to others becomes still more complicated. Maturation combined with experience brings about changes in the child's psychologic organization, his rhythms, abilities, feelings and interests. His mastery of walking and of doing many other things independently goes hand in hand with progress in cognitive development that makes him more aware of his own separate body and mental self as well as the world of objects and persons. He has developed strong enough attachments to the important adults in his life to want to please them and win their approval much of the time. Another characteristic of the toddler has been described as negativism. Perhaps, as Fraiberg suggests, *oppositional behavior* is a better term than *negativism* in that it suggests that his protest at adult instructions is a normal developmental step and part of the process through which he establishes himself as a separate person. As he becomes more aware of himself as distinct from others, as a person with his own wishes and ideas, he also wants to do more for himself. He asserts this wish and intention strongly. He also develops a greater capacity for fun and pleasure. He is intense and passionate in his expressions of joy, anger, disappointment, excitement and disgust. Pleasure and budding pride in autonomy are also readily seen. There is no doubt that such feelings now have an ideational content as well as an affective charge.

Fraiberg, S.: *The Magic Years.* New York, Charles Scribners' Sons, 1959.

Behavior that reflects the inner struggle between independent and dependent feelings and ambivalence of attitudes is especially vivid and dramatic in the second year. Clinging and rejecting, holding on and casting out, assertions of mastery and of helplessness are conspicuous. Regression is an everyday occurrence when the child becomes tired, ill, hungry or upset for any reason. These characteristics make living with toddlers both delightful and taxing, and many parents find this period a time of stress.

The toddler's attachment to people and his wish to please them are powerful influences in the adult's effort to help him learn to conform to some of society's expectations. It is generally accepted among early childhood specialists that a society and culture transmits its standards and customs through the way in which its representatives, usually the parents, provide the guidance needed for negotiating the various developmental phases. Our society usually assigns a toddler the task of at least beginning to learn to feed himself and control his sphincters. He is also expected to learn to respect certain prohibitions that are necessary either for his safety or to satisfy the preferences of his parents. The toddler increasingly recognizes the parents' importance to him, not only in providing comfort and protection but also because he enjoys them and wants to be involved in their activities. Separation from the parents at such times often upsets the child. This may show itself in disturbances in feeding, sleep, toilet habits or play. He may appear apathetic, depressed or bereaved. The extent of the reaction will depend on many things: the length of the separation, the conditions that led up to it, who the substitute caretakers are and the child's state of physical health at the time. Specific adults have special meaning for the child, and they cannot be casually exchanged for others. One has only to look at the child of one to two years to be impressed both with this growing self-reliance and his continued need for an adult. The toddler joyfully walks across the room and plays for a while with his toys, but he soon looks up to find the familiar adult with his eyes, or comes back and sits near her or leans against her for a few moments before he resumes his play. This common event is like a "recharging of the battery"; a few minutes of closeness to the adult permits the child to return contented to his play. A little later, when he is almost two, he may leave his play and come in from out-of-doors to find the adult. This may be when he is hurt or upset and needs comfort, but the behavior also occurs when there is no obvious trouble, reflecting the child's need to re-establish contact and to reassure himself that the adult is still around and cares about him. It is another sign of intellectual and emotional growth and progress in socialization: the child now has developed enough awareness of the importance of the adult to become concerned not only about whether she is there for him but also whether she approves or disapproves of his behavior. His reading of her responses and that of other emotionally important adults markedly influences whether he can approve or disapprove of himself. The child's awareness of himself as a thinking, acting and feeling person is shown in his behavior. The appearance of reactions that suggest feelings of disgust or shame implies that the child begins to internalize parental standards for his behavior and, as it were, to react to his own behavior with judgments about his goodness, naughtiness, dirtiness, etc. These feelings are phase characteristic in their emergence and are necessary steps in the process of self-regulation of behavior and the development of his own standards. They are also stimulate adaptive responses that assist the child in dealing with those internal psychic conflicts and move him toward more mature behavior. The child of around two who does not begin to show some signs of concern about his own behavior should raise questions in the mind of the clinician.

Another healthy step in development seen in the second and third years is an increase of aggressive behavior. Aggressive feelings are a normal part of human development. All human relationships are permanently influenced by the fact that the earliest love relationships are formed between the child and the adults who both gratify and limit him. The child has both positive and negative feelings about the emotionally important persons. Learning to control and channel aggressive energies is a gradual process that extends over many years, but one notes its beginnings in the very young child. This learning and other controls over behavior develop most favorably when the necessary education and guidance take place in an atmosphere in which there is a continuity of affectionate care, when adults communicate interest and tenderness as well as guidance and when the prohibitions and requirements placed on the child are not dominanted by sadism, anger, hostility or abuse. Unhappily, one not infrequently sees children who are too harshly dealt with during this time of their lives. The child who shows no anger or aggressive behavior is in trouble, just as is the one who is excessively aggressive and destructive.

In the second and third years one also sees much imitation and signs of identification with the adult. This will continue to expand as time passes. In many of the child's actions he does what he sees adults doing. For example, one notes his interest in doing household tasks: he wants to dust, sweep or wash the dishes. In play with a doll he may enact what is done to and for him or what he begins to wish for or to fear. He also copies the adults' tone of voice and at times their attitudes: disgust at messiness, shame at misbehavior, pleasure at the arrival of a friend and sympathy for a person in distress. These attitudes are still in their nascent state and quickly vanish when the child's own inclinations lead him in the opposite direction. But they illustrate one of the processes through which the child incorporates the models provided by the adults and how these gradually become a part of his own personality and standards. The child participates in the reaction of the adults and emulates their methods of solving problems and coping with events. In assuming the attitudes of adults and their methods, he strengthens his own ability to control his impulses.

Between his second and third year, the child with growing knowledge of himself as a person separate from others may show signs of increased vulnerability based on a new awareness of wishes and of his limited power coupled with an emerging sense of shame and guilt. Striving for a more solid image of his body and a sex identity, the boy talks about his penis and perhaps implies a fear of losing it. The girl may express her fantasy of having a hidden penis or about having lost it. Her brother may agree with her. Ideas of power, of bigness and of control of others or oneself are conspicuous. Anticipation of punishment and feelings of guilt may now become related to sex differences. The wish for bigness and power will at times lead the child to competitive feelings toward the parent and toward the peer group. Aggressive assertiveness, competitive measuring of strength, jealous harboring of possessions and emerging friendships are generally quite conspicuous as a part of the child's life at the end of the third year.

During the third year also the child is even more aware that he must share his mother with other adults, with his father or with siblings. He knows that he is important, but that he is not the only pebble on the beach. This is an important aspect of his social adaptation. He also learns increasingly to differentiate between the permanent people in his life and those who may be substitutes or additional people, ones who are available for certain activities (e.g., teachers). One must ask whether a child is emotionally ready to do without his parents when he is physically able to move away from them. Whether the child equates physical separation with a feeling of loss of the parent will very much depend on the extent to which he has achieved the stable, reliable relationship with them that permits the kind of continuing mental representations that he can carry with him as images when they are not directly available. It will also depend upon his belief that they will be available on his return. Such a consideration is important, for example, in decisions about nursery school and other separations. There is a wide range of activity between the age of two and three in which the child experiments with the task of being able to move away from the parents and tests their trustworthiness and the permanency of the relationship. During this time the child's growing cognitive abilities lead him to relinquish some of his earlier feelings of omnipotence, his belief in the magic of his wishes and his egocentrism. He is highly individual and interested in himself; at the same time he is much more aware of others as individuals. If reasonably well cared for he will have most or all of the characteristics of a three-year-old described earlier in this chapter.

# CHAPTER 26

# THE NERVOUS SYSTEM

## GENERAL APPROACH

The neurologic examination in infants and in young children requires patience, flexibility and time. For an accurate appraisal it may be necessary to see the child on a number of occasions. Observation of spontaneous behavior and play may be part of the neurologic appraisal. A few simple toys such as a ball, blocks and crayons are facilitative. Young children may be examined best, at least in part, sitting in their mother's lap.

Children should be asked to walk, perhaps down a hall, while the examiner observes for asymmetrical use of the upper or lower extremities and presence of truncal ataxia on turning. Children over four or five years can walk on toes, in a tandem along a line and hop. Evaluation of a gait is often best accomplished if the child is unaware of being watched.

Amiel-Tison, C.: A method for neurologic evaluation within the first year of life. *Cur. Probl. Pediatr.* 7:3 (Nov.) 1976.

Paine, R.S. and Oppe, T.E.: *The Neurological Examination of Children.* London, William Heinemann, Ltd., 1966.

## NEUROLOGIC INJURY IN THE NEWBORN INFANT

**Brachial Plexus Injuries.** The *Erb-Duchenne* type of brachial plexus injury involves the fifth and sixth cervical cords. The fingers can be used for grasping, but the arm is flaccid and lies in a position of adduction and internal rotation with pronation of the forearm. There is extension of the elbow and flexion of the wrist (waiter's tip position). Extension of the arm at the elbow may be possible, but the shoulder is functionless. Movements of the fingers and wrist are unaffected. Most of the function that is destined to return will have done so by the age of three months; however, slow improvement may continue up to two years of age. Concomitant injury to the *phrenic nerve* may occur with resultant unilateral paralysis of the diaphragm.

The *Klumpke* type of paralysis, due to involvement of C8 and T1, does not have as favorable a prognosis as the Erb-Duchenne type. The arm is held flexed at the elbow and the musculature of the hand is paralyzed so that the infant is unable to grasp objects with his fingers. Edema of the involved hand may occur. The first thoracic vertebra and its accompanying sympathetic fibers may also be injured with a resultant Horner's syndrome. Rarely, the entire arm is paralyzed.

Eng, G.D.: Brachial plexus palsy in newborn infants. Pediatrics 48:18, 1971.

**Spinal cord injury** in the newborn infant is characterized by flaccid paralysis, loss of the deep tendon reflexes and absence of sweating below the site of the lesion.

Although all extremities are involved, some function is frequently retained in the uppers. Abdominal breathing with intercostal reaction may be noted. Flaccidity persists in these infants and is not replaced by spasticity.

Byers, R.K.: Spinal-cord injuries during birth. *Dev. Med. Child Neurol.* *17*:103, 1975.

**Paralysis of the facial nerve** occasionally occurs in newborn infants. Birth injury, abnormal intrauterine position or a congenital absence of the nucleus of the facial nerve may be etiologic.

**Intracranial hemorrhage** in the newborn may be intraventricular or subarachnoid, the former occurring on the first and second day and the latter on the second to tenth. Both cause neonatal seizures and bloody spinal fluid. Intraventricular hemorrhage, which usually occurs in a premature infant, causes the baby to be severely depressed and flaccid or restless and opisthotonic. The fontanel bulges, and the infant has a high-pitched cry.

**Cerebral Damage.** The prediction of the future neurologic status of the newborn based on an assessment in the first days of life is an uncertain exercise. The rapidity with which a baby demonstrates recovery from an impaired neurologic status over the first days or weeks of life seems to be of prognostic significance. Findings in the neurologic examination depend on the gestational age of the infant, his state of arousal and the examiner's skill and experience.

Clinical manifestations of brain damage may not be evident at birth, especially in premature infants. It is usually not possible to differentiate the clinical picture caused by cerebral hemorrhage from that caused by anoxia or developmental defect. A history of maternal hemorrhage or maternal hypotension during spinal anesthesia makes cerebral anoxia a likely diagnosis.

Cerebrally injured infants may be pale or cyanotic. The fontanel may be tense and bulging. Ocular palsies, inequality in the size of the pupils, nystagmus, failure of the pupils to react to light and a wandering gaze may be noted. The Moro reflex may disappear, and the grasp reflex may be absent or weak. The infant may be apathetic and sleep almost constantly, or he may be constantly or intermittently restless and irritable. Term newborn infants lie in a position of flexion. With hypotonia the extremities are extended; with hypertonia they are excessively flexed.

Intracranial damage should be suspected in newborn infants who have a persistent, open-eyed stare. The normal tremulousness of the newborn may be increased. While hypertonicity, localized muscular twitchings, tremors and reflex extension or flexion of the extremities may occur, muscle tone and resistance may be diminished or absent. In addition to the mass type of reflex response that may occur after tapping of the patellar tendon, a "jumping jack" response may be noted in infants who are cerebrally injured. This response consists of a sudden and simultaneous jerk of all extremities when the sternum or the muscles of the chest or thigh are tapped sharply. Nuchal rigidity, retraction of the head and opisthotonus are also characteristic. A rhythmic protrusion of the tongue, the so-called Foote's sign, may occur. Cerebral injury is the most important cause of convulsions in the newborn infant. The cry may be feeble and whiny or intermittent, shrill, sharp, piercing and plaintive. Infants with cerebral injury may be colicky and cry excessively.

The respiratory rhythm may be abnormally irregular and Cheyne-Stokes. The pulse rate may be increased or decreased. Hyperpyrexia may result from impairment of temperature control. The cerebrally damaged infant often does not feed well since his sucking and swallowing reflexes are poorly developed or absent. Feeding proceeds slowly, and 45 or more minutes may be required for a 1½- to 2-ounce feeding. The somnolence of the baby, the protrusion of the tongue and gagging may make feeding difficult. Vomiting, at times forceful, may also occur.

In the *placing reaction*, normally present from birth through the first year of life, the infant is held upright around his chest and with one lower extremity flexed, and the anterior tibial surface or the dorsum of the foot of the other extremity is lightly touched to the edge of a table. The normal baby brings his foot up to the top of the table. This response is absent in brain-damaged infants and in those with infantile spinal atrophy and spinal cord injury and is asymmetrical in hemiplegia.

Zappela, M.: The placing reaction in the first year of life. *Dev. Med. Child Neurol.* 8:393, 1966.

**Kernicterus** is a complication of neonatal hyperbilirubinemia. In premature infants with severe respiratory problems and acidosis, kernicterus may occur with bilirubin levels under 20 mg. per cent. The condition is evident during the first week of life; affected infants are listless, unresponsive, feed poorly, have a high-pitched cry and may regurgitate or vomit. Opisthotonus, irritability and seizures may occur. In patients who survive beyond the first week, athetosis, particularly in the arms and in the head and neck, appears in the latter half of the first or in the second year. Neurosensory deafness is commonly present. There may also be an inability to move the eyes upward or downward.

The *Crigler-Najjar syndrome* is a congenital, familial disorder characterized by nonhemolytic jaundice. Kernicterus usually develops in the type I syndrome but unusually in type II. The infants may be persistently jaundiced from a few days after birth. Rigidity, athetosis and an expressionless facies may appear between two weeks and three months of age.

## CEREBRAL PALSY

Usually the term *cerebral palsy* implies aberrations in motor behavior arising from central nervous system damage. Hearing impairment, visual problems, mental retardation, speech defects, convulsive disorders and psychologic problems may also occur.

The clinical manifestations of cerebral palsy may not be apparent until the latter half of the first year or later. Usually, however, developmental and neurologic appraisal permits the diagnosis to be suspected or made in many infants in the first six months. Cerebral palsy should be considered with abnormal persistence of primitive reflex patterns such as the tonic neck reflex, delayed gross motor performance or atypical developmental patterns such as preferential use of one hand before the age of one and one-half to two years, atypical crawling patterns or alterations in muscle tone.

The *parachute reaction*, normally present by six to eight months of life, may be delayed or abnormal in infants with cerebral palsy. In this maneuver, the child held in ventral suspension is suddenly tilted forward toward the floor. Normally, abduction of the arms and extension of the elbows, wrists and fingers occur in a protective fashion. There is an asymmetric response in spastic hemiplegia. Absence of the parachute reaction is not significant until after eight to nine months of age.

## Types of Neuromuscular Disability

**Spasticity.** Muscle stiffness is the chief clinical feature of spastic cerebral palsy. Occasionally this is preceded or accompanied by muscular hypotonia and flaccidity. Spasticity usually becomes apparent within the first six months of life, somewhat later if hypotonia has been extensive. Early findings related to motor development appear either as retardation or alteration in normal patterns. The normal extremities are used preferentially, and the affected parts participate less in such activities as kicking, reciprocation and grasping. The mother may report that it is difficult to spread the infant's thighs when changing diapers. Spasticity of the abductors and internal rotators of the thighs and of the flexors of the hip accounts for this limitation of abduction and for the tendency of the lower extremities to scissor or cross over when the child is supported erect, stands or begins to walk. Infants with spastic paraplegia usually keep their knees in flexion when supine. In the supported standing position, the lower extremities are usually rigidly extended and the feet in equinus. The affected child stands or walks on his toes.

When babies up to four months are held upright under the axilla, flexion of the lower extremities will occur. With spastic diplegia, the lower extremities remain extended and perhaps adduct or scissor. Involvement of the upper extremities may be characterized by adduction of the arm, pronation of the forearm and flexion of the elbow, wrist and interphalangeal joints. The lower extremities are more commonly and severely involved than the upper. The normal infant, when suspended by his heels and lowered so that his head touches the examining table, drops his arms below his head (parachute reaction). With spasticity or athetosis this does not occur. Instead, the involved arm is rigidly extended outward, and the forearm is pronated. With spasticity of the hip extensors, the baby cannot be pulled to sit but rather is lifted board-like from the supine position. Increased extensor tone is also reflected in opisthotonic posturing of the baby.

The *stretch reflex* is a pathognomonic finding of spasticity. Rapid passive stretching of a spastic muscle leads to a powerful contraction of the muscle, and a sudden resistance to and blocking of the movement. The reflex is not elicited if the motion is performed slowly. This increased resistance (clasp-knife spasticity) is transient, however, and the movement can then be completed. If the child cries or voluntarily tenses his muscles, it may be difficult to be sure about a stretch reflex. Although often delayed in patients with mild spasticity or hypotonia, the stretch reflex usually appears within the first year of life. With severe involvement, it may be present within the first month.

Voluntary motor acts that require coordination may be accompanied by an "overflow" with participation by muscles not primarily concerned. This may be manifested by facial contortions, compression of the lips, increased extension of the lower extremities, a more rapid respiratory rate and the production of guttural sounds. Such manifestations may simulate athetosis.

Children with spastic cerebral palsy may also have hyperactive deep tendon reflexes, ankle clonus, muscle clonus when the muscle is quickly stretched and positive Babinski's sign. Strabismus, convulsive seizures and mental retardation occur more commonly than in other types of cerebral palsy. Contractures may develop if preventive measures are not taken.

Hypotonia, often an early finding in infants with cerebral palsy, is replaced over a period of months by other neurologic findings such as spasticity. Muscle tone is dynamic and varies with the position of the baby and turning of the head.

The terms *atonic spastic diplegia* or *flaccid spasticity* may be applied to patients who demonstrate muscular hypotonia and weakness but who do not have a true flaccid paralysis. Hypotonia may be limited to the muscles that oppose the action of the spastic muscles, or it may be so generalized as to simulate the "floppy infant" syndrome. The presence of normal or increased deep tendon reflexes, however, is a differentiating feature. Good muscle tone is apparent when voluntary motor activity is attempted. Another difference may be demonstrated by lifting the infant with muscular hypotonia by his armpits. The lower extremities of patients with benign muscular hypotonia remain extended while those of patients with atonic spastic diplegia are flexed at the hips and knees. A positive Babinski's sign and ankle clonus are present in some of these children. Muscle stiffness, spasticity and a stretch reflex may appear later. The hypotonia becomes less evident as the child grows older. Though hyperflexibility of the joints may be present early, many of these patients eventually have flexion contractures.

Spasticity develops in children with Schilder's disease.

**Dyskinesias** are characterized by involuntary, nonpurposeful, incoordinated movements often accompanied by increased muscle tone. The movements decrease during sleep or periods of motor inactivity and increase during voluntary activity. The manifestations of the dyskinesias are more distinct in the upper than in the lower extremities. The following subgroups frequently overlap.

CHOREA is characterized by spasmodic, involuntary, nonpurposeful, quick and jerky movements.

ATHETOSIS is manifested by continuous or spasmodic, bizarre, twisting, writhing and wormlike muscular movements, which are slower and more tortuous than in chorea. Athetosis is usually most evident in the fingers and wrists. Occasionally both types of dyskinesia are present in an individual patient (choreoathetosis). When the motions are of large amplitude, athetosis is readily apparent. In many patients, however, findings may be evident only when voluntary efforts are made. This is especially true in patients with muscular hypotonia. In reaching for an object, involuntary extension of the wrist and extension of the fingers may occur. Athetoid movements may be accentuated by asking the child to lie quietly on the examining table in the supine position. Although it may be suspected earlier, athetosis is not fully apparent until the end of the first or in the second year. The appearance of increased muscular tension in infants during voluntary motor activities suggests incipient dyskinesia. Such tension may be manifested as intermittent stiffening spells or extensor spasms that occur spontaneously or in response to minimal stimuli. When the extensor thrust reflex occurs, the involved portion of the body, commonly the trunk, is suddenly thrust into extension.

Attempts to suppress involuntary athetoid movements result in tension, which is confused, at times, with spasticity. The heightened muscle tone in patients with tension athetosis disappears with passive motion. The converse may occur in the patient with spasticity. The stretch reflex is absent in the former but present in the latter. Tension decreases in the athetoid child when the involved extremity is rapidly shaken but increases in the child with spasticity. Some intermittent resistance may, however, be encountered upon slow joint movement in the patient with tension athetosis. When voluntary motor activity of one extremity is attempted, athetoid movements may overflow into other parts of the body. Nonpersistent scissoring of the lower extremities and ankle clonus may occur. Dystonic, athetoid and choreiform movements occur in the Lesch-Nyhan syndrome and in 1–glutaric aciduria.

Nyhan, W.L.: The Lesch-Nyhan syndrome. *Dev. Med. Child. Neurol. 20*:376, 1978.
Whelan, D.T., Hill, R., Ryan, E.D. and Spate, M.: 1–Glutaric acidemia: investigation of a patient and his family. *Pediatrics 63*:88, 1979.

DYSTONIA.   The first symptom, usually appearing between six and ten years of age, is an intermittent, eventually constant, plantar flexion-inversion movement of the foot and ankle while walking. This is followed by involuntary flexion or extension of the wrist. The child may experience an involuntary flexion of the wrist and fingers when attempting to hold a pencil. Later, muscle contractions, torsion spasm and distortions of the neck and trunk may occur while walking. These patients are often initially misdiagnosed as hysterical.

Cooper, I.S.: Dystonia musculorum deformans: natural history and neurosurgical alleviation. *J. Pediatr. 74*:585, 1969.

RIGIDITY.   The musculature in patients with rigidity is stiff, hypertonic and plastic. Rigidity may be constant, variable or intermittent. These patients are often intellectually retarded and usually lie in a position of opisthotonus. Passive movement of a joint, especially when slowly performed, may meet with a constant "lead pipe" or an interrupted "cogwheel" resistance. These findings may be less notable with rapid movement of the joints. Deep tendon reflexes are not increased.

**Ataxia.**   In children with ataxia, the movements of the extremities are incoordinated and clumsy. These patients walk late and with a wide-based, unsteady gait. Muscular atony or hypotonicity with hyperactive deep reflexes is characteristic. Nystagmus may be present.

**Mixed Forms.**   Many patients present features characteristic of more than one group.


LOCALIZATION OF INVOLVEMENT

**Paraplegia** indicates neuromuscular dysfunction, usually spastic, limited to the lower extremities.

**Diplegia** is the term used in patients whose major involvement is in the lower but who also have some involvement of the upper extremities. Infants with spastic diplegia, often prematurely born, may be seen because of inability to sit up or an atypical crawling pattern in which the arms are used to propel the infant forward in a kind of "bunny hop."

**Quadriplegia,** or quadriparesis, is characterized by changes in all extremities, most prominent in the lower with spasticity and in the upper with dyskinesia. The term *double hemiplegia* may be used in patients with spastic cerebral palsy in whom involvement is greater in the upper than in the lower extremities.

**Hemiplegia** indicates involvement of one half of the body, usually spastic in type, and more pronounced in the upper than in the lower extremities. With walking, the involved lower extremity may be dragged along or circumducted, and the child may walk on his toes. In infants with congenital hemiplegia, a definite hand preference may be noted by six months of age. The crawling pattern in these babies is also abnormal. Mild hemiparesis may be detected by observing asymmetric associated movements of the upper extremities when the child walks or runs. The involved arm is carried in more of a hemiparetic posture while running than while walking. There is also an asymmetric response to the *lateral propping reaction* in which the child in the sitting position is pushed to one side. The normal response is for the arm on that side to extend to prevent the child from falling. This reaction is asymmetric in spastic hemiplegia. Absence of the lateral propping reflex is abnormal only after eight or nine months. Growth retardation, perhaps more extensive in the upper extremity, may occur on the involved side. Sensory modalities such as two-point discrimination and stereognosis are often impaired.

Molnar, G.E. and Taft, L.T.: Pediatric rehabilitation, Part I: cerebral palsy and spinal cord injuries. *Curr. Probl. Pediatr.* 7:3 (Jan.) 1977.
Taft, L.T.: Cerebral palsy. *In* Green, M. and Haggerty, R.J. (eds.): *Ambulatory Pediatrics II.* Philadelphia, W. B. Saunders Co., 1977, p. 294.

## EXAMINATION OF THE CRANIAL NERVES

I. The olfactory nerve may be tested by the recognition of odors such as peppermint and cloves. Each nostril is tested separately.

II. In the functional examination of the optic nerve the eyes are tested individually and then together for visual acuity, color recognition and ability to follow objects. An ophthalmologic examination and delineation of the visual fields are also indicated.

III, IV and VI. These cranial nerves control movement of the eyes. Defects in this innervation may be detected by having the patient follow objects up and down and from side to side while the head is held in a fixed position. The innervation of the muscles of the eye is reviewed on page 59.

III. Since the oculomotor nerve supplies the levator palpebrae superioris, a peripheral lesion of this nerve causes ptosis of the eyelid and narrowing of the palpebral fissure. The sphincter of the pupil and the ciliary muscle are also supplied by the oculomotor nerve so that dilatation of the pupil and failure to react to light or accommodation are additional findings. Divergent strabismus is also noted. The ptosis and pupillary changes may not occur in patients who have a nuclear lesion of the oculomotor nerve.

IV. The trochlear nerve is rarely affected alone but usually along with the oculomotor nerve.

V. The sensory division of the trigeminal nerve is responsible for sensation over the face and tongue. The *corneal reflex* is elicited by touching the cornea with a wisp of cotton after the patient has been directed to look away from the examiner. The normal response is bilateral blinking, the motor component of the reflex being mediated through the facial nerve. If the lesion involves the trigeminal nerve, neither eye blinks. With a lesion involving the ipsilateral facial nerve the other eye blinks. The corneal reflex is absent in comatose and anesthetized patients. It may also be absent in hysteria and familial dysautonomia.

Involvement of the motor division of the trigeminal nerve causes the jaw to deviate to the paralyzed side when the patient opens his mouth. When he clenches his teeth, contraction of the masseter and temporal muscles on the involved side is feeble.

VI. When the abducens nerve is involved, lateral movement of the eye is not possible so that internal strabismus and diplopia result. Since paralysis of the abducens nerve is often caused by a generalized increase in intracranial pressure, its presence may not help localize intracranial disease. Abducens paralysis developing in the absence of signs of increased intracranial pressure suggests a pontine tumor, especially if lateral conjugate movements of the eyes are abolished and other cranial nerves are involved. An isolated, benign VI nerve palsy may also occur in some children.

Knox, D.L., Clark, D.B. and Schuster, F.F.: Benign VI nerve palsies in children. *Pediatrics* *40*:560, 1967.

Robertson, D.M., Hines, J.D. and Rucker, C.W.: Acquired sixth-nerve paresis in children. *Arch. Ophthalmol. 83*:574, 1970.

**VII. Peripheral or Nuclear Paralysis of the Facial Nerve.** Asymmetry of the face due to peripheral facial paralysis is especially noticeable when the patient laughs or cries. The involved side is flat, drooped and expressionless. The angle of the mouth sags, and the nasolabial fold is obliterated or less prominent than normal. The patient cannot frown, wrinkle his forehead or close his eyelids tightly. When the child attempts to close his eyelids, the eye on the involved side is seen to roll upward (*Bell's phenomenon*). The sense of taste on the anterior two-thirds of the tongue may be lost and salivary secretion decreased. Facial paralysis may be demonstrated by asking the patient to talk, whistle, smile, inflate his cheeks or show his teeth.

Peripheral facial nerve paralysis is an occasional cause for facial asymmetry in the newborn. It also occurs acutely and unilaterally as Bell's palsy. Bilateral facial weakness may be present with the Guillain-Barré syndrome. The Ramsay Hunt syndrome due to herpetic involvement of the ear and the geniculate ganglion is characterized by vesicles involving the ear and external auditory canal, facial paralysis, tinnitus, vertigo, severe pain in the external auditory canal and pinna and impaired hearing. Facial diplegia is also seen in congenital myotonic dystrophy.

Partial facial paralysis, involving only a single branch of the facial nerve, may cause marked asymmetry of the lower lip during crying. Pouting and drawing of the unaffected side downward and outward is noted.

Pape, K.E. and Pickering, D.: Asymmetric crying facies: an index of other congenital anomalies. *J. Pediatr. 81*:21, 1972.

*Melkersson-Rosenthal syndrome* consists of recurrent peripheral facial paralysis, edema of the lips and face and a furrowed tongue.

*Möbius's syndrome*, due to incomplete or complete unilateral or bilateral weakness of the facial musculature, is characterized by a masklike facial expression. Other cranial nerves, especially VI, may also be involved. Anomalies of the brachial and thoracic muscles and the extremities may occur.

Facial nerve palsy may be due to embryonal rhabdomyosarcoma of the middle ear cleft. A conductive hearing loss, refractory otitis media and a mass in the external auditory canal may also be present.

Leviton, A., Davidson, R. and Gilles, F.: Neurologic manifestations of embryonal rhabdomyosarcoma of the middle ear cleft. *J. Pediatr. 80*:596, 1972.

Facial paralysis may also occur in children with hypertension.

Lloyd, A.V.C., Sewitt, D.E. and Still, J.D.L.: Facial paralysis in children with hypertension. *Arch. Dis. Child. 217*:292, 1966.

**Supranuclear Paralysis.** Supranuclear paralysis of the facial nerve may be caused by cerebral hemorrhage or other central nervous system lesions. Because of their bilateral cortical innervation, the upper facial muscles are not involved in patients with unilateral supranuclear facial paralysis. The eye can usually be closed to some extent and the forehead wrinkled.

VIII. The testing of auditory acuity is discussed on page 64. Involvement of the cochlear branch of the auditory nerve causes neurosensory deafness. Lesions of the vestibular branch of the auditory nerve may be demonstrated by vestibular function tests. The rotational test can be performed with the child sitting in his mother's lap. The normal response in the child after turning is a broad, roving type of nystagmus with fast and slow components. If nystagmus does not occur after rotation, labyrinth damage is present. If nystagmus is not obtained on the rotational test, the caloric test, which provides a unilateral stimulus to the labyrinth, may be done. Absence of nystagmus in the caloric test indicates that the labyrinth being tested is not functioning. The sensitivity and reliability of the rotational test are greater than that of the caloric test.

IX. Difficulty in swallowing and loss of the pharyngeal reflexes may occur with lesions of the glossopharyngeal nerve. Usually, however, isolated involvement of this nerve does not occur.

X. Lesions of the vagus nerve may cause difficulty in swallowing so that the patient chokes when feeding. Foods and liquids may be regurgitated through the nose. Pooling of mucus in the posterior pharynx may cause a loose, "bulbar" cough. The voice has a nasal quality. With a unilateral lesion of the vagus nerve the uvula deviates to the uninvolved side. With bilateral paralysis, elevation of the palate does not occur during phonation. The gag reflex may be absent.

XI. Contraction of the sternocleidomastoid and trapezius muscles may be impaired in patients with involvement of the spinal accessory nerve. There may be an inability to shrug the shoulders, and a torticollis may develop.

XII. Deviation of the tongue toward the affected side occurs in patients with hemiplegia.

**Bulbar involvement** may be characterized by pooling of secretions in the posterior pharynx. The pharyngeal muscles may continue to contract in response to touch with a tongue blade. Poliomyelitis may cause paralysis of the ninth, tenth, eleventh and twelfth cranial nerves.

The infantile form of Gaucher's disease may be characterized by a "pseudobulbar syndrome" with dysphagia and laryngospasm.

Dysphagia, regurgitation, poor sucking ability and pooling of saliva may occur in infants with Pompe's disease or type II glycogenosis.

In patients with rabies, painful, severe spasms of the pharynx and larynx are precipitated by attempts to swallow liquids or solids or by air blowing across the face. Later, spasms may be initiated by the sight or sound of liquids.

Diphtheritic neuritis may cause pharyngeal paralysis or weakness with dysphagia and difficulty in coughing. Bulbar symptoms may also be noted in tick paralysis and with the Guillain-Barré syndrome.

Bulbar symptoms may result from phenothiazine toxicity.

Cranial nerve involvement may also occur in patients with tuberculous meningitis, encephalitis and the demyelinating diseases.

Multiple involvement of the cranial nerves suggests a pontine glioma.

**Examination of the reflexes** in infants and children is performed much as in adults except that the response is more variable in infants. Unsustained ankle clonus is not a significant finding in infants. Abdominal reflexes may not be obtained in infants, especially during the first six months. When testing the patellar reflexes, the head should be in the midline since the reflex is modified by the tonic neck reflex. Adduction of the thighs as an overflow of the knee jerk reflex is normal in the first six months. Slight increases or decreases in the deep tendon reflexes are not clinically significant. In deep coma, all reflexes, muscle tone and meningeal signs are absent.

*Kernig's sign*, which denotes meningeal irritation, is elicited by extension of the knee with the patient in the supine position and the thigh flexed to 90 degrees. When Kernig's sign is positive, the knee can be extended only slightly, and the attempt is painful. A positive sign is usually not present early in young infants with meningitis. Kernig's sign may also be elicited with transverse myelitis.

*Brudzinski's sign* is adduction and flexion of the lower extremities when an attempt is made to flex the head.

**Plantar Reflexes.** *Babinski's sign* may be positive in normal infants, perhaps as a reflection of immaturity of the nervous system. It does not become clinically significant until the end of the second year. *Chaddock's sign* with extension of the big toe is obtained by stroking along the lateral malleolus and dorsolateral aspect of the foot. *Oppenheim's sign* is characterized by dorsiflexion of the toe when the examiner strokes downward along the medial aspect of the tibia. *Gordon's sign* consists of extension of the toe when the calf muscles are squeezed. These signs indicate the presence of a pyramidal tract lesion.

## ALTERATION OF TENDON REFLEXES

**Diminished Tendon Reflexes.** Although the deep reflexes may be diminished or absent in patients with the *Guillain-Barré syndrome*, the superficial reflexes are usually not involved.

In *pseudohypertrophic muscular dystrophy*, the deep reflexes gradually disappear.

The tendon reflexes in the lower extremities in *Friedreich's ataxia* gradually disappear.

Although the deep tendon reflexes may be hyperactive for a time in patients with *Werdnig-Hoffmann disease*, they eventually diminish.

Diminution or absence of the deep tendon reflexes is characteristic of patients with *peripheral neuritis*. Similar findings are present during episodes of *familial periodic paralysis*. The deep tendon reflexes may be absent or decreased in *familial dysautonomia*.

*Cerebellar tumors* are usually accompanied by a diminution in the deep tendon reflexes. Occasionally, increased tendon reflexes may occur with a medulloblastoma because of compression of the pyramidal tracts. Hyperactive tendon reflexes are commonly present with tumors of the brain stem.

**Hyperactive deep reflexes** are present with Tay-Sachs disease, spastic cerebral palsy, platybasia and the demyelinating encephalopathies.

## SENSORY CHANGES

Determination of sensory loss in infants and young children is difficult. This is especially true of two-point discrimination and temperature differences. It is usually possible, however, to test for pain by a pinprick. In the absence of paralysis, this stimulus causes withdrawal of the extremity.

Position and vibratory senses in the lower extremities are impaired with *Friedreich's ataxia*.

*Hyperesthesia* may occur in the Guillain-Barré syndrome and in meningococcal meningitis. *Paresthesia* may occur with the Guillain-Barré syndrome, lupus erythematosus, transverse myelopathy, tick paralysis. Refsum's disease and reflex sympathetic dystrophy.

Sensory changes ranging from anesthesia to hyperesthesia may occur with *hysteria*.

In *congenital indifference to pain* the children do not cry or demonstrate pain in response to painful stimuli or injury, but other sensation is not lost. Bizarre skeletal lesions may occur. In *congenital sensory neuropathy*, pain, temperature and touch sensibility is absent or diminished in the extremities and parts of the trunk. A relative indifference to pain occurs with *familial dysautonomia*.

Dancis, J. and Smith, A.A.: Familial dysautonomia. *J. Pediatr.* 77:174, 1970.

Sensory loss in the affected extremity may occur in children with hemiplegia.

## TREMORS

Brief, coarse tremors along with some stiffening of the extremities often occur in normal newborn infants when they are picked up, their extremities are moved or they experience other sudden postural changes. Tremors may also occur in response to loud noises and chilling. The significance of these startle responses in infants with possible cerebral injury may be difficult to establish in the neonatal period. Since these findings normally disappear in a few weeks, their persistence probably indicates a cerebral lesion.

*Tetany* of the newborn may cause a coarse tremor of the extremities.

A slow, involuntary, rhythmic tremor may be present in some children with *cerebral palsy*. This tremor may be present at rest but is most prominent during voluntary motor activity.

An *intention or action tremor* may occur in patients with cerebellar and brain stem tumors and with Wilson's disease. Tremor associated with lesions of the cerebellar hemispheres is absent at rest but present with action (intention) and increases in amplitude as the object or end point is approached (e.g., in the finger-to-nose test).

*Essential, hereditary or familial tremor* may begin in childhood. Most noticeable in the fingers and hands when the upper extremities are extended in front of the patient, it increases in amplitude as the hand approaches an object. The tremor also becomes worse when the child attempts to write.

The severity of the tremor in children with *hyperthyroidism* is variable. It may be fine or coarse and present in the hands, tongue and extremities. Usually the tremor is most prominent during voluntary motor activity and best demonstrated when the patient extends his upper extremities and spreads his fingers. The tongue may also show a fine tremor if protruded at this time.

*Anxiety* may cause a fine to coarse, rapid tremor of the forearms and hands. The tremor is present at rest and increases with voluntary movement. Bizarre tremors may be noted in children who live in stressful home environments.

Encephalitis may cause a tremor.

Hypoglycemia may cause a tremor.

*Wilson's disease* may begin with an action tremor and poor coordination especially apparent in fine motor performance such as handwriting. While the tremor may be present at rest, it is usually accentuated with purposeful movements and emotional stress. The tremor varies from fine to coarse, slow or choreoathetoid. At times localized to one hand, it may be general in some instances and involve the head, tongue and upper extremities. Asterixis may be present. Other findings include awkwardness, slurred speech, excessive salivation, dystonia, an unusual laugh and deterioration in school performance.

Slovis, T.L., Dubois, R.S., Rodgerson, D.O. and Silverman, A.: The varied manifestations of Wilson's disease. *J. Pediatr.* 78:578, 1971.

Involuntary movements, especially wing-beating tremors of the arms or *asterixis*, are seen in *hepatic, pulmonary and renal failure* and in Wilson's disease when the patient is asked to touch his nose with his index finger. Sudden movements of flexion and extension occur at the wrists, producing a flapping movement of the hands and sometimes the entire upper extremity.

Thallium poisoning may cause tremor, ataxia, paresthesias and alopecia. Hydantoin toxicity is characterized by an intention tremor.

Tremor, rigidity, dystonia, oculogyric crises and fixed stare may be caused by *phenothiazine toxicity*. The findings may be episodic and to some extent subject to voluntary control.

Gupta, J.M. and Lovejoy, F.H., Jr.: Acute phenothiazine toxicity in childhood: a five-year survey. *Pediatrics 39*:771, 1967.

Flapping, excited movements are made by some retarded children. Blind children may rub at their eyes or flutter their hands in front of their face (blindisms).

## TETANY

Tetany may be characterized by laryngospasm, twitching, tremors, restlessness, muscular rigidity, unsteadiness and convulsions. *Carpopedal spasm* begins with flexion and adduction of the thumb across the cupped palm of the hand. The fingers then become flexed at the metacarpophalangeal joints and extended at the interphalangeal joints. Flexion and some ulnar deviation of the wrist may also occur. Plantar flexion of the feet in a varus or equinus position may appear along with cupping of the sole and flexion of the toes. Both the upper and lower extremities may be held in flexion and adduction. Carpopedal spasm may be a manifestation of hysteria as well as tetany. The *peroneal sign* is obtained by tapping the peroneal nerve over the head of the fibula. Dorsiflexion and eversion of the foot occur when this sign is positive. *Chvostek's sign* is obtained by tapping over the facial nerve just anterior to the tragus. Contraction of the facial muscles occurs with blinking of the eyelids, twitching of the alae nasi and elevation of the corner of the mouth. Although a manifestation of tetany during infancy and early childhood, it can be elicited in normal newborn infants.

## RIGIDITY

*Tetanus* is characterized by muscle spasm and rigidity. Opisthotonus, clenching of the fingers and extension of the lower extremities and feet may occur.

The musculature in *cerebral palsy* of the rigid type is stiff, hypertonic and plastic. The rigidity may be constant or intermittent.

*Decerebrate* rigidity is characterized by the constant or paroxysmal occurrence of rigid extension of the extremities with hyperpronation of the forearms, flexion of the wrists, fingers, feet and toes, extension of the head and opisthotonus. Coma, pinpoint pupils and bilateral Babinski's signs may also be present. Decerebrate rigidity may occur with tumors in the region of the midbrain or the third ventricle or as a result of increased intracranial pressure due to other lesions such as hemorrhage into the brain stem, extradural hematoma, severe hypoxemia due to cardiorespiratory arrest, encephalitis and meningitis. Decerebrate rigidity occurs terminally in infants with Tay-Sachs disease and late in Schilder's disease.

NUCHAL RIGIDITY may occur with the following disorders:

Subarachnoid hemorrhage
Brain abscess
Poliomyelitis
Meningitis. Nuchal rigidity is often not present in young infants with meningitis.
Meningismus
Leptospirosis
Infantile Gaucher's disease
Spinal cord tumors
Intracranial tumors, especially cerebellar tumors with herniation. Nuchal rigidity is occasionally present in patients with supratentorial tumors.
Transverse myelopathy
Encephalitis
Aseptic meningitis
Phenothiazine toxicity. Severe retractional and rotational spasms of the neck may occur.
Arnold-Chiari malformation
Behçet's syndrome

In struggling infants, involuntary nuchal rigidity may be differentiated from voluntary rigidity by placing the supine infant with his shoulders at the edge of the table and his head supported by the examiner's hand. Involuntary rigidity will persist in this position when an attempt is made to flex the head.

OPISTHOTONUS may occur in

Tetanus
Meningitis
Encephalitis
Cerebral hemorrhage and anoxia
Acute infantile Gaucher's disease
Kernicterus
Tay-Sachs disease
l–glutaric aciduria
Rabies

HYPERACTIVITY   See Chapter 46.

## SOFT NEUROLOGIC SIGNS

A number of so-called *soft neurologic signs* may occur during normal development. These include choreiform movements of the arms, hyperactivity, short attention span, synkinesis (involuntary mirror movements of fingers on opposite hand), poor motor coordination, inability to hop or tandem walk, failure to appreciate simultaneous touch to face and hands, poorly performed alternating movements, mixed or confused laterality and inability to appreciate numbers drawn on the hand. While these signs may have a statistical relationship to learning problems, they are not clinically helpful in the individual child.

Barlow, C.F.: "Soft signs" in children with learning disorders. *Am. J. Dis. Child. 128*:605, 1974.
Page-El, E. and Grossman, H.J.: Neurologic appraisal in learning disorders. *Pediatr. Clin. N. Am. 20*:599, 1973.

## ATAXIA

Detection of ataxia in children under the age of two years may be difficult. The history of a change in gait is significant. An important part of the examination is observation of the child's spontaneous activity, retrieving a ball or coming for a toy. Patients old enough to cooperate should be asked to stand with their feet together, walk in tandem fashion, hop on one foot and turn quickly while walking. In the older child, the finger-to-nose and heel-to-knee tests may be used to evaluate coordination and balance. Vestibular ataxia due to bilateral labyrinthine disease or secondary to disturbances in proprioception (sensory ataxia) is accentuated when the eyes are closed whereas this is less marked with cerebellar ataxia. The more common disease states characterized by ataxia include:

Primary cerebellar ataxia

Acute, intermittent familial cerebellar ataxia

White, J.C.: Familial periodic nystagmus, vertigo and ataxia. *Arch. Neurol. 20*:276, 1969.

Cerebral palsy

Intracranial tumors, especially those involving the cerebellum

Cerebellar abscess

Encephalitis

Friedreich's ataxia and other degenerative spinocerebellar disorders. A staggering ataxic gait begins between the ages of 5 and 14 years. Later, clumsiness in writing, nystagmus, dysarthria, pes cavus and loss of position and vibratory senses are noted. The deep tendon reflexes are absent.

Tick paralysis

Pernicious anemia

Hydantoin sensitivity or intoxication

Lead poisoning

Guillain-Barré syndrome

$G_{m1}$ gangliosidosis

Schilder's disease, metachromatic leukodystrophy, Pelizaeus-Merzbacher and other degenerative diseases

Hartnup syndrome causes intermittent ataxia, diplopia and a pellagra-like rash.

Fisher's syndrome

Von Hippel-Lindau syndrome with retinal and cerebellar angiomas

Marinesco-Sjögren's syndrome with ataxia, cataracts, mental retardation and skeletal anomalies

Drug intoxication

Argininosuccinicaciduria

Maple syrup urine disease in older children may be characterized by episodes of ataxia.

Pyruvate decarboxylase deficiency may cause intermittent cerebellar ataxia.

Blass, J.P., Kark, R.A. and Engle, W.K.: Clinical studies of a patient with pyruvate decarboxylase deficiency. *Arch. Neurol.* 25:449, 1971.

Metachromatic leukodystrophy

Hysteria. In the Romberg test, the patient is more likely to sway from the hips than from the knees. Asked to perform another simultaneous task, e.g., finger-to-nose, the hysterical patient may stop swaying whereas the child with a true ataxia would not.

Acute labyrinthitis

Multiple peripheral neuropathy

Ataxia-telangiectasia. Neurologic symptoms and signs are usually the first to appear when the child begins to walk. Choreiform and athetoid movements may be noted in addition to ataxia.

Acute bacterial meningitis. Ataxia may be a prominent presenting clinical finding.

Schwartz, J.F.: Ataxia in bacterial meningitis. Neurology. 22:1071, 1972.

Occult neuroblastoma may present with ataxia.

Solomon, G.E. and Chutorian, A.M.: Opsoclonus and occult neuroblastoma. *N. Engl. J. Med.* 279:475, 1968.

Refsum's syndrome, along with neurosensory deafness and retinitis pigmentosa.

The myoclonic movements in *Kinsbourne's myoclonic encephalopathy* may simulate ataxia.

*Acute cerebellar ataxia* is characterized by the sudden onset of ataxia in a young child. Intention tremor, nystagmus and other cerebellar signs may be present.

*Perilymphatic fistula of the oval window region* may cause ataxia, neurosensory hearing loss and episodic vertigo.

Healy, G.B., Friedman, J.M. and DiTroia, J.: Ataxia and hearing loss secondary to perilymphatic fistula. *Pediatrics 61*:238, 1978.

*Abetalipoproteinemia* is characterized by ataxia, retinitis pigmentosa, acanthocytosis (thorny red cells) and celiac syndrome.

Bell, W.E.: Ataxia in childhood. *Lancet 85*:1, 1965.

## CHOREA

Patients with *Sydenham's chorea* demonstrate emotional lability. Restlessness may be so great that the child cannot sit still. Involuntary movements that are sudden, jerking, irregular, asymmetrical, uncoordinated and purposeless are the most prominent feature of this disorder. Choreiform movements, especially notable in the arms and face, cause grimacing. In hemichorea, the manifestations are predominantly unilateral. Occasionally, temporary paresis of an extremity may occur. The movements decrease or disappear after rest or during sleep and increase if the child is aware of being observed or is asked to sit still. The patient has difficulty counting up to ten and back again rapidly. Speech and writing may be almost unintelligible. If the child is asked to smile, the expression fades rapidly. The patient is able to protrude his tongue only for a short time and cannot maintain a tight hand grasp. A "hung-up" patellar reflex is occasionally observed. When the arms are extended and the fingers spread apart, flexion of the wrist and hyperextension of the fingers may occur. When the arms are extended above the head, pronation occurs so that the backs of the hands touch. Chorea may be a manifestation of rheumatic fever or of lupus erythematosus.

Aron, A.M., Freeman, J.M. and Carter, S.: The natural history of Sydenham's chorea. *Am. J. Med. 38*:83, 1965.
Herd, J.K., Medhi, M., Uzendoski, D.M. and Saldwar, V.A.: Chorea associated with systemic lupus erythematosus: report of two cases and review of the literature. *Pediatrics 61*:308, 1978.

While the *choreiform twitch,* in which choreiform movements are seen in the fingers when the forearms are extended and supinated, occurs in many otherwise normal children, boys with this twitch have a disproportionately high incidence of reading and spelling disabilities.

Prechtl, H.F.R. and Stemmer, C.J.: The choreiform syndrome in children. *Dev. Med. Child Neurol. 4*:119, 1962.
Wolff, P.H. and Hurwitz, J.: The choreiform syndrome. *Dev. Med. Child Neurol. 8*:160, 1966.

The *Lesch-Nyhan syndrome* is a familial disorder characterized by mental retardation, choreoathetosis, spasticity, opisthotonic spasms, dysphagia, self-multilative biting of lips and fingers and aggressive behavior toward others. Hyperuricemia is a constant finding. Clinical gout may also occur.

Nyhan, W.L.: Clinical features of the Lesch-Nyhan syndrome. *Arch. Int. Med. 130*:186, 1972.

*Huntington's chorea* becomes manifest in childhood in about one per cent of patients. The initial findings may include seizures, articulatory speech defects, rigidity, slow voluntary movements, intention tremor, dystonic posturing, behavioral problems, parkinsonian tremor and progressive dementia. Later, choreiform movements appear with facial grimacing and random jerks that may initially simulate tics.

Byers, R.K. and Dodge, J.A.: Huntington's chorea in children. *Neurology 17*:587, 1967.
Markham, C.H. and Know, J.W.: Observations on Huntington's chorea in childhood. *J. Pediatr. 67*:46, 1965.

Familial paroxysmal choreoathetosis of Mount and Reback occurs rarely as severe transient chorea.

Williams, J. and Stevens, H.: Familial paroxysmal choreoathetosis. *Pediatrics 31*:656, 1963.

Other familial, nonprogressive choreas may occur.

Chun, R.W.M., Daly, R.F., Mansheim, B.J. and Wolcott, G.J.: Benign familial chorea with onset in childhood. *JAMA 225*:1603, 1973.

## TICS

*Tics or nervous spasms* usually present no problem in differential diagnosis. Such repeated, rapid, involuntary contractions of isolated muscles or muscle groups include blinking of the eyelids, sniffing, wrinkling of the nose or forehead, twisting of the mouth, turning of the head to one side, shaking or nodding of the head, coughing, clearing of the throat, twisting of the neck, shrugging of the shoulders and jerking of the extremities. Though the involuntary facial grimacing of chorea may superficially resemble habit spasms, the two are sufficiently dissimilar to permit ready differentiation. Tics are most frequent between the ages of six and ten years. Tic-like mannerisms are also frequent in children who stutter.

*Gilles de la Tourette's syndrome*, which usually begins before the age of ten years, is characterized by tics, initially of the face or head with eye twitching and head jerking, but later involving the rest of the body with complex movements such as kicking and jumping. Involuntary noises are a central feature with barking, grunting, hissing and single words, including obscenities (coprolalia).

Bruun, R.D. and Shapiro, A.K.: Differential diagnosis of Gilles de la Tourette's syndrome. *J. Nerv. Ment. Dis. 155*:328, 1972.

## HYPOTONIA, MUSCLE WEAKNESS

The *"floppy"* or *hypotonic infant* presents a syndrome of many etiologies. Accurate diagnosis often requires electromyographic and other sophisticated muscle studies.

*Atonic cerebral palsy* is probably the most common cause of the floppy infant syndrome.

The term *benign congenital hypotonia* has been suggested for the clinical disorder in which symmetrical, generalized muscular weakness, hypotonia and flaccidity is apparent at birth or in the first year of life. The tendon reflexes are normal. Although these findings are especially notable in the lower extremities, the trunk and the arms are also often involved. Muscular activity is decreased, and motor development is delayed. Gradual improvement, at times complete, is the rule. In other cases, however, there is some residual disability.

Paine, R.S.: The future of the floppy infant: a follow-up study of 133 patients. *Dev. Med. Child Neurol. 5*:115, 1963.
Rabe, E.F.: The hypotonic infant. *J. Pediatr. 64*:422, 1964.

*Werdnig-Hoffmann disease,* or *progressive spinal muscular atrophy,* is characterized by generalized muscular hypotonia, weakness, fibrillation and atrophy. The onset may be prenatal with generalized weakness present at birth. In another group of patients, the onset is between the second and twelfth month while other patients become symptomatic in the second year. The later the onset, the more localized the initial weakness and the longer the life span. Fasciculations in the muscles may be obscured by the infant's subcutaneous fat. Fibrillation and wasting may involve the muscles of the tongue and palate. Breathing becomes diaphragmatic with paradoxical movement of the chest on inspiration due to intercostal weakness. Joint contractures may also occur. Although hyperactive at first, the tendon reflexes gradually diminish. Tremor of the fingers, hands and arms may occur.

Almost any metabolic disorder may cause symptomatic hypotonia (e.g., hypercalcemia, Lowe's syndrome, hypothyroidism, fluid and electrolyte disturbances, mental retardation, inborn errors of metabolism, malnutrition, Pompe's disease and cerebral degenerative disorders). Some infants who appear hypotonic have ligamentous relaxation and cutis hyperelastica. Hypotonia in infants is commonly due to cerebral factors (e.g., hypoxia, hemorrhage, Down's syndrome, and Prader-Willi syndrome). Many hypotonic infants later develop spasticity or athetosis.

*Leigh's syndrome,* or *subacute necrotizing encephalomyelopathy*, is characterized by exacerbations and remissions with hypotonia, ocular palsies, weakness, lethargy, feeding difficulties, failure to thrive, periodic acidosis, nystagmus and progressive motor deterioration. Intermittent hyperventilation, sobs and sighs may also occur.

Eisengart, M.A., Powers, J.M. and Rose, A.L.: Subacute necrotizing encephalomyelopathy. *Am. J. Dis. Child. 217:*730, 1974.
McCandless, D.W. and Hodgkin, W.E.: Subacute necrotizing encephalomyelopathy (Leigh's disease). *Pediatrics 60:*935, 1977.

*Myasthenia gravis*, characterized by muscular weakness and fatigability, may rarely be present at birth (congenital myasthenia gravis) or in infancy. Symptoms and signs include generalized hypotonia; weakness, especially of the facial muscles; feeble cry; cranial nerve palsies; and difficulty in sucking, swallowing and handling secretions. In infants born to affected mothers myasthenia may be transitory. Sudden strabismus, diplopia or ptosis in an older child may be the initial manifestation. Dysphagia and dysarthria may also occur. Muscular weakness is greatest late in the day and after activity. Weakness in the lower extremities, occasionally sudden in onset, may be the most prominent symptom in older children and adolescents. External ophthalmoplegia may also occur.

Drachman, D.B.: Myasthenia gravis. *N. Engl. J. Med. 298:*136, 186, 1978.

*Familial periodic paralysis* is characterized by periodic episodes of flaccid paralysis usually involving the extremities but occasionally generalized. Death may result from respiratory paralysis. Manifestations usually do not appear until adolescence. *Adynamia episodica hereditaria,* or *hyperkalemic familial periodic paralysis,* is characterized by episodes of paralysis accompanied by elevation of the serum potassium.

Rigidity of the back, or "poker spine," due to spasm of the muscles of the back is common with *poliomyelitis*. To sit up from the supine position the child first turns and raises one side on his elbow and forearm. He then places the other hand on the bed behind his back and raises himself into the so-called tripod position, still maintaining a stiff back. If the child is pulled from the supine to the sitting position along with some support underneath his head, the head, neck and back move as an almost inflexible unit. Both maneuvers may be accompanied by pain due to muscle spasm. If head support is not provided, the head may fall backward ("head-drop" sign). Sitting with his lower extremities flexed, the child cannot touch his knees with his forehead. Moderate stiffness of the neck may be present. Lateral movement of the head may be possible to a limited extent. It is difficult or impossible for the child to flex the neck so that his chin touches his chest.

## NEUROPATHY

The *Guillain-Barré syndrome* may be characterized by acute, progressive, symmetrical distal muscular pain and weakness or paralysis and by segmental sensory changes such as paresthesia, hyperesthesia or anesthesia. Stocking or glove hyperesthesia with preservation of position sense may be noted. Tendon reflexes are diminished or absent. Muscle tenderness may be extreme. The manifestations often begin in the feet and progress steadily upward over a period of days. Paralysis of the respiratory musculature and bulbar involvement with difficulty in swallowing and speaking may occur. Some patients demonstrate unilateral or bilateral facial paralysis. Elevation of the optic disk may occur. *Fisher's syndrome*, which may be a variant of Guillain-Barré syndrome, is characterized by external ophthalmoplegia, ataxia, decreased or absent deep tendon reflexes, seventh nerve involvement and an increase in spinal fluid protein. *Tick paralysis* causes progressive motor neuropathy with possible involvement of bulbar and respiratory musculature. An ascending paralysis may be caused by rabies, especially when due to a bat bite.

Marks, H.G., Augustyn, P. and Allen, R.J.: Fisher's syndrome in children. *Pediatrics* 60:726, 1977.

The *floppy infant* syndrome may be caused by polyneuropathy.

*Myeloradiculitis* has occurred after rubella vaccination. Brachial involvement causes paresthesias in the finger tips and shooting pains from the arms to the hands lasting from a few seconds to 30 minutes. Lumbosacral involvement causes aching and pain in the lower extremities, worse on arising. The child walks on his toes with his hips and knees flexed.

Gilmartin, R.C., Jr., Jabbour, J.T. and Duenas, D.A.: Rubella vaccine myeloradiculoneuritis. *J. Pediatr. 80*::406, 1972.

In *infant botulism*, over a period of 24 to 48 hours there is loss of the ability to suck and swallow and progressive weakness. Within one to two weeks the infant is profoundly weak, has no head control and only a feeble cry. Cranial nerve involvement is manifested by ptosis, pupils that react poorly to light and a decreased or absent gag reflex. Botulism in older children begins 18 to 36 hours after ingestion of the toxin with diplopia, photophobia and blurring of vision followed by dysphagia and generalized weakness.

Arnon, S.S., Midura, T.F., Clay, S.A., Wood, R.M. and Chin, J.: Infant botulism. *JAMA* 237:1946, 1977.
Berg, B.O.: Syndrome of infant botulism. *Pediatrics 59*:321, 1977.

*Tick paralysis* is characterized by the sudden onset of irritability, weakness, an ataxic gait, paresthesia, an ascending symmetrical flaccid paralysis and disappearance of the deep reflexes. Bulbar involvment may also occur.

*Peripheral neuritis*, or *multiple neuritis*, is characterized by symmetrical muscular weakness that is more marked distally, tenderness and gradually progressive paralysis. In some cases, proximal weakness affecting the shoulder or hip girdle and simulating muscular dystrophy may occur. Pain and tenderness may be present along the nerves. Paresthesia may also be a complaint. Wrist and foot drop often develop. Respiratory distress may be caused by intercostal or diaphragmatic involvement. Bulbar symptoms may follow pharyngeal paralysis. Involvement of the peripheral autonomic nervous system may be manifested by distal cutaneous redness, pallor, acrocyanosis and hyper- or hypohidrosis. Refsum's disease, lupus erythematosus, polyarteritis and rheumatoid arthritis may be accompanied by a peripheral neuritis. Rapidly developing multiple neuropathy occurs in botulism. Chronic interstitial polyneuropathy may become manifest in childhood and adolescence. Palpable enlargement of peripheral nerves may be noted. Diphtheria toxin may cause paralysis of the palate and blurred vision due to ciliary paralysis.

Watters, G.V. and Barlow, C.F.: Acute and subacute neuropathies. *Pediatr. Clin. N. Am.* *14*:997, 1967.

*Neurogenic limb-girdle muscular atrophy syndrome* (Kugelberg-Welander disease) is characterized by slow progressive muscle atrophy, which simulates that seen in limb-girdle muscle atrophy. There is electromyographic and muscle biopsy evidence of a neurogenic etiology. A form of neurogenic muscle atrophy simulating the facioscapulohumeral form of muscular dystrophy has also been described.

Furukawa, T. and Peter, J.B.: The muscular dystrophies and related disorders. II. Diseases simulating muscular dystrophies. *JAMA 238*:1654, 1978.

*Brachial plexus neuropathy* may be idiopathic or hereditary, unilateral or bilateral, acute or recurrent. A portion of the entire brachial plexus may be involved. Shoulder pain is a prominent initial symptom, followed by rapid, progressive weakness, paresis and atrophy of muscles of the shoulder, arm and perhaps the hand.

Guilozet, N. and Mercer, R.D.: Hereditary recurrent brachial neuropathy. *Am. J. Dis. Child. 125*:884, 1973.
Shaywitz, B.A.: Brachial plexus neuropathy in childhood. *J. Pediatr. 86*:913, 1975.

*Pack* or *rucksack paralysis*, due to traumatic compression of the brachial plexus, is characterized by pain or sensory symptoms in the shoulder or arm followed by weakness or muscle atrophy in the shoulder girdle. The child may be unable to use the involved arm.

Rothner, A.D., Wilbourn, A. and Mercer, R.D.: Rucksack palsy. *Pediatrics 56*:822, 1975.
White, H.H.: Pack palsy: a neurological complication of scouting. *Pediatrics 41*:1001, 1968.

*Sciatic nerve injury* may be caused by injection of antibiotics and other materials in the buttocks of infants. The risk is greatest in premature or small infants and with multiple injections. Neurologic findings include paralytic drop foot, sensory loss and absence of sweating over the distribution of the involved branches. The color and temperature of the foot are abnormal and edema may be present.

Gilles, F.H. and Matson, D.D.: Sciatic nerve injury following misplaced gluteal injection. *J. Pediatr. 76*:247, 1970.

Foot drop, with the child either dragging his foot or developing a steppage gait, may also be due to lead poisoning.

*Fabry's disease* is characterized by acral pain and paresthesias.

*Meralgia paresthetica* causes numbness, burning, itching and paresthesia over the distribution of the lateral femoral cutaneous nerve on the anterolateral aspect of the thigh.

*Peroneal muscular atrophy* (Charcot-Marie-Tooth disease), a familial disorder, may begin in adolescence. Weakness and atrophy of the peroneal and anterior tibial muscles cause early instability of the foot. Foot drop, clawing deformity of the toes, pes cavus and inversion of the foot (stork-like foot) develop bilaterally. Involvement of the hands and forearms occurs later with atrophy first of the thenar and then the hypothenar prominences.

*Reflex sympathetic dystrophy* in an extremity is characterized by persistent burning or aching pain. Hyperesthesia, hypesthesia or paresthesia occur in a glove, stocking or nerve distribution. Discoloration, edema and hyperhidrosis also occur.

Fermaglich, D.R.: Reflex sympathetic dystrophy in children. *Pediatrics 60*:881, 1977.

## PARALYSIS

In infants and young children the degree and extent of paralysis may be difficult to ascertain. The mother usually first notices that the child is not using his extremities normally. Failure to withdraw an extremity in response to appropriate stimuli is also helpful diagnostically if sensation is unimpaired. When raised and then permitted to drop, a paralyzed extremity falls more rapidly than normally. Paralysis due to central nervous lesions is usually flaccid with loss of tone in the paralyzed muscles and an absence of the tendon reflexes. After a week or two, spasticity develops, and the reflexes are hyperactive.

*Causes of flaccid paralysis:*

Poliomyelitis
Guillain-Barré syndrome
Neuromyelitis optica
Postdiphtheritic neuritis
Transverse myelitis
Familial periodic paralysis
Tick paralysis
Myasthenia gravis
Peripheral neuritis
Porphyria
Spinal cord injury at birth
Werdnig-Hoffmann disease
Platybasia
Organic phosphate poisoning
Idiopathic paroxysmal myoglobinuria
Rabies

*Infant botulism* is characterized by profound weakness, hypotonia, ophthalmoplegia, ptosis, absence of the gag reflex and sluggish pupillary light reflex.

McKee, K.T., Jr., Kilroy, A.W., Harrison, W.W. and Schaffner, W.: Botulism in infancy. *Am. J. Dis. Child. 131*:857, 1977.

Muscle pain, weakness and paralysis are features of *idiopathic myoglobinuria.* Acute episodes are characterized by muscle involvement and red or burgundy-colored urine. Striated muscle anywhere in the body may be affected, and widespread motor impairment may be noted. Involvement of the lower extremities is a constant feature. Swallowing, respiration and speech may be affected. Muscle pain usually precedes urinary findings by several hours.

HEMIPARESIS

Epidural, subdural and intracerebral hematomas

Extradural hematoma

Sturge-Weber syndrome

Myxomas of the heart with embolization

Cerebral thrombosis and hemorrhage

Arteritis (Takayasu's disease)

Acute infantile hemiplegia. Usually, no exact cause can be determined for an acute hemiplegia. Encephalitis due to such viral agents as herpes simplex, Coxsackie A–9, herpes zoster, measles and rubella may be etiologic. The onset of acute hemiplegia is usually preceded by generalized or focal seizures, fever of 101° or 103° F. (38.3° to 39.5° C.), coma and hemiplegia. Status epilepticus may persist for hours or days.

Gold, A.P. and Carter, S.: Acute hemiplegia of infancy and childhood. *Pediatr. Clin. N. Am. 23*:413, 1976.

Hilai, S.K., Solomon, G.E., Gold, A.P. and Carter, S.: Primary cerebral arterial occlusive disease. Part I: acute acquired hemiplegia. *Radiology 99*:71, 1971.

Isler, W.: *Acute Hemiplegias and Hemisyndromes in Childhood. Clinics in Developmental Medicine.* Nos. 41, 42. Philadelphia, J. B. Lippincott Co., 1971.

Todd's paralysis. Hemiparesis may follow a convulsive seizure.

Tuberculous meningitis

Fat embolism as a complication of a long-bone fracture

Sickle cell disease

Portnoy, B.A. and Herion, J.C.: Neurological manifestations in sickle-cell disease. *Ann. Int. Med. 76*:643, 1972.

Cyanotic congenital heart disease

Phornphutkul, C., Rosenthal, A., Nadas, A.S. and Berenberg, W.: Cerebrovascular accidents in infants and children with cyanotic congenital heart disease. *Am. J. Cardiol. 32*:329, 1973.

Brain abscess

Subacute bacterial endocarditis

Carotid artery thrombosis may cause an acute contralateral hemiplegia or hemiparesis and an ipsilateral Horner's syndrome. Occlusion of the internal carotid artery may follow nonpenetrating trauma to the head or neck (e.g., blunt trauma to the peritonsillar area as a result of falling on an object carried in the mouth). A 24-hour delay may occur between injury and complication. Palpation of the carotid artery is indicated in these patients, and angiography is required for proof of arterial occlusion.

Faris, A.A., Guth, C., Youmans, R.A. and Poser, C.M.: Internal carotid artery occlusion in children. *Am. J. Dis. Child. 107*:188, 1964.

Pitner, S.E.: Carotid thrombosis due to intraoral trauma. *N. Engl. J. Med. 274*:764, 1966.

Moyamoya syndrome. This angiographic pattern may occur in neurocutaneous syndromes and sickle cell anemia.

Carlson, C.B., Harvey, F.H. and Loop, J.: Progressive alternating hemiplegia in early childhood with basal arterial stenosis and telangiectasis (Moyamoya syndrome). *Neurology 23*:734, 1973.

Hysterical paralysis

Intermittent alternating hemiplegia may occur in early childhood as a familial migraine variant. Recovery occurs in hours to days. As the patient becomes older, a more characteristic pattern of migraine evolves. Although some patients do not experience headaches, there is usually a family history of migraine.

Verret, S. and Steele, J.C.: Alternating hemiplegia in childhood: a report of eight patients with complicated migraine beginning in infancy. *Pediatrics 47*:675, 1971.

## BRAIN TUMORS

Brain tumors enter into the differential diagnosis of many symptoms and signs, including:

Vomiting

Headache

Enlargement of the head
Convulsions
Stupor, coma
Unsteady gait
Eyes
    Diplopia
    Ptosis
    Strabismus
    Papilledema
    Optic atrophy
    Nystagmus
    Failing vision
    Visual field defects
Endocrine disorders
    Precocious puberty
    Hypogenitalism
    Obesity
    Gigantism
    Understature
Cranial nerve palsies
Paresis of extremities
Tremor
Failure to thrive
Muscular hypotonia
Reflex changes
Abnormal neurologic signs
Stiffness of the neck
Torticollis
Behavioral disturbances – listlessness, irritability, change in behavior, deterioration in school performance

Some of the common diagnostic considerations are reviewed below. Brain scanning and computerized axial tomography are the preferred methods of diagnosis of focal or expanding intracranial lesions.

Bachman, D.S., Hodges, F.J., III and Freeman, J.M.: Computerized axial tomography in neurologic disorders of children. *Pediatrics 59*:352, 1977.
McCullough, D.C., Kufta, C., Axelbaum, S.P. and Schellinger, D.: Computerized axial tomography in clinical pediatrics. *Pediatrics 59*:171, 1977.
Yalaz, K. and Treves, S.: Brain scanning and cerebral radioisotope angiography (CRA) in children. *Pediatrics 54*:696, 1974.

**Tumors of the Posterior Midline of the Cerebellum.** An important clinical feature is a staggering, unsteady, swaying, wide-based ataxic gait. The ataxia is more truncal than appendicular. Truncal ataxia is also manifested by swaying or gradual tilting of the trunk in the sitting position. Though incoordination is usually only mild or moderate in the upper extremities, it is particularly prominent in the trunk and lower extremities. Adiadochokinesis and an intention tremor may be present. Muscular hypotonia and hypoactive tendon reflexes are usually found. Hyperactive reflexes and a positive Babinski's sign occur if pressure is exerted upon the pyramidal tracts. Nuchal rigidity is occasionally present. Nystagmus, usually horizontal but occasionally vertical, is seen in most patients. Strabismus is frequent. If the vermis of the cerebellum is symmetrically involved, nystagmus may not occur, and muscle tone may not change.

**Tumors of Cerebellar Hemispheres.** The initial symptom may be headache, vomiting, unsteady gait or a change in behavior. Pain in the neck, failing vision or strabismus may also be presenting complaints. Cerebellar signs may be absent early and only demonstrated by testing the gait. Truncal ataxia may become evident as unsteadiness when the child is asked to walk a straight line or change his direction quickly or may be manifested as swaying of the trunk when the child is sitting or standing still. The tendency to move or fall toward the involved side may be elicited by having the child walk around a chair or take a few steps forward and then backward. The shoulder on the side of the tumor may be hunched upward as the child walks, and the automatic swinging action of the ipsilateral arm may not occur. The finger-to-nose test, the heel-to-knee test and adiadochokinesis may all demonstrate incoordination. An intention tremor may also be noted. Nuchal rigidity and retraction of the head may occasionally be seen, and the head may be tilted so that the occiput points toward the shoulder on the involved side. Muscular hypotonia and hypoactive reflexes are common, especially on the side of the tumor.

Nystagmus, especially on horizontal gaze, is common, usually evident when the patient focuses upon some point (fixation nystagmus). The nystagmus is slow and coarse on looking toward the side of the tumor and quick and minimal or absent when the gaze is to the opposite side. Headache, vomiting and paralysis of the lateral rectus muscles are also frequent.

**Tumors of the Fourth Ventricle.** Vomiting, the most frequent manifestation of tumors in this area, may persist for several months before other signs appear. Findings are similar to those with tumors of the cerebellar vermis.

**Tumors of the Brain Stem.** Cranial nerve involvement, especially of nerves V, VI and VII, is characteristic of tumors of the pons and medulla. Bulbar symptoms may include difficulty in swallowing. Nystagmus is often noted on horizontal and, occasionally, on upward gaze. Ptosis may also be present. The gait is often ataxic. Tendon reflexes are frequently hyperactive, and ankle clonus and a positive Babinski's sign commonly are present. Cerebellar signs often occur. Signs of increased intracranial pressure may not be present.

Panitch, H.S. and Berg, B.O.: Brain stem tumors of childhood and adolescence. *Am. J. Dis. Child. 119*:465, 1970.

**Tumors Involving the Hypothalamus and Optic Chiasm.** These lesions cause increased intracranial pressure, including headache, vomiting, and visual field defects. Involvement of the hypothalamus may cause endocrinopathy with obesity, diabetes insipidus, understature and sexual precocity or infantilism. Hyperthermia may also occur.

*Increased intracranial pressure* due to cerebral edema, neoplasm, abscess or other cause is characterized by headache, vomiting, personality and mood changes and papilledema. Lethargy, stupor, coma and systolic hypertension may occur later.

Batzdorf, U.: The management of cerebral edema in pediatric practice. *Pediatrics 58*:78, 1976.
Bell, W.E. and McCormick, W.F.: *Increased Intracranial Pressure in Children*. 2nd ed. Philadelphia, W. B. Saunders Co., 1978.
Rosman, N.P.: Increased intracranial pressure in childhood. *Pediatr. Clin. N. Am. 21*:483, 1974.

*Pseudotumor cerebri*, or benign intracranial hypertension, is usually characterized by papilledema, abducens palsy, sudden headache, vomiting and diplopia. Other symptoms of increased intracranial pressure may be present.

*Brain abscess* is to be considered in the differential diagnosis of an intracranial mass, localized neurologic findings, headache or fever. Patients with congenital heart disease are predisposed to develop a brain abscess.

*Platybasia or basilar impression of the skull* is usually congenital. Flattening of the base of the skull leads to a decrease in the size of the posterior fossa. A Klippel-Feil syndrome may also be present. Compression of the cerebellum, medulla and other structures in that area may cause suboccipital pain, stiffness of the neck and hyperextension of the head and neck. Later, unsteady gait, weakness of the extremities, cerebellar ataxia, nystagmus and involvement of the cranial nerves may occur.

In the *Arnold-Chiari malformation*, the child may present with dizziness, ataxia, syncope, gait disturbance and poor coordination. The lower cranial nerves may also be involved. Spastic paraparesis may eventually occur.

## SPINAL CORD

*Spina bifida occulta*, or incomplete closure of the vertebral laminae, is present usually in the lumbosacral region in about 25 per cent of children. While often asymptomatic, this defect may occur along with myelodysplasia in patients with an abnormal gait, urinary incontinence due to impaired sphincter tone or muscular and sensory changes in the lower extremities. Cutaneous lesions that may occur along the midline of the back in patients with spina bifida occulta, spinal dysraphism or diastematomyelia include tufts of hair, dimples or dermal sinuses, subcutaneous lipomas, pigmented nevi, hemangiomas, bony protrusion and scoliosis.

Occult spinal dysraphism or myelodysplasia represent developmental variants in the most distal portion of the neural tube. Clinical manifestations include impaired urinary control, fecal incontinence, deformities of the feet and delay or awkwardness in walking. With a tight filum terminale, disturbances in gait such as limping and stumbling are common. Weakness and atrophy of muscles and aching pain occur in the lower extremities. Tightness of the hamstrings and the achilles tendon is present. Urinary incontinence is frequent.

Anderson, F.M.: Occult spinal dysraphism: a series of 73 cases. *Pediatrics 55*:826, 1975.

The *meningocele* is a spherical, membranous or skin-covered cystic protrusion anywhere along the spinal column but most common in the lumbar or lumbosacral area. With a meningocele, nervous tissue is not evident within the protruding sac and signs of neurologic dysfunction such as muscular weakness or paralysis of the lower extremities, loss of sphincter tone or changes in cutaneous sensation are not seen. An anterior meningocele may be palpated on rectal or vaginal examination as a smooth, resilient pelvic mass. Persistent constipation may begin in infancy. With a *myelomeningocele*, nervous tissue is involved and neurologic findings are present, including flaccid paralysis, sensory deficits and neurogenic bowel and bladder dysfunction. When fatty tissue accompanies these defects, the terms *lipomeningocele* and *lipomyelomeningocele* are used. The Arnold-Chiari malformation is frequently associated with a myelomeningocele.

Current approaches to evaluation and management of children with myelomeningocele. Action Committee on Myelodysplasia, Section on Urology, American Academy of Pediatrics. *Pediatrics 63*:663, 1979.

The *myelocele* is the most extreme of these defects with neural tissue directly exposed at the site of the lesion or covered by moist granulation tissue. *Encephaloceles* are meningoceles and myelomeningoceles that occur through bony defects in the skull (cranium bifidum) or at nasal, nasopharyngeal, frontal, parietal or occipital sites. The occipital location is the most common, and lesions there usually contain neural tissue.

Molnar, G.E. and Taft, L.T.: Pediatric rehabilitation, Part II: spina bifida limb deficiencies. *Cur. Prob. Pediatr. 7*:3 (Feb.) 1977.

*Syringomyelia and hydromelia* may accompany other developmental anomalies of the neuroaxis. The clinical manifestations, which are initially unilateral and later bilateral, include numbness of the fingers and weakness of the shoulder girdle, paravertebral, hand and finger muscles; muscle atrophy, and thoracic scoliosis.

*A congenital dermal sinus* is an epithelial-lined tract that extends inward from the skin to the subcutaneous tissue, the meninges or into the spinal cord or brain. An epidermoid or dermoid cyst along the course of the sinus may produce neurologic symptoms due to compression or infection. Bacterial contamination may lead to meningitis or an abscess with Staphylococcus aureus as the most likely etiologic agent.

The sinus opening may be pinpoint or dimple-like and surrounded by a small pigmented nevus or capillary hemangioma. While it may be present anywhere along the midline of the scalp or back, it is most frequent in the occipital, cervical, thoracic or lumbar region. The opening may be best seen in bright light or through a plus ophthalmoscopic lens. A congenital dermal sinus in the scalp may not be evident until the head has been shaved. Hairs may project from the sinus, and occasionally a sebaceous or other discharge may cause local excoriation of the skin. There may be a localized thickening of the scalp or a palpable subcutaneous mass at the site. A roentgenogram may demonstrate an underlying osseous defect.

Prompt recognition of an *epidural abscess* is of utmost importance. The earliest clinical findings are back pain and tenderness over the spinous processes in the involved area. The patient may be unwilling to lie down. The presence of an accompanying pyogenic skin lesion makes the diagnosis presumptive. Sensory impairment, weakness and paralysis of the lower extremities are late findings.

**Spinal Cord Tumors.** The early diagnosis of spinal cord tumors in children, especially in infants, is difficult. Intraspinal tumors are most common in the first four years of life. Symptoms are often insidious with pain in the back, neck and extremities; weakness of the extremities, most commonly the lower; alteration of reflexes; and diminution in sensation below the involved level. Unexplained, intermittent or persistent pain in the neck, back, trunk or extremities should always suggest an intraspinal tumor. Pain due to a spinal cord tumor may be precipitated or accentuated by coughing, sneezing, jumping, flexion of the neck or back, being picked up or by straight leg raising. The infant with a tumor may be unable to kick one lower extremity or use one hand. There may be a history of constipation and urinary retention or incontinence. Stiffness of the neck and back due to paraspinal muscle spasm is a frequent complaint. Torticollis, scoliosis, or kyphosis may occur. Flexion of the back may be so restricted that the child does not bend over to pick up an object but rather keeps a poker spine and flexes his knees. In some instances the onset may be sudden with weakness of the extremities, stiff neck, fever and an increased number of cells in the cerebrospinal fluid. Roentgenograms should be taken of the *entire* spine when a spinal cord tumor is suspected.

> Matson, D.D. and Tachdjian, M.O.: Intraspinal tumors in infants and children. *Postgrad. Med. 34*:279, 1963.

Spinal cord injury at birth is discussed on page 168.

*Transverse myelopathy* may be characterized by back or root pain and paresthesia or sensory loss below the level of the lesion. While in some patients paresis of the arms occurs first, in others the process begins in the lower extremities and moves upward. Flaccid initially, the muscle weakness may in time become spastic. Urinary and fecal incontinence or retention occasionally occur. Motor and sensory impairment may demonstrate laterality. Transverse myelitis may be caused by accidental retrograde intra-arterial injection of penicillin

> Altrocchi, P.H.: Acute transverse myelopathy. *Arch. Neurol. 9*:111, 1963.
> Shaw, E.B.: Transverse myelitis from injection of penicillin. *Am. J. Dis. Child. 11*:548, 1966.

*Neuromyelitis optica* is characterized by impairment of vision and neurologic symptoms, which may simulate transverse myelopathy or multiple sclerosis.

In *diastematomyelia* a bony or fibrocartilaginous septum produces a sagittal division and transfixation of the spinal cord or cauda equina. The clinical picture includes delay or difficulty in walking, an abnormal gait, muscle atrophy and weakness, shortening of the lower extremities, absence of tendon reflexes, deformities of the feet and urinary incontinence.

The *caudal regression syndrome* consists of sacral agenesis with associated defects that may include a neurogenic bladder, paralysis of the lower extremities and defects of the feet, especially equinovarus deformities. The baby may lie in a frog-leg position.

> Passarge, E. and Lenz, W.: Syndrome of caudal regression in infants of diabetic mothers: observations of further cases. *Pediatrics 37*:672, 1966.

*Herniation of the lumbar intervertebral disc* leads to back pain and sciatica. Findings include a slight scoliosis, decreased lumbar lordosis, paravertebral muscle spasm and positive straight leg raising. Sensory and deep tendon reflex changes are variably present. A history of trauma is frequent.

> Bradford, D.S. and Garcia, A.: Herniations of the lumbar intervertebral disk in children and adolescents. *JAMA 210*:2045, 1969.

## MENINGITIS

Young infants with meningitis may not demonstrate the nuchal rigidity, extension of the head, opisthotonus and positive Kernig's and Brudzinski's signs characteristically present in older infants and children. A tense or bulging fontanel is an especially important sign. Fever, vomiting and diarrhea may occur or the infant may be unusually irritable or drowsy. A convulsion may be the first symptom.

Symptoms of meningeal irritation may occur with leptospirosis.

The *Vogt-Koyanangi-Harada syndrome* (uveomeningoencephalitic syndrome) is characterized by meningoencephalitis, uveitis, pigment loss in the skin, alopecia and dysacousia.

Riehl, J-L. and Andrews, J.M.: The uveomeningoencephalitic syndrome. *Neurology 16*:603, 1966.

Swartz, M. and Dodge, P.: Bacterial meningitis — a review of selected aspects. I. General clinical features, special problems and unusual meningeal reactions mimicking bacterial meningitis. *N. Engl. J. Med. 272*:779, 1965.

*Behçet's disease* may cause a meningoencephalitis syndrome with stiff neck and headache or brain stem symptoms such as extraocular nerve palsies, nystagmus, ataxia and extensor toe signs.

## MENINGISMUS

Acute infectious diseases such as pneumonia, pyelonephritis, salmonellosis, typhoid fever and bacillary dysentery may be accompanied by headache, nuchal rigidity, opisthotonus, a positive Kernig's sign and convulsions even though a true meningitis may not be present. Since meningitis cannot be excluded clinically in these instances, a lumbar puncture is necessary. Meningismus may occur in patients with rabies.

## GENERAL REFERENCES

Bell, W.E. and McCormick, W.F.: *Neurologic Infections in Children.* Philadelphia, W. B. Saunders Co., 1975.

Ford, F.R.: *Diseases of the Nervous System in Infancy, Childhood and Adolescence.* 4th ed. Springfield, Charles C Thomas, 1959.

Ingraham, F.C. and Matson, D.D.: *Neurosurgery of Infancy and Childhood.* Springfield, Charles C Thomas, 1954.

Menkes, J.H.: *Textbook of Child Neurology.* Philadelphia, Lea & Febiger, 1974.

Weiner, H.L., Bresnan, M.J. and Levitt, L.P.: *Pediatric Neurology for The House Officer.* Baltimore, Williams & Wilkins Co., 1977.

# CHAPTER 27

# THE SKELETAL SYSTEM

## CONSTITUTIONAL DISEASES OF BONE

The skeletal dysplasias constitute several dozen distinct syndromes with a wide variety of clinical presentations. Because of their wide heterogeneity, classification is difficult. The International Nomenclature for Constitutional Diseases of Bone, revised in 1977, classifies these disorders into *osteochondrodysplasias* (abnormalities of cartilage or bone growth and development or both); *dysostoses* (malformation of individual bones, singly or in combination); *idiopathic osteolyses*; and *chromosomal aberrations: primary metabolic abnormalities*. Some of the more common osteochondrodysplasias are discussed in this section.

International nomenclature of constitutional diseases of bone. Revision of May, 1977. *J. Pediatr. 93*:614, 1978.

McKusick, V.A.: *Heritable Disorders of Connective Tissue*. 4th ed. St. Louis, C. V. Mosby Co., 1972.

Sillence, D.O., Rimoin, D.L. and Lachman, R.: Neonatal dwarfism. *Pediatr. Clin. N. Am. 25*:453, 1978.

Spranger, J.W., Langer, L.O. and Wiedemann, H-R.: *Bone Dysplasias: An Atlas of Constitutional Disorders of Skeletal Development*. Philadelphia, W. B. Saunders Co., 1974.

### OSTEOCHONDRODYSPLASIAS

*Achondroplasia* is usually diagnosed readily by inspection but differentiation from other causes of short limb dwarfism may be difficult. While the characteristic skeletal features may be present at birth, occasionally the manifestations are incomplete or atypical. In the latter event roentgenographic examination of the long bones may be helpful. The extremities, especially the thighs and upper arms, are short and wide with their normal curvatures exaggerated. The hands, often of the trident type, may not extend below the waist. Usually, the patient cannot approximate his fingers when extended, especially the third and fourth. Enlargement of the epiphyses may limit extension at the shoulder, supination of the forearm and abduction of the hip. The head is relatively large and the forehead and mandible prominent. The bridge of the nose is depressed, the tip broad and turned up. The length of the vertebral column is relatively normal. Lordosis, protrusion of the abdomen and prominent buttocks are other characteristic features.

In *hypochondroplasia*, only a slight degree of rhizomelic (root of the extremities) dwarfism is present, and understature is not marked.

*Metaphyseal chondrodysplasia type McKusick (cartilage-hair hypoplasia)* is characterized by short-limbed dwarfism simulating achondroplasia without the head enlargement or depressed nasal bridge. Additional features include ligamentous relaxation in the fingers and hands and sparse, fine, silky, light-colored scalp hair, eyebrows and eyelashes. The hair fractures easily. The patient may be almost completely bald.

McKusick, V.A., Eldrige, R., Hostetler, J.A., Ruangwit, U. and Egeland, J.A.: Dwarfism in the Amish. II. Cartilage-hair hypoplasia. *Bull. Johns Hopkins Hosp. 116*:285, 1965.

*Diastrophic dysplasia* is manifested by severe dwarfism with shortening of the limbs more proximally than distally, club feet, ulnar deviation of the hands, short fingers with extension contracture and fusion of proximal interphalangeal joints, hypermobile "hitchhiker" thumbs, scoliosis at times associated with kyphosis, tendency to subluxation and dislocation of the joints, limitation of motion of large joints with flexion contraction of knee and hip, and cyst-like masses on the ears.

Langer, L.O., Jr.: Diastrophic dwarfism in early infancy. *Am. J. Roentgenol. Radium Ther. Nucl. Med. 93*:399, 1965.
Walker, B.A. et al.: Diastrophic dwarfism. *Medicine 51*:41, 1972.

*Chondrodysplasia punctata* (*congenital stippled epiphyses*), which occurs as an autosomal dominant (Conradi's syndrome), an autosomal recessive (rhizomelic type) and an X-linked form, is characterized by shortening of the extremities, most pronounced proximally in the rhizomelic type, and by other skeletal anomalies such as joint contractures, dislocated hips and club feet. Involvement may be limited to one extremity or one side of the body in the dominant form. Flat face, saddle nose, optic atrophy and mental retardation are other findings. Congenital cataracts are frequently present. Failure to thrive may occur in the severe form of the disorder. Roentgenologic examination may reveal multiple punctate calcific deposits in the epiphyses.

Tasker, W.G., Mastri, A.R. and Gold, A.P.: Chondrodystrophia calcificans congenita: (dysplasia epiphysalis punctata). *Am. J. Dis. Child. 119*:122, 1970.

*Chondroectodermal dysplasia* (the *Ellis–van Creveld syndrome*) is characterized by features of both chondrodystrophy and ectodermal dysplasia. The extremities are decreased in length, relatively more distally than proximally. Genu valgum is regularly present. Polydactyly is also found with a sixth digit on the ulnar aspect of each hand. Ectodermal defects include fine, sparse hair; small, deformed nails; defective teeth; and fusion of the upper lip to the underlying gum. Congenital heart disease may be present.

McKusick, V.A., Egeland, J.A., Eldridge, R. and Krusen, D.E.: Dwarfism in the Amish. I. The Ellis–van Creveld syndrome. *Bull. Johns Hopkins Hosp. 115*:306, 1964.

*Spondyloepiphyseal dysplasia congenita* is characterized by a normal-shaped head and short neck, varus deformity of the feet, barrel-shaped chest, pectus carinatum, cleft palate, genu valgum, deformity of the knees, marked shortening of the spine, exaggerated lumbar lordosis and a waddling gait. Myopia and retinal detachment may also occur. As the child becomes older, the clinical appearance resembles Morquio's disease.

Spranger, J.A. and Langer, L.O., Jr.: Spondyloepiphyseal dysplasia congenita. *Radiology 94*:313, 1970.

In *pseudoachondroplasia*, sometimes called a type of spondyloepiphyseal dysplasia and usually not diagnosed until the child is one to two years of age, the extremities are affected more than the spine. Mild kyphoscoliosis develops. The head and face are normal. The child is generally dwarfed.

In *metaphyseal chondrodysplasia* the joints are enlarged, the upper extremities are shorter than the lower, and the child is severely dwarfed. Severe anterior bowing of the legs may occur along with a waddling gait.

*Multiple epiphyseal dysplasia* is characterized by epiphyseal dysgenesis, stubby digits and dwarfism. The patients experience joint pain, stiffness and difficulty in walking. A waddling gait is present if the hip joints are involved.

*Enchondromatosis* (*Ollier's disease*) becomes clinically manifest early in life, owing to the presence of enchondromas near the end of the shafts. Usually unilateral in distribution, the lesions may be single or multiple. Minimal involvement may occur on the contralateral side. Shortening of the involved bones results, and facial asymmetry may develop. Rarely, a few cartilaginous exostoses may be present.

Occasionally, the localization of multiple enchondromata may be confined to the hands and feet, especially the phalanges, causing macrodactyly. *Maffucci's syndrome*, a variant of this process, is characterized by deformities of the hands and feet, hypertrophy and cutaneous cavernous angiomas.

*Multiple cartilaginous exostoses* is characterized by single or multiple hard, irregular bony projections that grow from the epiphyseal region of the bone toward the diaphysis. Exostoses usually appear in the preschool age or later. There is a familial incidence in most cases. The lesions are usually bilateral and vary considerably in form. Although most frequently occurring around the knees, they may also involve the phalanges, ribs, vertebrae, scapulae and the base of the skull. Occasionally, some shortening in height does occur.

## PRIMARY METABOLIC ABNORMALITIES

*Hurler's syndrome* may first be suspected because of a dorsolumbar kyphosis in a young infant. Similar kyphosis may be seen in patients with fucosidosis, mannosidosis and the mucolipidoses. Other clinical characteristics become evident over time. There is usually a large head with a broad, turned-up or pug-shaped nose; coarse facial features; large bushy eyebrows; prominent supraorbital ridges; and a short neck. The fingers are held in partial flexion, and the hands are claw-like. The fourth and fifth fingers may be incurved. Both the hands and feet are relatively broad and short. Limitation of motion, chiefly of extension, may occur at the shoulder, elbow, knee and other joints. Other manifestations include corneal clouding, mental retardation and hepatosplenomegaly.

*Morquio's disease* (mucopolysaccharidoses IV) usually does not become clinically manifest until the end of the first year of life or later. The head is relatively large, and the base of the nose may be flat and broad. The most significant physical findings occur in the trunk. The vertical height of the chest is shortened, and the anteroposterior diameter is elongated. Anteriorly the sternum bulges forward to an almost horizontal position. Posteriorly, there is thoracic kyphosis. Shortening of the extremities is not marked. Characteristically, the epiphyses are enlarged, and flexion deformities may be present at the hip and knees. Genu valgum and pes planus also occur. The child stands in a "jump" or crouching posture. Because of this position and the shortening of the trunk, the patient's hands extend to the level of the knees. Cataracts are a later complication.

## EXTREMITIES

During infancy the extremities appear relatively short. Until puberty the rate of growth of the extremities, particularly the lower, exceeds that of the trunk. At puberty, the rate is about the same. After puberty, owing to the earlier epiphyseal closure in the long bones, the growth of the extremities decelerates more rapidly than that of the trunk. Premature growth arrest may occur in an epiphysis secondary to trauma or infection.

*Amelia* refers to a congenital absence of all extremities; *ectromelia* indicates absence of an individual extremity; and *hemimelia* denotes defects of the distal portions of the extremities. *Congenital constriction bands* (Streeter's dysplasia) may encircle the digits, feet, hands or other parts of the extremities.

Baker, C.J. and Rudolph, A.J.: Congenital ring constrictions and intrauterine amputations. *Am. J. Dis. Child. 121*:393, 1971.
Hall, C.B., Brooks, M.B. and Dennis, J.F.: Congenital skeletal deficiencies of the extremities. Classification and fundamentals of treatment. *JAMA 181*:590, 1962.

*Hemihypertrophy*, characterized by enlargement of one half of the body or by enlargement of one or both extremities and the adjoining parts, may be idiopathic or occur in the Beckwith-Wiedemann and the Russell-Silver syndromes. When accompanied by aniridia, a Wilms' tumor may also be present. *Neurofibromatosis* may also be associated with hypertrophy of a body part.

*Congenital arteriovenous fistula* may cause enlargement of an extremity along with increased skin temperature, varices, pain and a local bruit.

Patients with *arachnodactyly*, homocystinuria and the mucosal neuroma syndrome have long, thin extremities, hands, feet, fingers and toes.

*Infantile cortical hyperostosis (Caffey's syndrome)* is characterized by deep, diffuse, firm and, at times, exquisitely tender, nonpitting swellings over bones with cortical hyperostosis. Swelling of the face, especially over the mandible, is characteristic. The clavicles, ribs, scapulae and the long bones of the extremities may be involved, but those of the hands and feet are usually not. Fever and irritability may be associated symptoms. Caffey's syndrome is usually limited to the first six months of life.

A similar clinical picture may occur in infants with *vitamin A poisoning* in the latter half of the first year or later. Pressure over the long bones causes pain. Facial or mandibular swelling does not occur.

*Congenital bowing deformities* and thickening of the long bones, probably attributable to abnormal intrauterine positioning, with cutaneous dimpling over the center of the curvatures, may occur. These deformities usually disappear during infancy. Skin dimples over the extremities may also occur with hypophosphatasia and over the knees in congenital rubella.

*Rickets*, today usually due to familial hypophosphatemic vitamin D resistance, vitamin D dependency or chronic anticonvulsant therapy, causes epiphyseal enlargement at the wrists and ankles. Epiphyseal enlargement, angulation and deformity of the extremities along with costochondral beading may occur early with *hypophosphatasia*.

Beale, M.G., Chan, J.C.M., Oldham, S.B. and DeLuca, H.F.: Vitamin D: the discovery of its metabolites and their therapeutic applications. *Pediatrics 57*:729, 1976.

Epiphyseal enlargements also occur in Morquio's syndrome, chondrodystrophy and primary hyperparathyroidism.

Infants with *scurvy* experience severe pain when their extremities are handled, owing to exquisitely tender swellings over the femurs and other long bones. In addition to a pseudoparalysis of the lower extremities, the infant lies supine in the frog-leg position with the lower extremities flexed at the knees and hips and the thighs abducted and externally rotated.

Osteochondritis due to *congenital syphilis* may occur during the first three months of life. Physical findings include local swelling and pain on passive motion. The extremity is not moved voluntarily.

The early symptoms of *osteomyelitis* include pain and localized tenderness over the involved bone. Point tenderness, an especially suggestive diagnostic sign, is by no means common. Occasionally, the pain and tenderness are diffuse and actual bone pain difficult to elicit. Muscle spasm may also be noted in the surrounding area. Soft tissue swelling and redness may not be present initially but often develop within a short time. Tenderness on deep palpation between the ischial tuberosity and greater trochanter is an early finding in osteomyelitis of the femoral neck. Osteomyelitis of the pelvic bones may present with fever, abnormal gait and point tenderness. Bone scanning is indicated if osteomyelitis is suspected.

Dich, V.Q., Nelson, J.D. and Haltalin, K.C.: Osteomyelitis in infants and children. *Am. J. Dis. Child* 129:1273, 1975.

Edwards, M.S., Baker, C.J., Granberry, W.M. and Barrett, F.F.: Pelvic osteomyelitis in children. *Pediatrics* 61:62, 1978.

Weissberg, E.D., Smith, A.L. and Smith, D.H.: Clinical features of neonatal osteomyelitis. *Pediatrics* 53:505, 1974.

Exquisitely painful, tense and slightly warm swellings may occur over one or more extremities in *sickle cell anemia*. Frequently, an early osteomyelitis cannot be excluded.

*Traumatic separation of an epiphysis* may occur in the newborn infant, causing tenderness and local swelling. The affected extremity is not used, and manipulation causes the infant to cry. Although the upper humeral epiphysis is probably most frequently involved, similar separation may occur at the elbow, wrist, knee or ankle. If the upper extremity is involved, the infant can still flex his arm, though this may be painful. This movement is not possible with a brachial plexus injury.

*Subluxation of the head of the radius* occurs frequently in preschool children, especially between the ages of two and four years. Traction on the extended arm of the child causes the head of the radius to be displaced distally. The child complains of pain that may be localized in the wrist rather than in the elbow. The extremity is not used but held at the side with the elbow slightly flexed and the hand pronated. Passive motion of the elbow joint is possible and painless in all directions except supination. Limitation of supination is diagnostic. Roentgenographic examination of the elbow joint may rule in or out a fracture or dislocation but not a subluxation. At times, the subluxation corrects itself spontaneously during sleep. Active reduction may be accomplished by flexion of the child's elbow to about a right angle followed by supination of the forearm past the point of resistance while pressure is maintained on the head of the radius with the examiner's thumb. An audible or palpable click and the ability of the child to supinate his arm indicate that the subluxation has been corrected.

Subluxation or dislocation of the radial head occurs in the *nail-patella syndrome*.

*Madelung's deformity* may appear in adolescent children, usually bilaterally. Radial deviation of the hand occurs along with dorsal bowing of the ulna and prominence of the ulnar styloid. Dorsiflexion of the wrist is limited. Dyschondrosteosis is the most common cause of Madelung's deformity; this deformity may also occur in Turner's syndrome or as an isolated congenital deformity. Curving of the radius may be due to multiple cartilaginous exostoses.

Herdman, R.C., Langer, L.O., Jr. and Good, R.A.: Dyschondrosteosis. *J. Pediatr. 68*:432, 1966.

*Cubitus valgus*, or increased carrying angle of the arm, may be present in Turner's syndrome.


## FRACTURES

The humerus and the femur are occasionally fractured during birth. Local tenderness may occur without much swelling and the infant does not move the extremity. Fractures in infants and young children should always raise the suspicion of *physical abuse*.

Most fractures in children are accompanied by local pain, swelling and tenderness. Deformity, crepitation and a point of false motion are not present in greenstick fractures.

Fractures that extend into or through an epiphyseal line are always a source of concern because of the possibility of partial or complete premature arrest of epiphyseal growth. Fractures through the distal femoral epiphysis without displacement are often overlooked.

Fractures about the elbow, especially supracondylar or intercondylar fractures, are difficult to manage. A complicating Volkmann's ischemic contracture is always a possibility.

Rang, M.C. and Willis, R.B.: Fractures and sprains. *Pediatr. Clin. N. Am. 24*:749, 1977.

*Osteogenesis imperfecta* is characterized by frequent fractures. Intrauterine fractures account for the deformities present at birth. In osteogenesis imperfecta tarda, fractures do not occur during infancy. Fractures of the long bones are a complication of *hypophosphatasia*. *Fibrous dysplasia* is a diagnostic consideration when a pathologic fracture occurs in a patient with *cafe-au-lait* lesions.

The early findings in *wringer-arm injury* may be deceptively minimal. The injured extremity, which initially appears only mildly swollen or ecchymotic, may within hours become edematous due to extensive subcutaneous and subfascial extravasation of blood.


## HANDS

During much of the first two months of life, the hands remain closed or fisted. A palmar grasp reflex is present. During the third and fourth months the infant may bring both arms toward the midline, at first somewhat uncertainly, but later with enough coordination to grasp a rattle or other object placed in the midline (raking motions). With further maturation the infant begins to use the radial aspect instead of a raking motion or his entire hand to grasp objects. He may then change from a somewhat simultaneous and bilateral to a more lateralized approach. True handedness is not definitely established until the early preschool period.

The development of more advanced prehensile ability with the use of the thumb and index finger occurs at the age of about nine months. A little later, neuromuscular progress permits the infant to release and then to throw objects. The 15-month-old child can do this in the sitting position and a few months later while standing.

Skill in the use of the hands may be delayed with cerebral palsy. With spasticity, the clenched position of the fingers is retained much longer than normal, and the fingers are not easily extended to grasp objects. Each upper extremity can be checked in an infant suspected to have a hemiparesis by placing a cloth over the baby's face and alternately restraining each extremity while observing his ability to remove the cloth with the contralateral hand.

In *Hurler's syndrome* the hand is broad and short. The fingers are held in a clawlike position with limitation of extension. The fourth and fifth fingers are incurved.

The whistling face syndrome or craniocarpotarsal dysplasia is characterized by contractures and ulnar deviation of the fingers.

*Campodactlyly*, or flexure contractures of the fingers, may occur on a genetic or sporadic basis.

Goodman, R.M., Katznelson, M.B-M. and Manor, S.: Campodactyly: occurrence in two new genetic syndromes and its relationship to other syndromes. *J. Med. Genet.* 9:203, 1972.

*Clinodactyly* is the term applied to medial or lateral deviation of a finger.

*Marchesani's syndrome* is characterized by short, stubby fingers, thick palms and a spade-like hand. Understature, spherophakia, severe myopia, glaucoma and ectopia lentis are other features.

The *Aarskog syndrome* is characterized, in part, by brachydactyly with clinodactyly of the fifth fingers.

Patients with *chondrodystrophy* may have a trident hand with spaces between the thumb and first finger and between the third and fourth fingers. The hands and feet are short and broad, and the index, middle and fourth fingers are about equal in length.

*Clubbing of the fingers* occurs most commonly in children with chronic pulmonary disease such as cystic fibrosis, bronchiectasis, empyema and lung abscess; cyanotic congenital heart disease; chronic liver disease; and long-standing gastrointestinal disorders characterized by diarrhea. Rarely, clubbing may be familial. While advanced clubbing is readily evident, assessment of early changes may be difficult. One method for differentiation is the ratio of the distal phalangeal depth (DPD) of the index finger at the base of the nail to the distal interphalangeal joint depth (IPD). If by simple visual estimation from the side of one or both index fingers, the DPD exceeds the IPD, the patient has clubbing.

Waring, W.W., Wilkinson, R.W., Wiebe, R.A., Faul, B.C. and Hilman, B.C.: Quantitation of digital clubbing in children. *Am. Rev. Resp. Dis.* 104:166, 1971.

Short, stubby fingers and toes with a drumstick appearance and spoon-shaped nails along with short stature, osteopetrosis and bossing of the skull are seen in *pycnodysostosis*. When the distal phalanges are absent, the soft tissues appear telescoped.

Elmore, S.M.: Pycnodysostosis: a review. *J. Bone Joint Surg.* 49-A:153, 1967.

Infants with *Down's syndrome* have short digits, low-set thumbs, incurved little fingers and often a simian palmar crease.

*Shortening of the digits*, particularly the thumb and big toe, occurs in many patients with progressive myositis ossificans. The metacarpals are often shortened in patients with pseudohypoparathyroidism, pseudo-pseudohypoparathyroidism, Turner's, Larsen's and the nevoid basal cell carcinoma syndromes and in some normal children. As a result, there is apparent shortening of the thumb and the fourth and fifth fingers. In the presence of a short fourth metacarpal, a dimple is present over the metacarpal-phalangeal joint (Albright's sign).

Slater, S.: An evaluation of the metacarpal sign (short fourth metacarpal). *Pediatrics* 46:468, 1970.

The "thumb sign," protrusion of the thumb beyond the palm when the hand is fisted, is characteristic of Marfan's syndrome.

One or more extra creases on the fingers is seen in *Larsen's syndrome*.

*Dactylitis*, characterized by a painless, red, firm and spindle-shaped swelling of a digit, may be due to tuberculosis, syphilis, coccidioidomycosis or sickle cell anemia.

*Polydactyly* with a sixth digit on the ulnar aspect of each hand occurs in chondroectodermal dysplasia (Ellis–van Creveld syndrome), Lawrence-Moon-Biedl syndrome and trisomy 13.

*Syndactylism*, fusion or webbing of the toes or fingers, may appear as an isolated defect or accompany other anomalies such as premature synostosis of the cranial sutures. When the three middle fingers are fused, a common nail may be present (mitten hand) as in Apert's syndrome. Syndactyly occurs in Poland's anomaly and in Pfeiffer's, Carpenter's, the frontodigital, Smith-Lemli-Opitz, orofaciodigital and focal dermal hypoplasia syndromes.

*Macrodactylism*, or enlargement of a digit, is usually idiopathic but may occur with neurofibromatosis, Ollier's disease, Maffucci's syndrome and congenital lymphedema. Large hands and feet occur in cerebral gigantism.

*Arachnodactyly* occurs in Marfan's syndrome, homocystinuria and the mucosal neuroma syndrome.

*Anomalies of the hands and radius*, such as absence or hypoplasia of the thumb and the radius, may be associated with an atrial septal defect of the secundum type (Holt-Oram syndrome) or a ventricular septal defect. Fanconi's pancytopenia may be accompanied by similar defects.

Carroll, R.E. and Louis, D.S.: Anomalies associated with radial dysplasia. *J. Pediatr.* 84:409, 1974.
Harris, L.C. and Osborne, W.P.: Congenital absence or hypoplasia of the radius with ventricular septal defect: ventriculoradial dysplasia. *J. Pediatr.* 68:265, 1966.

Short, broad terminal phalanges of the thumbs and great toes, mental retardation, prominent nose and high arched palate are seen in the *Rubinstein-Taybi syndrome*. Broad toes and thumbs may also occur in Pfeiffer's, Apert's, Carpenter's, the frontodigital and Leri's pleonostosis syndromes. Patients with Larsen's syndrome have broad thumbs.

Marshall, R.E. and Smith, D.W.: Frontodigital syndrome: a dominantly inherited disorder with normal intelligence. *J. Pediatr.* 77:129, 1970.

Rubinstein, J.H. and Taybi, H.: Broad thumbs and toes and facial abnormalities. *Am. J. Dis. Child.* 105:588, 1963.

Temtamy, S.A.: Carpenter's syndrome: acrocephalopolysyndactyly. *J. Pediatr.* 69:111, 1966.

*Diastrophic dwarfism* is characterized by broad, short hands with an ulnar deviation. The interphalangeal joints show contractures either in flexion or contraction, and the thumbs demonstrate a proximal insertion as well as being often subluxated in a "hitch-hiker" position.

*Snapping or trigger thumb* is usually fixed in flexion; however, it may be possible to force the thumb into extension accompanied by a snapping sensation. Limitation of movement is due to a nodular enlargement of the long flexor tendon of the thumb in the presence of a narrowed tendon sheath. A small swelling may be palpable on the palmar aspect of the metacarpophalangeal joint.

Flexion of the fingers with the index finger overlapping the third finger occurs in patients with trisomy 18. Flexion deformity of the fingers and retroflexed thumbs occur in trisomy 13.

In *symphalangism*, the first and second phalanges of the fingers are ankylosed. The little finger is always affected. If additional digits are involved, there is preference for those on the ulnar side of the hand. There is no skin wrinkling over the involved joints. The medial and lateral malleoli are prominent, and the patient may be unable to invert and evert the foot. Conduction deafness may be an associated defect.

Strasburger, A.K., Hawkins, M.R., Eldridge, R., Hargrove, R.L. and McKusick, V.A.: Symphalangism: genetic and clinical aspects. *Bull. Johns Hopkins Hosp.* 117:108, 1965.

*Triphalangeal thumbs* and other anomalies of the thumb may be associated with congenital hypoplastic anemia.

Alter, B.P.: Thumbs and anemia. *Pediatrics* 62:613, 1978.

Contractures of one or more fingers with variable limitation of active and passive flexion and extension of the metacarpophalangeal joints, wrists, elbows, toes, ankles, knees and hips occur in many children with long-standing *diabetes*. Affected children may not be able to touch a flat surface with their entire palm.

Grgic, A., Rosenbloom, A.L., Weber, F.T., Giordano, B. and Malone, J.I.: Joint contracture in childhood diabetes (letter to the editor). *N. Engl. J. Med.* 292:372, 1975.

Rosenbloom, A.L. and Frias, J.L.: Diabetes, short stature and joint stiffness — a new syndrome. *Clin. Res.* 22:92A, 1974.

*Digital neurofibrosarcoma* usually presents early in infancy as a nontender, firm, glistening, pea-sized tumor fixed to the overlying skin, most frequently the lateral or dorsal surface of the distal phalanx of a finger or toe. Multiple tumors may be present.

*Juvenile aponeurotic fibromas* occasionally occur as infiltrative or discrete tumors involving the palms and/or the soles.

Painful swelling of the dorsa of the hands, fingers, feet and toes (*hand-foot syndrome*) may be the earliest clinical manifestation of sickle cell disease in infants.

Watson, R.J.: The hand-foot syndrome in sickle cell disease in young children. *Pediatrics* *31*:975, 1963.

## LOWER EXTREMITIES

Whether shortening of the lower extremities is actually present or not may be determined by measuring the distance from the anterior superior spine to the lower end of the medial malleolus bilaterally. If muscle atrophy appears to be present, the circumference of each thigh or calf may be measured at the same level above and below the patella.

*Shortening* of an extremity may occur with a congenitally short femur or tibia, congenital dislocation of the hip, slipped femoral capital epiphysis, coxa plana, poliomyelitis, Ollier's disease and premature arrest of epiphyseal growth due to infection or trauma. The involved extremity in infants with hemiplegia may be short and poorly developed. These changes are usually greater in the upper than in the lower extremities.

*Enlargement of an extremity* may be associated with hemangiomas, hemihypertrophy, arteriovenous fistula, neurofibromatosis, lymphangiectasia and stimulation of epiphyseal growth following ostoemyelitis or a fracture near an epiphysis.

**Bowing (Genu Varum).** The tibias of infants normally appear to be bowed. Such mild bowing is normal up to the age of two or three years. Internal or medial torsion of the tibia is also present in the majority of newborn and young infants and accounts for their pigeon-toed or toeing-in gait. Tibial rotation decreases gradually over a year or two.

Lateral bowing of the tibias may be due to rickets or unilateral or bilateral osteochondrosis of the medial tibial condyle (Blount's disease). Early differentiation between marked physiologic bowing and Blount's disease may be difficult.

*Congenital pseudarthrosis* is characterized by anterior bowing of the lower tibia evident in the newborn period or not until later infancy.

Bilateral or unilateral *anterior bowing of the tibia* may be a prenatal occurrence. Cutaneous dimpling may be present in the center of the curvature. Such dimpling and anterior angulation of the leg may be associated with congenital absence of the fibula.

**Knock-Knee (Genu Valgum).** Just as mild bowing is a normal finding in infants and children before two or three years of age, mild knock-knee or genu valgum is common in children between two and one-half and four years of age. Genu valgum may occur with rickets, hypophosphatasia, Morquio's disease, Hurler's syndrome and pes valgus.

*Genu recurvatum*, hyperextension or "back" knee, which occurs not uncommonly in newborn infants, is attributable to generalized ligamentous relaxation and to abnormal fetal posture. Spontaneous correction occurs in a few weeks. Occasionally, congenital dislocation of the knee occurs with the tibia lying anterior and lateral to the femur with the knee hyperextended.

Congenital lateral dislocation of the patella occurs rarely.

Hypoplasia of the patella occurs in the *nail-patella* syndrome.

A *popliteal hernia* (Baker's cyst) appears as a smooth, transilluminable cystic mass in the popliteal space accompanied, at times, by swelling of the knee joint.

*Congenital discoid lateral cartilage* may cause a palpable and audible clicking or snapping sound with movement of the knee joint, especially at the limits of flexion and extension. Localized tenderness may be present over the cartilage.

Osteochondrosis of the tibial tubercle or *Osgood-Schlatter disease* occurs in adolescent children. Physical findings include local pain, tenderness on deep pressure and swelling of the tibial tubercle. Pain may be especially severe after physical activity such as kicking, prolonged kneeling, running or forceful extension of the knee against resistance. A light limp may appear.

*Subluxation of the patella*, with the patella slipping partially out of the intercondylar groove when the quadriceps contracts with the knee flexed and the foot placed on the ground in a position of external rotation, may cause buckling of the knee or a popping sensation. With the patient sitting and the knees flexed to 90 degrees, the patella should face anteriorly and its anterior surface should be vertical; otherwise, the patella may be regarded as unstable. This may be checked by the Fairbanks test, in which the patella is pushed laterally while the knee is flexed 30 degrees, the foot supported and the quadriceps relaxed. Normally, the patella can be displaced laterally a centimeter or so. In the presence of excessive laxity, the test is positive — that is, if the patella can be moved up on the lateral femoral condyle, leading to a reactive contraction of the qudriceps and extension of the knee to move the patella medially. Dislocation of the patella is more likely in girls with genu valgum. Athletes may dislocate the patella after vigorous quadriceps contraction when knees are flexed and in a valgus position or in jumping for a basketball shot.

The *popliteal pterygium syndrome* consists of a skin web or pterygium, usually bilateral, which extends from the heel to the ischial tuberosity; anomalies of the hand and feet; genitourinary defects; cleft lip and cleft palate; and lip pits.

Gorlin, R.J., Sedano, H.O. and Cervenka, J.: Popliteal pterygium syndrome. *Pediatrics* *41*:503, 1968.
Smith, J.B.: Knee problems in children. *Pediatr. Clin. N. Am. 24*:841, 1977.

## FEET

*Congenital clubfoot*, or *talipes equinovarus*, is characterized by adduction of the forefoot, inversion of the hindfoot and an equinus position (plantar flexion) of the heel. Muscular resistance and pain are encountered when an attempt is made to correct this fixed deformity. Full dorsiflexion of the foot is possible with metatarsus varus but not with a true clubfoot. Many newborn infants hold their feet in a somewhat inverted position, but this position can be readily overcorrected. With a clubfoot the space between the navicular tubercle and the medial malleolus is much diminished and the two bony landmarks may be in complete apposition. Normally, the little finger may be placed in this space.

Clubfoot may be a manifestation of arthrogryposis, craniocarpotarsal dysplasia, Larsen's syndrome, diastrophic dwarfism, meningomyelocele, spinal cord tumor, cerebral palsy, caudal regression syndrome and the peroneal type of progressive muscular atrophy.

*Metatarsus varus*, characterized by adduction and inversion of the forefoot and often due to abnormal intrauterine position, differs from a clubfoot in the absence of an equinus deformity and in the ability to dorsiflex the foot fully. The heel may be neutral, varus or valgus in position. If the hindfoot is held in a fixed position, the forefoot cannot be brought to the midline by manipulation. If inversion is absent, the term *metatarsus adductus* should be used.

Metatarsus varus is to be differentiated from the common internal rotation of the tibia that occurs in young children and that may account for a pigeon-toed or toeing-in gait. These children may stumble over their feet if they walk rapidly or run. Differentiation can readily be made by placing the child supine so that the patellas point straight up. In patients with metatarsus varus the forefoot will be held in adduction and the hindfoot will be straight in line with the patella. With tibial rotation, both the forefoot and the hindfoot are held in the pigeon-toe position and not in line with the patella. In-toeing may also be due to increased femoral anteversion. In walking, patients with anteversion will turn their knees in. They tend to sit with the legs under them in a "W" position rather than in a tailor, cross-legged or "M" posture.

Internal rotation may be measured by having the child lie prone with his knees flexed and the pelvis held level. The legs are allowed to fall laterally into full internal rotation by gravity. Normally, the angle they assume from the vertical (the angle of internal rotation) will be less than 70 degrees. When the angle is greater than this, increased femoral anteversion is usually present. The anteversion is mild between 70 and 80 degrees and severe over 85 degrees.

Staheli, L.T.: Torsional deformity. *Pediatr. Clin. N. Am. 24*:799, 1977.

Infants and young children may walk with the forefoot in abduction or toeing out, owing to external rotation contractures of the hips or external tibial torsion. Other infants and children walk with a pigeon-toed or in-toed gait. Pronated feet are a common cause of toeing-in gait as is limitation of external rotation of the hip in extension.

*Talipes calcaneovalgus* is characterized by eversion, abduction and dorsiflexion of the foot. The heel is the most dependent portion of the foot, and the dorsum of the foot may touch the anterolateral aspect of the tibia. Usually, the soft tissues on the lateral aspect of the foot are tight. This position is easily corrected by passive manipulation. A small depression may be present just anterior to the lateral malleolus. Equinovalgus also occurs in Larsen's syndrome.

In many normal infants the foot can be acutely dorsiflexed because of a congenitally long Achilles tendon.

An *equinus position* of the foot may develop with spastic cerebral palsy. Heel cord shortening is also a relatively early finding in pseudohypertrophic muscular dystrophy. Tightness of the Achilles tendon may be checked by slightly inverting the foot to lock the heel before the foot is dorsiflexed. If the foot cannot be flexed more than 30 degrees, the heel cord is tight.

*Pes cavus* or high longitudinal arch may be congenital or may develop with Friedreich's ataxia, spina bifida, a cauda equina lesion, metatarsus varus, diastematomyelia, peroneal muscular atrophy and Hurler's syndrome.

*Pes planus or flat feet* are normal during infancy. Because of the fat pad present in the arch of the infant foot, the longitudinal arch does not become apparent until around the third year. Flat feet are often accompanied by pronation or eversion of the forefoot and, at time, by a hallux valgus. The medial malleolus is prominent in pronated feet, and an unusual amount of wear occurs on the medial surface of the heel.

Flat or pronated feet may be congenital or acquired. The congenital type is frequently hereditary. The acquired type of pronated foot may occur along with knock knees in children who have generalized ligamentous relaxation.

*Congenital "rocker-bottom" foot,* or *congenital vertical talus,* causes a severe, rigid flat foot with a boat-shaped deformity of the sole of the foot. The talus and calcaneus are in equinus. The heel points downward and the forefoot is dorsiflexed on the hindfoot and abducted. Rocker-bottom feet occur with trisomy 18.

*Tarsal coalition* with a bony bridge between two of the bones causes peroneal muscle spasm and a rigid, spastic foot, which may become painful early in adolescence. On inversion of the foot, pain occurs in the region of the peroneal tendons on the lateral aspect, accounting for the synonym *peroneal spastic flatfoot.*

An *accessory navicular bone* may cause a severe flatfoot.

Ehrlich, M.G.: Foot disorders in infants and children. *Cur. Probl. Pediatr. 4:*3 (May) 1974.

*Osteochondrosis of the tarsal navicular* (Köhler's disease), most common between four and six years of age, may also appear during school age or adolescence. Tenderness, redness, swelling and, occasionally, pain occur over the tarsal navicular bone. Pain and limping may be accentuated by walking and jumping.

Osteochondrosis of the *head of the second metatarsal,* which usually appears during adolescence, is characterized by local pain and, at times, redness, swelling and a slight limp.

*Achilles tendinitis,* usually unilateral, is characterized by swelling, tenderness and, perhaps, pain over the insertion of the Achilles tendon, especially after running and jumping. Limping may occur. Achilles tendinitis and tenosynovitis, occurring in episodes of two or three days' duration, may be an early manifestation of familial type II hyperlipoproteinemia.

Shapiro, J.R., Fallat, R.W., Tsang, R.C. and Glueck, C.J.: Achilles tendinitis and tenosynovitis. *Am. J. Dis. Child. 128:*486, 1974.

*Apophysitis of the os calcis,* which occurs in adolescents, is characterized by swelling and tenderness on pressure over the apophysis of the os calcis. The heel cord may also be tight. Involvement is usually bilateral.

Calluses or corns are produced by thickening of the skin in areas subjected to abnormal pressure as a result of improperly fitting shoes or foot abnormalities. Plantar warts may also occur in children.

## TOES

*Polydactylism* is characterized by accessory toes and fingers. *Syndactylism* represents fusion or webbing of the toes or fingers. *Macrodactyly,* or enlargement of a digit, is usually idiopathic.

The term *varus toe* may be used when one of the toes lies above or below the adjoining medial toe. A *hammer toe,* one held in position of flexion, may be congenital, occur with trisomy 18 or develop with acquired pes cavus. In patients with *Friedreich's ataxia* the proximal phalanx of the large toe is dorsiflexed while the distal phalanx is plantar flexed.

*Hallux varus,* or medial deviation of the large toe, is common in infants. In *hallux valgus,* the large toe points laterally. The majority of children with *myositis ossifi-*

*cans progressiva* demonstrate hallux valgus with the large toes held underneath the second toes. Both the large toes and the thumbs may also be abnormally short.

In *Pfeiffer's syndrome*, the middle phalanges of all toes are absent.

In young infants the ends of the toenails are often slightly elevated from their nail beds. In infants with Down's syndrome the cleft between the first and second toes is wider than normal and may extend backward as a shallow crease.

Marked swelling, redness and edema of a distal portion of a toe or finger may be due to constriction by a hair or a fine thread from a garment.

Narkewitz, R.M.: Distal digital occlusion. *Pediatrics 61*:922, 1978.

## GAIT

There are many variations in the gait of children who are beginning to walk. A change in gait, especially the report of ataxia, staggering or walking into door frames, requires careful evaluation. Gait is best observed by having the child walk up and down a well-lighted corridor for about 20 feet or so and observing his gait when he does not know he is being watched.

An *atalgic gait*, due to a painful extremity, is characterized by a short stance phase, the time that the extremity bears the body weight.

A *waddling gait* may be seen in:
Exstrophy of the bladder due to separation of the pelvic bones
Bilateral dislocation of the hips
Pseudohypertrophic muscular dystrophy
Bilateral slipped epiphysis
Bilateral coxa vara
Achondroplasia
Morquio's disease
Engelmann's disease (progressive diaphyseal dysplasia)
Myelodysplasia

An *equinus gait* may occur with spastic cerebral palsy, pseudohypertrophic muscular dystrophy or other disorders characterized by shortening of the Achilles tendon. *"Toe walking,"* a normal phase in some children, is also observed with autism.

A *scissors gait* may occur with spastic cerebral palsy and in slipped femoral epiphysis.

The *hemiplegic gait* is characterized by abduction and internal rotation of the thigh, flexion of the hip and knee and walking on the toes with the heel not touching the floor. In the upper extremity, the elbow is flexed and the shoulder abducted. The gait abnormality is accentuated when the child runs or walks fast.

The *steppage gait* seen in patients with foot drop is characterized by the involved foot being raised higher than the contralateral one so that the toe clears the floor.

Chronically ill children may have a *shuffling gait*. A similar gait may occur in dermatomyositis. Patients with tetralogy of Fallot characteristically *squat* to rest for a few minutes after they have walked a short distance.

Unusual types of gait may be seen with *hysteria*.

Dubowitz, V. and Hersov, L.: Management of children with nonorganic (hysterical) disorders of motor function. *Dev. Med. Child. Neurol. 18*:358, 1976.

Diagnostic considerations with an *ataxic* gait are presented on page 181.

## THE ETIOLOGIC CLASSIFICATION OF LIMP

I. Trauma is the most frequent cause of limp in young children.
   A. Sprains
   B. Fractures, especially the greenstick variety, involving the lower extremities
   C. Traumatic periostitis. The periosteum in young children is not firmly attached to the underlying bone. Minor trauma to the tibia or femur may result in subperiosteal hemorrhage with local tenderness and, at times, fullness, along with limp or refusal to walk. Symptoms may persist for several days. Roentgenograms when the child is first seen are negative. On films taken a week or two later, subperiosteal ossification is often evident.
   D. Contusions
   E. Splinter or other foreign body in the foot, stone bruises, improperly fitted shoes
II. Osteochondroses. Along with local tenderness, pain and, perhaps, swelling, patients with an osteochondrosis may have a limp.
   A. Osteochondrosis of the tarsal navicular (Köhler's disease)
   B. Osteochondrosis of the head of the second metatarsal
   C. Osteochondrosis of the patella
   D. Osteochondrosis of the tibial tubercle
   E. Osteochondrosis of the femoral capital epiphysis
   F. Calcaneal apophysitis
   G. Osteochondritis dissecans
   H. Avascular necrosis of bone occurs in systemic lupus erythematosus

Bergstein, J.M., Wiens, C., Fish, A.J., Vernier, R.L. and Michael, A.: Avascular necrosis of bone in systemic lupus erythematosus. *J. Pediatr. 85*:31, 1974.

III. Joint diseases
   A. Arthritis (see page 212)
   B. Diseases of the hip
      1. Congenital dislocation of the hip.
      2. Osteochondrosis of the femoral capital epiphysis (coxa plana, Legg-Calvé-Perthes disease) occurs between four and ten years of age. The onset is insidious with an almost imperceptible limp. A bone scan may be diagnostically helpful.
      3. Slipped femoral epiphysis. Pain in the knee or in the medial aspect of the thigh above the knee is the *earliest* sign of a slipped epiphysis. The diagnosis should be made at that time. Limp does not develop until later.
      4. Coxa vara. With a congenital coxa vara a painless limp is noted shortly after the child has begun to walk. With an acquired coxa vara the time of appearance of limp depends on the primary etiology.
      5. Otto's pelvis, in which there is an abnormally deep acetabulum, becomes symptomatic during adolescence. The patient begins to limp and may complain of pain in the inguinal region or inner aspect of the knee. Motion of the hip joint, especially rotation and abduction, is limited.
      6. Transient synovitis of the hip joint ("observation hip"). The presenting complaints in this common condition are pain, which may be mild or

severe, and limp. Patients are usually under ten years of age. The onset may be acute or insidious. Pain is present in the region of the hip or referred to the thigh or knee. Low-grade fever may be recorded. There is limitation in motion at the hip, and the lower extremity is held in flexion, external rotation and adduction. Internal rotation and abduction are restricted. Symptoms persist from a few days to several weeks. Differential diagnosis includes septic arthritis, Legg-Calvé-Perthes disease, early osteomyelitis of the femur, tuberculosis, osteoid osteoma, slipped femoral capital epiphysis and rheumatoid arthritis.

Jacobs, B.W.: Synovitis of the hip in children and its significance. *Pediatrics* 47:558, 1971.

    7. Hemarthrosis
IV. Tumors and neoplastic disease
    A. Leukemia. A limp is often an early finding with leukemia.
    B. Metastases from neuroblastoma
    C. Osteoid osteoma. The neck of the femur is a common site.
    D. Ewing's tumor
    E. Osteogenic sarcoma
 V. Other orthopedic disorders
    A. Leg length discrepancies
    B. Osteomyelitis
    C. Progressive diaphyseal dysplasia
    D. Calcaneal bursitis
    E. Cerebral palsy
    F. Vertebral disorders
    G. Infections of the intervertebral disc
    H. Herniated intervertebral disc
 VI. Neurologic disorders
    A. Tight filum terminale
    B. Spinal cord tumor
    C. Muscle weakness or paralysis
 VII. Muscle
    A. Muscular dystrophy
VIII. Miscellaneous
    A. An anal fissure may rarely cause a young child to limp.
    B. Iliac adenitis
    C. Appendicitis with irritation of the psoas muscle
    D. Hysteria
 IX. Leg pain
    A. The presence of leg pain may cause a child to limp. See Chapter 68.

## JOINTS

The term newborn infant lies with his elbows, hips and knees in partial flexion. There is frequently some resistance to passive movement at the joints, and full extension of the upper extremities at the elbows and lower extremities at the hips and knees may not be possible.

Joint disease may be manifested by swelling, redness, heat, pain and limitation of motion. To detect excessive fluid in the knee joint, the fluid may be expressed from the capsular reflections into the main joint space by placing one's palms above and below the knee and pushing downward and upward. With the joint so compressed, depression of the patella by one index finger followed by rebound indicates the presence of excessive fluid. The examiner may also place his index fingers opposite each other just beyond the edge of the patella. In the presence of joint effusion, downward pressure by one finger causes the other to be pushed upward by transmitted pressure.

## ETIOLOGIC CLASSIFICATION OF ARTHRITIS

Schaller, J.G.: Arthritis and infections of bones and joints in children. *Pediatr. Clin. N. Am.* 24:775, 1977.
Wedgwood, R.J. and Schaller, J.G.: The pediatric arthritides. *Hosp. Pract.* 12:83 (June) 1977.

I. Infectious arthritis
   A. Pyogenic or septic arthritis may be caused by the Staphylococcus aureus, hemolytic streptococcus, pneumococcus, meningococcus, Hemophilus influenzae, brucella organisms, Escherichia coli, dysentery bacillus and Eberthella typhosa. Gonococcal arthritis may be characterized by migratory polyarthritis with later localization in one or more joints. Joint penetration by an object such as a thorn may cause bacterial arthritis. All suspicious joints should be tapped and the synovial fluid cultured.

Fink, C.W.: Gonococcal arthritis in children. *JAMA 194*:237, 1965.

In pyogenic arthritis usually only one of the larger joints is involved. Systemic sysmptoms such as fever, chills, irritability and malaise may be prominent, or the complaints may be mainly confined to the joint. Pain and exquisite local tenderness may be early findings, followed by redness, swelling, protective muscle spasm and limitation of motion. Both active and passive motion of the joint is extremely painful. When peripheral joints are involved, inflammatory changes are more apparent than with joints such as the shoulder and hip. Pyogenic arthritis of the hip may be followed by dislocation. Suppurative arthritis of the hip is frequently overlooked in infants since early recognition is often difficult. Diagnostic needle puncture of the hip joint may be indicated in the presence of swelling of the upper part of the thigh in young infants. Flexion contracture and limitation of abduction of the hip are other suggestive signs. Osteomyelitis presents many of the signs and symptoms of septic arthritis; however, joint motion in this disorder is moderately good and less painful.

Transient synovitis of multiple joints may occur early in meningococcemia with pain and, perhaps, tenderness and redness. Monarticular arthritis, usually sterile, may appear late in the first week of the illness. Brucellosis may cause arthralgia and, rarely, inflammatory changes. The hip joint is most commonly involved.

Nelson, J.D.: The bacterial etiology and antibiotic management of septic arthritis in infants and children. *Pediatrics 50*:437, 1972.

B. Arthritis may be associated with many viral diseases: rubella, hepatitis, mumps, chickenpox, infection from adenovirus and Epstein-Barr virus.

Rahal, J.J., Millian, S.J. and Noriega, E.R.: Coxsackie virus and adenovirus infection. Association with acute febrile and juvenile rheumatoid arthritis. *JAMA 235*:2496, 1976.

Two types of arthralgia syndromes developed after rubella immunization when dog kidney virus was used: the "arm syndrome" with pain and paresthesia in the wrists and hands that awakened the child at night and the "leg syndrome" or "catcher's crouch" with pain in the knees, especially on awakening, a crouching gait and toe walking.

Kilroy, A.W., Schaffner, W., Fleet, W.F., Jr., Lefkowitz, L.B., Karzon, D.T. and Fenichel, G.M.: Two syndromes following rubella immunization. *JAMA 214*:2287, 1970.

C. Acute, painful swelling and redness of the joints may occur with rat-bite fever and Haverhill fever.
D. Toxic arthritis characterized by pain, redness and swelling, usually of a single joint, may occur with pharyngitis, scarlet fever and other acute infections, especially those due to the streptococcus. Arthritis occurring in patients with chronic ulcerative colitis and Crohn's disease may simulate either rheumatoid or pyogenic arthritis.
E. Lyme arthritis, presumably caused by a tick, occurs chiefly in the summer or early fall in patients who live in wooded areas. Sudden joint swelling occurs, usually of the knee but perhaps of the elbow or wrist. Migratory joint pains may involve the small joints of the fingers and toes. Fever, malaise, weakness and myalgia are other symptoms. Attacks lasting a week to months recur, followed by remissions usually of several months. A rash that progresses from a papular lesion to a large ring with a clearing center may precede the arthritis.

Steere, A.C. et al.: Lyme arthritis: an epidemic of oligoarthritis in children and adults in three Connecticut communities. *Arthritis Rheum. 20*:7, 1977.

F. In Scandinavia, episodes of polyarthritis have been associated with Yersinia enterocolitica infections. Diarrhea and abdominal pain are most common accompanying symptoms.

Jacobs, J.C.: Yersinia enterocolitica arthritis. *Pediatrics 55*:236, 1975.

G. Tuberculous arthritis is usually monarticular with swelling and a thickened, doughy consistency of the periarticular tissues. Effusion and inflammatory changes usually do not occur, although some warmth and redness may be present early. Joint pain is not prominent at this time. Spasm of the adjacent muscles may be severe, and muscle atrophy may rapidly develop. A negative tuberculin test almost completely excludes tuberculosis as an etiologic possibility. The diagnosis can be established by culture or guinea pig inoculation of the synovial fluid or biopsy.

II. Collagen diseases
A. Rheumatic fever may be characterized by an acute migratory arthralgia, usually of larger joints such as the ankles, knees, hips, wrists, elbows and shoulders. Involved joints may be swollen, tender, red, hot and painful. Involvement lasts only one to three days and joint residuae do not occur.

B. Lupus erythematosus may be characterized by migratory, transient joint involvement with arthralgia or redness, swelling and stiffness of joints. The manifestations may simulate those in rheumatic fever or early rheumatoid arthritis.

C. Serum sickness may be characterized by redness, swelling, pain, stiffness and considerable joint effusion. Arthralgia may be part of a serum sickness-like syndrome caused by penicillin sensitivity.

D. Juvenile rheumatoid arthritis usually begins during the preschool years but may occur at any age. A disorder of protean manifestations, juvenile rheumatoid arthritis has four chief modes of onset: (1) systemic with high, spiking fever, pericarditis, pleuritis, leukemoid reaction, hepatosplenomegaly with arthritis appearing concurrently or later; (2) polyarticular with involvement of more than four joints; (3) pauciarticular with two or three joints; and (4) monarticular.

The onset is frequently insidious with pain and swelling of the knee or ankle and a limp. The involved joints may be slightly warm, and passive motion is often painful and limited. Easy fatigability, morning stiffness, anorexia and poor growth progress may be present, or the symptoms may be completely confined to the joints. Fever may be the earliest manifestation. This may be low grade or spiking, persistent or intermittent. *Rheumatoid arthritis is to be considered a definite possibility in children with spiking fever of undetermined origin.* The fever, at times accompanied by chills, may be over 105°F (40.5°C) and may persist for weeks. It is quotian in type with wide swings from hyperpyrexia to normal or subnormal temperatures once or twice a day. In other patients, the onset of joint involvement is acute. A transient and migratory polyarthritis may occur along with fever. The differential diagnosis between rheumatoid arthritis and rheumatic fever may be difficult. In some cases, the arthralgia may be transitory and not accompanied by signs of inflammation.

In children, the knees, ankles or elbows are commonly the first joints to be involved. Except for the cervical spine, the vertebral column usually remains normal. The joint manifestations are often monarticular at the onset. Other joints, including those of the hands and feet, may later become involved. When involvement is monarticular, diagnostic confusion with infectious arthritis, particularly tuberculosis, may occur; however, infectious arthritis other than tuberculosis generally demonstrates more prominent manifestations of acute inflammation than does rheumatoid arthritis.

Muscle atrophy, especially around the joints, may be severe. The combination of joint effusion and muscle atrophy causes the fusiform swelling often evident in the spindle-shaped proximal and distal interphalangeal joints characteristic of this disease. The overlying skin may be red, shiny, smooth and atrophic.

Other manifestations of rheumatoid arthritis include a transient, usually nonpruritic erythematous or salmon-pink, macular or maculopapular skin rash chiefly on the trunk, face, neck and inner aspects of the extremities, especially during febrile periods. Slight hepatomegaly and splenomegaly may occur in a few patients. Children with young-age onset of pauciarticular arthritis have a 1:4 to 1:2 chance of developing iridocyclitis whether or not the rheumatoid process is active. With older-age onset pauciarticular arthritis, involvement of the hip girdle and sacroiliac joints is common and acute iridocyclitis occurs in 5 to 10 per cent of patients.

Grossman, B.J. and Mukhopadhyay, D.: Juvenile rheumatoid arthritis. *Cur. Probl. Pediatr.* 5:3 (Oct.) 1975.

Schaller, J.G., Kupfer, C. and Wedgwood, R.J.: Iridocyclitis in juvenile rheumatoid arthritis. *Pediatrics 44*:92, 1969.

Schaller, J.G. and Wedgwood, R.J.: Is juvenile rheumatoid arthritis a single disease? A review. *Pediatrics 50*:940, 1972.

E. Patients with dermatomyositis may have joint involvement suggestive of rheumatoid arthritis. *Mixed connective tissue disease* of childhood has features of systemic lupus erythematosus, scleroderma and polymyositis. Polyarthritis and Raynaud's phenomenon are commonly present at the onset.

Singsen, B.H., Bernstein, B.H., Kornreich, H.K., King, K.K., Hanson, V. and Tan, E.M.: Mixed connective tissue disease in childhood. *J. Pediatr. 90*:893, 1977.

F. Ankylosing spondylitis may begin with peripheral joint involvement that simulates rheumatoid arthritis. Later, the spine and sacroiliac joints are affected with pain in the lower back, hips or thighs. Initially, symptoms may be mild and intermittent.

Schaller, J., Bitnum, S. and Wedgwood, R.J.: Ankylosing spondylitis with childhood onset. *J. Pediatr. 74*:505, 1969.

III. Other causes of arthritis

A. Arthritis-like symptoms and signs may precede by months other manifestations of malignancies, especially leukemia and neuroblastoma. Interphalangeal as well as larger joints may be exquisitely painful, warm and swollen.

Fink, C.W., Windmiller, J. and Sartain, P.: Arthritis as the presenting feature of childhood leukemia. *Arthritis Rheum. 15*:347, 1972.

Schaller, J.: Arthritis as a presenting manifestation of malignancy in children. *J. Pediatr. 81*:793, 1972.

B. Some patients with immunodeficiency have polyarthritis that is indistinguishable from rheumatoid arthritis.

McLaughlin, J.F., Schaller, J. and Wedgwood, R.J.: Arthritis and immunodeficiency. *J. Pediatr. 81*:801, 1972.

C. Disseminated lipogranulomatosis, or Farber's disease, simulates rheumatoid arthritis to some extent. Painful joint enlargement in infants is followed by fixation of the involved joints. Subcutaneous and periarticular nodules are also present along with hepatomegaly, lymphadenopathy and hoarseness.

Moser, H.W.: Farber's lipogranulomatosis. *Am. J. Med. 47*:869, 1969.

D. Sickle cell disease. Acute pain, swelling and warmth of one or many joints may occur with sickle cell disease. Both large and small joints may be involved. Pain is often extreme and spasm of the muscles adjacent to the joints often occurs.

Espinoza, L.R., Spilberg, I. and Osterland, C.K.: Joint manifestations of sickle cell disease. *Medicine 53*:295, 1974.

E. Reiter's syndrome, characterized by nonspecific arthritis, conjunctivitis and urethritis, rarely occurs in childhood.

Vergnani, R.J. and Smith, R.S.: Reiter syndrome in a child. *Arch. Ophthalmol. 91*:165, 1974.

F. Gout rarely occurs in infants and children.
G. Psoriasis may be a rare cause of arthritis in children.
H. Familial osteolysis of the carpal and tarsal bones begins at about five years of age with symptoms that suggest an acute arthritis of the wrists and ankles. This is followed by slow, progressive, painless dissolution of the carpal and tarsal bones.

Gluck, J.: Familial osteolysis of the carpal and tarsal bones. *J. Pediatr. 81*:506, 1972.

I. Intermittent hydarthrosis or recurrent effusion involving the knees occasionally occurs in adolescent girls.
J. Schönlein-Henoch purpura may be characterized, in part, by arthralgia, usually of the ankle or knee, with redness, tenderness, swelling and heat. Multiple joints may be involved in a migratory fashion, with arthralgia at times being the first manifestation of this syndrome.
K. Pigmented villonodular synovitis may cause intermittent pain and swelling, usually of the knee, in older children and young adults after minimal trauma or activity. Aspirated synovial fluid is dark brown or serosanguineous.
L. Arthritis may occur with periodic neutropenia and in familial Mediterranean fever. In the latter, arthritis may be the predominant symptom. Involvement is usually monarticular at first, but then other joints, including the sacroiliac, are involved.

Lehman, T.J.A. et al.: HLA-B27–negative sacroilitis: a manifestation of familial Mediterranean fever in childhood. *Pediatrics 61*:423, 1978.

M. Sarcoid arthritis is characterized by extensive joint swelling, effusion and boggy synovial thickening of both joints and tendon sheaths. Little or no pain or limitation of motion occurs. Wrists, ankles, knees and elbows are involved.

North, A.F., Jr. et al.: Sarcoid arthritis in children. *Am. J. Med. 48*:449, 1970.

N. Behçet's disease may be associated with synovitis, arthritis or arthralgia affecting the larger joints.
O. Chronic active hepatitis may be accompanied by arthralgia or arthritis involving single or multiple large joints.
P. Inflammatory bowel disease may be preceded or accompanied by arthritis involving large joints or the spine.

Lindsley, C.B. and Schaller, J.G.: Arthritis associated with inflammatory bowel disease in children. *J. Pediatr. 84*:16, 1974.
Haslock, I. and Wright, V.: The musculoskeletal complications of Crohn's disease. *Medicine 52*:217, 1973.

Q. Stickler syndrome may be suspected at birth on the basis of bony enlargement of ankles, knees and wrists and hyperextensibility of the knees, elbows and fingers. Some infants may present with the Pierre Robin syndrome or with spondyloepiphyseal dysplasia. Progressive myopia may be followed by retinal detachment or cataracts.

Stickler, G.B. et al.: Hereditary progressive arthroophthalmopathy. *Mayo Clin. Proc. 40*:433, 1965; *42*:495, 1967.

IV. Traumatic arthritis
   A. Sprain
   B. Hemarthrosis is common with hemophilia.
   C. Acute traumatic synovitis occurring after an acute knee injury is characterized by distention of the joint capsule, discomfort and restriction of motion. In contrast to hemarthrosis, in which swelling is noted in 30 to 60 minutes, distention in acute traumatic synovitis is delayed for 6 hours after the injury.
   D. "Little league elbow" in young baseball pitchers may be characterized by pain, tenderness and swelling over the involved medial epicondyle.

Collins, H.R. and Evarts, C.M.: Injuries to the adolescent athlete. *Postgrad. Med.* 49:72, 1971.
Torg, J.S., Pollack, H. and Swelterlitsch, P.: The effect of competitive pitching on the shoulders and elbows of preadolescent baseball pitchers. *Pediatrics* 49:267, 1972.

## HYPEREXTENSIBLE JOINTS

*Hyperextensibility of joints* may occur in Ehlers-Danlos syndrome, Marfan's syndrome, osteogenesis imperfecta and primary hyperparathyroidism. Hypotonia and unusual mobility of the joints are often present in Down's syndrome and in infants with cerebral hypotonia. Hyperextensibility of the fingers and hands is marked in the cartilage-hair hypoplasia syndrome.

The generalized relaxation and pliability of newborn infants during the first week of life permit them to be "folded" into a position that simulates the intrauterine posture.

*Larsen's syndrome* may be characterized by multiple joint dislocations, including those of the knee, elbow and, most commonly, the hip. Other anomalies include a low nasal bridge, abnormalities of the fingers and short metacarpals.

Latta, R.J., Graham, C.B., Aase, J., Scham, S.M. and Smith, D.W.: Larsen's syndrome: a skeletal dysplasia with multiple joint dislocations and unusual facies. *J. Pediatr.* 78:291, 1971.

In diastrophic dysplasia, there is a tendency to dislocation of many joints, especially the hip.

## LIMITATION OF JOINT MOTION

Limitation of joint motion occurs with arthralgia, arthritis, synovitis and osteomyelitis.

After the first year of life, flexural contractures may develop with spastic *cerebral palsy*.

In *Morquio's disease* extension of the lower extremities at the hip is limited. The child walks in a crouched position with the hips and knees partially flexed.

Limitation of extension, especially at the elbow, may occur in *Hurler's syndrome*.

Patients with acquired paralysis may develop joint contractures unless preventive measures are taken.

In its late stages *dermatomyositis* is characterized by joint contractures.

*Volkmann's ischemic contracture* may complicate fractures about the elbow, especially the supracondylar type. Once the contracture has developed, the involved extremity is held in flexion at the elbow, wrist and interphalangeal joints; the forearm is pronated; and the metacarpophalageal joints are hyperextended.

Contractures also occur in children with arthritis, particularly rheumatoid arthritis.

Joint motion is restricted in *diastrophic dysplasia*.

*Arthrogryposis multiplex congenita* is a congenital syndrome of diverse neuropathic or myopathic etiology that is characterized by complete or moderate limitation of motion at one or many joints. Usually all four extremities are involved. Joint fixation may occur in either flexion or extension. Talipes equinovarus is frequently present. Dislocation of the hip and knees may occur. The periarticular and subcutaneous tissues around the joints may appear thickened, and the extremities may taper from the hip to the ankle and from the wrists to the shoulders. Skin dimpling may be present over the patella, the styloid process of the ulna and other joints. The normal skin creases are absent. Muscles of the extremities are often hypotonic or hypoplastic. The Pierre Robin syndrome may be an accompanying defect.

Beckerman, R.C. and Buchino, J.J.: Arthrogryposis multiplex congenita as part of an inherited symptom complex: two case reports and a review of the literature. *Pediatrics* 61:417, 1978.

With *iliac adenitis* the child may keep the lower extremity on the affected side flexed at the hip because of spasm of the iliopsoas muscle.

Older children and adolescents, especially boys, may have *osteochondritis dissecans* with limp, intermittent pain and stiffness of a joint. Usually one or both knees are involved, but other joints may also be affected. The patient may be aware of something moving within the joint, and the knee may intermittently "give way." Clicking and locking of the joint may occur on movement. Joint effusion and periarticular muscular atrophy may develop. The medial femoral condyle is most commonly involved. Localized tenderness may be present when the knee is flexed.

## HIP JOINT

**Congenital Dislocation of the Hip.** The diagnosis of congenital dislocation of the hip should be established early. If overlooked at that time, it may not be made until the child begins to walk with a limp. Screening examinations for the detection of congenital dislocation of the hip are an *essential* part of the physical examination in all infants.

In the newborn, the *Barlow test* may be used to diagnose an unstable or potentially dislocatable hip. This sign is usually not present after six weeks of age. With the infant supine, the hip flexed to 90 degrees and the knee fully flexed, the examiner places his palm over the infant's knee, his thumb in the femoral triangle opposite the lesser trochanter and his index or middle finger over the greater trochanter. The hip is then brought into mid-abduction with the thumb exerting gentle pressure laterally and posteriorly while posterior and medial pressure is exerted by the palm on the knee. In the presence of a dislocatable hip, the femoral head can be felt to click as it dislocates across the posterior lip of the acetabulum. When the thumb pressure is released, the femoral head returns to the acetabular socket.

In the *Ortolani test* for hip dislocation, the knee of the baby is fully flexed while the hip is flexed to 90 degrees and fully abducted. As the femoral head moves across the posterior rim of the acetabulum into the socket, the examiner can hear or feel a click. Likewise, redislocation can be detected with adduction of the hip.

If the hips and knees are flexed so that the soles are placed flat on the table, the knee on the affected side is lower than the normal one.

In infants with unilateral dislocation of the hip, the inguinal and gluteal folds are higher on the involved side. An extra skin crease on the involved side below the gluteal fold is not of diagnostic help since such creases also occur normally, especially in obese infants.

Normally, when an infant is placed in the supine position with the thighs flexed to 90 degrees, the knees may be abducted 160 degrees or so. After the second or third month of life, limitation of abduction of the hip may be noted in congenital dislocation of the hip. Such limitation of abduction may not be present during the first weeks of life. A normal, crying infant may offer considerable resistance to abduction as may the infant with spastic cerebral palsy. Limitation may also be caused by arthrogryposis multiplex or coxa plana. An acquired dislocation of the hip may occur in spastic cerebral palsy.

Although dislocation of the hip should be detected early in infancy, the diagnosis is occasionally overlooked until the child is noted to limp on beginning to walk. A waddling gait and lordosis are present with bilateral dislocation of the hip. A positive Trendelenburg sign may also be present if the child is old enough to stand. When a child with a unilateral dislocation uses the involved extremity for weight bearing, a downward tilt or sinking of the pelvis occurs on the normal side. When the normal extremity is used for weight bearing, elevation of the pelvis occurs on the other side. These are late findings, however, and the orthopedic correction obtained at this time is unsatisfactory.

Ritter, M.A.: Congenital dislocation of the hip in the newborn. *Am. J. Dis. Child. 125*:30, 1973.

**Legg-Calvé-Perthes disease,** or osteochondrosis of the femoral capital epiphysis, occurs most commonly in boys between the ages of four and ten years. The onset is insidious with an almost imperceptible limp that may be painless but that is usually accompanied by pain in the groin, lateral hip or referred along the distribution of the obturator nerve to the medial aspect of the thigh and knee. The pain is usually relatively slight, simulating that of myalgia or muscle stiffness and may increase with activity. Symptoms may be intermittent initially. Limitation of motion is usual, particularly extension, abduction and internal rotation. That muscle spasm is absent or minimal may be helpful in differentiation from inflammatory disorders of the hip joint. Muscle atrophy about the hip and shortening of the lower extremity may develop later.

**Slipped Capital Femoral Epiphysis.** Slipping of the femoral capital epiphysis occurs most commonly between the ages of 12 and 15 years. While the incidence is greatest in obese children and in tall, thin children who have recently undergone rapid growth, children of normal physique may also be affected.

Pain in the knee or along the medial aspect of the thigh above the knee, referred along the course of the obturator nerve from the hip, is usually the earliest symptom. Actual hip pain is a late complaint. Minimal early pain may be accentuated by activity and alleviated by rest. A slight limp without pain may be the presenting complaint. When a limp develops, the child walks with his foot in external rotation. Limitation of abduction may cause adduction of the lower extremities. As a result, the child may have to cross his lower extremities in order to sit, and he may walk with a scissors gait. Limitation of internal rotation of the hip, an early finding, is best demonstrated with the child in the prone position and his knee flexed. The range of extension may, however, be greater than on the uninvolved side. Another characteristic finding can be elicited at times by having the supine patient flex the knee and hip. As the knee is elevated, in the neutral position, it will block before a 90-degree angle is reached. With further flexion, the hip will externally rotate and move out to abduction. The difference between the involved and uninvolved sides is striking. Patients with bilateral involvement have a waddling gait and a lumbar lordosis. A positive Trendelenburg sign may be present in advanced cases.

Early diagnosis is necessary if orthopedic correction is to be satisfactory. This disorder should be considered, therefore, whenever a patient complains of pain in the knee. *Anteroposterior and lateral roentgenograms of both hips are indicated in all patients who have unexplained pain in the knee.*

**Cox Vara.** Normally, an angle of approximately 135 degress is present between the shaft and the head and neck of the femur. Coxa vara due to a decrease in this angle may be congenital or acquired, the latter being more common.

Shortly after beginning to walk, the child may be seen because of a painless, lurching limp. Later, pain, perhaps referred to the knee, may be associated with the limp.

Acquired coxa vara may follow or be associated with slipped femoral epiphysis, Legg-Calvé-Perthes disease, osteomyelitis, tuberculosis, pyogenic arthritis, rickets, chondrodystrophy, osteogenesis imperfecta, hypothyroidism, spastic cerebral palsy, trauma to the epiphyseal plate, congenital dislocation of the hip and fractures.

In addition to a painless or minimally painful limp, limitation of abduction and internal rotation are also present. Muscle atrophy, shortening and external rotation of the involved extremity may appear, and the greater trochanter may be elevated and more prominent than normal. A positive Trendelenburg sign is present on the involved side. Children with bilateral coxa vara have a waddling gait and a lumbar lordosis.

## SHOULDERS

In *Sprengel's deformity* the scapula is higher than normal and may be rotated so that its lower angle is directed toward the spine. An omovertebral bone may extend as an osseous bridge between the medial aspect of the scapula and a cervical vertebra. Abduction of the arm on the involved side is limited to about 90 degrees. Scoliosis and torticollis with tilting of the head to the affected side may also be present.

## CLAVICLE

Children with *cleidocranial dysostosis* have drooping shoulders and can approximate their shoulders in the midline. Delayed cranial ossification, large fontanels, open suture lines and fontanels and parietal and occipital bossing may also be present.

The clavicle is fractured more frequently than any other bone during birth. The arm on the involved side may not be used, or its motion may be limited. The Moro reflex causes an unilateral rather than a bilateral response. Crepitus, angulation and irregularity at the fracture site may be detected by palpation. Callus formation proceeds rapidly, and a lump may be palpable within a few weeks.

*Pseudoarthrosis* of the clavicle is extremely rare.

## PELVIS

Diastasis of the symphysis pubis occurs with exstrophy of the bladder.

Prominence of the anterior superior spine or horn-like projections from the iliac crests are seen in the *nail-patella syndrome*.

## BACK

In the newborn infant there is a slight convexity of the spine in the thoracic and sacral regions. Cervical and lumbar curves do not appear until the end of the first year of life when the infant assumes a standing posture. In this position infants and young children have a physiologic lumbar lordosis that is accentuated by a prominent abdomen. A slight lumbar kyphosis may be apparent in the sitting position.

*Scoliosis* is characterized by a lateral curvature of the spine. A rotary deformity is usually associated. The initiating or primary curve is balanced by the secondary or compensatory one.

Children between the ages of 8 and 15 years should be regularly screened for scoliosis. Unclothed except for shorts and halter, the child should be examined in the following three positions:

(1) From the back with the child standing erect and feet together, the examiner should look for unilateral elevation of shoulder, prominence or elevation of a scapula, deeper crease on one side at the waistline, prominence of one hip, asymmetrical arm-flank distance, asymmetry of the hips or pelvis or curvature of the spine. The occiput should be aligned over the intergluteal cleft. Curves of under 30 per cent may not be detected in this position.

(2) The child bends 90 degrees forward at the hips with the knees straight and the arms dangling from the shoulders or pressed together in the prayer position. Looking parallel to the back from either end, the examiner inspects for a thoracic rib or lumbar paravertebral prominence or hump. The two sides should be symmetrical.

(3) Standing upright, the child is examined from the side for excessive thoracic kyphosis or lumbar lordosis.

Standing anteroposterior and lateral x-rays of the entire spine should be obtained when scoliosis or kyphosis is suspected on the screening examination. Functional scoliosis disappears when the patient lies down, sits or bends over. Persistent scoliosis does not.

## ETIOLOGIC CLASSIFICATION OF SCOLIOSIS

I. Functional scoliosis may result from poor postural habits. This mild type of scoliosis, characterized by a long C curve, may be present in patients who have a shortened lower extremity. The pelvis is tilted to the affected side.

II. Idiopathic scoliosis occurs most commonly in the dorsal and dorsolumbar regions as an S-shaped curve with the primary curvature to the right in 85 per cent of cases. Idiopathic scoliosis usually occurs between 10 and 14 years of age and is more common in girls than boys. Infantile scoliosis occurs in the first three years of life and juvenile idiopathic scoliosis between 4 and 10 years of age. In excluding known causes of scoliosis, the examiner may measure the lower extremities to determine if they are of equal length. If the scoliosis progresses rapidly, a compensatory curvature does not develop; therefore, the shoulders and pelvis are not aligned parallel as in patients with a compensated scoliosis.

III. Acquired scoliosis
    A. *Neurofibromatosis* produces an acutely angulated scoliosis, usually in the thoracic area. The etiology may be suggested by *cafe-au-lait* lesions. Usually, the scoliosis progresses rapidly and is compensated.
    B. Muscle imbalance due to paralysis of the muscles of the back is another cause of scoliosis. Scoliosis may occur with spastic cerebral palsy, muscular dystrophy and other myopathies due to involvement of the back muscles.
    C. Syringomyelia
    D. Hemihypertrophy
    E. Marfan's syndrome
    F. Friedreich's ataxia and other spinocerebellar degenerative disorders
    G. Dystonia musculorum deformans
    H. Tuberculosis and other inflammatory disease of the spine
    I. Diastematomyelia
    J. Spinal cord tumor
    K. Noonan's syndrome
    L. Familial dysautonomia
IV. Congenital scoliosis
    A. Hemivertebrae cause an acutely angulated scoliosis.
    B. Congenital torticollis may be followed by a compensatory scoliosis.
    C. Pectus excavatum may be associated with a kyphoscoliosis.
    D. Myelomeningocele
    E. Chondrodysplasia punctata
    F. Diastrophic dysplasia (kyphoscoliosis)
    G. Spondyloepiphyseal dysplasia congenita
    H. Metatropic dysplasia is characterized by the development of a rapidly progressing kyphoscoliosis when the child becomes older.
    I. Pseudoachondroplasia
*Kyphosis* denotes a pronounced posterior curvature of the spine.

## ETIOLOGIC CLASSIFICATION OF KYPHOSIS

    I. A mild functional kyphosis may be caused by poor posture. The normal rounding of the lumbar spine present in infants when they first begin to sit may be especially pronounced in those with muscular atony and ligamentous relaxation. Functional kyphosis disappears when the infant is prone.
    II. Hemihypertrophy
    III. Generalized skeletal disorders
        A. Kyphosis (gibbus) of the dorsolumbar spine may be an early physical finding in infants with Hurler's syndrome, in Sandhoff's disease and spondyloepiphyseal dysplasia congenita.
        B. The kyphosis in Morquio's disease usually does not appear until late infancy or the preschool years.
        C. Kyphosis may develop in hypophosphatasia.
        D. A mild thoracolumbar kyphosis may appear wtih achondroplasia.
    IV. Vertebral epiphysitis (Scheuermann's disease) occurs during adolescence. Involvement of the epiphyses of the vertebral bodies with consequent anterior wedging causes kyphosis of the thoracic or upper lumbar spine that may

progress over a period of several years. This disorder is largely asymptomatic except for the postural defect.

V. Tuberculous spondylitis (Pott's disease). Tuberculous involvement of the spine develops insidiously, usually during the first decade. Because of paravertebral muscle spasm, the child characteristically demonstrates a "poker spine," walking stiffy erect or on tiptoe and squatting to pick up objects from the floor rather than flexing the spine to bend over. Depending on the level of involvement, pain may be referred to the arms, the abdomen or the lower extremities.

VI. Kyphoscoliosis may occur with pectus excavatum.

VII. Tumors of the spinal cord

VIII. Noonan's syndrome

*Lordosis* denotes an exaggeration of the normal anterior curvature of the lumbar spine. The abdomen may also be protuberant and the buttocks prominent. Some degree of lordosis is normal in older infants and young children and with poor posture. Thoracic kyphosis may lead to a compensatory lumbar lordosis. Lordosis may accompany congenital dislocation of the hips, pseudohypertrophic muscular dystrophy, spondylolisthesis, achondroplasia, spondyloepiphyseal dysplasia congenita and congenital deficiency or absence of abdominal muscles.

*Flattening* of the normal curvatures of the spine or a mendicant, stooped posture may occur in asthma, bronchiectasis, cystic fibrosis, other chronic and debilitating diseases and hysteria.

*Stiffness* of the back occurs with tetanus, poliomyelitis and tuberculus spondylitis, spinal cord tumors and discitis.

*Infections of the intervertebral disc (discitis)* occurs in young children, primarily in the lumbar region. Symptoms include irritability; refusal to sit, stand or walk; limp; crying at night; stiffness of the back; vague back pain; abdominal pain; mild fever and occasionally localized tenderness. Movement of the pelvis or thigh causes pain. A positive Kernig's or Brudzinski's sign may be present. Roentgenographic changes may not occur for two to four weeks.

Rocco, H.D. and Eyring, E.J.: Intervertebral disk infections in children. *Am. J. Dis. Child.* *123*:448, 1972.

*Herniated intervertebral disc* is a rare cause of low back pain in older children and adolescents. The most frequent physical findings are pain on deep pressure between the fifth lumbar and the first sacral vertebrae, limited ability to elevate the extended lower extremity, unilaterally or bilaterally, restriction of back movement and flattening of the lumbar spine.

*Calcification of the intervertebral discs*, usually involving the cervical spine in children between 5 and 10 years of age, may be accompanied by pain, spasm, tenderness and torticollis.

Swick, H.M.: Calcification of intervertebral discs in childhood. *J. Pediatr. 86*:364, 1975.

*Vertebral osteomyelitis* may be characterized by localized back pain and fever.

*Spondylolisthesis*, caused usually by L5 slipping forward on S1, and *spondylolysis* are rare causes of low back pain in adolescents. The pain may radiate into the buttocks, legs or groins and may be accompanied by tight hamstrings and limited ability for straight leg raising. Scoliosis may be present. The patient is less symptomatic when leaning forward.

*Winging of the scapulae* may occur with juvenile muscular atrophy or facioscapulohumeral muscular dystrophy.

The *Klippel-Feil syndrome* is characterized by limitation of movement and shortening of the neck due to congenital anomalies of the cervical vertebrae that may be decreased in number, abnormally wide, fused or irregularly segmented. Hemivertebrae may also be present.

*Ankylosing spondylitis* may present after the age of 15 with recurrent, transient stiffness and pain involving the lumbosacral spine, sacroiliac joints, buttocks, and thighs and hips. Pain may radiate into the lower extremities. Tenderness may be present over the sacroiliac joints and lumbar spine. Anterior flexion of the lumbar spine may be limited. Peripheral arthritis may precede or accompany complaints referable to the back.

Schaller, J., Bitnum, S. and Wedgwood, R.J.: Ankylosing spondylitis with childhood onset. *J. Pediatr. 74*:505, 1969.

Pain, stiffness and limitation in motion of the neck may be an early manifestation of *juvenile rheumatoid arthritis*.

*Tuberculous spondylitis* may present with back pain, stiffness and limitation of motion.

*Bone tumors* of the spine such as aneurysmal bone cyst, osteoid osteoma, Ewing's sarcoma, osteogenic sarcoma, neuroblastoma, lymphomas and leukemia may cause back pain.

*Spinal cord tumors* may present with neck, back or extremity pain exacerbated by coughing, sneezing, straining or straight leg raising; motor weakness; muscle atrophy; paraspinal muscle spasm; positive Babinski's sign and change in bladder or bowel habits.

Hayden, J.W.: Back pain in childhood. *Pediatr. Clin. N. Am. 14*:611, 1967.
Hoppenfeld, S.: Back pain. *Pediatr. Clin. N. Am. 24*:881, 1977.
Tachdjian, M.O. and Matson, D.D.: Orthopaedic aspects of intraspinal tumors in infants and children. *J. Bone Joint Surg. 47-A*:223, 1965.

Back pain may be due to vertebral collapse and compression with *leukemia* or *chronic corticosteroid therapy*.

Back pain or pain over the coccyx (coccyadynia) in adolescents may have a psychological etiology.

*Agenesis of the sacrum, caudal dysplasia* or the *caudal regression* syndrome due to congenital deformities of the lower lumbar, sacral, and coccygeal vertebrae and related portions of the spinal cord is characterized, depending on the extent of the defect, by neurologic impairment of the bladder and lower extremities and orthopedic deformities.

Thompson, I.M., Kirk, R.M. and Dale, M.: Sacral agenesis. *Pediatrics 54*:236, 1974.

## BONE TUMORS

Clinical and roentgenographic differentiation between benign and malignant bone tumors is frequently not possible. The diagnosis must be made by biopsy.

I. *Ewing's tumor* is the most common bone tumor in young children. Systemic symptoms such as fever and malaise occur along with local pain, swelling and tenderness. The clinical picture may simulate osteomyelitis.

II. *Osteogenic sarcoma* may be characterized by local pain, swelling and increased warmth. Chondrosarcoma is usually a low-grade malignancy.

III. *Osteochondroma*, the most common bone tumor in children, is a benign tumor generally first discovered after trauma. It most frequently occurs at the distal end of the femur or proximal end of the tibia and humerus. Multiple osteochondromas occur in hereditary multiple exostoses.

IV. *Osteoid osteoma*, a benign tumor, may cause chronic, boring or aching bone pain. Limp may be present if the tumor is in the lower extremity. Muscle atrophy may also be noted. Pain is usally intermittent and worse at night, often awakening the child. Episodes last an hour or two. Long bones are the most common site, but any bone in the body may be involved. If the affected area of bone is superficial, a fusiform swelling and inflammatory changes may be noted in the overlying skin. Pain may be localized or referred (e.g., from the proximal or middle femur to the thigh or knee). Striking relief of pain follows aspirin therapy.

Orlowski, J.P. and Mercer, R.D.: Osteoid osteoma in children and young adults. *Pediatrics* 59:526, 1977.

### GENERAL REFERENCES

Ferguson, A.B.: *Orthopedic Surgery in Infancy and Childhood*. 4th ed. Baltimore, Williams & Williams Co., 1975.
Lovell, W.W. and Winter, R.B.: *Pediatric Orthopaedics*. Vols. I and II. Philadelphia, J.B. Lippincott Co., 1978.

CHAPTER **28**

# THE MUSCULAR SYSTEM

In general, muscular development corresponds to the state of nutrition and activity of a child. A rapid increase in the amount of muscle tissue is a characteristic feature of the late adolescent period, especially in boys.

Muscle tone varies considerably even among normal newborn and young infants. It is influenced by the type of delivery, duration of labor, amount of anesthesia and the status of the central nervous system. Muscle tone is absent in infants who are asphyxiated secondary to central respiratory depression associated with narcosis or central nervous system injury.

The clinical implications of the various degrees of muscle tonus in the young infant are not entirely clear. The so-called hypertonic infant demonstrates heightened muscle tone and tenseness. These infants frequently have colic, cry excessively and vomit some of their feedings.

*Generalized ligamentous relaxation* may be present in many otherwise normal children. Congenital laxity of the ligaments may be accompanied by extreme hypotonia of the muscles. Characteristically, many of the joints are hyperextensible. The feet may be dorsiflexed, and genu valgum and flat, everted feet are often present. These children may walk relatively late, fall frequently and complain of leg pains after exercise.

*Benign congenital myopathies* are characterized by mild generalized or proximal, nonprogressive muscle weakness noted in early infancy. The serum enzymes are normal. Syndromes included in this group include central core disease, nemaline myopathy, mitochondrial myopathy, congenital fiber-type disproportion, myotubular myopathy, multicore myopathy, reducing body myopathy, fingerprint body myopathy and familial myopathy with probable lysis of myofibrils in type I fibers.

Saper, J.R.: Benign congenital myopathy. *Am. J. Med. 57*:157, 1974.

*Muscular hypotonia* may occur in patients with hypopotassemia, hypothyroidism, primary hypoparathyroidism, hyperparathyroidism, glycogenosis type II (Pompe's disease, acid maltase deficiency), arthrogryposis, Werdnig-Hoffmann disease, Marfan's syndrome, platybasia, gliomas of the hypothalamus and optic chiasm, medulloblastoma and astrocytoma. Muscular hypotonia associated with tumors of the cerebellar hemispheres may be generalized or present only on the involved side. The muscular hypotonia in patients with idiopathic hypercalcemia may be striking. Generalized muscle weakness with the infant becoming floppy may occur in infantile botulism. Severe malnutrition is usually characterized by muscular hypotonia, although hypertonia may occur in marasmic infants. Muscle atony and hypotonia may be present in children with cerebral palsy of either the spastic or athetoid type. Tay-Sachs disease is characterized by a generalized hypotonia of muscles but with hyperactive deep reflexes. Similar findings may be present in patients with tumors of the brain stem. Infants with congenital myotonic dystrophy may demonstrate marked floppiness.

In patients with hyperthyroidism the presence of otherwise inapparent muscle weakness may be demonstrated by having the patient sit on an examining table or in a chair and extend his lower extremities straight out. Normally, they can be maintained extended for over two minutes. Easy fatigability and some muscle atrophy may accompany the weakness.

Rosman, N.P.: Neurological and muscular aspects of thyroid dysfunction in childhood. *Pediatr. Clin. N. Am. 23*:575, 1976.

Muscular weakness may also be a manifestation of Addison's disease and is frequently present with Cushing's syndrome. Periodic, severe muscular weakness is a manifestation of primary aldosteronism. Other findings include paresthesias, intermittent tetany, polyuria, polydipsia, hypertension, hypokalemia and metabolic alkalosis. Hyperparathyroidism may cause proximal muscle weakness, wasting, hypotonia, muscle pain and cramps. Myopathy may be a complication of prolonged corticosteroid therapy. Profound generalized weakness may occur along with pain in patients with rhabdomyolysis and myoglobinuria.

*Periodic paralysis and muscle weakness* may be associated either with hypo- or hyperkalemia. With *primary hypokalemic periodic paralysis,* episodes of weakness and flaccid paralysis, which is predominantly proximal and mild or extends to complete quadriplegia, usually begin early in the morning and last from 2 to 24 hours. The extent and duration of the paralysis varies. In *hyperkalemic periodic paralysis* (adynamia episodica hereditaria), a familial disorder, the episodes are briefer and less severe. They occur during the day, especially on resting after exercise. Muscles of the trunk, pelvic girdle and extremities are predominantly involved. Myotonia may be elicited in the eyelids, tongue, forearm extensors and thenar eminences. In *paramyotonia congenita,* myotonia secondary to exposure to cold is a dominant feature. The attacks of paralysis in this disorder are similar to those in hyperkalemic periodic paralysis.

Painful muscle cramps followed by transient myoglobinuria, weakness and stiffness may be brought on by physical exertion in patients with *McArdle's syndrome* (phosphorylase deficiency) and in those with muscle phosphofructokinase or carnitine palmital transferase deficiency.

Fattah, S.M., Rubulis, Ā. and Faloon, W.W.: McArdle's disease. *Am. J. Med. 48*:693, 1970.

In the exercise-induced type of *idiopathic rhabdomyolysis* and *myoglobinuria,* muscle pain, cramps, weakness and myoglobinuria occur within a few hours after exercise.

Roelofs, R.I. and Engel, W.K.: Myopathies associated with systemic diseases. *Postgrad. Med. 50*:95, 1971.

*Clostridial myositis* or gas gangrene is characterized by severe pain, crepitance, edema and discoloration. The patient may be very toxic.

**Dermatomyositis.** Muscle weakness, which may range from mild to severe, stiffness, tenderness, firmness and edema may develop early and insidiously in patients with dermatomyositis, along with systemic symptoms such as easy fatigability, fever and malaise. Involvement may be extensive and symmetrical. Pharyngeal and esophageal muscles may be involved. Eventually, swallowing, speech and respiration are affected. Although muscle weakness is generalized, it is predominantly proximal, involving the limb girdle and anterior neck flexors rather than peripheral. Muscle atrophy, fibrosis and "woody" induration develop later along with joint contractures and periarticular swelling. The skin manifestations of dermatomyositis are reviewed on p. 259. The skeletal muscle enzymes, especially creatine phosphokinase, are elevated.

Banker, B.Q. and Victor, M.: Dermatomyositis (systemic angiopathy) of childhood. *Medicine 45*:261, 1966.
Schaller, J.G.: Dermatomyositis. *J. Pediatr. 83*:699, 1973.
Sullivan, D.B., Cassidy, J.T., Petty, R.E. and Burt, A.: Prognosis in childhood dermatomyositis. *J. Pediatr. 80*:555, 1972.

*Polymyositis* presents with clinical manifestations that, except for the skin involvement, simulate dermatomyositis. Many of these patients demonstrate Raynaud's phenomenon. Chronic polymyositis may closely resemble muscular dystrophy.

Bohan, A. and Peter, J.B.: Polymyositis and dermatomyositis. *N. Engl. J. Med. 292*:344–403, 1975.

*Chronic myositis* may accompany other connective tissue or collagen-vascular diseases such as lupus erythematosus, periarteritis nodosa and, occasionally, rheumatoid arthritis. Proximal muscle weakness may be noted.

*Acute myositis* may also be associated with influenza B infection, following two to four days of fever, headache and other systemic symptoms. There is a sudden onset of severe pain and tenderness in the gastrocnemius and soleus muscles bilaterally and, occasionally, in the thighs. On physical examination, tenderness and, at times, swelling are noted in the calf muscles, and the feet are held in plantar flexion.

Dietzman, D.E., Schaller, J.G., Ray, C.G. and Reed, M.E.: Acute myositis associated with influenza B infection. *Pediatrics* 57:255, 1976.
Sirinavin, S. and McCracken, G.H.: Primary suppurative myositis in children. *Am. J. Dis. Child.* 133:263, 1979.

Myalgia occurs with leptospirosis and with Rocky Mountain spotted fever. Bubonic plague may cause myalgia.

Congenital *muscular hypertrophy* has been described in association with mental deficiency and cerebral palsy. Idiopathic benign congenital muscular hypertrophy may also occur. Rarely, generalized muscular hypertrophy may be observed in patients with hypothyroidism (the Kocher-Debré-Semelaigne syndrome).

Hopwood, N.J., Lockhart, L.H. and Bryan, G.T.: Acquired hypothyroidism with muscular hypertrophy and precocious testicular enlargement. *J. Pediatr.* 85:233, 1974.

*Myositis fibrosa generalista,* a rare disease in childhood, is characterized by painless muscle stiffness, induration, atrophy and contractures. The extent of involvement initially is usually slight, but the process gradually progresses until entire muscles are affected, most commonly those of the lower extremities. Except for the masseter muscles, the face is uninvolved.

*Progressive myositis ossificans* begins most commonly in the muscles of the neck and back as localized, tender, pliable or firm masses. Transient edema and erythema of the skin may appear over the involved area. Remissions occur, but over a period of months calcification develops in the connective tissue of the muscle, and the induration is replaced by a bony hardness. As the process gradually extends to involve most of the striated musculature of the body, limitation of movement and ankylosis of joints appear. Shortening of the digits, particularly of the thumb and large toe, hallux valgus and other digital anomalies may also occur.

Lutwak, L.: Myositis ossificans progressiva. *Am. J. Med.* 37:269, 1964.

*Localized myositis ossificans* may be caused by trauma. Swelling, tenderness and pain on use of the involved muscle may occur. The brachialis anticus is the most frequently affected muscle. This complication may also appear in the quadriceps femoris after a thigh injury.

*Myotonia congenita* is a familial disease that usually begins early in childhood with myotonia and hypertrophy of the muscles. The patient has difficulty in initiating muscular action, especially after a period of inactivity or quickly releasing his grip as in a handshake. Muscular relaxation occurs slowly. Local contraction and dimpling occur when a muscle such as the deltoid or the thenar eminence is struck with a reflex hammer and may persist for 30 to 60 seconds. Symptoms are exacerbated by cold, fatigue or excitement.

*Paramyotonia congenita* is characterized by myotonia following exposure to cold. Attacks of muscle weakness and stiffness may occur with or without exposure to cold. Elevation of the serum potassium may occur in some instances.

Muscular stiffness and twitching may occur in *tetany.*

**Muscular Dystrophy.** In addition to clinical evaluation of muscle involvement, other diagnostic procedures include serum aldolase, creatinine phosphokinase, transaminase (SGOT and SGPT), electromyography and muscle biopsy. Muscle testing and electromyography help select the appropriate muscle for biopsy. In the clinical differentiation between myopathy or neuropathy as causes for muscle weakness, muscle fasciculations suggest the latter. The deep tendon reflexes are never increased with a myopathy although they may be increased with neurogenic weakness associated with involvement of the corticospinal tracts. The serum enzymes do not always allow etiologic differentiation. They are, however, always elevated in the severe form of Duchenne dystrophy.

Munsat, T.L., Baloh, R., Pearson, C.M. and Fowler, W., Jr.: Serum enzyme alterations in neuromuscular disease. *JAMA 226*:1536, 1973.
Evans, O.B.: Polyneuropathy in childhood. *Pediatrics 64*:96, 1979.

*Pseudohypertrophic muscular dystrophy* may become manifest during infancy or early childhood, predominantly in boys. The progression of the disease is variable with many children becoming wheelchair-bound in adolescence while in the more benign type, the patient remains ambulatory 25 to 30 years after the onset of the disease. Symptoms, usually first noted when the child begins to walk, include inability to run well, difficulty in climbing stairs, a waddling gait and a history of frequent falls. The gastrocnemius, soleus, gluteus, deltoid and triceps muscles are most commonly involved. Weakness and atrophy may also occur in the muscles of the abdomen, pelvis, thighs and back, but usually not those of the face. Early, many of the affected muscles, especially those of the calves, the triceps and the deltoid, are enlarged, with a firm, doughy or rubbery texture. As the disease progresses, however, muscular atrophy develops, initially at the musculotendinous insertions. The tendon reflexes gradually diminish and are eventually unobtainable. Atrophy is not preceded by pseudohypertrophy in the Leyden-Möbius type of progressive muscular dystrophy. The Achilles tendon becomes shortened and flexural contractures develop at the hips, knees and elbows along with a lumbar lordosis. Because the Achilles tendon is short, the child walks on his toes. The gait is waddling with the trunk swaying from side to side.

The muscles of the shoulder girdle are extremely weak so that the patient seems to slip through the examiner's hands when an attempt is made to pick him up by the axillae. Winging of the scapulae also occurs.

Involvement of the flexors of the neck makes it difficult or impossible for the patient to elevate his head from the supine position. The loss of strength in the abdominal and other trunk musculature also makes it difficult to sit or stand from the supine position. The manner in which the patient achieves the standing position by "climbing up himself" has been called *Gower's sign*. The child first turns on his side, flexes his hips and knees and uses his extended arm as a pivot to assume a kneeling position. The feet are then brought forward and the lower extremities straightened by extension at the knee. Finally, the hands are lifted from the floor and placed sequentially over the tibias, the knees and the thighs until the child is standing upright. This sign is consistently present with progressive muscular dystrophy, but it may also occur in patients with pelvic girdle weakness due to other causes.

The *facioscapulohumeral* type of muscular dystrophy begins between 12 and 20 years of age with weakness of the facial muscles and lack of facial expression (myopathic facies). The patient has difficulty closing his eyelids, elevating his eyebrows, frowning, raising the corners of his mouth on smiling and puckering his lips to whistle. Progression of the disease leads to weakness and atrophy of the muscles in the scapulohumeral and pectoral areas. Generalized involvement similar to that of the pseudohypertrophic type may eventually result. A form of neurogenic muscle atrophy may simulate the FSH form of muscular dystrophy (page 187).

*Limb-girdle dystrophy* is intermediate between the Duchenne and facioscapulohu-meral forms. Pseudohypertrophy of the calves and marked elevation of the serum enzymes usually do not occur. The pelvic girdle is principally involved with the shoulder girdle less often affected. The onset is usually between 10 and 40 years of age. Children with late onset *acid maltase deficiency* may demonstrate chronic progressive proximal muscle weakness that may simulate limb-girdle dystrophy. A neurogenic form of muscle atrophy may also simulate limb-girdle dystrophy (page 187). Dermatomyositis and polymyositis may have a similar distribution.

Jackson, C.E. and Strehler, D.A.: Limb-girdle muscular dystrophy. *Pediatrics 41*:495, 1968.

Tanaka, K. et al.: Muscular form of glycogenosis Type II (Pompe's disease). *Pediatrics 63*:124, 1979.

*Juvenile muscular atrophy,* or Erb's type of muscular dystrophy, which begins at puberty or somewhat later, is characterized by weakness of the shoulder girdle. The facial muscles are uninvolved.

*Congenital muscular dystrophy,* a rare cause of the "floppy infant" syndrome, is present at birth and rapidly progressive.

*Myotonic muscular dystrophy,* a familial disorder, may be present at birth or first noted between 10 and 15 years of age. In newborn infants manifestations include facial diplegia that resembles Möbius's syndrome, sucking, swallowing and breathing difficulties, muscle weakness, hypotonia with deep tendon reflexes preserved and retardation of motor development. On chest x-ray, the ribs appear to be abnormally slender. Myotonia usually appears later. Patients with early onset of myotonic dystrophy also demonstrate lumbar lordosis and weakness of proximal muscles. Arthrogryposis, talipes deformities or other joint immobility may be noted. In the older child and adolescent, the involvement begins distally in the hands and feet. Myotonia, characterized by slow relaxation of a muscle after contraction, may be the initial manifestation when the onset is in early childhood.

Dodge, P.R., Ganstorp, I., Byers, R.K. and Russell, P.: Myotonic dystrophy in infancy and childhood. *Pediatrics 35*:3, 1965.

Dyken, P.R. and Harper, P.S.: Congenital dystrophia myotonica. *Neurology 23*:465, 1973.

Sarnat, H.B., O'Connor, T. and Byrne, P.A.: Clinical effects of myotonic dystrophy on pregnancy and the neonate. *Arch. Neurol. 33*:459, 1976.

Vignos, P.J., Jr.: Diagnosis of progressive muscular dystrophy. *J. Bone Joint Surg. 49-A*: 1212, 1967.

Zatz, M.: Diagnosis, carrier detection and genetic counseling in the muscular dystrophies. *Pediatr. Clin. N. Am. 25*:557, 1978.

## GENERAL REFERENCE

Dubowitz, V.: *Muscle Disorders in Childhood.* Philadelphia, W. B. Saunders Co., 1978.

# CHAPTER 29

# THE SKIN

Frequently, the diagnosis of a dermatologic disorder is immediately apparent, especially if it has been previously encountered. When the diagnosis is less obvious, it is generally helpful to identify the individual lesion as a macule, papule, vesicle, bulla, wheal, pustule, petechia, nodule or erythema. Pruritus may be reported in the history or may be indicated by scratch marks. Attention to the distribution of lesions may also be helpful diagnostically (i.e., whether localized or generalized, on flexural or extensor, exposed or covered surfaces).

## SKIN OF THE NEWBORN INFANT

Easterly, N.B. and Solomon, L.M.: Neonatal dermatology. II. Blistering and scaling dermatoses. *J. Pediatr.* 77:1075, 1970.

Hodgman, J.E., Freedman, R.I. and Levan, N.E.: Neonatal dermatology. *Pediatr. Clin. N. Am. 18*:713, 1971.

Solomon, L.M. and Easterly, N.B.: *Neonatal Dermatology.* Philadelphia, W. B. Saunders Co., 1973.

Solomon, L.M. and Easterly, N.B.: Neonatal dermatology. I. The newborn skin. *J. Pediatr.* 77:888, 1970.

*Premature infants* have little subcutaneous tissue, and their skin is delicate, almost transparent, with vessels visible through the skin. The skin of the term infant is soft, smooth and velvety, especially during the first few days of life. The hands and feet are often cold, bluish-red and sometimes glossy. A few hours after birth, the skin becomes intensely red, and this color persists for several hours.

In the *postmature infant* the vernix caseosa is minimal in amount or absent. The skin is dry, cracked and parchment- or collodion-like. Peeling is noted at birth. With greater postmaturity the umbilical cord and skin are stained green or golden yellow.

The *vernix caseosa* is a soft, cheesy, clay-colored material that covers the skin of newborn infants. The amount varies considerably, being almost absent at times, especially in postmature infants. Meconium or yellow staining of the vernix caseosa, abnormal except in breech presentations, may occur in hemolytic disease of the newborn, postmature infants and fetal distress.

Branny or flaky *desquamation* of the skin, including that of the palms and soles, occurs to some extent in nearly all term infants during the first few days of life, but in premature infants not until the second or third week. In some, however, the desquamation is more extensive and sheetlike, especially over the trunk, with transverse creases or cracks. Babies subjected to acute intrauterine hypoxia show desquamation at birth. The soles of premature infants are smooth. Only 1 or 2 creases are present at 32 weeks. The creases appear distally and gradually extend toward the heels. Two-thirds of the sole has creases at 37 weeks while the entire sole, including the heels, is creased in term infants. The postmature infant has deeper *sole creases*.

*Lanugo*, a fine, downy kind of hair, is usually present over the face, ear lobes, back and shoulders of premature babies but practically absent in term infants.

The skin of newborn infants reacts to pressure and irritation with erythema, tiny papules and nonspecific eruptions. The terms *flea bite dermatitis* and *toxic erythema of the newborn* have been used for one type of nonspecific, transient, blotchy and erythematous lesion commonly seen in the newborn. These lesions have tiny, central, yellow or white vesicles or wheals, most evident when the skin is stretched. The so-called pustular form of toxic erythema is characterized by yellow or white papular or pustular lesions, 1 to 3 mm. in size, which contain eosinophils rather than neutrophils as in impetigo. The lesions are usually found in skin creases. Clinical differentiation from pyoderma may not be possible.

*Pustular melanosis*, more common in black than in white newborn infants, is vesicular-pustular lesions without surrounding erythema or pigmented macules on the chin, neck, lower back, pretibial region or palms and soles. The vesicopustules fade in one to two days, and the macules disappear in a few weeks.

Ramamurthy, R.S., Reveri, M., Esterly, N.B., Fretzin, D.F. and Pildes, R.S.: Transient neonatal pustular melanosis. *J. Pediatr.* 88:831, 1976.

Newborn infants who are very active sometimes develop abrasions over their elbows, knees, ankles, heels, toes and other pressure areas. Scratch marks are not infrequently seen on the face.

*Cutis marmorata*, a purplish mottling of the skin, may occur in healthy infants and young children and is especially prominent in premature, hypothyroid and debilitated infants.

*Shock or hypotension* in the newborn infant is manifested by pallor, gray or cyanotic skin color, clammy skin, respiratory distress, lethargy and hypotonia. The systolic blood pressure in neonatal hypotension is under 40 mm. Hg in prematures and under 50 mm. Hg in term infants. Disorders causing neonatal shock include blood loss; sepsis, especially from group B streptococcus; and asphyxia.

*"Harlequin" color change.* In an occasional newborn infant, more commonly of low birth weight, one half of the body suddenly becomes pale or reddened with a sharp line of demarcation exactly down the midline. These episodes, which last seconds to minutes, are without pathologic significance. Episodes of flushing, pallor or cyanosis may accompany *neonatal hypoglycemia*.

*Acne*, with papules, pustules and comedones due to maternal hormonal stimulation, may occur in newborn infants about the first week of life.

*Milia* are yellowish-white, pinpoint-sized or larger, usually grouped, somewhat shiny vesicles caused by plugging and distention of sebaceous ducts. Milia may be noted during the first or second week of life on the forehead, nose, nasolabial folds, chin and cheeks.

*Intertrigo,* or *chafing*, refers to the moist, erythematous areas in creases of the skin. Folds of the neck, axillae, inguinal region and perineum are commonly involved. Seborrheic dermatitis and moniliasis may be etiologic.

*Subcutaneous fat necrosis* may occur during the neonatal period as single or multiple, indurated, button-like lesions, 1 to 2 cm. in diameter or larger. Sites of predilection are the back, cheeks, buttocks and extremities. The overlying skin may be reddened or purplish. Usually the lesions are not attached to the underlying subcutaneous tissue. Gradual disappearance over a period of weeks or months is the rule, but fluctuation and external drainage occasionally occur. Subcutaneous calcification and hypercalcemia may develop.

Michael, A.F., Jr., Hong, R. and West, C.D.: Hypercalcemia in infancy. *Am. J. Dis. Child.* *104*:235, 1962.

*Sclerema neonatorum* is an intense, nonpitting hardening of subcutaneous tissues, usually of the trunk and proximal portions of the extremities, which occurs rarely in premature or debilitated newborn infants. A nonspecific finding, this disorder usually accompanies a life-threatening disorder such as septicemia, pneumonia, peritonitis or severe gastroenteritis. The process may begin on the buttocks, cheeks, thighs, calves or trunk and extend to much of the body. The overlying skin is cold, hard, bound down and colored a mottled reddish-purple or waxy white.

Warwick, W.J., Ruttenberg, H.D. and Quie, P.G.: Sclerema neonatorum — a sign, not a disease. *JAMA 184*:984, 1963.

*Scleredema* is an extremely rare brawny, pitting edema that usually appears first on the lower extremities and then extends to involve the entire body. Premature or debilitated infants may be affected during the first or second week of life. Findings include feeble respiratory movements, a weak pulse, a subnormal temperature and listlessness.

*Impetigo neonatorum* is usually characterized by single vesicles or pustules surrounded by an erythematous areola. The vesicle is easily ruptured, leaving a red, moist base with a wrinkled fringe. The lesions occur most commonly in skin folds and over the lower abdomen but may be more extensive. Bullae appear suddenly, coalesce and become widespread. Large areas of skin may become denuded. With *Ritter's disease*, a generalized erythema of the skin develops rapidly. The skin then becomes wrinkled, loose and exfoliates in sheets, leaving large, bright red, raw patches. Nikolsky's sign is positive (i.e., the skin separates in sheets as a result of friction by the examiner's finger).

The eruption of *congenital viral infections* such as cytomegalovirus and rubella has been called a "blueberry muffin" rash. The individual lesions are round, slightly raised, firm, dark blue to magenta in color and last three to four weeks. Dark red, gray-purple or copper brown macular lesions may also occur.

Brough, A.J., Jones, D., Page, R.H. and Mizukami, I.: Dermal erythropoiesis in neonatal infants. A manifestation of intrauterine viral disease. *Pediatrics 40*:627, 1967.

*Congenital syphilis* is a diagnostic consideration whenever an eruption occurs on an infant's palms or soles. The lesions are thickened, diffuse and either moist or covered by shiny, desquamating scales. Bullae may also occur on the palms and soles. The face and much of the body may be involved. Individual leisons are usually small, slightly elevated, annular, shiny, reddish-brown maculopapules. Moist, flat condylomas may appear in the perianal and genital resions. The moist fissures that occur around the mouth and nose heal with rhagades or linear scars that radiate from the corners of the mouth.

*Neonatal neuroblastoma* with subcutaneous metastasis is characterized by "blueberry muffin" skin lesions that become erythematous on rubbing and then blanch.

Pachedly, C.: The broad clinical spectrum of neuroblastoma. *Postgrad. Med. 51*:79, 1972.

Flat, light red *capillary hemangiomas* occur commonly over the base of the nose, upper eyelids, upper lip and nape of the neck. These lesions blanch on pressure and are more prominent during crying. They usually fade over a period of months and unless intensely red, completely disappear. A prominent facial flame nevus over the center of the forehead and upper eyelids occurs in Beckwith's syndrome and in trisomy 13. Petechiae may appear on the head along with cyanosis and edema when a baby is born with the umbilical cord wrapped around his neck.

*Mongolian blue spots* are irregularly shaped, bluish or bluish-gray pigmented areas over the buttocks, sacrum, upper back and extremities, more commonly seen in black, Indian and Oriental but occasionally also in white babies. The pigmented area, which may be 10 cm. or more in diameter, gradually disappears during infancy.

Rarely, *localized defects of the hair, skin and subcutaneous tissue* may be present at birth. Such defects, ½ to 1 inch in diameter, most commonly involve the scalp, especially the vertex. While they are usually unassociated with other anomalies, the *focal dermal hypoplasia syndrome* is characterized by areas in which the skin or scalp is absent or very thin, hyper- or hypopigmented and covered by telangiectasia. Additional striking features are reddish or brownish-yellow herniations of fat through the dermis (or linear hamartomas) and multiple wart-like papillomas involving the skin or mucous membrane of the mouth, genitalia or general skin surface. Anomalies of the hands, eyes and teeth may occur.

Goltz, R.W., Henderson, R.R., Hitch, J.M. and Ott, J.E.: Focal dermal hypoplasia syndrome. *Arch. Dermatol. 101*:1, 1970.

## DERMATOGLYPHICS

The arches, loops and whorls of the fingers may be examined either from fingerprints or by a magnifying lens. Unusual dermatoglyphic markings or patterns may be found in various syndromes such as trisomy 21, trisomy 13, trisomy 18 and 5p syndrome, but they are not specific for a given syndrome. Patients with Down's syndrome have a distal axial triradius of the palms, ulnar loops on all fingers, a simian line and a single flexion crease of the fifth finger along with clinodactyly.

Preus, M. and Fraser, F.C.: Dermatoglyphics and syndromes. *Am. J. Dis. Child. 124:933*, 1972.

## PIGMENTATION

**Jaundice.** The symptom of jaundice is discussed in Chapter 38. Jaundice appears more readily in some patients and in some areas of the skin than in others. Although there is some correlation with the serum bilirubin, there is no critical level at which clinical jaundice appears. Jaundice may persist in tissues for some time after plasma levels have begun to fall. The affinity of elastic fibers for biliary pigments may explain the early appearance and persistence of pigmentation in the sclera and other areas of the body in which elastic tissue is plentiful. In the presence of edema, jaundice is less evident. Its clinical detection may be difficult in the black patient except by inspection of the sclera. The greenish component sometimes noted in jaundiced patients is thought to be due to biliverdin. Increased melanin pigmentation may occur in patients with chronic jaundice as a result of pruritus and scratching.

*Bronze pigmentation* may occur as a complication of phototherapy for hyper-bilirubinemia.

Kopelman, A.E., Brown, R.S. and Odell, G.B.: The "bronze" baby syndrome: a complication of phototherapy. *J. Pediatr. 81*:466, 1972.

*Cyanosis* is discussed in Chapter 56.

*Carotenemia* and *carotenoderma* account for the lemon-yellow coloration of the skin frequently observed in infants, especially along the nasolabial folds, over the forehead, on the palms and soles, around the nails, periorbitally, along body folds and over pressure areas. The sclerae and mucous membranes are not pigmented. Carotenoderma may be especially prominent in infants who perspire profusely since some of the pigment is excreted in the sweat and then deposited in the stratum corneum. Carotenemia may also occur in hypothyroid children.

A lemon-yellow tint of the skin may be present in patients with thalassemia. A dusky, brown or grayish pigmentation may develop in children with a chronic hemolytic or hypoplastic anemia who have received large numbers of transfusions. Dark yellow to brown coloration of the skin is sometimes noted in patients with Niemann-Pick disease. This pigmentation may be more prominent over joints and exposed parts, especially the lower extremities.

*Addison's disease* may be characterized by dirty brown, tan or bluish-black pigmentation, especially around the genitalia, breast areolae, umbilicus, in the skin folds and over the joints and exposed parts. This pigmentation may occasionally be more generally distributed over the body in the form of freckle-like lesions. Depigmented areas within a zone of increased pigmentation have been described. Pigmented spots may also appear on the oral and buccal mucous membrane.

The *Rothmund-Thomson syndrome* is characterized initially in early infancy by redness and swelling of the cheeks and ears with the residual of areas of pigmentation, depigmentation, atrophy and telangiectasia along with hyperkeratoses over the joints, palms and soles. Bilateral cataracts occur.

A generalized brown pigmentation of the skin may be seen with *adrenoleukodystrophy*.

Under the age of five years, up to five *cafe-au-lait spots* over ½ inch in diameter may be within normal limits. In white children, the lesions are light brown, while they are brown in black children. Large, often unilateral, flat, brown cafe-au-lait spots are present in patients with *Albright's syndrome* along with polyostotic fibrous dysplasia and sexual precocity. The lesions may be present at birth or develop soon thereafter. The edges of these lesions are more irregular than those of neurofibromatosis.

*Cafe-au-lait* lesions are often the first manifestation of neurofibromatosis. Numerous freckle-like spots may occur in the axillae, inguinal or cervical regions. Neuromas in the skin and subcutaneous tissue are small, soft, boggy, raised or penduculated tumor masses. *Cafe-au-lait* spots also occur in Gaucher's disease, tuberous sclerosis and Fanconi's syndrome.

Holt, J.F.: Neurofibromatosis in children. *Am. J. Roentgenol. 130*:615, 1978.

Thalassemia and hemolysis due to an unstable hemoglobin may be accompanied by a gray cast to the skin or by a diffuse tan discoloration.

*Melanin spots* have been noted on the lips, mouth and fingers in patients with generalized intestinal polyposis (Peutz-Jeghers syndrome). These macules range in size from 0.2 to 5 mm. and are light brown to deep blue-black in color. The patient is usually asymptomatic until adolescence, when intussusception may occur.

*Acanthosis nigricans*, which rarely appears in children at puberty, is characterized by thickened, reddish-brown or black, verrucous, scaling lesions with small papillomatous tumors in the axillary and inguinal folds and around the nipples. Glucose intolerance and insulin resistance may also be present.

Kahn, C.R. et al.: The syndromes of insulin resistance and acanthosis nigricans. *N. Engl. J. Med. 294*:739, 1976.

*Incontinentia pigmenti* is characterized in about 80 per cent of cases by the appearance at birth or early in infancy of bullous or vesicular lesions. These are followed by a keratotic or warty stage in about 70 per cent and then by development of irregular, sharply outlined, nonelevated brownish or slate-colored areas. These areas, which have been likened to the irregular veins present in marble or to the splashing of brown spray on a light-colored surface, are found chiefly over the trunk and extremities in 100 per cent. The bullous and keratotic stages do not occur in all patients. Other ectodermal anomalies and neurologic disorders may be present.

Jackson, R., and Nigam, S.: Incontinentia pigmenti: a report of three cases in one family. *Pediatrics 30*:433, 1962.

In *albinism* the skin and hair are devoid of pigment. Partial albinism is characterized by patches of congenital hypopigmentation that do not enlarge. A white forelock of depigmented hair may occur.

*Vitiligo* refers to acquired white depigmented areas, encircled at times by a zone of increased pigmentation. These areas tend to spread. The etiology is unknown. The uveomeningoencephalitic syndrome (*Vogt-Koyanangi-Harada*) may be characterized by vitiligo and loss of hair pigment. Vitiligo may also occur in juvenile diabetes mellitus, sometimes preceding other clinical manifestations, and in collagen vascular disease.

Lerner, A.B. and Nordlung, J.J.: Vitiligo: what is it? Is it important? *JAMA 239*:1183, 1978.
Macaron, C. et al.: Vitiligo and juvenile diabetes mellitus. *Arch Dermatol. 113*:1515, 1977.

*Pityriasis alba*, probably a form of atopic dermatitis, causes patches of depigmentation and minimal dermatitis, 2 or 3 cm. in diameter, on the cheeks and extensor surfaces of the forearms.

Dull, white, ash leaf macules, may be the initial manifestation of *tuberous sclerosis*. These 1- to 3-cm. well-demarcated, oval lesions are rounded at one end and taper at the other (lance-ovate). Present at birth or appearing in early infancy predominantly on the trunk, the lesions may be few or may number more than 100. The Wood's light may accentuate the hypopigmentation.

Hurwitz, S. and Braverman, I.M.: White spots in tuberous sclerosis. *J. Pediatr. 77*:587, 1970.

## PIGMENTED NEVI

*Junctional nevi*, small brown or black lesions, absent at birth or present in only about 3 per cent of newborn infants, appear usually between 3 and 5 years of age and gradually increase until there are a maximal number of 20 to 40 in adolescence.

*Giant hairy or bathing trunk nevus*, present at birth, may cover 15 to 35 per cent of the skin surface, commonly the trunk, buttocks or an extremity. Light brown to deep black in color, the nevus may contain hairs, warty lesions and have a leathery feel. Malignant melanoma may occur as a complication.

*Compound nevi* are discrete, hairy, pigmented, usually raised verrucous or dome-shaped lesions, 2 to several centimeters in diameter, present at birth or appearing as the child becomes older.

*Spindle and epitheloid nevi* generally appear before puberty, usually on the face but at times on the extremities or trunk as 1 to 3-cm. dome-shaped, usually smooth but occasionally rough, pink or reddish lesions.

*Nevus unius lateris (linear nevus)* may be present at birth as dark brown papules, usually unilaterally, in longitudinal streaks and tending to become verrucous over time. Mental retardation may be present and seizures may occur.

*Nevus linearis sebaceus* consists of slightly raised yellow-brown, warty lesions, present at birth, occurring partially in a linear distribution over the forehead or body and, at times, accompanied by yellow or dark brown skin plaques. Mental retardation and seizures may be associated findings.

*Ichthyosis hystrix* is a light brown or dark gray marbling or brush stroke hyperkeratosis.

*Halo nevus* refers to a depigmented halo around a nevus that tends to develop in adolescence. Involution of the nevus then occurs over time.

*Blue nevus*, an oval, raised, dome-shaped, usually single, gray or steel-blue lesion may occur at birth or in early infancy on the face, hands or extremities.

*Malignant melanoma* may rarely occur in children.

Esterly, N.B. and Solomon, L.M.: Neonatal dermatology. III. Pigmentary lesions and hemangiomas. *J. Pediatr. 81*:1003, 1972.

Holden, K.R. and Dekaban, A.S.: Neurological involvement in nevus unis lateris and nevus linearis sebaceus. *Neurology 22*:879, 1972.

Trozak, D.J. Rowland, W.D. and Hu, F.: Metastatic malignant melanoma in prepubertal children. *Pediatrics 55*:191, 1975.

Walton, R.G.: Pigmented nevi. *Pediatr. Clin. N. Am. 18*:897, 1971.

The *multiple lentigenes (leopard) syndrome* is comprised of multiple defects in addition to the Lentingenes. These include Electrocardiographic conduction defects, Ocular hypertelorism, Pulmonary stenosis, Abnormalities of the genitalia, Retardation of growth and Deafness. The skin lesions are small, less than 5 mm. in diameter, oval or round dark brown spots that occur anywhere except the mucosal surfaces and are most concentrated on the neck and upper trunk. They may be present at birth but usually develop when the patient is between two and five years of age.

Gorlin, R.J., Anderson, R.C. and Blaw, M.: Multiple lentigenes syndrome. *Am. J. Dis. Child. 117*:652, 1969.

*Xeroderma pigmentosa*, a rare and serious disorder, may become evident late in infancy as numerous freckle-like lesions, especially prominent on the face, neck and extremities. The skin is abnormally sensitive to sunlight. Atrophic depigmented areas may develop along with scattered telangiectasia and flat verrucous lesions. Superficial ulcerations of the skin, which may appear most commonly about the facial orifices during the course of the disease, heal with scarring and contractures. Finally, malignant epitheliomas develop.

Siegelman, M.H. and Sutow, W.W.: Xeroderma pigmentosum. *J. Pediatr. 67*:625, 1965.

*Striae* sometimes appear in adolescent children who have gained weight rapidly. These children are usually obese but not always. The striae may be light pink or white. Prominent red or purple striae, perhaps 1 cm. in width and a few centimeters in length, may occur in infants and children with Cushing's syndrome, chiefly on the lower part of the abdomen, over the hips, the upper part of the chest and the extremities. Striae may also occur in children treated with corticosteroids.

## EDEMA

The discussion here will be concerned with localized edema. Edema as a symptom is discussed in Chapter 67.

In young infants minimal edema may be chiefly evident on the dorsum of the hands and feet. This localization has been described in tetany of the newborn.

Nonpitting edema of the hands and feet has been reported in infants with *Turner's syndrome*.

Patients with pertussis who have frequent severe paroxysms of coughing may demonstrate puffiness of the face.

*Angioneurotic edema* may be localized to the face, tongue, lips, larynx, ear, periorbitally or the extremities as a pale, tense, brawny, nonpruritic, nonpitting swelling. Recurrent episodes of edema or abdominal pain occur in hereditary angioneurotic edema and may be precipitated by physical trauma or emotional stress.

Frank, M.M. et al.: Hereditary angioedema: the clinical syndrome and its management. *Ann. Int. Med. 84*:580, 1976.

With *Schönlein-Henoch purpura*, migratory massive areas of edema may involve an extremity, part of the abdominal wall, the face or the scalp and may precede the appearance of purpura by one or more days. *Insect bites* often lead to local edema in infants and children, usually on the face or ear. *Serum sickness* may be characterized by facial or periorbital edema. The lips, tongue, buccal mucous membrane, larynx or external genitalia may also be involved. Edema may be a component of the serum sickness-like reaction that may occur after penicillin administration. Edema, especially of the face, may be a rare side effect of insulin treatment. Presternal edema has been noted in patients with mumps, usually with swelling of the submaxillary glands. Edema appears five to eight days after swelling of the salivary glands and lasts two to three days. Edema of the hands and feet occurs in *Kawasaki disease*.

Doughy edema of the skin is a common manifestation of *dermatomyositis*. This swelling may be either generalized or localized to the lower eyelids and involved areas of the body.

Periorbital edema is common in *acute glomerulonephritis*.

Massive edema of an extremity may occur in infants with osteomyelitis.

The physical findings caused by congenital or acquired obstruction of the inferior vena cava depend upon the site. When this is distal to the hepatic veins, a superficial collateral circulation develops over the lower part of the chest, abdomen and the inguinal regions. The lower extremities may or may not become edematous. Hepatomegaly and ascites develop with obstruction proximal to the hepatic veins. Patients with Chiari's syndrome or obliterative endophlebitis of the hepatic veins demonstrate hepatomegaly, ascites, abdominal pain and hepatic insufficiency. Obstruction of the superior vena cava (the superior vena caval syndrome) causes dilatation of the superficial tributary veins. Edema is localized to the arms, head and neck. Dyspnea and localized cyanosis may be evident. Minimal collateral circulation develops when the obstruction is distal to the azygos vein. Obstruction below the azygos vein is followed by a prominent superficial collateral circulation over the chest and abdomen, and the blood returns through the inferior vena cava. Thrombosis of the inferior vena cava may occur in children with cyanotic congenital heart disease.

Kuehl, K.S., Perry, L.W. and Scott, L.P.: Thrombosis of the inferior vena cava in patients with cyanotic congenital heart disease. *J. Pediatr. 79*:430, 1971.

Edema of the face, including the eyes and lips, may occur in the *Melkersson-Rosenthal* syndrome along with a furrowed tongue and recurrent peripheral facial paralysis.

Roseman, B. and Mulvihill, J.J.: Melkersson-Rosenthal syndrome in a 7-year-old-girl. *Pediatrics 61*:490, 1978.

Myxedema usually is nonpitting. The skin is thickened and puffy.

## LYMPHEDEMA

*Congenital lymphedema* may occur with lymphangiectasis or lymphangiomas. This swelling usually pits readily and may be either soft or firm. Lymphedema may be chiefly localized to one or more extremities, with less conspicuous involvement of the body generally. Deep creases are present in the region of the joints. *Milroy's disease* is a familial disorder evident at birth. The edema is usually confined to the lower extremities and does not pit except with firm pressure. Lymphangiectatic edema of the hands and feet, pterygium colli and other congenital anomalies may accompany Turner's syndrome in infants. The edema involves the dorsa of the hands and feet and may extend up the leg. The edema gradually disappears as the child becomes older.

*Lymphedema praecox* or *late-onset lymphedema*, a primary disorder of lymphatic drainage of the lower extremities, may appear at adolescence, usually in girls. Initially, the swelling involves the foot or ankle and may be intermittent, subsiding with rest. Usually, the edema proceeds proximally and, in time, may no longer pit. The skin over the involved areas may become thickened and have a "pigskin" appearance.

One form of hereditary lymphedema beginning in childhood is characterized by recurrent streptococcal lymphangitis. Another type is associated with distichiasis (extra eyelashes) and a widened spinal canal. In the lymphedema with yellow nails syndrome, the nail deformity may precede the lymphedema by a period of years.

Fonkalsrud, E.W. and Coulson, W.F.: Management of congenital lymphedema in infants and children. *Ann. Surg. 177*:280, 1973.
Holmes, L.B., Fields, J.P. and Zabriskie, J.B.: Hereditary late-onset lymphedema. *Pediatrics 61*:575, 1978.
Kleiman, P.K.: Congenital lymphedema and yellow nails. *J. Pediatr. 83*:454, 1973.
Robinow, M., Johnson, G.F. and Verhagen, A.D.: Distichiasis lymphedema: a hereditary syndrome of multiple congenital defects. *Am. J. Dis. Child. 119*:343, 1970.

Most instances of acquired lymphedema are postinfectious. Cat-scratch disease may cause secondary lymphedema in an extremity.

Filler, R.M., Shwachman, H. and Edwards, E.A.: Lymphedema after cat-scratch fever. *N. Engl. J. Med. 27*:244, 1964.

Acquired lymphedema involving one lower extremity may be due to a pelvic or retroperitoneal neoplasm or retroperitoneal fibrosis.

Peterson, A.S., Besecker, J.A. and Hutchison, W.A.: Retroperitoneal fibrosis and gluteal pain in a child. *J. Pediatr. 85*:228, 1974.

## PURPURA

Purpura refers to hemorrhage into the skin or mucous membranes. Pinpoint or pinhead-sized, scarlet or bluish-purple extravasations of blood are referred to as *petechiae*. Larger areas are usually termed *ecchymoses*. At first the lesions are bluish-purple, and the color does not fade on pressure. With local conversion of the extravasated hemoglobin to hemosiderin, the color gradually changes to brownish-green and then to yellow. Petechiae or larger purpuric spots may first occur about the ankles, wrists and neck folds. *Meningococcemia must always be immediatley ruled out with unexplained petechiae and purpura even in the absence of evidence of arthritis or meningitis.* Although the rash of meningococcemia is frequently petechial or purpuric, it may consist only of faint pink macules. Petechiae may occur in scarlet fever, streptococcal pharyngitis and echovirus infections. In the Waterhouse-Friderichsen syndrome the skin may appear mottled and livid or cyanotic. Petechial embolic lesions may be present in patients suspected of having subacute bacterial endocarditis.

In addition to hemorrhage into the skin, *anaphylactoid or Henoch-Schönlein purpura* may be accompanied by a variety of cutaneous lesions symmetrically distributed over the extensor surfaces of the extremities, the buttocks and the lower back. The lesions may be pink or brownish-red macules or maculopapules, 0.25 to 2 cm. in diameter. They remain small and slightly nodular or coalesce to become large. Hemorrhage common occurs into the center of the lesion. The erythema and elevation of the lesions may then disappear. Purpura disappears more slowly over a period of one to two weeks, the color changing gradually from purple to brown to yellow. Urticarial and vesicular lesions, either very small or large and bullous, may precede or accompany this eruption. Hemorrhage may also occur into these lesions, which resemble erythema nodosum. The cutaneous lesions tend to occur in crops for several weeks or months. Swelling of the hands, feet and joints and localized angioneurotic edema, especially in the scalp, often occur.

Borges, W.H.: Anaphylactoid purpura. *Pediatr. Clin. N. Am. 56*:201, 1972.

*Purpura fulminans* (purpura gangrenosa) is characterized by the sudden occurrence and rapid progression of extensive areas of ecchymosis and gangrene usually involving the extremities in a symmetrical fashion. There may be a preceding infectious disease such as scarlet fever, chickenpox, measles or meningococcemia.

Bouhasin, J.D.: Purpura fulminans. *Pediatrics 34*:264, 1964.

Purpuric and seborrheic skin lesions occur as manifestations of *Letterer-Siwe disease* (histiocytosis X) and can be almost pathognomonic. The patient may have crusted papular lesions, petechiae and a scaling eruption that resembles seborrheic dermatitis. The scalp, external auditory canals and trunk may be predominantly affected.

Tests of capillary fragility permit a crude evaluation of vascular integrity. In the *Rumpel-Leede test* a pressure midway between systolic and diastolic is maintained by a cuff wrapped around the upper arm for 5 to 10 minutes. Five minutes later, the skin distal to the cuff is examined for petechiae. If none are found, the procedure is repeated on the other arm, using a pressure of 100 mm Hg for 10 minutes. Normally, not more than 15 petechiae should appear in a circular area 5 cm. in diameter on the flexor surface of the forearm.

## HEMANGIOMAS

*Capillary hemangiomas* occur commonly in young infants in the form of a *nevus flammeus.* These nevi are poorly defined, flat, diffuse, pink to dark blue lesions usually present over the root of the nose, upper eyelids, upper lip and nape of the neck. They blanch upon pressure and become more evident during crying. A prominent nevus flammeus is present in trisomy 13 and the Beckwith syndromes. These hemangiomas become faint and often disappear over time. The *port wine stain,* another type of capillary hemangioma, is flat and pale pink to slate or reddish-blue. A vascular nevus present on the face over the distribution of the trigeminal nerve may be accompanied by involvement of the underlying meninges. The grouping of facial nevus, convulsions and intracranial calcifications is known as the *Sturge-Weber syndrome. von Hippel-Lindau disease* is characterized by hemangiomas in the skin, retina and cerebellum.

*Strawberry capillary hemangiomas* are sharply outlined, raised, moderately soft, smooth or irregularly lobulated lesions, a few millimeters to several centimeters in diameter and a bright strawberry or raspberry in color. They may be present at birth or appear during infancy and increase in size over the next 6 to 12 months. These lesions blanch with pressure. Gray patches appear on the hemangioma as the lesion begins to involute. At times a deep cavernous hemangioma may be palpable below and beyond the superficial strawberry nevus.

*Cavernous hemangiomas* may be small and localized above or beneath the skin, or they may be deep, diffuse and extensive. These lesions may be noted at birth or in early infancy. When extensive, local hypertrophy of the part may occur. Cavernous hemangiomas are usually moderately soft, lobulated and compressible. The overlying skin may appear normal, purplish or cloudy blue in color. *Giant hemangiomas* may involve much of an extremity in an infant and may be accompanied by thrombocytopenia.

Jacobs, A.H.: Birthmarks: I. Vascular nevi. *Pediatr. Rev. 1*:21, 1979.

*Angiokeratomas* begin to appear between 7 and 10 years of age on the buttocks, genitalia, lower back, abdomen, umbilicus and thighs in *Fabry's disease.* These lesions are 2 to 4 mm., round, purple or bluish-red and blood-filled macules or papules. Burning, lightning-like pain, warmth and perspiration occur in the hands and feet, especially the fingers and toes.

The *spider nevus* consists of dilated capillaries that radiate from a slightly raised, pinpoint center that does not disappear on pressure. Sites of predilection are the dorsum of the hands and the face. Although spider angiomas may occur in patients with chronic hepatitis and with cirrhosis, they are not of diagnostic significance in otherwise healthy children. Groups of dilated capillaries or telangiectasia are not uncommonly present in infants and children, especially on the face, over the nose and below the eyes and over the upper back. These benign lesions, which have a familial predisposition, may simulate spider nevi.

Wenzl, J.E. and Burgert, E.O., Jr.: Spider nevus in infancy and childhood. *Pediatrics* *33*:227, 1964.

*Telangiectasia* of the skin and conjunctiva may be accompanied by ataxia, respiratory disease and other findings in the ataxia-telangiectasia syndrome. Telangiectatic erythema of the face, photosensitivity and understature occur in *Bloom's syndrome.* Telangiectasia is also present in the focal dermal hypoplasia syndrome and in moya-moya.

## LYMPHANGIOMA

*Cavernous lymphangiomas*, or cystic hygromas, are soft, boggy, somewhat compressible, poorly demarcated, thin-walled tumors in the skin, subcutaneous or muscle tissue, most commonly in the neck. Cystic hygromas may also occur in the tongue and in the mediastinum.

*Lymphangioma circumscriptum* consists of closely and irregularly grouped, glistening or crusted, flesh-colored, thick-walled and deep-seated vesicles that contain a colorless liquid. Scattered, raisin-sized, wartlike, brown shiny papules may also occur.

*Lymphangiectasias*, or enlarged lymph spaces in the subcutaneous tissue, may cause enlargement of an extremity. Generalized lymphangiectasia may involve the bone and be associated with chylothorax.

## PERSPIRATION

Visible perspiration usually does not appear during the first day or two of life but may begin on the face on the third day and on the palms somewhat later, especially in the premature. Hyperhidrosis persisting for hours or days occurs in both term and premature infants experiencing *heroin withdrawal. Miliaria,* or *heat rash,* is due to keratinous plugging of sweat glands. Perspiration that occurs about the head and causes moistening of the underlying sheet is not uncommon in normal infants. *Miliaria crystallina*, due to sweat retention, consists of numerous fine, pinhead-sized, clear vesicles unaccompanied by inflammatory changes in the skin. *Miliaria rubra* consists of discrete erythematous papular lesions caused by sweat retention in the dermis.

*Excessive perspiration* may occur in children who are chronically ill and in patients with cystic fibrosis, hyperthyroidism, pheochromocytoma, hypoglycemia and febrile illnesses. Children with labile vasomotor control become flushed and perspire excessively with little provocation. Excessive perspiration occurs in children with *familial dysautonomia.* Increased sweating may occur in infants and children in congestive heart failure.

Behrendt, H. and Green, M.: Nature of the sweating deficit of prematurely born neonates. *N. Engl. J. Med. 286*:1376, 1972.
Morgan, C.A. and Nadas, A.S.: Sweating and congestive heart failure. *N. Engl. J. Med. 268*:580, 1963.

Excessive sweating of the palms along with nailbiting and dilatation of the pupils usually indicates anxiety.

"Sweaty sock" dermatitis is due to hyperhidrosis and the wearing of socks made of synthetic fibers.

Gibson, W.B.: Sweaty sock dermatitis. *Clin. Pediatr. 2*:175, 1963.

*Ectodermal dysplasia* of the anhydrotic type is a familial disease characterized by absence of visible perspiration. The skin may be dry, thin, white, glossy and eczematoid in the flexural areas and around the base of the nose. The children have a characteristic facies. Anodontia, absence or dysplasia of the nails and atrophic rhinitis may be present.

Absence of sweating below the site of the lesion may be seen in spinal cord injury.

## SKIN TEXTURE

*Tissue turgor* is poor in patients with significant dehydration and in malnourished infants, owing to loss of subcutaneous fat. In patients with *hyperosmolarity* or *hypernatremia* the tissue turgor may be fair, but the skin and subcutaneous tissue may feel firm and doughy.

The earliest clinical signs of dehydration usually reflect an acute volume loss equivalent to 5 per cent of weight. Babies who have lost 10 per cent of their body weight show early circulatory impairment while those with 15 per cent loss are in shock and near death.

Finberg, L.: Dehydration in infants and children. *N. Engl. J. Med. 276*:458, 1967.

The skin may be warm and moist in hyperthyroidism and dry, coarse and scaly in hypothyroidism. In dehydrated and malnourished patients, the skin is dry.

Premature wrinkling of the skin about the eyes and mouth occurs in older adolescents with pituitary dwarfism (IGHD, type I).

Thickening and brawny texture of the skin occur in children with Hurler's syndrome. Patients with chronic idiopathic hypoparathyroidism may also have a thickened and roughened skin texture. *Shagreen patches,* raised, flat plaques simulating sharkskin or demonstrating horizontal wrinkling and ranging in diameter from a few millimeters to several centimeters, may occur with tuberous sclerosis, especially on the face and trunk. The lesions are light brown or skin-colored.

A collodion-like covering of the skin may rarely be observed in the newborn. This brownish-yellow, shiny "varnished" appearance may be generalized or localized to the hands and feet. In those with *lamellar desquamation of the newborn* the skin is normal after completion of desquamation, which occurs in large sheets. On the other hand, in some infants collodion skin represents the first manifestation of *sex-linked ichthyosis* or *bullous* or *nonbullous congenital ichthyosiform erythroderma.*

All of the ichthyoses are characterized by scaly skin that desquamates. *Ichthyosis vulgaris,* the most common form that is inherited in an autosomal dominant manner, is not usually noted in the early months of life. The scales are fine, whitish or brown and occur primarily on the back and extensor surfaces. Hyperkeratoses may be present on the elbows, knees and ankles. Keratosis pilaris and chapping of hands and feet may be noted. In the other ichthyosiform dermatoses the scales, which periodically desquamate, are large, yellow or dark brown. Hyperkeratoses involve portions of the skin, palms and nails. Redness of the underlying skin occurs in two of these disorders and one is characterized by crops of large or small bullae that rupture and leave a raw surface. The term *harlequin fetus* has been applied to infants with the most severe form of nonbullous congenital ichthyosiform erythroderma. Such infants demonstrate on "O" shaped mouth, diamond-shaped or triangular hyperkeratotic plaques on the trunk and extremities and deep fissures.

The *Sjögren-Larssen syndrome* is characterized by nonbullous congenital ichthyosis, spasticity and mental retardation. Ichthyosis also occurs in *Refsum's syndrome*.

Esterly, N.B.: The ichthyosiform dermatoses. *Pediatrics 42*:990, 1968.

During the winter months, many children show dryness and follicular hyperplasia to a mild extent. Too frequent bathing and synthetic clothing finishes may be contributory in some instances.

*Vitamin A deficiency* results in a dry, scaly, rough skin with "goose pimple" hyperkeratosis over the extensor surfaces of the arms and thighs, the flexor surfaces of the legs and over the shoulders and buttocks.

*Keratosis pilaris,* pinhead-sized keratotic papules on the sides of the arms and thighs, and dry skin occur in atopic dermatitis and ichthyosis. Follicular psoriasis with "horny spikes" may require differentiation.

*Keratosis palmaris et plantaris* is a rare familial disorder characterized by a yellowish-brown, dry, fissured thickening of the palms and soles. Hyperkeratosis of the palms and soles may be associated with periodontoclasia with premature loss of the deciduous and permanent teeth. Similar involvement of the palms and soles may occur with *pityriasis rubra pilaris* and in the *Rothmund-Thomson syndrome*. Thickening of the skin of the palms, soles, elbows and knees may be accompanied by ring-like constrictions of the middle phalanx of the digits and profound congenital deafness. Hyperkeratosis of the palms and soles, accompanied at times by bullae, often occurs in *pachyonychia congenita*.

*Keloid* formation with excessive formation of scar tissue may complicate wounds and operative scars.

*Seborrheic dermatitis* is a moist, greasy, scaly, dirty yellow or yellowish-red crusting eruption ("potato chip" scales) that usually begins over the scalp, chiefly over the anterior fontanel ("cradle cap"), eyebrows, the sternal region, flexural areas and behind the ears. The diaper area and the skin folds are commonly involved. Fissuring or intertrigo in the skin creases is often present. Lesions may also appear on the trunk. Infants with Letterer-Siwe disease, or histiocytosis X, may have a seborrheic type of dermatitis over the scalp, face, neck and trunk. This brown, scaly, papular and vesicular rash may have both petechial and crusting components. Extensive involvement of the skin with seborrheic dermatitis occurs in *Leiner's disease* (page 247).

Winkelmann, R.K.: The skin in histiocytosis X. *Mayo Clin. Proc. 44*:535, 1969.

*Cutis laxa* may appear at birth or later. The loose skin may form large folds that can be drawn out from the body. The neck may appear webbed. The drooping eyelids and cheeks give the child a bloodhound appearance.

Smith, D.W.: Redundant skin folds in the infant — their origin and relevance. *J. Pediatr. 94*:1021, 1979.

In *cutis hyperelastica* a fold of skin may be grasped and stretched several inches. When released, the skin returns without folds. Hyperelasticity may be limited to localized areas of the skin. The mucous membrane of the mouth may also be involved. The skin feels thin and is fragile with a tendency to split with slight trauma. The resultant gaping wounds heal with shiny, white, wrinkled, thin and perhaps pigmented scars that may bulge or balloon out from the skin. Capillary hemorrhage occurs readily in these patients, and large hematomas may develop. These findings are present in *Ehlers-Danlos syndrome* along with subcutaneous lipomas.

> Hollister, D.W.: Heritable disorders of connective tissue: Ehlers-Danlos syndrome. *Pediatr. Clin. N. Am. 25*:575, 1978.

*Calcification* may occur in the skin and underlying tissues in cavernous hemangiomas, dermatomyositis and other connective tissue disorders and progressive myositis ossificans. Necrosis and ulceration of the skin may follow with discharge of gritty, chalk-like material.

> Leistyna, J.A. and Hassan, A.H.I.: Interstitial calcinosis. *Am. J. Dis. Child. 107*:96, 1964.

*Scleredema adultorum,* which usually follows a respiratory infection, is characterized by a hard, nonpitting induration of the skin first noted along the sides of the neck and then extending to the face, scalp, arms, neck and chest. The skin cannot be wrinkled or picked up in a fold. The facial expression may be masklike.

> Bradford, W. D., Cook, C. D., Vawter, G. F. and Berenberg, W.: Scleredema of childhood. *J. Pediatr. 68*:391, 1966.
> Robinow, M.: Scleredema adultorum — a children's disease. *Am. J. Dis. Child. 105*:81, 1963.

In the *stiff skin syndrome,* stony-hard, localized lesions develop in the skin, especially over the buttocks and upper thighs, along with mild hirsutism and limitation of joint motion. The dermis in these patients contains an abnormal amount of mucopolysaccharide.

Skin changes in the Hurler, Hunter, Morquio and Scheie type of mucopolysaccharidoses include thickened, roughened skin and papular or nodular plaques on the trunk and upper extremities. These have an orange peel texture.

> Esterly, N.B. and McKusick, V.A.: Stiff skin syndrome. *Pediatrics 47*:360, 1971.

## ATOPIC DERMATITIS

Atopic dermatitis in infancy begins usually on the cheeks and forehead. Later, the scalp and the extremities may also be involved. Eczema rarely appears on the back and in the diaper area.

The lesions of eczema may be acute, subacute or chronic. These may occur sequentially or concomitantly in different parts of the body. During the acute phase a rough, orange-red, glossy erythema of the skin occurs, especially over the cheeks, along with fine scales. This is usually followed by an intensely pruritic, papulovesicular eruption. Itching is always present with atopic dermatitis whereas it is often absent or minimal in seborrheic dermatitis. Rupture and coalescence of the minute vesicles produce raw, weeping and crusted lesions. In the subacute stage the weeping lesions begin to dry. Epithelization, thickening and scaling of the skin follow. In older infants and children, thickening, drying and lichenification of the skin occurs with involvement of the flexural areas and skin folds. The child scratches and rubs his skin relentlessly. Lighter and darker areas of pigmentation may develop and persist. The eyelids may appear wrinkled.

Eczema is also seen, at times in infants with phenylketonuria and in some children with ectodermal dysplasia of the anhydrotic type.

Atopic dermatitis with papular and petechial lesions may involve the scalp and trunk in Letterer-Siwe disease. It may need to be differentiated from seborrheic dermatitis. At times, seborrheic dermatitis may precede eczema. Weeping of the skin and severe or persistent pruritus is more characteristic of atopic dermatitis.

Norins, A.L.: Atopic dermatitis. *Pediatr. Clin. N. Am. 18*:801, 1971.

*Kaposi's varicelliform eruption,* a vesicular eruption caused by herpes or coxsackie A16 virus, may occur in infants with atopic eczema. The lesions, which appear in crops for several days, progress through vesiculation, umbilication, rupture and desiccation with various kinds of lesions present at one time.

The *Wiskott-Aldrich syndrome,* a sex-linked recessive disorder, is characterized by eczematoid dermatitis, draining ears, bloody diarrhea and petechiae due to thrombocytopenia.

*Contact dermatitis* may be due to innumerable substances: scented or strongly alkaline soaps, skin lotions, cosmetics, wool clothing, plastic toys and so forth. Involvement occurs chiefly on the exposed areas of skin, though in reactive persons the eruption may become widespread. Acute involvement is characterized by erythema, edema and vesiculation. The lesion is usually sharply demarcated. Chronic involvement results in drying and lichenification.

*Circumoral dermatitis* may occur in infants who drool excessively.

*Dermatitis venenata* due to contact with poison ivy or similar agents is characterized by erythema, edema and an intensely pruritic vesicular eruption over the exposed parts of the body, especially along scratch marks.

*Infectious eczematoid dermatitis* may occur as the result of irritation produced by a purulent discharge in patients with chronic rhinitis, suppurative otitis media and other draining lesions. Occasionally, the term *infectious eczematoid dermatitis* is applied to raised, infiltrated, sharply marginated patches covered with scales, tiny papules, vesicles or a purulent and crusting exudate.

## ERUPTIONS IN THE DIAPER AREA

*Primary irritant dermatitis* is a bright erythematous or papulovesicular eruption over the diaper area, occasionally so severe as to simulate a first-degree burn. Most commonly caused by the presence of ammonia, the eruption may also be caused by putrefactive bacterial enzymes acting on urinary amino acids to produce irritant by-products.

In *monilial diaper dermatitis* the characteristic lesions on the glabrous skin begin as small papules that transform into vesicles; on rupture these leave a denuded erythematous patch surrounded by a "white collar." The small patches may fuse into one larger beefy-red patch with pea- to dime-sized satellite lesions around the periphery. A psoriasiform *id* reaction (napkin psoriasis) may occur. Oral thrush is usually present.

*Seborrheic diaper dermatitis* usually begins at three or four weeks of age in the inguinal skin creases and then extends to adjacent areas with a sharp demarcation from normal skin. Intertrigo with greasy scales may be noted in other skin folds along with cradle cap. Satellite lesions may occur — small erythematous papules or pustules with peripheral scaling — due to secondary infection with Candida albicans.

*Psoriasis* in infants may first present in the diaper region, including the skin folds. "Napkin" psoriasis may also be due to infection by Candida albicans.

*Granuloma gluteale infantum* appears as firm, round or oval, painless, cherry or plum-sized, bluish-red, slightly protruding nodules on the buttocks. Spontaneous resolution slowly occurs.

Bazex, A. et al.: Infantile gluteal granuloma. *Ann. Dermatol. Syphilol. 99*:121, 1972.
Jacobs, A.H.: Eruptions in the diaper area. *Pediatr. Clin. N. Am. 25*:209, 1978.

*Acrodermatitis enteropathica* appears in early infancy with erythematous, vesiculobullous, pustular and eczematoid skin lesions present around the body orifices, scalp and the distal extremities along with persistent diarrhea and alopecia. Zinc deficiency secondary to prolonged *parenteral* alimentation may cause similar findings.

Neldner, K.H. et al.: Acrodermatitis enteropathica. *Arch. Dermatol. 110*:711, 1974.

*Nummular eczema* is characterized by round or oval, discrete plaques, ½ to 2 inches in diameter, covered by minute vesicles, exudate and crusts and occurring chiefly on the extensor aspects of the extremities.

*Circumscribed neurodermatitis* occasionally occurs in older children as a sharply defined, slightly raised, lichenified patch, probably produced by chronic pruritus and scratching.

*Leiner's disease,* which occurs during the first few months of life, is characterized by severe seborrheic dermatitis, intractable diarrhea, recurrent infections and failure to thrive. Affected infants have a deficiency of C5 or serum opsonic activity.

Jacobs, J.C. and Miller, M.E.: Fatal familial Leiner's disease: a deficiency of the opsonic activity of serum complement. *Pediatrics 49*:225, 1972.

## SKIN INFECTIONS

*Impetigo contagiosa,* usually due to staphylococcus or group A beta-hemolytic streptococcus, begins as purulent vesicles, bullae or pustules that rupture quickly with the formation of a sticky, purulent honeycomb crust. The staphylococcus is more likely to cause bullae whereas the streptococcus tends to cause crusting. Peripheral extension may then occur. Lesions are most frequent on the hands, lower extremities and around the nose and mouth. Some children have recurrent crops of boils.

*Periporitis staphylogenes* may occur as a complication of miliaria due to infection with the staphylococcus. There may be a few or many small to pea-sized papules and pustules with a predilection for the scalp, forehead, neck and upper trunk.

*Ecthyma* is characterized by deep-seated, pustular lesions covered by a thick, sticky crust. The lower extremities, the buttocks and the forearms are most frequently involved. The lesions may be primary or may occur secondary to pruritus and scratching as in patients with scabies and insect bites. Healing may be followed by brownish pigmentation or scarring.

*Furunculosis,* which results from suppuration involving the follicles and sebaceous glands of the skin, is characterized by large, elevated, exquisitely tender, erythematous patches.

*Pyoderma gangrenosum,* which begins as a tender erythematous nodule and progresses to a pustule followed rapidly by ulceration and extension of the lesion, occurs in patients with leukemia and inflammatory bowel disease.

Lewis, S.J., Poh-Fitzpatrick, M.B. and Walther, R.R.: Atypical pyoderma gangrenosum with leukemia. *JAMA 239*:935, 1978.

*Pseudomonas infections* of the skin may appear in clusters as vesicular lesions that have an inflammatory base and contain an opalescent fluid. These quickly become green, purulent and hemorrhagic blebs that on rupture leave round, indurated, ulcerated areas with necrotic black centers and bright red areolae (ecthyma gangrenosa), most commonly in the anogenital area. Areas of cellulitis with hemorrhage, necrosis and erythematous or violaceous nodules with or without fluctuation may also occur.

Reed, R.K., Larter, W.E., Sieber, O.F., Jr. and John, T.J.: Peripheral nodular lesions in Pseudomonas sepsis: the importance of incision and drainage. *J. Pediatr. 88*:977, 1976.

The cutaneous manifestations of *tuberculosis* are extremely protean. Primary tuberculous infection of the skin is characterized by a papular, granulomatous or ulcerated lesion ranging in size from a few millimeters up to 2 cm. Regional lymphadenopathy constitutes the other component of this primary complex. Scrofuloderma results from involvement of the skin overlying tuberculous lymph nodes or osseous tuberculosis. The cervical region is most frequently involved. Purplish discoloration, thinning and ulceration of the skin are followed by draining sinuses. Lupus vulgaris is a chronic, slowly growing, discrete, tuberculous skin lesion that appears most commonly on the face but may occur elsewhere. Solitary lesions are the rule, but occasionally a wider distribution is noted. Lupus vulgaris begins as a discrete, small, flat, red or brown plaque that does not fade on pressure. The classic apple butter color is noted when pressure is applied with a glass slide. The lesion then becomes elevated and extends peripherally, up to an area of several centimeters, accompanied by central clearing. Ulceration, crusting and scaling finally appear, followed by incomplete central scarring. The papulonecrotic type of tuberculid is a superficial, small, red papule that appears acutely in crops. These lesions, which may be a few or numerous, persist for a few weeks and then either disappear spontaneously or become crusted and heal with central umbilication.

*Erysipelas* occurs as a bright red, hot, slightly elevated lesion over the butterfly area of the face, the genitalia, about the umbilicus or on the hands and feet. The border is usually sharply circumscribed except in infants when it may be less well demarcated. Central clearing and peripheral extension of the lesion occur. Erysipeloid lesions occasionally occur in patients with nephrosis.

*Blistering distal dactylitis* is characterized by a superficial blister containing thin, white pus over the anterior fat pad at the end of a finger or thumb.

Hays, G.C. and Mullard, J.E.: Blistering distal dactylitis: a clinically recognizable streptococcal infection. *Pediatrics 56*:129, 1975.

*Human scabies* is a diagnostic consideration in patients with chronic, marked pruritus. The lesions consist of tiny, 1 to 2 mm. papulovesicles, slightly raised papules or burrows. Because of scratching and secondary infection, the primary lesions may be obscured by excoriations and pustular, crusted lesions that may be mistaken for infantile eczema. Areas most commonly involved are the flexor surfaces of the wrists, the interdigital spaces, nipples, axillae, groin, umbilicus, around the waist, the genitalia in boys and the buttocks. In infants, the palms, soles and sometimes the face are sites of predilection. The diagnosis may be confirmed by scraping the lesion gently with a Number 15 scalpel blade after a drop of mineral oil has been placed on a suspected lesion and examining the scrapings microscopically. Animal scabies usually is contracted by young children who have had skin contact with a puppy that has mange.

Orkin, M. and Maibach, H.I.: Scabies in children. *Pediatr. Clin. N. Am. 25*:371, 1978.

## FUNGUS INFECTIONS

Tinea capitis is discussed on p. 34.

*Tinea corporis* appears as circular, pinkish patches about 1 to 2 cm. in diameter. The lesions begin as small red macules. Peripheral spread with central clearing produces a ringlike effect. Small vesicles or scales may be present about the margin. The etiology of this lesion as well as others suspected to be due to tinea should be confirmed by culture and KOH examination.

*Tinea versicolor,* caused by Pityrosporum orbicular (formerly Malassezia furfur), is characterized by yellowish-brown, almost skin colored (either lighter or darker in pigmentation than the surrounding skin), finely scaling macular or irregular patches. Some large lesions occur over the upper part of the back in older children and adolescents who perspire profusely and do not change shirts frequently. The neck and chest may also be involved.

*Tinea cruris* is a brownish, erythematous, clearly demarcated lesion over the upper medial surfaces of the thighs usually first noted in adolescent males. Peripheral spreading may extend down the thigh. Central clearing and fine scaling along the border may be present. The scrotum is not affected.

*Tinea pedis,* or athlete's foot, usually involves the interdigital spaces, especially between the fourth and fifth toes and may cause the skin to be erythematous, vesicular, scaling, macerated or fissured. Patches of vesicles or thickened, scaly, dry areas may occur on the soles and sides of the feet.

*Dermatophytids* or secondary fungus eruptions may consist of pinkish maculopapules, tiny vesicles or scaly, eczematoid patches. Slight pruritus may be present. This eruption may develop on the sides of the fingers, palms, legs and trunk of children with ringworm infection.

Chronic *monilial infection* of the skin may occasionally result in hyperkeratoses with hornlike lesions or verrucous plaques on the face and scalp. Chronic monilial infections of the skin, mucous membranes and nails may accompany hypoparathyroidism and Addison's disease. Chronic mucocutaneous candidiasis may complicate immunodeficiency disorders such as DiGeorge's syndrome, Hodgkin's disease, sarcoidosis and leukemia.

Landau, J.W.: Chronic mucocutaneous candidiasis — associated immunologic abnormalities. *Pediatrics 42*:227, 1968.
Schlegel, R.J. et al.: Severe candidiasis associated with thymic dysplasia, IgA deficiency, and plasma antilymphocyte effects. *Pediatrics 45*:926, 1970.

In patients with *sporotrichosis,* subcutaneous nodules occur in linear distribution along the lymphatic channels from the primary indolent ulcer at the inoculation site to the enlarged regional lymph nodes. The primary lesion is a firm, painless red papule that slowly enlarges to become a 2- to 4-cm. violaceous, ulcerated nodule with undermined or raised border and crusting. *Actinomycosis* may involve the face, neck, or abdomen with hard, nodular masses and sinus tracts draining pus, which contains yellow granules. *Blastomycosis* proceeds slowly from a papular stage to a chronically ulcerated, crusted lesion.

Lynch, P.J. and Botero, F.: Sporotrichosis in children. *Am. J. Dis. Child. 122*:325, 1971.
Orr, E.R. and Riley, H.D., Jr.: Sporotrichosis in childhood: report of ten cases. *J. Pediatr. 78*:951, 1971.

## VASCULAR MANIFESTATIONS

*Capillary pulsation* may be observed in the lips or fingernails of patients with increased pulse pressure.

*Livedo reticularis* is a reddish-blue mottling or reticular pattern of the skin, chiefly over the extremities and the trunk, most evident on exposure to cold. *Cutis marmorata,* the mildest form of this disorder, occurs transiently in young infants and in some older children. *Cutis marmorata telangiectatica congenita* is a benign condition characterized at birth by a reticulate, bluish mottled appearance, phlebectasia, telangiectasia and ulceration with crust formation. Episodes of mottling of the skin may be the first manifestation of hereditary angioneurotic edema. *Acrocyanosis* is a persistent cyanotic discoloration involving the hands or feet, accompanied perhaps by livedo reticularis.

South, D.A. and Jacobs, A.H.: Cutis marmorata telangiectatica congenita (congenital generalized phlebectasia). *J. Pediatr. 93*:944, 1978.

In *familial dysautonomia* blotching of the skin occurs with crying, eating and excitement.

*Gangrene,* usually of part of an extremity, occurs rarely in infancy. Severe dehydration, shock, sepsis or femoral puncture may be etiologic. Often, the cause is unknown. Gangrene of the skin may occur rarely with chickenpox, meningococcemia and other infectious diseases. Pseudomonas infection may also lead to skin necrosis. Massive areas of gangrene occur in purpura fulminans.

Smith, E.W.P. et al.: Varicella gangrenosa due to Group A beta-hemolytic Streptococcus. *Pediatrics 57*:306, 1976.

*Vascular thrombosis* may occur with homocystinuria, with paroxysmal nocturnal hemoglobinuria, in patients on corticosteroid therapy or spontaneously. Gangrene may follow peripheral arterial injuries. Disseminated intravascular coagulation may occur in a wide variety of disease states.

Abildgaard, C.F.: Recognition and treatment of intravascular coagulation. *J. Pediatr. 74*:163, 1969.
Kitterman, J.A., Phibbs, R.H., and Tooley, W.H.: Catheterization of umbilical vessels in newborn infants. *Pediatr. Clin. N. Am. 17*:895, 1970.
Knowles, J.A.: Accidental intra-arterial injection of penicillin. *Am. J. Dis. Child. 111*:552, 1966.
White, J.J., Talbert, J.L. and Haller, J.A., Jr.: Peripheral arterial injuries in infants and children. *Ann. Surg. 167*:757, 1968.
Wise, R.C. and Todd, J.K.: Spontaneous, lower-extremity venous thrombosis in children. *Am. J. Dis. Child. 126*:766, 1973.

Ulcers on the lower legs may occur in adolescent children who have sickle cell anemia.

*Brown recluse spider (Loxosceles reclusus)* bites produce little immediate reaction; however, in a few hours, intense pain and erythema, at times extensive, and vesiculation occur along with fever, chills, nausea and vomiting. Acute hemolysis and thrombocytopenia may also develop. Necrosis begins at about 24 hours and continues over 5 to 6 days.

Dillaha, C.J., Jansen, G.T., Honeycutt, W.M. and Hayden, C.R.: North American loxo-scelism. *JAMA 188*:33, 1964.

*Acute necrotizing fasciitis,* a serious bacterial infection of subcutaneous tissue and fascial sheaths, may occur in a surgical wound, after trauma or secondary to bacteremia. Swelling, erythema, pain and warmth occur over involved areas, usually the trunk or an extremity, followed by cyanosis of the skin and the appearance of bullae.

Wilson, H.D. and Haltalin, K.C.: Acute necrotizing fasciitis in childhood. *Am. J. Dis. Child. 125*:591, 1973.

*Gas gangrene* is characterized by crepitance in the affected tissues.

*Raynaud's phenomenon* is characterized by intermittent, transient attacks of pallor or cyanosis and erythema of the digits, most commonly the fingers, precipitated by cold or emotion. This disorder may accompany lupus erythematosus, polymyositis, scleroderma, mixed connective tissue disease and polyarteritis.

Guntheroth, W.G., Morgan, B.C., Harbinson, J.A. and Mullins, G.L.: Raynaud's disease in children. *Circulation 36*:724, 1967.

*Redness of the fingers and toes* and occasionally of the cheeks and nose may be noted in patients with arterial desaturation. Redness of the fingers and toes is also a nonspecific finding in some intellectually retarded children.

*Reflex neurovascular dystrophy* is characterized by soft tissue swelling and/or vasomotor instability (e.g., mottled bluish or erythematous discoloration, decrease in skin temperature or alteration in perspiration along with tenderness and pain in an extremity).

*Pruritus* may be marked in patients with infantile atopic eczema, scabies, hypervitaminosis A, fungus infections of the skin, lichen urticaria and dermatitis herpetiformis.

## ERYTHEMA

*Toxic erythema,* characterized by blotchy, erythematous areas or a reddish, macular eruption, may occur in patients with pharyngitis, rheumatoid arthritis and other illnesses. A diffuse erythematous eruption may appear in patients with rat-bite fever. During periods of excitement sharply demarcated blotches occur in children with familial dysautonomia. Flushing of the skin occurs in patients with atropine and Jimson weed poisoning.

An evanescent rash may frequently be noted in patients with *rheumatoid arthritis* during febrile periods. The lesions are salmon pink, discrete maculopapules or erythematous blotches.

In patients with *pellagra,* a symmetrical, erythematous eruption, often accompanied by scaling, bleb formation and pigmentation, occurs over the exposed areas of the body. A pellagra-like rash on skin exposed to sunlight occurs in the Hartnup syndrome along with ataxia and mental retardation.

*Toxic epidermal necrolysis,* or the *scalded skin syndrome,* is characterized by the abrupt onset of diffuse erythema, perhaps with periorbital edema. This disorder occurs primarily in infants and young children. Exquisite tenderness of the skin is a prominent early feature. The patient does not want to be touched. Involvement spreads rapidly followed by loosening and separation of the epidermis and the formation of bullae, at times very large, which contain clear fluid. The skin is wrinkled and separates with slight stroking or trauma (Nikolsky sign) leaving extensive raw, red and oozing scalded-appearing areas, especially in the skin folds. Healing begins with disappearance of erythema at the end of one week, loss of irritability, scaling and desquamation.

A nonstreptococcal scarlatiniform rash associated with coagulase-positive staphylococci may simulate the scalded skin syndrome or streptococcal scarlet fever. After 24 to 48 hours of erythema, cracks occur in the skin creases, especially around the eyes and mouth, followed by large, thick flakes of dried skin and then desquamation. No enanthem or strawberry tongue develops.

Melish, M.E. and Glasgow, L.A.: Staphylococcal scalded skin syndrome: the expanded clinical syndrome. *J. Pediatr.* 78:958, 1971.

The lesions of *erythema multiforme* are polymorphous with erythema, macules, papules, vesicles, bullae and wheals. Usually, the lesions are predominantly of one type. The papular lesions may show peripheral spread and central clearing. Iris or cockade lesions may be noted. In the former, a purplish center is surrounded by a light red margin; in the latter, concentric colored rings (red, white and blue) are evident. At times, coalescence of lesions occurs, and the aggregate is surrounded by an annular or serpiginous border. Erythema multiforme may be caused by drugs, infections, collagen-vascular disease and malignancy.

In the *Stevens-Johnson syndrome* or *erythema multiforme exudativum pluriorificialis,* the lesions of erythema multiforme are complicated by involvement of the mucous membranes. Stomatitis and pharyngitis may be accompanied by bullae, ulcers, pseudomembrane formation and hemorrhagic crusting. Mucopurulent conjunctivitis and uveitis may also be present. The anal, vaginal and urethral orifices are often involved.

*Erythema chronicum migrans* appears to be a diagnostic feature of *Lyme arthritis.* Beginning on the proximal portion of an extremity or the trunk as a red macule or papule, the lesion enlarges to form a large, round area (5 to 50 cm.). The outer border is intensely red and flat, the center is indurated and deep red and there is clearing in between. Subsequent lesions are usually smaller. The rash, which often causes a burning sensation and is hot to touch, fades after three weeks or so. Fever and systemic symptoms may be present. Arthritis may accompany the rash or appear months later.

Steere, A.C. et al.: Erythema chronicum migrans and Lyme arthritis. The enlarging clinical spectrum. *Ann. Int. Med.* 86:685, 1977.

*Erythema nodosum* is characterized by painful, tender, firm, raised yet deep-seated, round or oval subcutaneous nodules 2 to 4 cm. in diameter. The lesions may appear in crops. Most commonly, they occur over the anterior thighs and tibiae, but they may also appear on the extensor aspects of the arms, the lateral aspect of the thighs and elsewhere. The overlying skin is tense and, at first, bright red. In a few days, these areas become lusterless and change to a bluish-purple and then a reddish-brown color. Erythema nodosum may occur in patients with streptococcal infections, tuberculosis, sarcoidosis, coccidioidomycosis, blastomycosis, lupus erythematosus, cat-scratch fever, regional enteritis, histoplasmosis, chronic active hepatitis, chronic ulcerative colitis, Behçet's syndrome, Yersinia enterocolitica infection and, rarely, in rheumatic fever.

*Erythemalgia* is characterized by intermittent episodes of burning pain involving the extremities, usually the fingers and toes or hands and feet, along with redness and increased skin temperature.

Mandell, F., Folkman, J. and Matsumoto, S.: Erythromelalgia. *Pediatrics 59*:45, 1977.

*Tache cérébrale,* a dermatographic streak observed after drawing a fingernail or other sharp object across the skin, may be elicited in patients with encephalitis, meningitis and other acute inflammatory diseases of the central nervous system.

*Photosensitivity* on exposure to sunlight or ultraviolet light may be due to systemic drugs, e.g., phenothiazine; topical agents, e.g., perfumes and cosmetics; photoallergy, e.g., deodorant soaps; biochemical disorders, e.g., porphyrias; and genetic diseases such as Bloom's syndrome. Symptoms include burning, itching, vesiculation, weeping, eczema and crusting.

Willis, I.: Sunlight and the skin. *JAMA 217*:1088, 1971.

*Erythropoietic porphyria* is characterized by severe photosensitivity with the development of erythema followed by vesicles, bullae and weeping lesions on exposed areas with pigmented scars on healing. *Erythropoietic protoporphyria* is characterized by the onset of intense burning and itching on exposure to ultraviolet light for a few hours. Severe erythema, edema, vesicles and bullae develop. With a chronic reaction, thickening, scaling and scarring occur. *Hepatic porphyria* may be accompanied by abdominal, neurologic and hematologic symptomatology.

Chisolm, J.J., Jr.: Pediatric aspects of the porphyrias. *J. Pediatr. 64*:159, 1964.
DeLeo, V., Poh-Fitzpatrick, M., Mathews-Roth, M. and Harber, L.: Erythropoietic protoporphyria. *Am. J. Med. 60*:8, 1976.

The *Cockayne syndrome,* characterized by microcephaly, disproportionately large ears and nose, sunken eyes, mental retardation and dwarfism, is also associated with photosensitive skin. Sensitivity to sunlight also occurs in the Rothmund-Thomson and Bloom's syndromes.

Schmickel, R.D., Chu, E.H.Y., Trosko, J.E. and Chang, C.C.: Cockayne syndrome: a cellular sensitivity to ultraviolet light. *Pediatrics 60*:135, 1977.

Although *rheumatic erythemas* occur chiefly with rheumatic fever, these lesions are not diagnostic of rheumatic activity. They may merely represent a "toxic" eruption. Erythematous papules are discrete, dull red lesions, usually 2 to 4 mm. in diameter, which appear transiently for a few hours or days in some patients with rheumatic fever. Most commonly affecting areas surrounding the joints and on extensor surfaces, the eruption may occur in crops and, at times, has an urticarial as well as papular component. *Erythema marginatum* is characterized by transient, annular, erythematous patches with raised, dull red, discrete edges and brownish, flat centers. The lesions usually appear on the trunk but are occasionally also present on the extremities. Wide size variation is characteristic, some lesions being many centimeters in diameter. Coalescence may occur with the formation of polycyclic forms. A brownish pigmentation of the skin may persist after fading of the lesions. *Erythema annulare* is similar to erythema marginatum except that the lesions are flat, undergo rapid change in form and outline and recur frequently.

## OTHER PAPULAR LESIONS

The lesions of *molluscum contagiosum* are shiny, pearly white, firm, rounded papules that range in size from 2 to 5 mm. They have a central umbilication from which a white, cheesy material can be extruded upon pressure.

*Papular urticaria* usually occurs during the spring and summer. The lesions are small, indurated, intensely pruritic, pale red papules 3 to 10 mm. in diameter. They are distributed chiefly over the extensor surface of the extremities, the buttocks, face and neck. Early, the lesions have a vesicular component. Later, because of itching and scratching, secondary infection, crusting and pigmentation may be noted. The lesions often persist for weeks, and recurrences are frequent.

The *Gianotti-Crosti syndrome,* which occurs especially in young children, consists of crops of papules — usually large, nonpruritic and at times hemorrhagic and infiltrative — on the face, extremities, including the palms and soles, buttocks and back. The lesions, which persist for two to eight weeks, become confluent to form plaques of flat-topped papules. Generalized lymphadenopathy and some hepatomegaly persist for up to three months. Liver enzymes are elevated and the hepatitis B surface antigen is often present.

Rubenstein, D., Esterly, N.B. and Fretzin, D.: The Gianotti-Crosti syndrome. *Pediatrics 61*:433, 1978.

*Granuloma annulare* is characterized by deep-seated waxy, whitish or pinkish, flat-topped papules arranged in a raised circle about $2\frac{1}{2}$ cm. or more in diameter or in a crescent around a center that is clear, erythematous or demonstrates atrophy. The sides of the fingers and the dorsum of the hands or feet, the knees and the buttocks are sites of predilection, although other areas of the body may be involved.

*Insect bites* are common, especially over exposed parts. Examination usually reveals a small punctum or elevation in the center of the lesion. Local edema may occur secondary to an insect bite. The lesions are usually grouped. Flea bites are especially likely to produce pruritic papules around the ankles.

The lesions associated with *pityriasis rosea* are salmon-pink, irregular, maculopapular, oval patches usually distributed along lines of cleavage (especially over the covered part of the body), the trunk, proximal portions of the extremities and the scalp. Individual lesions are 1 to 4 cm. in diameter and are characterized by a yellowish-brown central clearing ("crinkly cigarette paper center"). Thin, flaky scales are attached along the peripheral border of the lesion. The generalized eruption consists of about 100 lesions with new lesions continuing to appear over a 5- or 6-week period. This rash is usually preceded some 10 days before by one or more "herald" patches, annular or oval lesions, 1 to 5 cm. in diameter without a raised border or central clearing.

*Psoriasis* is characterized by sharply defined, round or oval, elevated plaques in which the primary lesion is an erythematous papule covered by a shiny silvery or mica scale. Bleeding points may be noted on removal of the scale. The lesions coalesce to form plaques, up to several centimeters in diameter, with discrete borders. Although psoriasis may appear anywhere, the sites of predilection are the scalp, elbows, knees and the presacral and intergluteal regions. Acute *guttate psoriasis* may appear suddenly as round to oval lesions, 2 mm. to 1 cm. in diameter, principally over the trunk and proximal extremities. Pitting of the fingernails may be noted. In the diaper area, psoriasis has an eczematous appearance. Differentiation between seborrheic dermatitis, pityriasis rosea and psoriasis may be difficult.

Watson, W. and Farber, E.M.: Psoriasis in childhood. *Pediatr. Clin. N. Am. 18*:875, 1971.

*Pityriasis rubra pilaris*, which may be mistaken for seborrheic dermatitis or psoriasis, is characterized by orange to deep red, very dry papular lesions that give a grater sensation when the skin is stroked. Patches of yellowish scales occur on the face, knees, elbows, wrists and buttocks. Palmar and plantar hyperkeratosis also occurs.

Huntley, C.C.: Pityriasis rubra pilaris. *Am. J. Dis. Child. 122*:22, 1971.

## VESICLES

*Urticaria* may occur either as white, pink or red macular wheals or as edematous, vesicular lesions that have pseudopodia and, perhaps, an erythematous flare. The lesions, which range from several millimeters to over an inch in diameter, may be present for only a few minutes or may persist for several hours. Pruritus may be intense. Urticaria may occur on exposure to cold.

Halpern, S.R.: Chronic hives in children: an analysis of 75 cases. *Ann. Allergy 23*:589, 1965.

*Urticaria pigmentosa* begins in infancy as red, urticarial, macular or papular lesions, $\frac{1}{2}$ to 1 cm. in diameter. These gradually change to a yellowish-red or deep brown color and become predominantly macular. Wheals or bullae may form on stroking macular lesions with a tongue blade. Vesicular and bullous lesions may also occur spontaneously. Dermatographia may be noted. There may be 30 or 40 lesions, or the skin may be more generally involved. The eruption tends to disappear at puberty. Urticaria pigmentosa may be associated with generalized mast cell infiltration of other tissues.

*Dyshidrotic dermatitis* or *pompholyx* consists of tiny, deep, slightly pruritic vesicles that seem to be embedded in the palms and along the lateral aspects of the fingers. The lateral aspects of the feet may also be involved. Excessive palmar perspiration is common.

*Epidermolysis bullosa* is characterized by bullae and large vesicles that form either spontaneously or as a result of slight trauma. In the simple form, the lesions occur chiefly on the hands and feet, and healing proceeds without scarring. Involvement of the mucous membranes does not occur in this type, nor are there associated ectodermal anomalies. The dystrophic form is characterized by involvement of the mucous membrane and by large bullae. The most serious form of the disease, epidermolysis bullosa hereditaria letalis, is characterized by progressive lesions and usually leads to early death. Rupture of the bullae, some of which are hemorrhagic, produces a raw surface that may be extensive. Healing occurs with scar formation. The nails may be lost, and secondary infection of the skin becomes a major problem. Epidermolysis bullosa in the newborn must be differentiated from bullous impetigo.

*Herpes simplex* is usually present on the lips as single or grouped lesions, but may occur elsewhere on the skin either in patients with infantile eczema or as a primary skin infection. The lesion usually begins as an erythematous area, rapidly becomes papular and is capped by a minute, painful vesicle. Crusting and secondary infection may follow rupture of the vesicle. In generalized skin infections with herpes simplex virus, the lesions appear in crops for eight to nine days.

*Herpes zoster* begins as erythematous, papular and sometimes painful patches over the cutaneous distribution of cranial and spinal nerves. Vesicular lesions then develop, followed by crusting.

Feldman, S., Hughes, W.T. and Kim, H.Y.: Herpes zoster in children with cancer. *Am. J. Dis. Child. 126*:178, 1973.
Rogers, R.S., III and Tindall, J.P.: Herpes zoster in children. *Arch. Dermatol. 106*:204, 1972.

*Hydroa aestivale* is a rare eruption that begins in late infancy or early childhood. Photosensitivity of the skin to sunlight is present, and characteristic lesions recur throughout the summer. Remissions occur in winter and usually after puberty. Lesions begin as small reddish macules that become vesiculated, last for a few days and then become crusted. These manifestations are preceded by pruritus. After separation of the crusts, a pigmented, pitlike scar remains. Involvement is confined to exposed surfaces such as the face and hands. Many of these patients have congenital porphyria.

*Dermatitis herpetiformis* is a rare skin disease in childhood characterized by frequent relapses and remissions. The eruption, which is polymorphous but usually bullous or papulovesicular, may persist for two or three months at a time. It may be confined to the forearms and hands or generally distributed over the extremities, trunk and perineum with a tendency toward symmetry. The bullous or vesicular lesions appear suddenly, usually on the trunk, pelvis and thighs. Clear and tense, they range in size from 0.5 to 2 to 4 cm. or more. They may be confluent, grouped like herpetic lesions or arranged in an annular fashion. Rupture of the lesions eventually occurs, leaving a raw surface that may become crusted and secondarily infected. The papulovesicular lesions are usually on the elbows, knees and thighs. The maculopapular lesions may demonstrate peripheral spreading with central clearing. Pruritus may be absent or mild in the bullous form and severe in the papulovesicular type. Healing may be followed by pigmentation of the skin. Intestinal malabsorption may be an associated finding.

Bean, S.F., Jordon, R.E., Winkelmann, R.K. and Good, R.A.: Chronic nonhereditary blistering disease in children. *Am. J. Dis. Child. 122*:137, 1971.
Hertz, K.C., Katz, S.I. and Aaronson, C.: Juvenile dermatitis herpetiformis. *Pediatrics 59*:945, 1977.

## NODULES, PLAQUES AND TUMORS

*Subcutaneous nodules* (antigen cysts) may occur after routine immunization.

Subcutaneous nodules occur with *rheumatic fever* and *rheumatoid arthritis*. Those associated with rheumatic fever are of much shorter duration than those with rheumatoid arthritis. The latter may persist for months or years. The oval, hard nodules are usually about ½ cm. in diameter but may be smaller. The nodules in rheumatoid arthritis may be slightly larger than those of rheumatic fever. They may appear in crops: in the scalp, especially over the occiput; over the scapula; spinous processes of the vertebral column; elbows; malleoli; patellae; and the dorsum of the hands and feet. Since the lesions lie deeply in the subcutaneous tissue, they are, at times, more easily palpated than seen. They may become apparent, however, if the overlying skin is made taut.

*Rheumatic-like nodules* in the subcutaneous tissues on the scalp, face, feet and elsewhere or in association with fascia or tendons may represent an unusual reaction to trauma.

Simons, F.E.R. and Schaller, J.G.: Benign rheumatoid nodules. *Pediatrics 56*:29, 1975.

Subcutaneous nodules are present in *disseminated lipogranulomatosis.*

*Sporotrichosis* may be characterized by nodules in a linear distribution along the lymphatics draining from the ulcer at the site of entrance of the fungus to the regional lymph nodes.

Extremely tender, indurated and erythematous subcutaneous nodules, occurring in crops, may present on the soles of the feet, calves and pretibial surfaces in patients with *periarteritis nodosa.* Fever and other systemic symptoms may be present.

Magilavy, D.B., Petty, R.E., Cassidy, J.T. and Sullivan, D.B.: A syndrome of childhood polyarteritis. *J. Pediatr. 91*:25, 1977.

*Lymphosarcoma* in the skin and scalp may take the form of pinkish or purplish plaques.

The lesions of *leukemia cutis* may be small or moderate-sized, discrete or confluent, livid red or purple papules and plaques. These appear most commonly around the eyes or elsewhere on the face.

*Mucosal neuromas,* white nodules that appear on the anterior tongue, palpebral conjunctiva or commissures of the lips, along with a characteristic facies, occur in the syndrome of *multiple mucosal neuromas and medullary thyroid carcinoma.*

Brown, R.S., Colle, E. and Tashjian, A.H., Jr.: The syndrome of multiple mucosal neuromas and medullary thyroid carcinoma in childhood, *J. Pediatr. 86*:77, 1975.

The *Gardner syndrome* consists of multiple soft tissue tumors (inclusion cysts, lipomas, fibromas), bone tumors (usually in the mandible) and intestinal polyps that may undergo malignant change.

Duncan, B.R., Dohner, V.A. and Priest, J.H.: The Gardner syndrome: need for early diagnosis. *J. Pediatr. 72*:497, 1968.

The *nevoid basal cell carcinoma syndrome* consists of cutaneous tumors, skeletal anomalies and cysts of the jaw. The nevoid basal cell cancers appear in the first years of life, usually in crops of flesh-colored or pigmented papules. The most frequent site is the face, especially around the eyes, the eyelids, the nose, the malar region and upper lid. The trunk and upper extremities may also be involved. Tiny pits, diagnostic of this syndrome, appear on the hands and feet in young adults.

Howell, J.B., Anderson, D.E. and McClendon, J.L.: Multiple cutaneous cancers in children: the nevoid basal cell carcinoma syndrome. *J. Pediatr. 69*:97, 1966.

*Juvenile fibromatosis* is the general designation given to connective tissue tumors that may appear as localized soft tissue masses in or around the muscles, especially of the neck or extremities, or as more diffuse and generalized involvement. Keloids represent one kind of fibromatosis. In *juvenile aponeurotic fibroma,* small to moderate-sized poorly marginated tumors may gradually develop on the hand, wrist or sole of a young child. *Recurring digital fibrous tumors* are smooth, dome-shaped nodules on the distal extensor surface of a digit.

Beckett, J.H. and Jacobs, A.H.: Recurring digital fibrous tumors of childhood: a review. *Pediatrics 59*:401, 1977.

Goslee, L., Clermont, V., Bernstein, J. and Woolley, P.V., Jr.: Superficial connective tissue tumors in early infancy. *J. Pediatr. 65*:377, 1964.

Levkoff, A.H., Gonzalez, C.G. and Neher, J.L.: Congenital diffuse fibromatosis: a case report. *Pediatrics 35*:331, 1965.

Sprecht, E.E. and Konkin, L.A.: Juvenile aponeurotic fibroma. *JAMA 234*:626, 1975.

*Nodular panniculitis,* characterized by firm, usually pruritic and tender subcutaneous nodules, may develop after massive corticosteroid therapy.

*Relapsing, nodular, febrile panniculitis* (Weber-Christian disease) is characterized by a chronic febrile course with recurrent crops of elevated, sometimes tender, nodular subcutaneous lesions ranging in diameter from 0.5 to 10 cm. The overlying skin may be erythematous or normal. The lesions disappear slowly, followed by atrophy of the subcutaneous tissue and, at times, by changes in pigmentation.

## SARCOIDOSIS

The cutaneous manifestations of sarcoidosis include papules, nodules and plaques. The papules, which are the most common manifestation, are usually small, firm but elastic, well circumscribed and round or oval. They may be brown, bluish or yellowish-red. The number of lesions ranges from a few to many. Sites of predilection include the face, especially around the margins of the eyelids and nose, the neck, shoulders and back and the extensor aspects of the arms. The surface of the lesions may be smooth and covered by delicate telangiectasia or by small scabs. Although in some cases resolution is complete, atrophy and depigmentation of the skin may persist.

## XANTHOMAS

Xanthomatous lesions may appear as yellow, orange or brownish-red papules, plaques, nodules, striae or pigmentation.

### CUTANEOUS XANTHOMAS ASSOCIATED WITH NORMAL SERUM CHOLESTEROL

*Xanthoma disseminatum (juvenile xanthogranuloma)* occurs predominantly in infants. There may be over 100 lesions. Sites of predilection include the trunk, face, scalp and the axillary and inguinal folds. The mucous membranes may also be involved. Individual lesions are bright orange, reddish-yellow or golden brown, discrete macules or papules that range in size from pinhead to several millimeters. The lesions are usually benign and disappear after a time.

### CUTANEOUS XANTHOMAS ASSOCIATED WITH ELEVATION OF SERUM CHOLESTEROL

Patients with *xanthoma tuberosum* or *planum* demonstrate elevated serum cholesterol. Their close relatives often have similar cholesterol findings, if not xanthomatous lesions. The lesions of xanthoma tuberosum are usually large, brownish-yellow or golden papules, nodules, infiltrated plaques or yellow striae and are most frequently distributed over the extensor surfaces and around the large joints. Areas of predilection include elbows, knees, hip, heels, palms and knuckles. Tendons may also be involved.

Primary type I hyperlipoproteinemia is often characterized in infants by crops of xanthomas. In the type II homozygote, xanthomas often occur at birth or appear in a few years.

Levy, R.I. and Rifkind, B.M.: Diagnosis and management of hyperlipoproteinemia in infants and children. *Am. J. Cardiol. 31*:547, 1973.

Xanthomatous lesions may appear transiently in disease states associated with prolonged hyperlipemia. These xanthomas are small, reddish-yellow or orange papules or plaques. They occur especially on the extensor aspects of the extremities and on the palms and soles.

## COLLAGEN-VASCULAR DISEASES

*Lupus erythematosus* most commonly involves the butterfly area of the face, over the cheeks and across the nose with well-circumscribed, maculopapular, violaceous or reddish-brown patches that can range from 1/2 to 1 cm. in diameter. Adherent, thin, whitish scales may be present over the lesions. Varying degrees of erythema and edema may occur. Capillary telangiectases are, at times, noted over involved areas. Lesions may also occur along the nails, on the palms and other exposed parts. Bullae may appear if inflammatory changes are severe. Though some lesions recede rapidly and without residua, the more persistent ones result in local atrophy and pigmentation of the skin. There may be a history of photosensitivity or Raynaud's phenomenon. A few patients never have a skin eruption. *Discoid lupus erythematosus,* characterized by red, elevated, indurated lesions on the face and exposed areas often followed by scarring, does not have systemic manifestations.

Raymond, D.A., Peterson, M.D., Vernier, R.L. and Good, R.A.: Lupus erythematosus. *Pediatr. Clin. N. Am. 10*:941, 1963.

Patients with *rheumatoid arthritis* often have widespread, blotchy erythematous lesions or a migratory, reddish macular eruption. The rheumatoid rash may be pruritic. *Koebner's phenomenon* in these patients may be evoked by making scratch marks on the skin. After several minutes, maculopapules appear along the scratch mark.

Calabro, J. J. and Marchesano, J. M.: Rash associated with juvenile rheumatoid arthritis. *J. Pediatr. 72*:611, 1968.

The skin eruption associated with *serum sickness* may be characterized by dermatographia, pruritus and urticarial wheals. Occasionally, the skin manifestations may be erythematous, morbilliform, scarlatiniform or purpuric. Angioneurotic edema may also occur.

*Dermatomyositis* may be accompanied by a variety of skin manifestations, including erythema and morbilliform, purpuric or urticarial lesions. Brawny induration or doughy edema are common. A dull red or deep crimson (heliotrope) color and scaling dermatitis may be present on the upper eyelids along with periorbital edema. An erythematous, scaling dermatitis and telangiectasia over the knees, elbows, knuckles, interphalangeal joints and malar prominences is virtually pathognomonic. Generalized edema may occur in some children. As the disease progresses, the tight, glossy and bound-down skin gives an indurated, thickened and leathery feel. The skin breaks down easily. Atrophy of the skin in involved areas may occur along with calcification of subcutaneous tissue. Gritty calcium deposits may occasionally extrude through the skin. Joint contractures occur over time.

Cook, C.D., Rosen, F.S. and Banker, B.Q.: Dermatomyositis and focal scleroderma. *Pediatr. Clin. N. Am. 10*:979, 1963.

In *periarteritis nodosa,* presenting symptoms may be subcutaneous nodules, calf pain and spiking fever.

*Scleroderma* may be *systemic* or *localized.* In the former, rare before puberty, involvement may be of the distal extremities or face *(acrosclerosis)* with loss of subcutaneous tissue. With generalized involvement, affected areas are bound down, tight, shiny and indurated without sharp demarcation from uninvolved skin. Raynaud's phenomenon may be the presenting complaint. Dysphagia may occur secondary to esophageal involvement.

*Focal* scleroderma may occur in the form of sharply demarcated plaques *(morphea)* or linear bands. These are often unilateral. The underlying subcutaneous tissue, muscle and bone may atrophy. Lesions may become pigmented and many have a violaceous edge. Linear scleroderma commonly involves the face or extremities. The term *en coup de sabre* is applied to lesions that involve the scalp and face.

Kass, H., Hanson, V. and Patrick, J.: Scleroderma in childhood. *J. Pediatr. 68*:243, 1966.
Tuffanelli, D.L. and LaPerriere, R.: Connective tissue diseases. *Pediatr. Clin. N. Am. 18*:925, 1971.

## SUBCUTANEOUS TISSUE

The thickness of the skin and subcutaneous tissue may serve as an index of nutritional status. Except for premature infants, well-nourished babies have a firm layer of subcutaneous fat. Bony landmarks such as the ribs, clavicles, scapulae and the interspaces of the chest are not as prominent on physical inspection as in prematures, malnourished infants and many older children. It is normal for both the infant during most of the first year and for the adolescent to have a greater thickness of subcutaneous tissue than does the preschool or school child.

*Partial* or *progressive lipodystrophy* is a rare disorder of childhood in which subcutaneous fat is gradually lost from the upper half of the body, especially from the cheeks, while the lower half of the body remains normal or becomes obese. There is a high incidence of renal disease in these patients.

Poley, J.R. and Stickler, G.B.: Progressive lipodystrophy. *Am. J. Dis. Child. 106*:356, 1963.

*Total lipodystrophy* is characterized by generalized loss of subcutaneous fat, either present at birth or appearing later, hyperglycemia, hepatomegaly, hyperlipemia, hirsutism, hyperpigmentation or acanthosis nigricans, muscle hypertrophy, increased stature, advanced bone age, enlarged genitalia, renal and central nervous system problems and insulin-resistant but nonketotic diabetes mellitus. In the congenital form, patients may have an acromegalic appearance with large hands and feet.

Huseman, C., Johanson, A., Varma, M. and Blizzard, R.M.: Congenital lipodystrophy: an endocrine study in three siblings. I. Disorders of carbohydrate metabolism. *J. Pediatr. 93*:221, 1978.
Senior, B. and Gellis, S.S.: The syndromes of total lipodystrophy and of partial lipodystrophy. *Pediatrics 33*:593, 1964.

*Insulin atrophy* with loss of subcutaneous adipose tissue or local subcutaneous fat hypertrophy may complicate sites of insulin injection.

*Cold panniculitis,* characterized by tender, slightly reddened, disc-like subcutaneous lesions usually involving the cheeks or submental region, may occur on exposure to severely cold weather.

Lowe, L.B., Jr.: Cold panniculitis in children. *Am. J. Dis. Child. 115*:709, 1968.

Patients with *progeria* have little subcutaneous fat.

Subcutaneous plaques and calcification of tendons may occur in *pseudohypoparathyroidism.*

*Subcutaneous emphysema* produces a crinkling, crepitant and crunching sensation on palpation of the skin. Involvement may include the neck, the upper thorax and the axillae. With extension, the trunk and genitalia may also be involved. Subcutaneous emphysema may be secondary to mediastinal emphysema or pneumothorax.

*Gas gangrene* causes crepitation in the tissues.

## SOME LESIONS FOUND ON THE FACE

*Adenoma sebaceum* consists of shiny, waxy, skin-colored, discrete or grouped papules, 2 to 6 mm. in diameter, or red seed-like spots distributed over the butterfly area of the face and chin and sometimes accompanied by telangiectasia. Lesions may not appear until late childhood. Adenoma sebaceum, mental retardation, sexual precocity and convulsions may occur in *tuberous sclerosis.* These patients may also demonstrate a patch of dark, thickened, shark-like skin over the lumbosacral area or elsewhere.

The lesions of *acne,* which are erythematous macules, papules and pustules, are a common problem in adolescents. Preadolescent acne may occur with the adrenogenital syndrome. The openings of the skin follicles may appear enlarged. Comedones or "blackheads" are frequently associated findings. Scarring and pitting of the skin may occur.

Esterly, N.B. and Furey, N.L.: Acne: current concepts. *Pediatrics 62*:1044, 1978.
Hurwitz, S.: Acne vulgaris. *Am. J. Dis. Child. 133*:536, 1979.

*Steroid rosacea,* caused by the use of topical fluorinated glucocorticosteroids, is characterized by erythematous papules, pustules and telangiectasia on the eyelids, cheeks and chin.

Franco, H.L. and Weston, W.L.: Steroid rosacea in children. *Pediatrics 64*:36, 1979.

Hemophilus influenzae type B may cause a characteristic *cellulitis of the face.* The etiology may be suspected on clinical grounds. Involvement of the cheek begins with little in the nature of prodromata other than fever and irritability for 24 to 36 hours. A central indurated area develops, surrounded peripherally by a nonindurated edematous zone without elevated or sharply demarcated borders. The involved area is tender, warm to hot and has a dusky or reddish-purple color resembling a fading hematoma. The buccal mucosa is slightly edematous on the involved side.

Rapkin, R.H. and Bautista, G.: Hemophilus influenzae cellulitis. *Am. J. Dis. Child. 124*:540, 1972.

*Plexiform neurofibromas* appearing in the distribution of cutaneous nerves may give a thickened sensation or feel like a tangle of worms. The overlying skin may be normal, thickened or pigmented. Neurofibromas commonly appear on the head or neck, especially periorbitally.

A faint or prominent violaceous or erythematous discoloration of the upper eyelids and, at times, periorbital tissues along with periorbital edema is an early manifestation of *dermatomyositis.* These findings occasionally extend across the bridge of the nose to involve the malar prominences. In some cases the involvement is limited to the latter, perhaps accompanied by periorbital edema.

*Coarse facial features* may be noted in infants with one of the lysozymal storage diseases and the Coffin-Siris syndrome.

## VERRUCAE

*Verruca vulgaris* occurs commonly as single or multiple lesions over the hands and fingers and occasionally under the nails. The lesions are firm, discrete, gray or brownish-gray papules, up to 1 cm. in diameter. The surface may be flat and smooth early, but later becomes roughened and fissured. Multiple small, flesh-colored flat warts, which occur on the face, lips, tongue and neck as well as on the hands, are only slightly elevated, sharply circumscribed and round or polygonal. Millet-seed to pea size, these lesions are skin colored or yellow-brown. There may be an explosion of warts in children receiving chemotherapy or corticosteroids.

*Plantar warts* are thickened, firm, plaque-like, sometimes painful lesions on the soles and occasionally on the palms. Tiny black dots or seeds may be present on the surface.

*Verrucae acuminata (condylomata acuminata)* are filiform papular, sometimes coalescing, lesions in the perineal and genital areas usually associated with poor hygiene.

## NAILS

*Postmature infants* have long nails that extend beyond the tips of the digits.

*Fingernail biting* in older children may be correlated with other evidences of anxiety or tension.

*Spoon-shaped nails,* in which there is a concavity in the nail, may be congenital, associated with iron deficiency anemia in infants or, rarely, observed with hypo- or hyperthyroidism. The significance of longitudinal or transverse ridging is often obscure. These changes may occur with hyperthyroidism or rheumatoid arthritis and in other severe or chronic illness. *Pitting* of the nails may be noted in fungus infections and psoriasis along with thickening and ridging. *Brittleness* occurs with fungus infections, rheumatoid arthritis, hypoparathyroidism and chronic hypochromic anemia.

The clinical diagnosis of *fungus infections* of the nails *(onychomycosis)* may be difficult without studies of nail scrapings for fungi. Involved nails may be pitted, friable and scaly, with hypertrophy in some areas and atrophy in others. Ridging and fissuring may occur, as may separation of the nail from its bed. The nail becomes clouded, lusterless and dull yellow.

White spots or lines in the nails *(leukonychia)* may be due to trauma, nutritional deficiency and illness. Congenital leukonychia involving all the nails may be accompanied by knuckle pads over the interphalangeal joints of the digits and hearing loss.

*Hemorrhage* beneath the nail secondary to trauma may cause loss of the nail.

Hemorrhage may also represent embolic phenomena in patients with subacute bacterial endocarditis.

Firm, skin-colored subungual and periungual fibromas arising from the groove of the nail bed of the fingers and toes may occur in adolescents with *tuberous sclerosis*.

In patients with *hypoparathyroidism* the nails may be deformed, atrophic, brittle, thickened, and covered by overgrowing skin. Monilial infections of the nails and skin are also not uncommon in hypoparathyroidism.

The *Coffin-Siris syndrome* is characterized by bilateral absence of the nails of the fifth fingers and toes, sparse scalp hair, hypotonia and mental retardation.

Feingold, M.: The Coffin-Siris syndrome. *Am. J. Dis. Child. 132*:660, 1978.

*Paronychia* is characterized by an inflammatory swelling around the edge of the nails. Severe paronychia occurs in acrodermatitis enteropathica.

Nails may be congenitally absent in congenital ectodermal dysplasia.

In *pachyonychia congenita* the nails are congenitally thickened, hard and discolored. They have longitudinal striations and are elevated at their distal end. The undersurface of the nail contains a yellow-brown horny material. Other findings may include hyperhidrosis and hyperkeratosis of the palms and soles, follicular keratosis and leukokeratosis of the oral mucosa, especially the tongue.

*Yellow nails* may precede by many years the development of lymphedema.

Patients with chondroectodermal dysplasia have abnormally small, friable and deformed nails. Hereditary dysplasia of the nails may be accompanied by absence or hypoplasia of the patella, elbow dysplasia and iliac horns in the *nail-patella* or *hereditary onycho-osteodysplasia* (Hood) *syndrome*.

Lucas, G.L. and Opitz, J.M.: The nail-patella syndrome. *J. Pediatr. 68*:273, 1966.

The fingernails in *porphyria* may have a reddish-purple discoloration. Loss of the nails may occur.

Loss of nails also occurs in the dystrophic form of *epidermolysis bullosa* and as a complication of tetracycline therapy.

Lasser, A.E. and Steiner, M.M.: Tetracycline photo-onycholysis. *Pediatrics 61*:98, 1978.

## EXANTHEMS

**Rubeola.** Beginning behind the ears, along the hair line, over the forehead and the sides of the neck, the eruption of rubeola extends downward to the trunk on the second day and to the extremities by the third day. The rash lasts about five days. It begins to fade from the face on the third day and continues to disappear in the order of its appearance. Individual lesions begin as discrete, brownish-red macules, which later become papular or morbilliform, blotchy and confluent. Unusually, the lesions may become hemorrhagic. Unless deeply colored, the rash fades on pressure. The skin between confluent areas is normal. With fading of the eruption a brownish, coppery pigmented color and a powdery desquamation may be noted for a few days. A prodromal transient rash may be blotchy and erythematous, urticarial or scarlatiniform.

The occurrence of the rash on the face in rubeola and its characteristic absence there in scarlet fever is a point of differentiation. The lesions of scarlet fever are also more macular, and the intervening skin is erythematous. The appearance of Koplik spots just before and for 12 to 24 hours after the appearance of the rash of rubeola is also diagnostically helpful.

*Atypical measles,* occurring in children previously immunized with inactivated measles vaccine, is characterized by an erythematous, maculopapular rash that begins on the ankles, wrists, palms and soles and spreads to the upper extremities and trunk. The lesions often become petechial or vesicular. Edema may occur over the shins and dorsum of the hands and feet.

Hall, W.J. and Hall, C.B.: Atypical measles in adolescents: evaluation of clinical and pulmonary function. *Ann. Int. Med. 90*:882, 1979.

Martin, D.B., Weiner, L.B., Nieburg, P.I. and Blair, D.C.: Atypical measles in adolescent and young adults. *Ann. Int. Med. 90*:877, 1979.

**Rubella.** A rubelliform rash may be caused by many viruses, so a diagnosis on clinical grounds alone is usually unreliable. The rash of rubella usually begins on the face and extends over the body within a few hours. The eruption consists of fine, light pink, discrete macules. It may change rapidly, perhaps resembling rubeola during the first 24 hours and becoming punctate or scarlatiniform during the second day. The lesions may become confluent and produce erythematous, flushed areas that fade on pressure. When the rash begins to fade after two to four days, a fine desquamation may occur. Transitory pigmentation of the skin is not present after disappearance of the eruption. The presence of the eruption around the mouth in patients with rubella as contrasted with the characteristic circumoral pallor in scarlet fever is a differential feature. Enlarged and tender suboccipital and postauricular and suboccipital nodes may precede the rash or may persist for a week or more. Rubella may also occur without a rash.

**Scarlet Fever.** The rash of scarlet fever usually begins in the axillae, inguinal areas, around the neck and over the chest or back, and is frequently most evident along the skin folds. It extends over the body rapidly, reaching maximal intensity in one or two days, after which the rash begins to fade. Total duration of the eruption is usually four to seven days. Except for flushing of the cheeks and circumoral pallor, the face is usually not involved.

The rash is characterized by a generalized, bright red erythema and a fine, pinpoint, papular, "goose-flesh" eruption that blanches on pressure. The skin is hot and dry. At times the rash on the extremities is blotchy and morbilliform. In severe cases pinhead-sized blebs may be found over the chest. In black children the diagnosis may be difficult. The palms and soles may be brightly erythematous and covered by a pinpoint papular rash. A similar rash may be noted over the general skin surface.

*Pastia's sign* refers to the transverse hyperemic or petechial lines in the skin folds of the antecubital fossae, axillae and inguinal creases. These do not fade on pressure. Desquamation in the form of fine, branny or large flakes usually begins at the end of the first week over the neck, chest, around the nails and over the tips of the fingers and toes and may continue for weeks.

It is sometimes difficult to differentiate the rash of scarlet fever from so-called toxic eruptions. The latter are usually chiefly erythematous and do not have the fine, pinpoint papular or punctate characteristics of scarlet fever. Toxic eruptions are usually much briefer in duration. Transient erythematous rashes may occur during the prodromal period of scarlet fever.

**Roseola infantum** or *exanthem subitum* is a common exanthem in infants and young children, preceded by a three-day febrile course and appearing as the temperature begins to fall. Beginning over the trunk, the rash extends chiefly to the neck and arms with slight involvement of the face and lower extremities. The individual lesions are rose-pink, discrete, small macules or maculopapules that fade on pressure. The eruption usually begins to fade shortly after its appearance but may persist for one or two days. Residual pigmentation does not occur.

**Viral Exanthems.** The echo and coxsackie enteroviruses and, occasionally, the adenovirus and reovirus may cause a variety of exanthems and enanthems. The viral exanthems may be maculopapular, rubelliform, petechial, purpuric or vesicular. Papular, vesicular or ulcerated oral lesions may occur. Cervical or occipital lymphadenopathy and, occasionally, aseptic meningitis may also be present. Because of the great variability of lesions, a specific etiologic diagnosis is usually not possible clinically. It may also be difficult to differentiate viral from drug rashes.

Cherry, J.D., Lerner, A.M., Klein, J.O. and Finland, M.: Coxsackie A9 infections with exanthems. *Pediatrics 31*:819, 1963.
Forman, M.L. and Cherry, J.D.: Exanthems associated with uncommon viral syndromes. *Pediatrics 41*:873, 1968.
Horstmann, D.M.: Viral exanthems and enanthems. *Pediatrics 41*:867, 1968.
Lerner, A.M., Klein, J.O., Cherry, J.D. and Finland, M.: New viral exanthems. *N. Engl. J. Med. 269*:678, 736, 1963.

**Chickenpox** lesions begin in the scalp or on the trunk and spread centripetally to the face and, to a limited extent, to the extremities. The palms and soles may be minimally involved. Progression of the lesions is from macules to papules, vesicles, pustules and crusts. Since these appear in crops with new lesions for four days, various stages of progression may be represented at any one time. The papules appear as small, red, elevated lesions that continue to enlarge and rapidly develop into flat, unilocular vesicles. These simulate a "tear drop" surrounded, usually, by a ring of erythema $\frac{1}{2}$ to 1 cm. in diameter. The vesicles are soft, do not have the central umbilication characteristic of smallpox lesions and rupture easily with subsequent crusting. Regressing lesions may appear slightly umbilicated. There may be many or as few as 5 or 10 lesions. Pruritus is intense. Some papules do not progress to later stages, and vesicles may be noted in the absence of a preceding papule. The duration of the eruption is 8 to 14 days. Rarely, bullous lesions occur.

The exanthem in *Rocky mountain spotted fever* begins with discrete pink or bright red macular lesions, a few millimeters in diameter, which initially blanch with pressure. In a few hours the rash becomes papular. It first appears on the flexural surface of the wrists and around the ankles usually on the second to fourth febrile day and then spreads centripetally to the rest of the body during the next day or two. The eruption often becomes purpuric or petechial. The rash usually involves the palms and soles and is always most marked on the extremities. Nonpitting edema may develop around the eyes and on the face and extremities.

Haynes, R.E., Sanders, D.Y. and Cramblett, H.G.: Rocky mountain spotted fever in children. *J. Pediatr. 76*:685, 1970.

*Kawasaki disease* is characterized by fever of one to two weeks' duration, conjunctivitis, erythema of the lips and mouth, a "strawberry" tongue and cervical lymphadenopathy. An erythematous macular rash appears on the third to fifth day. Intense redness of the palms and soles and indurative swelling of the hands and feet is followed by desquamation at the juncture of the nails and skin of the tips of the toes and fingers.

Darby, C.P. and Kyong, C.U.: Mucocutaneous lymph node syndrome. *JAMA 236*:2295, 1975.

*Leptospirosis* may be accompanied by a maculopapular, petechial or purpuric rash followed by peripheral desquamation. The clinical manifestations may resemble those in Kawasaki disease.

Wong, M.L., Kaplan, S., Dunkle, L.M., Stechenberg, B.W. and Feigin, R.D.: Leptospirosis: a childhood disease. *J. Pediatr. 90*:532, 1977.

*Hand-foot-and-mouth disease,* usually caused by coxsackie A16 and other coxsackie strains, begins in the summer and fall with a sore mouth or throat followed by lesions on the hands and feet. The oral lesions, usually 5 to 10 in number, begin as macules and progress rapidly to vesicles and then ulcers with an erythematous halo. In some patients, tender and painful vesicles, 2 to 10 mm. in diameter, appear on the hands and feet preceded by a red macule. The papulovesicular lesion may be oval, angular or streaked. Occasionally, maculopapular lesions may develop elsewhere.

Tindall, J.P. and Callaway, J.L.: Hand-foot-and-mouth disease — it's more common than you think. *Am. J. Dis. Child. 124*:372, 1972.

**Rat-Bite Fever.** A diffuse erythematous eruption may occur in rat-bite fever in addition to induration and ulceration at the site of the bite.

**Erythema infectiosum** (fifth disease) usually, but not always, begins with a bright red, confluent eruption over the cheeks, malar prominences and bridge of the nose. The patient is otherwise asymptomatic. The involved area has a raised, sharply delimited edge. Lesions may then appear as macules over the lateral aspect of the extremities and the buttocks. These progress to papules that begin to fade on the sixth day with areas of central clearing, leaving a lace-like, reticular or geographic pattern. The eruption lasts seven to nine days and has a tendency to disappear and reappear for weeks. Constitutional symptoms are mild.

Ager, E.A., Chin, T.D.V. and Poland, J.D.: Epidemic erythema infectiosum. *N. Engl. J. Med. 275*:1326, 1966.
Balfour, H.H., Jr.: Fifth disease: full fathom five. *Am J. Dis. Child. 130*:239. 1976.

**Infectious mononucleosis** is occasionally accompanied by a morbilliform or scarlatiniform eruption.

**Rose spots** are small, reddish macules that blanch on pressure. These appear on the abdomen in typhoid, other salmonella infections and shigellosis and last about three days.

Goscienski, P.J. and Haltalin, K.C.: Rose spots associated with shigellosis. *Am. J. Dis. Child. 119*:152, 1970.

## DRUG RASHES

Drug rashes may be produced by atropine, penicillin, ampicillin, barbiturates, salicylates, phenobarbital, hydantoin and many other drugs. The lesions may be polymorphous or chiefly erythematous, papular, vesicular, pustular or purpuric. Therapeutic or "overtreatment" dermatitis, occurring after the use of some remedial agent on the skin, may be characterized by pruritus and erythema over the site of application. Occasionally, a generalized and severe dermatitis may result. The following chemicals and substances are frequently involved: local anesthetics, penicillin, phenol, tar, menthol, camphor, iodine and salicylic acid. Almost any chemical substance may cause a contact dermatitis.

## BURNS

Burns may be characterized according to their depth and the extent of the surface area involved. A *first degree burn* is limited to the epidermis and characterized by erythema. The *second degree burn,* which represents a partial thickness injury, is manifested by erythema, blisters and marked pain. *Third degree burns,* which are full thickness thermal injuries, are not painful. If less than 10 per cent of the skin surface area is involved by a second degree burn and less than 1 per cent by a third degree burn, the burn is characterized as minor. A severe burn is characterized by involvement of greater than 20 per cent of the surface area by a second degree and 10 per cent by a third degree burn. A moderate burn demonstrates intermediate involvement.

O'Neil, J.A., Jr.: Evaluation and treatment of the burned child. *Pediatr. Clin. N. Am.* 22:407, 1975.

*Electrical burns of the mouth* may be misleading because the initial minimal edema and white mucosal coagulum may be followed seven to ten days later by extensive loss of tissue and severe hemorrhage.

Cigarette burns that are round and uniform and well demarcated or scalding burns of the buttocks or feet without involvement of the hands raise the suspicion of *child abuse.*

## CHILD ABUSE

In addition to the burns just described, other cutaneous signs of *child abuse* include multiple burns in areas not usually traumatized, welts from a belt or multiple scars.

Schmitt, B.D.: Current pediatric roles in child abuse and neglect. *Am. J. Dis. Child. 133:* 691, 1979.

## HAIR

The fine, unpigmented *lanugo hair* present during the last trimester of fetal life gradually disappears over a period of weeks after birth. This type of hair is observed most commonly in the premature but occasionally is noted over the shoulders and upper arms in the term newborn infant. *Vellus* or *down hair,* which begins to appear shortly before birth and is similar to lanugo hair, is the predominant type seen during childhood. Eventually, gradual and partial replacement of vellus hair by the coarser, longer and more pigmented *terminal hair* occurs. During the preschool and school-age periods vellus and then terminal hair appears on the extensor surfaces of the extremities, along the spine, in the interscapular region, across the shoulders and sometimes in the pilonidal or sacral area. The prominence of body hair is variable, being extensive in some children but minimal in the majority. Fairly long, silken, blond hair may also appear on the sides of the face and over the upper lip in early childhood. The hair in children with albinism is nonpigmented, fine and silky.

*Hypertrichosis,* the excessive growth of body hair not primarily due to an endocrine disorder, is not synonymous with hirsutism. Hypertrichosis may be a genetic or familial characteristic. It may also appear in chronically ill patients. Patients with porphyria may have excessive hair growth over exposed areas. Hairiness may rarely occur as an idiosyncrasy to hydantoin. Hair on the side of the face may occur with the Treacher-Collins syndrome. Hair growth may be noticeably slowed in hypothyroidism and chronic illness.

Adrenal cortical androgens are responsible for the growth of axillary, pubic and facial hair. This growth is conditioned by the level of circulating androgen and the responsiveness of the hair follicles. The latter may show considerable normal variation.

In the Tanner maturational scale, *stage 1* is the preadolescent one in which vellus hair is present over the pubic area in prepubescent boys and over the labia in prepubescent girls. In the adolescent male, pubic hair appears after the growth of the testes and penis has begun. In Tanner *stage 2,* there is a sparse growth of long, slightly pigmented, downy hair on the pubis, chiefly at the base of the penis. In *stage 3,* the hair is darker, coarser and more curled. In *stage 4* the hair is more adult in type but covers a smaller area than in the mature adult. With *stage 5,* the adult quantity and type are achieved with extension of the hair growth to the adjacent medial surface of the thighs and upward to and around the umbilicus.

In the adolescent girl, the beginning of breast development usually antedates the appearance of pubic hair. Unpigmented down or *stage 1* usually appears between the ages of 10½ and 12½ years with long, sparse, slightly pigmented down hair present in *stage 2.* In *stage 3,* a few more pigmented, semiterminal darker and coarser hairs appear. In *stage 4,* full length, pigmented, wiry, sparse, terminal hairs appear, but the area covered is less than in adults. In *stage 5,* dense, fully mature terminal hairs appear.

In most adolescent children the pubic hair has a characteristic male or female distribution. There are, however, exceptions to this generalization. In the male the distribution is in the form of a diamond, the superior apex of which extends upward toward the umbilicus. In the female the pubic hair appears in the form of an inverted triangle.

Axillary hair usually does not appear until the second stage of pubic hair development has been attained. In general, its development is some six months behind that of pubic hair. In some children, however, axillary hair may appear concomitantly with or may even precede pubic hair. A small amount of axillary hair may be present in girls at the menarche.

In boys, facial hair appears shortly after axillary hair has been noted. Its distribution and other characteristics may reflect a familial pattern. Body hair becomes prominent in the male during adolescence and continues to develop throughout the postadolescent period. A greater amount of pubic and occasionally of axillary hair, at times coarse and curled, may occasionally be noted in young children, especially in girls, in the absence of other signs of sexual precocity or virilism. Termed *precocious adrenarche,* this development is due to an advanced maturation of the adrenal androgenic zone. Continued observation is important because of the possibility of an adrenocortical neoplasm, adrenocortical hyperplasia or isosexual precocity in the male. In the latter conditions, however, other secondary sex characteristics or additional evidences of excessive androgen secretion are concomitantly present or appear shortly.

Korth-Schutz, S., Levine, L.S. and New, M.I.: Serum androgens in normal prepubertal and pubertal children and in children with precocious adrenarche. *J. Clin. Endocrinol. Metab. 42*:117, 1976.

Sexual hair is decreased or absent in patients with hypopituitarism, in hypothyroidism and in adolescent girls with Addison's disease. It is decreased and may be delayed in girls with Turner's syndrome. While hirsutism, the appearance of hair on the face and chest with a male distribution of pubic hair with or without other virilizing signs, may be a manifestation of Cushing's disease and fibrocystic disease of the ovary (Stein-Leventhal syndrome), in most instances no specific cause can be determined.

Greenblatt, R.B.: Diagnosis and treatment of hirsutism. *Hosp. Pract. 8*:91 (June) 1973.
Leng, J-J. and Greenblatt, R.B.: Hirsutism in adolescent girls. *Pediatr. Clin. N. Am. 19*:681, 1972.

## GENERAL REFERENCES

Korting, G.W., Curth, W. and Curth, H.O.: *Diseases of the Skin in Children and Adolescents.* Philadelphia, W. B. Saunders Co., 1978.
Solomon, L.M., Esterly, N.B. and Loeffel, E.D. (eds.): *Adolescent Dermatology.* Philadelphia, W. B. Saunders Co., 1978.
Solomon, L.M. and Esterly, N.B.: *Neonatal Dermatology.* Philadelphia, W. B. Saunders Co., 1973.
Weinberg, S., Leider, M. and Shapiro, L.: *Color Atlas of Pediatric Dermatology.* New York, McGraw-Hill Book Co., 1975.

PART II

# SIGNS
# AND
# SYMPTOMS

# CHAPTER 30

# FEVER

## CLINICAL CONSIDERATIONS

Fever, one of the most common symptoms experienced by children, is in most instances due to a readily identifiable infection, usually a respiratory one. Not infrequently, however, the cause of fever is not immediately apparent, and further observation or laboratory examinations are required. This is especially true with recurrent or prolonged fever. Fever may be accompanied by delirium, convulsions and chills.

Constancy of body temperature is maintained by complex and incompletely understood physiologic mechanisms. The central thermoregulatory center in the hypothalamus is influenced by the temperature of the blood, skin and deep thermoreceptors and endogenous pyrogen. Depending upon the area involved, damage to the hypothalamus may result in either hyperthermia or hypothermia.

The maintenance of a constant body temperature requires that the expenditure of heat equals the production of heat by the basal metabolic processes and the digestion and assimilation of food. Proteins are particularly significant in the latter regard because of their high specific dynamic action. A slight physiologic rise in body temperature follows a meal. Exercise also has an important effect in the production of heat and may cause as much as a 1.1° C. (2° F.) rise in the body temperature. Heat is lost from the body by radiation, conduction, evaporation and convection. The mechanisms for heat loss are limited in the presence of a high environmental temperature, high humidity and in patients with congenital ectodermal dysplasia of the anhydrotic type in whom sweating does not occur.

During the first two years of life there is usually no significant diurnal variation in body temperature. Between the ages of 6 months and 2 years there may be some fluctuation, perhaps as much as 0.6° C. (1° F.). In children between the ages of 2 and 6 years the diurnal variation may be as much as 0.9° C. (1.6° F.). In children above this age, the variation may be as much as 1.1° C. (2° F.). Usually, the highest body temperature is recorded in the late afternoon or early evening. The body temperature is especially labile in certain children.

No one temperature reading can be given as *normal* for all children at all times. There is, instead, a *range* of normality. A rectal temperature of 38.5° C. (101.3° F.) usually is regarded as abnormal. The child should be at bed rest or physically inactive for 30 minutes before the temperature is taken. After exercise, the rectal temperature may be 37.8 to 38.3° C. (100 to 101° F.). The temperature should also not be taken within one hour after a meal. Oral temperatures are also affected by prior intake of cold or hot foods. In children under the age of 6 years the temperature may be taken rectally or by placing the thermometer in the axilla for three minutes. The oral recording of the temperature is usually satisfactory in children above 6 years of age. When the temperature is taken rectally, the thermometer should be inserted about 5 cm. into the rectum of an infant or up to 7 cm. in an older child. Since the thermometer may perforate the colon, axillary temperature may appropriately be substituted with the normal range being 36.5° C. (97.7° F.) to 37.2° C. (99° F.). The rectal temperature is often considered to be up to a degree higher (F.) than the oral temperature and the axillary reading correspondingly lower.

The temperature regulatory mechanisms of the premature infant are poorly developed. Anatomic and physiologic immaturity is manifested by an absence or inadequate amount of sweating, a minimal amount of insulating subcutaneous fat, a relatively large surface area and poor vasomotor control.

Not only does the premature infant have difficulty in balancing heat production with heat loss, but he also is easily overheated. Skin temperature on the anterior abdominal wall should be between 36 and 36.5° C. (96.8 and 97.7° F.).

Imperfect thermoregulatory mechanisms are also present in the term newborn infant, but to a lesser extent than in the premature infant. Little concern need be shown over rectal temperatures in the range from 36.1 to 37.8° C. (97 to 100° F.) in term infants who appear healthy.

Atkins, E. and Bodel, P.: Fever. *N. Engl. J. Med. 286*:27, 1972.
Sinclair, J.C. (ed.): *Temperature Regulation and Energy Metabolism in the Newborn.* New York, Grune and Stratton, 1978.

Since fever is such a common manifestation of disease, a comprehensive etiologic classification of fever would be impractically long. The classification given here is of disease states in which fever may be the presenting or prominent complaint. In many instances, the febrile course is acute and self-limited; in others, it is intermittent, recurrent or chronic. Patients with unexplained fever should be re-examined daily since new physical findings may have become evident.

## ETIOLOGIC CLASSIFICATION OF FEVER

    I. Infections. Infections, especially those of the upper respiratory tract, are by far the most common cause of fever in childhood.
        A. Respiratory infections and disease
            1. Common cold
            2. Acute sinusitis may contribute to acute fever in children. While sinusitis may account for chronic fever, it is not a significant consideration in most cases.
            3. Pharyngitis is probably the most frequent cause of fever in childhood. Fever occasionally precedes by some hours the other symptoms and signs of pharyngitis.
            4. Streptococcosis
            5. Otitis media, mastoiditis
            6. Pneumonia. The etiologic classification of pneumonia is included on page 500.
            7. Pulmonary tuberculosis is an important diagnostic consideration in infants and children with unexplained fever. Roentgenographic examination of the chest is indicated in children with fever of undetermined origin. Since the chest x-ray and tuberculin skin tests may be normal, gastric cultures may be indicated in some children with fever of undetermined origin.

B. Urinary tract infections
1. Pyelonephritis. *The importance of including the possibility of a urinary tract infection in the differential diagnosis of fever cannot be overstressed.* Repeated urinalyses and urine cultures are an essential part of the work-up in children with acute or chronic fever, even though urinary symptoms such as frequency are not present.
C. Exanthems. Fever is a prominent symptom in the prodromal phase of the exanthematous diseases, especially in the presence of a community epidemic or a history of recent exposure.
1. Exanthem subitum, or roseola infantum, is a diagnostic consideration in children with acute, unexplained fever, especially in infants between the ages of six months and two years. Although the child usually does not appear ill, the disease may be ushered in by hyperpyrexia, convulsions and a bulging fontanel. A leukopenia and a relative lymphocytosis may be present. The fever continues for three to four days to be followed by an evanescent rash.
D. Enteric infections. Although other symptoms may be more prominent, fever may be an important complaint in patients with these infections. Cultures and serologic tests are often helpful in arriving at a specific diagnosis.
1. Salmonellosis
2. Brucellosis

Street, L., Jr., Grant, W.W. and Alva, J.D.: Brucellosis in childhood. *Pediatrics* 55:416, 1975.

3. Trichinosis
4. Ascariasis
5. Amebiasis
E. Infections of the central nervous system
1. Meningitis. In the presence of fever and such physical findings as a bulging fontanel, nuchal rigidity, convulsions, altered sensorium and positive Kernig's sign, meningitis is, of course, a likely diagnostic possibility. *The possibility of meningitis exists in every infant with unexplained fever,* even though the fever has been present for several days. Irritability, unusual drowsiness or failure to feed well may also occur. Unusual irritability is, at times, the only indication that meningitis has developed in an infant. Fever may not be present when the patient is first seen. Meningitis due to Hemophilus influenzae is especially likely to have an insidious onset with fever the most prominent early symptom. Tuberculous meningitis is *always* a diagnostic consideration when irritability or unexplained fever occurs in a child with a positive tuberculin skin test or a known tuberculous infection. Examination of the cerebrospinal fluid is frequently indicated as a diagnostic measure in infants and children with an unexplained serious illness and in patients with unexplained fever. Persistence of fever 72 hours after initiation of adequate therapy in a patient with meningitis may be due to a complicating subdural effusion. Other complications include brain abscess, arthritis, ophthalmitis, phlebitis and drug fever. Because persistent meningeal infection is a possibility, repeated cerebrospinal fluid examinations are indicated.

Balagtas, R.C., Levin, S., Nelson, K.E. and Gotoff, S.P.: Secondary and prolonged fevers in bacterial meningitis. *J. Pediatr. 77*:957, 1970.

2. Encephalitis. The possibility of postinfectious encephalitis is to be considered whenever fever recurs during convalescence from measles, chickenpox or other exanthem. Primary encephalitis is, of course, another cause of fever.
3. Poliomyelitis. Unexplained fever of a few days' duration may precede the appearance of paralysis in patients with poliomyelitis.

F. Infections of the liver
   1. Infectious hepatitis
   2. Chronic active hepatitis
   3. Ascending cholangitis in a partially obstructed biliary tree may account for septic fever in patients with cystic fibrosis.
   4. Liver abscess
   5. Granulomatous hepatitis due to sarcoidosis, tuberculosis, histoplasmosis or brucellosis

Simon, H.B. and Wolff, S.M.: Granulomatous hepatitis and prolonged fever of unknown origin: a study of 13 patients. *Medicine 52*:1, 1973.

G. Infections involving the heart
   1. Rheumatic fever
   2. Subacute bacterial endocarditis
   3. Myocarditis. An electrocardiogram should be obtained in patients with unexplained fever when the tachycardia is greater than ordinarily attributable to the fever. The quality of the heart sounds in these patients may also be abnormal.

H. Systemic infections
   1. Bacteremia. *The practice of including bacteremia as a diagnostic consideration in infants and children with unexplained fever is essential, especially in newborn and young infants.* Blood cultures are of great diagnostic help, not only in the patient with spiking fever or chronic fever of undetermined etiology but also in patients with infectious diseases such as meningitis, pneumonia and diarrhea. A specific etiologic diagnosis can often be made in this manner. In patients with spiking fever, blood cultures should be drawn, if possible, an hour or two before the spike. If this cannot be done, several blood cultures may be obtained during 24 hours. The clinical picture of sepsis in young infants is particularly deceptive since fever may not be present.

     Bone marrow cultures may be diagnostic for fever of bacterial, fungal or mycobacterial etiology and should be pursued in addition to the examination for malignant and storage diseases. Serologic tests are also helpful.

     Pneumococcal bacteremia is especially a possibility in children under the age of 2 years seen with fever over 38.9° C. (102° F.); a WBC of 15,000/mm$^3$ or higher; evidence of pneumonia or upper respiratory tract infection; or no localized focus of infection. Blood cultures should be obtained in such children. If the culture is positive for Streptococcus pneumoniae, the child should be admitted for repeat blood cultures, lumbar puncture if clinically indicated and intravenous penicillin. Continued observation on an ambulatory basis is justifiable only if the child is afebrile and will be under close surveillance. The finding of otitis media or pharyngitis makes the presence of a bacteremia less likely.

Bratton, L., Teele, D.W. and Klein, J.O.: Outcome of unsuspected pneumococcemia in children not initially admitted to the hospital. *J. Pediatr. 90*:703, 1977.

McCarthy, P.L., Grundy, G.W., Spiesel, S.Z. and Doland, T.F., Jr.: Bacteremia in children: an outpatient clinical review. *Pediatrics 57*:861, 1976.

Teele, D.W. et al.: Bacteremia in febrile children under 2 years of age: results of cultures of blood of 600 consecutive febrile children seen in a "walk-in" clinic. *J. Pediatr. 87*:227, 1975.

2. Bacterial endocarditis. In patients with rheumatic or congenital heart disease, an adequate number of blood cultures should be drawn when subacute bacterial endocarditis is suspected. A small number of these patients consistently demonstrate negative blood cultures. Therefore, six blood cultures for both aerobic and anaerobic organisms should be obtained over several days. When bacterial endocarditis occurs in the postoperative cardiac patient, fever may be the only presenting finding. Bacterial endocarditis may occur in the absence of a murmur.

Johnson, D.H., Rosenthal, A. and Nadas, A.S.: A forty-year review of bacterial endocarditis in infancy and childhood. *Circulation 51*:581, 1975.

3. Infectious mononucleosis
4. Acute infectious lymphocytosis
5. Epidemic influenza
6. Echovirus infections. Fever may persist for 5 to 12 days or up to 3 weeks. Severe headache, abdominal pain, myalgia and stiff neck may be associated symptoms. A rubelliform rash may also occur. The clinical spectrum caused by the echovirus overlaps that of coxsackie disease.

Linnemann, C.C., Jr. et al.: Febrile illness in early infancy associated with echovirus infection. *J. Pediatr. 84*:49, 1974.

7. Colorado tick fever
8. Haverhill fever
9. "Spirillum" fever
10. Cytomegalovirus infection. Acquired cytomegalovirus infection may resemble infectious mononucleosis with atypical lymphocytes, fever, lymphadenopathy and hepatosplenomegaly. The heterophile test is negative.
11. Leptospirosis may present as a febrile illness or as fever of undetermined etiology.
12. Q fever may present as a purely febrile syndrome.
13. Rocky mountain spotted fever
14. Psittacosis. This may be considered if there is a history of exposure to psittacine birds and a pulmonary infiltration.
15. Epidemic myalgia
16. Tularemia

17. Histoplasmosis
18. Blastomycosis (nonpulmonary)
19. Visceral larva migrans
20. Malaria
21. Cat-scratch disease
22. Toxoplasmosis
23. Tuberculosis in nonpulmonary forms may be a cause of fever (e.g., disseminated tuberculosis or involvement of the peritoneum, pericardium, genitourinary tract or liver).

I. Abscesses, localized infections
1. Osteomyelitis. After initial evaluation of a patient considered to have acute osteomyelitis, a number of blood cultures should be obtained. The length of time during which therapy is withheld in an attempt to secure the etiologic organism depends upon the severity of the illness in each patient. No rigid schedule should be followed. It seems reasonable that even in the most toxic patients a minimum of two blood cultures may be obtained and that probably in no patient should therapy be withheld for more than 24 hours.
2. Intracranial abscess
3. Lung abscess
4. Retropharyngeal abscess
5. Alveolar abscess
6. Perinephritic abscess. Both the urinalysis and the intravenous pyelogram are usually normal.
7. Appendiceal abscess
8. A pelvic abscess should be looked for in children with fever of unknown cause.
9. Mediastinitis
10. Liver abscess
11. Subphrenic abscess
12. Nontuberculous spinal epidural infections
13. Purulent pericarditis
14. Empyema
15. Bronchiectasis
16. Agammaglobulinemia
17. Chronic granulomatous disease of childhood
18. Thrombophlebitis of the saphenous or other vein at the site of a cutdown may cause fever. Erythema, tenderness and induration are noted along the course of the vein. Edema of the lower extremity may also occur.

II. Collagen-vascular disease
A. Rheumatic fever. A low-grade fever is occasionally the earliest manifestation of rheumatic fever with major and minor manifestations appearing later.
B. Serum sickness
C. Dermatomyositis
D. Periarteritis nodosa
E. Polyarteritis nodosa of infancy is characterized by a prolonged febrile

illness, skin rash, conjunctivitis, convulsions, anemia and congestive heart failure.

Tang, P.H.L. and Segal, A.J.: Polyarteritis nodosa of infancy. *JAMA 217*:1666, 1971.

   F. Lupus erythematosus. Initially, some of these patients may demonstrate intermittent fever.

Fish, A.J. et al.: Systemic lupus erythematosus within the first two decades of life. *Am. J. Med. 62*:99, 1977.

   G. Juvenile rheumatoid arthritis is as an important diagnostic possibility in children with fever of undetermined origin. Fever, which may be the earliest manifestation of this disease, appearing before the onset of arthritis, may be low or spiking, persistent or intermittent. One or two spikes of 39° C. (102.2° F.) may occur each day with the temperature returning to normal between elevations. Occasional hyperpyrexia with temperatures above 40.6° C. (105° F.) may occur. Fever may persist for months before arthritis becomes evident.

Calabro, J.J. and Marchesano, J.M.: Fever associated with juvenile rheumatoid arthritis. *N. Engl. J. Med. 276*:11, 1967.

III. Neoplastic diseases
   A. Leukemia frequently presents with fever as the initial clinical symptom. Peripheral blood examination may show only slight anemia and leukopenia with few or no blast cells.
   B. Hodgkin's disease usually is manifested by lymphadenopathy by the time that fever occurs.
   C. Ewing's tumor
   D. Neuroblastoma with bone metastases

IV. Dehydration. Dehydration, especially in newborn and young infants, may cause fever and irritability.
   A. Hypertonic dehydration (hyperosmolarity) may also be accompanied by fever.
   B. Diabetes insipidus in infants may also cause fever.

V. Drugs, immunization
   A. Idiosyncrasy to a variety of drugs and antibiotics may cause drug fever.
   B. Atropine poisoning may be accompanied by hyperpyrexia.
   C. Immunization reactions
   D. Salicylate intoxication is frequently accompanied by fever, at times over 40.6° C. (105° F.). Young infants appear especially prone to hyperpyrexia due to salicylism.

VI. Central nervous system disturbances
   A. A number of central nervous system disorders may cause irregularities in control of body temperature resulting either in hyper- or hypothermia. Such disorders include intracranial hemorrhage, brain tumors, infections and surgical operations that involve the hypothalamus, the region of the third ventricle, the medulla or other areas. Since the anterior hypothalamus acts to prevent an abnormal elevation of the body temperature, injury to this structure may result in hyperthermia. The regulatory center for the prevention of excessive heat loss is thought to be in the posterior hypothalamus. Infants with intracranial hemorrhage due to birth trauma are

especially prone to hyperpyrexia or hypothermia. Neurogenic hyperthermia may also occur in patients with bulbar poliomyelitis and in those with encephalitis.

  B. The association of febrile states and infectious diseases with convulsive seizures in young children is well known. Fever may not only result from the muscular contractions that occur during a convulsion but may also, in rare instances, be the sole clinical manifestation of a paroxysmal seizure discharge from the hypothalamic region. Fever may develop in patients in status epilepticus.

  C. Infections of the central nervous system are discussed on page 275.

  D. Children with familial dysautonomia often have episodes of unexplained fever.

  E. Infants with congenital familial nonhemolytic jaundice with kernicterus have frequent febrile episodes, probably central in origin.

  F. Neurogenic fever may occur in Krabbe's disease.

  G. Fever has been described with cervical spinal cord tumors.

VII. Blood diseases

  A. Fever may be one of the primary manifestations of a hemolytic anemia, especially during a crisis.

  B. Fever may also be a manifestation of a transfusion reaction.

  C. Fever is a common manifestation of leukemia.

VIII. Hemorrhage

  A. The systemic hemorrhagic diseases may be characterized by fever if hemorrhage occurs into a viscera or other body tissue.

  B. Intracranial hemorrhage in the newborn infant may cause fever.

  C. Adrenal hemorrhage in the newborn infant is often accompanied by fever.

  D. Hemorrhage into a tumor may be accompanied by fever.

IX. High environmental temperature

  A. Premature infants readily develop elevation of body temperature when the environmental temperature is excessively high.

  B. Sustained elevation of the environmental temperature, as occurs in very hot weather, may also cause an elevation of body temperature in term infants. This response is more likely in very young infants but may be noted in those who are older. Heat stroke may develop in otherwise normal infants if the environmental temperature is high enough to overtax the ability of the body to dissipate heat.

  C. Infants with brain damage often tolerate high environmental temperatures poorly and may suffer hyperpyrexia and heat stroke.

  D. Patients with cystic fibrosis are also prone to heat prostration when subjected to a persistent high environmental temperature.

X. Miscellaneous causes for fever

  A. Some cases of fever of undetermined origin undergo spontaneous resolution with no cause established.

  B. Periodic disease may be characterized by the episodic occurrence of fever, sometimes accompanied by abdominal pain or arthralgia. Cyclic neutropenia is a rare disorder with neutropenia occurring at approximately 21- to 27-day intervals along with fever, malaise, mouth ulcers, sore throat, arthritis and headache.

C. Familial Mediterranean fever, or periodic polyserositis, an autosomal recessive disorder occuring primarily in Sephardic Jews and persons of Armenian descent, is a syndrome characterized chiefly by recurrent fever and abdominal pain but also by pleural, pericardial, meningeal and articular symptoms.

Cone, T.E., Jr.: Periodic diseases in children. *Postgrad. Med. 50*:242, 1971.
Siegal, S.: Familial paroxysmal polyserositis. *Am. J. Med. 36*:893, 1964.

D. Some evidence has been presented for a relationship between unconjugated etiocholanolone in the plasma and the occurrence of fever in periodic syndromes.

Bondy, P.K., Cohn, G.L. and Gregory, P.B.: Etiocholanolone fever. *Medicine* 44:249, 1965.

E. Virilizing adrenal hyperplasia. Episodes of periodic fever, headaches, abdominal pain and chills, cutaneous flushing and prostration have been described in a variant of virilizing adrenal hyperplasia.

F. Ectodermal dysplasia of the anhydrotic type may be responsible for episodes of unexplained fever in infants.

G. Infantile cortical hyperostosis may be characterized, in part, by fever that may range from 38.3 to 39.4° C. (101 to 103° F.). At times, fever is the initial symptom followed shortly by irritability and swelling over involved bones.

H. Regional enteritis and ulcerative colitis may be accompanied by fever. Regional enteritis, or Crohn's disease, may initially present as fever of undetermined origin.

I. Paroxysmal atrial tachycardia

J. Congestive cardiac failure. Although fever is known to be associated with congestive cardiac failure, the temperature usually does not exceed 37.8° C. (100° F.). Fever higher than this should be ascribed to some other cause.

K. Hyperthyroidism during toxic crises

L. Spurious fevers. When children are seen with recurrent or chronic fever of undetermined origin, it is important to determine what the mother considers to be "fever," whether she has read the thermometer correctly, whether the temperature was taken at rest or after exercise and whether the thermometer is accurate. The basis for so-called fever of undetermined etiology is frequently clarified on such questioning.

Murray, H.W.: Factitious fever updated. *Ann. Int. Med. 139*:739, 1979.

M. Masked school phobia should be considered in a history of continuing low-grade "fever" in a school-age child, especially when coupled with complaints of "sore throat," tiredness or recurrent abdominal pain. Although the child's absence from school, often for weeks, is usually not mentioned by the parents, it should be explored by the doctor by a question such as, "How much school has this illness caused Johnny to miss?"

N. Sarcoidosis. The chest film is abnormal in 95 per cent of children with sarcoidosis.

Schmitt, E., Appelman, H. and Threatt, B.: Sarcoidosis in children. *Radiology 106*:621, 1973.

O. The postpericardiotomy syndrome, which may occasionally follow pericardiotomy two or three weeks postoperatively, is characterized by persistent fever and precordial pain. A pericardial friction rub may be transiently heard.

Engle, M.A., Zabriskie, J.B., Senterfit, L.B. and Ebert, P.A.: Postpericardiotomy syndrome. *Mod. Concepts Cardiovasc. Dis. 44*:59, 1975.

P. A benign postperfusion syndrome, due to the cytomegalovirus and characterized by fever, splenomegaly and atypical lymphocytes, occasionally occurs after open heart surgery utilizing extracorporeal circulation. The fever is first noted 6 to 7 weeks after operation, and may persist for 7 to 21 days.

Riemenschneider, T.A. and Moss, A.J.: Postperfusion syndrome. *J. Pediatr. 69*:546, 1966.

Q. About one third of children may develop a transient elevation of body temperature up to 39° C. within 12 hours of cardiac catheterization and angiography.

Gilladoga, A.C., Levin, A.R., Deely, W.J. and Engle, M.A.: Cardiac catheterization and febrile episodes. *J. Pediatr. 80*:215, 1972.

R. Disseminated fat necrosis associated with pancreatitis may be characterized by fever, tender erythematous subcutaneous nodules, polyarthritis, soft tissue swelling, bone pain and eosinophilia.

## HYPERPYREXIA

Hyperpyrexia with elevation of the body temperature to 41.1° C. (106° F.) or above is uncommon in childhood. It may occur in patients with neurologic disorders, central nervous system infections, heat stroke, atropine poisoning, salicylate poisoning, bulbar poliomyelitis and terminally in tetanus. In the newborn, hyperthermia may be a manifestation of adrenal hemorrhage, intraventricular hemorrhage or toxoplasmosis. Hyperpyrexia also is a late manifestation in patients with metachromatic leukodystrophy and of subacute sclerosing panencephalitis. Hyperpyrexia may also occur in patients severely ill with fulminant infections, especially when accompanied by peripheral circulatory failure.

Pomerance, J.J. and Richardson, C.J.: Hyperpyrexia as a sign of intraventricular hemorrhage in the neonate. *Am. J. Dis. Child. 126*:854, 1973.

Malignant hyperpyrexia, a syndrome characterized by the rapid onset of hyperpyrexia during anesthesia, is also accompanied by cyanosis, tachypnea, tachycardia, muscle rigidity and severe metabolic acidosis. Susceptible patients have an underlying clinical or subclinical myopathy or neuropathy including myotonia congenita, central core disease and elevation of serum creatinine phosphokinase. There may be a progressive congenital myopathy associated with a characteristic phenotype: an understatured male with cryptorchidism, pectus carinatum, spinal defects, hypoplasia of the mandible, antimongoloid palpebral fissures, ptosis, low-set ears, webbed neck and weak serrati muscles. Malignant hyperpyrexia also occurs in the Schwartz-Jampel syndrome characterized by dwarfism, skeletal anomalies and muscular stiffness.

Kaplan, A.M., Bergeson, P.S., Gregg, S.A. and Curless, R.G.: Malignant hyperthermia associated with myopathy and normal muscle enzymes. *J. Pediatr. 91*:431, 1977.

King, J.O. and Denborough, M.A.: Anesthetic-induced hyperpyrexia in children. *J. Pediatr. 83*:37, 1973.

Seay, A.R. and Ziter, F.A.: Malignant hyperpyrexia in a patient with Schwartz-Jampel syndrome. *J. Pediatr. 93*:83, 1978.

## HYPOTHERMIA

Hypothermia may occur in premature infants and in infants with intracranial birth injury. If heat loss is not prevented, the body temperature of normal newborn infants may fall as much as 1.1 to 2.8° C. (2 to 5° F.) within the first hour after birth. Hypothermia in the newborn infant may cause tachypnea, apnea, acidosis, hypoglycemia and disseminated intravascular coagulation. Hypothermia refers to a body temperature under 35°C. (95°F.).

An abnormally low body temperature may also occur in patients in shock, in those who are severely or critically ill and in those who are heavily sedated. Encephalitis may also be accompanied by hypothermia. Hypothermia and instability of temperature is a persistent problem in patients with Menke's kinky hair syndrome.

Accidental hypothermia may be caused by wind chill, especially when the infant is wet, or by immersion in cold water.

Accidental hypothermia. Committee on Pediatric Aspects of Physical Fitness, Recreation and Sports, American Academy of Pediatrics. *Pediatrics 63*:926, 1979.

### GENERAL REFERENCES

Cone, T.E., Jr.: Diagnosis and treatment: children with fevers. *Pediatrics 43*:290, 1969.

Feigin, R.D. and Shearer, W.T.: Fever of unknown origin in children. *Cur. Probl. Pediatr. 6*:3 (Aug.) 1976.

Jacoby, G.A. and Swartz, M.N.: Fever of undetermined origin. *N. Engl. J. Med. 289*:1407, 1973.

Pizzo, P.A., Lovejoy, F.H., Jr. and Smith, D.H.: Prolonged fever in children: review of 100 cases. *Pediatrics 55*:468, 1975.

---

## ETIOLOGIC CLASSIFICATION OF FEVER

I. Infections, 274
  A. Respiratory infections and disease, 274
    1. Common cold
    2. Acute sinusitis
    3. Pharyngitis
    4. Streptococcosis
    5. Otitis media, mastoiditis
    6. Pneumonia
    7. Pulmonary tuberculosis
  B. Urinary tract infections, 275
    1. Pyelonephritis
  C. Exanthems, 275
    1. Exanthem subitum
  D. Enteric infections, 275
    1. Salmonellosis
    2. Brucellosis
    3. Trichinosis
    4. Ascariasis
    5. Amebiasis

  E. Infections of the central nervous system, 275
    1. Meningitis
    2. Encephalitis
    3. Poliomyelitis
  F. Infections of the liver, 276
    1. Infectious hepatitis
    2. Chronic active hepatitis
    3. Ascending cholangitis
    4. Liver abscess
    5. Granulomatous hepatitis
  G. Infections involving the heart, 276
    1. Rheumatic fever
    2. Subacute bacterial endocarditis
    3. Myocarditis
  H. Systemic infections, 276
    1. Bacteremia
    2. Bacterial endocarditis
    3. Infectious mononucleosis

# CHAPTER 31

# REGURGITATION AND VOMITING

## REGURGITATION

Regurgitation refers to nonforceful expulsion of food and secretions from the esophagus or stomach through the mouth. This symptom is usually not accompanied by nausea or forceful contractions of the abdominal muscles.

### ETIOLOGIC CLASSIFICATION OF REGURGITATION

I. "Physiologic" regurgitation. In the early weeks of life many normal babies regurgitate one or more times a day, bringing up a mouthful or two of food a short time after feeding. Mothers often refer to this as "spitting up." Frequently, the exact cause of this regurgitation cannot be determined. As long as normal weight gain continues, there is no cause for concern. Ordinarily, the frequency of regurgitation tends to diminish as the baby becomes older and ceases usually by seven to eight months of age.

II. Faulty feeding techniques. Frequently, the cause of regurgitation may be found in the feeding technique. Direct observation of the mother feeding the baby may be informative. Babies who nurse either vigorously or slowly may require burping more than once during a meal. If the baby is put down without being burped, eructation of air may cause regurgitation of milk.

Nipple holes that are too small unduly prolong the feeding time and increase the amount of air swallowed, leading to overdistention of the stomach and regurgitation. Retracted nipples may result in excessive air swallowing in the breast-fed infant. Bottle propping often leads to swallowing of air. If a baby's formula is inadequate calorically or if he is not fed frequently enough, he may swallow an excessive amount of air as a result of increased non-nutritive sucking; on the other hand, overfeeding may also cause regurgitation. Excessive handling of an infant immediately after feeding also facilitates regurgitation.

III. Gastroesophageal reflux (cardioesophageal relaxation; chalasia; incompetence of the gastroesophageal valve mechanism). Regurgitation in babies with this disorder may be severe enough to cause an abnormally slow weight gain or a weight loss. These babies remain hungry and refeed eagerly. Symptoms begin between the third and tenth days of life. Regurgitation, which usually does not occur until the infant is put down, may be prevented almost entirely if the baby is held or is set in an upright position for approximately 30 minutes after feeding. The clinical diagnosis of esophageal chalasia can be confirmed by fluoroscopic demonstration of esophageal reflux when the baby is in a horizontal position. Cardioesophageal relaxation continues for weeks or a few months with gradual disappearance of symptoms. Differentiation between chalasia and a hiatus hernia may not be possible in all instances. Relaxation of the cardia may occur in debilitated or developmentally retarded infants and in babies who ruminate. The presence of a hemangioma at the cardia may interfere with cardioesophageal closure. Gastroesophageal reflux may also cause night cough and recurrent pneumonia or bronchitis.

Bray, P.F. et al.: Childhood gastroesophageal reflux. *JAMA 237*:1342, 1977.

IV. Congenital esophageal obstructions
- A. Esophageal atresia with or without tracheoesophageal fistula. Symptoms begin shortly after birth. There may be a history of maternal hydramnios. *The presence of an excessive amount of mucus in a baby's mouth and throat should always suggest this diagnosis.* Prompt regurgitation, choking and, perhaps, cyanosis occur with the first and subsequent feedings attempted. Diagnosis may be made by failure in the attempt to pass a Number 8 or 10 French soft rubber radiopaque catheter into the stomach. Radiopaque material instilled through this catheter at fluoroscopy pools in the proximal esophageal pouch. Esophageal atresia may be a component of the VATER association, which includes vertebral defects, anal atresia, radial dysplasia, renal defects and, at times, ventricular septal defect and a single umbilical artery.
- B. Stenosis of the esophagus. A stenotic segment may be present in the midportion of the esophagus. Regurgitation may begin after the first week of life. When the stenosis is minimal, difficulty is not experienced until solid foods are begun. The infant may then be considered a "slow" or "fussy" eater. Less frequently, the diagnosis is not suspected until later when a foreign body lodges in the midesophagus.
- C. Congenitally short esophagus may cause dysphagia, regurgitation and hematemesis due to esophageal ulceration. Symptoms may occur in infancy but usually not until the late childhood or early adult years. These children are also "slow" eaters and present feeding problems. Gastric rugae can be visualized above the diaphragm on roentgenographic study. Rather than a congenital defect, this disorder may be the result of cicatricial contraction associated with a chronic esophagitis caused by gastroesophageal reflux. A true congenital short esophagus is rare.
- D. Esophageal hiatus hernia may cause "spitting up" or occasional projectile vomiting. If esophagitis is present, the vomitus may be coffee ground or blood flecked. Complications include tracheal aspiration with resultant pulmonary infiltration or peptic esophagitis. Contortions of the neck, including torticollis, opisthotonus and posturing of the trunk, may occur with esophageal reflux and hiatus hernia (Sandifer's syndrome). Rarely, laryngospasm following reflux and aspiration may cause apneic episodes, cyanosis and stiffening.

Blattner, R.J.: Hiatus hernia. *J. Pediatr. 72*:424, 1968.
Filler, R.M., Randolph, J.G. and Gross, R.E.: Esophageal hiatus hernia in infants and children. *J. Thorac. Cardiovasc. Surg. 47*:551, 1964.
Kinsbourne, M.: Hiatus hernia with contortions of the neck. *Lancet 1*:1058, 1964.
Sutcliffe, J.: Torsion spasms and abnormal postures in children with hiatus hernia, Sandifer's syndrome. *Prog. Pediatr. Radiol. 2*:190, 1969.

E. Webbing of the esophagus

F. Cardiospasm

G. Congenital vascular ring. In addition to respiratory symptoms, infants with this anomaly demonstrate hesitancy in swallowing, and choking and regurgitation. Dysphagia may first occur or become more notable after the introduction of solid foods.

H. Duplication of the esophagus may cause dysphagia, regurgitation, respiratory obstruction, cough and, occasionally, hematemesis. Symptoms often occur during the first two years of life. Esophageal duplications occur in the posterior mediastinum. Enterogenous duplications may occur elsewhere in the chest.

V. Acquired esophageal lesions

A. Esophagitis usually results from a transient inflammation of the esophagus. Occasionally, however, ulceration occurs, followed by stricture formation and obstruction. Esophagitis may occur in the following situations:

  1. Infectious diseases: pneumonia, moniliasis, scarlet fever, diphtheria, syphilis, typhoid fever and poliomyelitis

  2. Ingestion of corrosive agents

  3. Cardiac disease with chronic elevation of venous pressure

  4. Chronic pulmonary infections

  5. Reflux of gastric juice in patients with esophageal chalasia or hiatus hernia

B. Strictures

  1. Secondary to infectious diseases

  2. Scleroderma

  3. Corrosive agents. Chief offenders are lye, bleaches and ammonia. The reflux of gastric contents through a lax cardiac sphincter may cause peptic esophagitis, mucosal ulceration and, eventually, a stricture.

  4. Foreign body. Ulceration or inflammation due to a foreign body may be followed by scar formation.

C. Esophageal diverticulum. Rarely, a tracheobronchial lymph node, adherent to the esophagus after an inflammatory process, may cause a traction diverticulum.

D. Traumatic pseudodiverticulum of the pharynx in newborn infants may follow injury to the posterior pharyngeal wall. Because of the resultant cricopharyngeal spasm and functional high esophageal obstruction, nasogastric tubes cannot be passed or may perforate the pharyngeal wall. This acquired condition may be mistaken for esophageal atresia.

Girdany, B.R., Sieber, W.K. and Osman, M.Z.: Traumatic pseudodiverticulums of the pharynx in newborn infants. *N. Engl. J. Med.* 280:237, 1969.

E. Foreign body. Foreign bodies may cause esophageal obstruction either because of their size or the inflammatory reaction they initiate. Esophageal stenosis should be suspected whenever a foreign body stops at some level other than one of the three anatomically narrow points of the esophagus.

F. Retroesophageal abscess

  1. Extension of retropharyngeal abscess

    2. Esophageal perforation

    3. Foreign bodies

    4. Vertebral tuberculosis

    5. Ulceration from a tracheotomy tube

    6. Suppurating mediastinal lymph nodes

VI. Rumination usually begins between the third and sixth months of age as the regurgitation of previously swallowed food with rechewing and reswallowing. The baby protrudes his tongue and lower jaw, slightly extends his head, and then makes rhythmical chewing and swallowing motions until regurgitation occurs. Part of the food is then expelled and some reswallowed. Rather than being distressed, the infant appears to enjoy the process. Occasionally, the baby initiates regurgitation by inserting his fingers or a toy into his mouth. Babies who ruminate are often markedly visually alert — "radar-like." Rumination occurs primarily when the infant is left to himself. Weight loss may be severe. The term "spitting up" is rarely used in the presenting complaint; rather, the mother will report vomiting or failure to gain. Rumination results from a parenting disability with the mother usually depressed, uninvolved or fearful of the infant's vulnerability to illness. Recovery is usually prompt when increased mothering and developmentally appropriate nurturing care is provided by nurses. Persistent rumination may also occur in older infants and children who are severely mentally retarded or psychotic.

Fleisher, D.R.: Infant rumination syndrome. *Am. J. Dis. Child. 133*:266, 1979.

VII. Regurgitation may be the initial manifestation of pyloric stenosis, but vomiting soon supervenes.

VIII. Miscellaneous causes

    A. Dyspnea from any cause may lead to air swallowing and gastric overdistention.

    B. Ascites, abdominal cysts, organ enlargements and neoplasms may cause regurgitation as a result of increased intra-abdominal pressure.

    C. Eventration of the diaphragm can cause frequent regurgitation, probably as a result of angulation of the lower esophagus or stomach.

## VOMITING

### CLINICAL CONSIDERATIONS

Vomiting refers to the forceful expulsion of gastric contents through the mouth, usually accompanied by vigorous contractions of the abdominal muscles. This highly coordinated sequence of events is controlled by a medullary vomiting center that lies close to the dorsal nuclei of the vagus nerves and the respiratory center. Integration of the processes involved in vomiting appears to be accomplished in the medullary reticular formation. The vomiting center is influenced by both excitatory and inhibitory nervous and metabolic influences.

The act of vomiting begins with closure of the pylorus and constriction of the antrum. Concomitant relaxation of the stomach, cardia and esophagus then occurs. Respirations are inhibited, the glottis closes and the soft palate is elevated to close off the nasopharynx. Forceful contraction of the diaphragm and the abdominal muscles then causes vomiting. In infants and young children, vomitus often comes through the nose as well as the mouth. Because of their poor coordination and the danger of aspiration, vomiting is exceedingly hazardous in prematures or in infants with neuromotor disability.

The threshold of the vomiting center can be exceeded by emetic impulses from any sensory nerve. Stimuli come primarily from the labyrinth; pharynx; gastrointestinal, biliary and genitourinary tracts; heart; pelvic organs and peritoneum. Unpleasant sights, odors or tastes may cause vomiting, as may any sufficiently painful stimulus.

The threshold of the vomiting center can also be lowered so that the subthreshold stimuli that continually enter the center may result in vomiting. This may be the mechanism through which psychogenic causes and increased intracranial pressure operate. There is no conclusive evidence that drugs that evoke emesis have a direct action on the vomiting center. Rather, such agents may act on a central chemoreceptor trigger zone separate from but anatomically near the vomiting center. Abnormal body metabolites in patients with diabetic acidosis, liver disease, uremia and other disease states may act similarly.

Since nausea is a subjective sensation, its presence cannot be determined precisely in infants. Grimacing, restlessness, yawning, pallor, salivation, sweating, failure to suck the fist and refusal to refeed after vomiting suggest nausea in this age group. Older children may complain that their "tummy" or their "throat" hurts.

### Appearance of Vomitus

The appearance of the vomitus or stomach aspirate may be of diagnostic help.

**Gastric aspirate in the newborn** greater than 20 ml. or containing bile, especially in the presence of a history of maternal polyhydramnios, may suggest intestinal obstruction.

**Undigested Food.** Regurgitation of uncurdled milk in a newborn infant suggests esophageal atresia. Regurgitation of undigested food in older children suggests a stricture of the esophagus or other obstructive lesion at or above the cardia.

**Absence of Bile.** Absence of bile in the vomitus suggests an obstruction proximal to the ampulla of Vater. Bile may not be clinically apparent in freshly passed vomitus because its yellow color is often diluted with food and gastric juice. Shortly after exposure to air, however, oxidation of the bile pigments causes the pathognomonic green color.

**Bilious Vomiting.** In the term newborn infant, bilious vomitus should always be considered a sign of intestinal obstruction. It may occasionally occur in the premature infant with an immature pyloric sphincter and in infants with sepsis as a result of adynamic ileus.

**Fecal Vomiting.** When the vomitus has a fecal odor, peritonitis or an obstruction of the lowel bowel or colon is suggested.

### HEMATEMESIS

Bright red blood in the vomitus indicates that there has been little or no contact of the blood with gastric juice: that active bleeding is present at or above the cardia or in the stomach. Rapid or massive duodenal bleeding may also be manifested by the vomiting of bright red blood. "Coffee ground" emesis indicates that blood has been altered by gastric digestion and suggests slow or inactive bleeding from the esophagus, cardia, stomach or duodenum. Epistaxis is occasionally followed by the vomiting of fresh or altered swallowed blood. If blood is returned through a nasogastric tube introduced into the stomach, gastrointestinal bleeding may be assumed to be proximal to the ligament of Treitz; if there is no blood in the stomach, the bleeding is most likely distal to this point.

Hematemesis may be associated with the following disease states:

1. Peptic ulcer
2. Esophageal duplication
3. Esophageal varices (the most common cause of massive hematemesis).
4. Peptic esophagitis in patients with a hiatus hernia or chalasia
5. After repeated vomiting due to any cause, including pyloric stenosis.
6. Acute gastritis during the course of a severe infectious disease such as pneumonia
7. Poisoning due to ingestion of iron sulfate
8. Aminophylline toxicity
9. Hemangioma in the esophagus

Cox, K. and Ament, M.E.: Upper gastrointestinal bleeding in children and adolescents. *Pediatrics 63*:408, 1979.

## ETIOLOGIC CLASSIFICATION OF VOMITING

I. Mechanical vomiting is frequently due to obstructive lesions of the stomach or intestinal tract. Congenital anomalies are most often implicated. Intestinal obstruction occurs frequently in the newborn period and should be suspected in any newborn infant who has over 20 ml. of fluid in the gastric aspirate, especially if bile-stained; who vomits and has abdominal distention in the first 24 to 36 hours of life; and who does not pass stools. A history of maternal polyhydramnios raises the possibility of a high intestinal obstruction. Plain films of the abdomen in the upright and supine positions are important diagnostic aids.

A. Obstruction

1. Intestinal atresia. The ileum is the most common site of atresia. Symptoms due to obstruction begin in the first 24 hours of life. If the atretic area is proximal to the ampulla of Vater, the stools contain bile, but the vomitus does not. Distention is confined to the epigastrium or left upper quadrant, and gastric peristaltic waves may be seen. X-ray films show air in the stomach and duodenum, but none in the small bowel. Duodenal atresia occurs in an increased frequency in babies with Down's syndrome. If the atretic area is distal to the ampulla of Vater, the vomitus contains bile but the stools do not. Abdominal distention is generalized when the atresia is within or distal to the jejunum.

Holder, T.M. and Leape, L.L.: The acute surgical abdomen in the neonate. *N. Engl. J. Med. 278*:605, 1968.
Talbert, J.L., Felman, A.H. and DeBusk, F.L.: Gastrointestinal surgical emergencies in the newborn infant. *J. Pediatr. 76*:783, 1970.

2. Imperforate anus. Symptoms of obstruction begin within 24 to 36 hours after birth with abdominal distention and vomiting. Meconium is not passed. Findings vary with the anatomic variants of this anomaly. Most commonly, the anus is imperforate, and the proximal rectal pouch ends blindly somewhere above. The site of the anus is revealed by dimpling

or increased pigmentation of the skin. Stroking of the area causes visible puckering. In other infants, a normal anus is present but there is a blind rectal pouch. A digital rectal examination reveals the site of obstruction. In another type, a thin membrane separates the anus from the rectum. Dark meconium may be seen through the membrane, and the area may bulge when the baby cries. Anoperineal, rectovesical, rectourethral, rectovaginal and rectoperineal fistulas commonly accompany an imperforate anus. Meconium may be present in the urine of boys and the vagina of girls.

3. Meconium ileus. Symptoms of obstruction beginning within the first 24 to 36 hours represent the earliest manifestation of cystic fibrosis. If passed, meconium is thick, tenacious and tarry. Palpation may reveal firm, rubbery loops of bowel, giving the impression of a sausage-filled abdomen. A plain film of the abdomen reveals small bubbles throughout the meconium.

O'Neill, J.A., Jr., Grosfeld, J.L., Boles, E.T., Jr. and Clatworthy, H.W., Jr.: Surgical treatment of meconium ileus. *Am. J. Surg.* *119*:99, 1970.

4. Meconium plug. Inspissated meconium in the distal colon may cause abdominal distention, bile-stained vomiting and failure to pass meconium. The obstruction may be relieved by enemas or digital rectal examination. Meconium plug syndrome may be a manifestation of cystic fibrosis or Hirschsprung's disease.

5. Intestinal stenosis
   a. Duodenal. Symptoms of partial obstruction may begin in the first week of life, and obstruction may rapidly become complete. Differentiation from duodenal atresia is often difficult. If complete obstruction is not present, the baby may feed poorly, have frequent emeses and demonstrate poor weight gain.
   b. Jejunal or ileal. Complete obstruction may simulate atresia.
   c. Rectal. Symptoms of obstipation and megacolon present from birth may simulate aganglionic megacolon. Fecal impaction may cause intestinal obstruction.

6. Neonatal small left colon syndrome may be asymptomatic or associated with low intestinal obstruction. Uniform narrowing of the colon from the splenic flexure to the anus is demonstrated by barium enema. There is a high incidence of maternal diabetes.

Davis, W.S. and Campbell, J.B.: Neonatal small left colon syndrome. *Am. J. Dis. Child.* *129*:1024, 1975.

7. Malrotation of the bowel. In infants with malrotation of the bowel, the descending duodenum often becomes obstructed in the first three weeks of life. Obstruction may be due to peritoneal bands that cross the duodenum and bind the cecum to the posterior abdominal wall or to direct pressure from the malrotated cecum itself. The vomitus almost always contains bile. Since duodenal obstruction may be accompanied by midgut volvulus, immediate surgery is indicated. Infants with the syndrome of asplenia and congenital heart disease may also have malrotation.

8. Midgut volvulus. Incomplete fixation of the malrotated bowel may lead to volvulus of the midgut (duodenum to midtransverse colon). Delay in diagnosis is dangerous because of the threat of infarction of the bowel. Obstructive symptoms with bilious vomiting sometimes begin as early as three to four days after birth but may occur at any age. Gastric peristaltic waves may be noted. Distention may be epigastric or generalized but is often absent. Recurrent episodes of volvulus with spontaneous resolution occasionally cause cyclic vomiting in older children. Volvulus occurs, at times, around the atrophied cord of the omphalomesenteric duct. When an infant with the asplenic syndrome (cyanotic congenital heart disease and nucleated red blood cells in the peripheral blood) has obstruction, a midgut volvulus may be present.

Berdon, W.E., Baker, D.H., Bull. S. and Santulli, T.V.: Midgut malrotation and volvulus. *Radiology 96*:375, 1970.

9. Pyloric stenosis. Regurgitation in the first week of life is frequently the initial symptom in this disorder. Usually, vomiting gradually becomes evident in the second and third weeks. As mucosal edema is superimposed on the muscular narrowing of the pyloric canal, vomiting becomes increasingly projectile. If the baby is given a small amount of fluid by mouth and examined in an adequate light, vigorous gastric peristalsis is usually visible. The diagnosis depends upon an absence of bile in the vomitus and the presence of a palpable pyloric tumor.
10. Pylorospasm is a doubtful clinical entity.
11. Torsion of the stomach may cause vomiting in infants, beginning soon after birth and, at times, projectile in character. The diagnosis is established by roentgenographic examination.
12. Annular pancreas is an extremely rare cause of intestinal obstruction in children. Obstruction may be complete or partial and recurrent.
13. Diaphragmatic hernia. Dyspnea, cyanosis or vomiting may appear in newborn babies if a massive herniation of the abdominal viscera has occurred through a congenital diaphragmatic defect. Symptoms of esophageal hiatus hernia may begin at any age. Recurrent episodes of colicky lower thoracic or epigastric pain, ulceration of the herniated stomach with hematemesis, discomfort after eating and vomiting may occur.
14. Duplications of the alimentary tract may cause partial intestinal obstruction with colicky pain and vomiting.

Grosfeld, J.L., O'Neill, J.A. and Clatworthy, H.W., Jr.: Enteric duplications in infancy and childhood: an 18-year review. *Ann. Surg. 172*:83, 1970.

15. Incarcerated or strangulated hernias
16. Intussusception usually causes vomiting early. In the older child intussusception may be a complication of cystic fibrosis.

Holsclaw, D.S., Rocmans, C. and Shwachman, H.: Intussusception in patients with cystic fibrosis. *Pediatrics 48*:51, 1971.

17. Adhesive bands
18. Foreign bodies in the gastrointestinal tract
    a. Trichobezoar

b. Lactobezoar due to a milk coagulum. Intestinal obstruction may occur 5 to 14 days after birth due to inspissated milk curds. This disorder occurs primarily in premature infants who receive a high-calorie powdered milk formula. Abdominal x-rays reveal dense round or elongated masses in the bowel surrounded by air halos.

Erenberg, A., Shaw, R.D. and Yousefzadeh, D.: Lactobezoar in the low-birth-weight infant. *Pediatrics 63*:642, 1979.
Graivier, L., Harper, N.E. and Currarino, G.: Milk-curd bowel obstruction in the newborn infant. *JAMA 238*:1050, 1977.

19. Paralytic ileus
    a. Peritonitis
    b. Postoperative
    c. Acute infectious diseases such as pneumonia
    d. Severe hypokalemia
20. Intramural hematoma of the intestine secondary to even slight blunt abdominal trauma may cause nausea, bilious vomiting, abdominal pain, tenderness, ileus and, at times, fever. Acute symptoms and signs may follow immediately or be delayed several days. An abdominal mass may be palpable. A "coil spring" deformity on an upper gastrointestinal series is diagnostic.

Judd, D.R., Taybi, H. and King, H.: Intramural hematoma of the small bowel. *Arch. Surg. 89*:527, 1964.
Stewart, D.R., Byrd, C.L. and Schuster, S.R.: Intramural hematomas of the alimentary tract in children. *Surgery 68*:550, 1970.

21. Hirschsprung's disease may cause vomiting in the newborn infant.
22. Sigmoid volvulus, which may occur in patients with a large redundant sigmoid loop attached to a narrow mesenteric base, is usually a fulminant process with early necrosis of the bowel. Chronic constipation may be a contributing factor. A barium enema is required for diagnosis.

Carter, R. and Hinshaw, D.B.: Acute sigmoid volvulus in children. *Am. J. Dis. Child. 101*:631, 1961.
Hunter, J. G., Jr. and Keats, T.E.: Sigmoid volvulus in children. *Am. J. Roentgenol. Rad. Ther. Nuc. Med. 58*:621, 1970.

23. The chronic idiopathic pseudo-obstruction syndrome in infants and children is characterized by intermittent vomiting, distention, abdominal pain, diarrhea, constipation and failure to thrive. The upper gastrointestinal series reveals abnormal motility and dilated small bowel loops.

Byrne, W.J., Cipel, L., Euler, A.R., Hapin, T.C. and Ament, M.E.: Chronic idiopathic pseudo-obstruction syndrome in children — clinical characteristics and prognosis. *J. Pediatr. 90*:585, 1977.

24. Ascariasis may cause vomiting due to mechanical obstruction by masses of parasites.
B. Mechanical vomiting due to nonobstructive causes
    1. Severe cough. The vigorous contractions of the abdominal muscles and diaphragm that occur during episodes of severe coughing frequently result in vomiting.

II. Reflex causes
   A. Reflex vomiting due to stimuli from the gastrointestinal tract
      1. Swallowing of amniotic fluid. Often, no definitive cause can be found for retching and vomiting in the first two to three days of life. Excessive swallowing of amniotic fluid has been suggested as an explanation.
      2. Postnasal drip and pharyngeal mucus may stimulate the gag reflex and lead to vomiting, especially in the morning on arising.
      3. Edematous uvula. Rarely, a long uvula that has become inflamed during a respiratory infection may stimulate gagging and retching.
      4. Gastritis. Vomiting may occur during almost any acute parenteral infection.
         a. Respiratory infections. Many babies and young children vomit in association with respiratory infections. Whether this is due to simultaneous infection of the gastrointestinal and respiratory tracts or to the irritant effect of swallowed secretions is not known.
         b. Acute viral or bacterial gastroenteritis
         c. Epidemic nausea and vomiting (winter vomiting disease, "intestinal grippe"). Vomiting may occur with epidemic incidence in children during the fall and winter with rotavirus as a frequent etiologic agent. The onset is often explosive with vomiting recurring every 10 to 30 minutes for the initial 4- to 8-hour period. Diarrhea usually persists for 6 to 12 hours after the vomiting. Muscular aching and weakness are often severe and fever is frequent. Symptoms subside in 24 to 48 hours.

   Webb, C.H. and Wallace, W.M.: Diagnosis and treatment: epidemic gastroenteritis, presumably viral. *Pediatrics 38*:494, 1966.

         d. Moniliasis
         e. Scarlet fever
         f. Diphtheritic pseudomembranous gastritis
         g. Corrosive gastritis: lye, bleaches, ammonia
      5. Spontaneous gastric perforation may occur during the first week of life in the newborn infant. Findings include bilious vomiting, rapid abdominal distention, lethargy and shock.
      6. Gastrointestinal allergy may rarely cause vomiting.
      7. Peptic gastric or duodenal ulcer. The presenting symptom in premature, debilitated or acutely ill infants may be vomiting, at times simulating that of pyloric stenosis. In others, colic, vomiting, loose stools and, occasionally, melena occur. Early in childhood, anorexia and abdominal pain are the predominant complaints, and vomiting is infrequent. Occasionally, however, vomiting occurs without abdominal pain.
      8. Enterocolitis. (See discussion of diarrhea.)
      9. Necrotizing enterocolitis is characterized by poor feeding, bilious vomiting, respiratory distress, abdominal distention, jaundice, diarrhea, apnea, lethargy, hypothermia and blood in the stools. The infant appears septic and in shock. X-rays reveal free peritoneal air, pneumatosis intestinalis or hepatic portal venous gas. Necrotizing enterocolitis occurs most frequently in premature infants on the third to fifth day of life, especially those who have experienced perinatal stress. It may also

occur in the term infant and in the second and third weeks of life. Signs of peritonitis (e.g., resistance, induration and edema of the abdominal wall) may be present.

Santulli, T.V. et al.: Acute necrotizing enterocolitis in infancy: a review of 64 cases. *Pediatrics* 55:376, 1975.

10. In patients with celiac disease, vomiting may be the initial manifestation. Although it may be mild and inconstant, vomiting is more frequently forceful and severe.
11. Appendicitis. Vomiting usually preceded by pain is the rule in children who have acute appendicitis. A history of pain may not be elicited in infants and young children, and vomiting may be the only early symptom. An appendiceal abscess may cause bowel obstruction.
12. Acute peritonitis. Fecal vomiting often occurs due to ileus.
13. Hemorrhagic diseases producing bleeding of the upper gastrointestinal tract.
14. Superior mesenteric artery syndrome is characterized by intermittent duodenal dilatation and stasis without evidence of mechanical obstruction. Symptoms include frequent vomiting, abdominal cramps, poor weight gain and weight loss. In the so-called cast syndrome severe vomiting occurs after the application of a body cast.

Burrington, J.D.: Superior mesenteric artery syndrome in children. *Am. J. Dis. Child.* 130:1367, 1976.
Shandling, B.: The so-called superior mesenteric artery syndrome. *Am. J. Dis. Child.* 130:1371, 1976.

15. Mesenteric vascular occlusion leads to vomiting, abdominal distention, intermittent abdominal pain, blood in the stools and diarrhea or constipation. Appropriate small bowel x-ray studies are diagnostically helpful.

B. Reflex vomiting due to stimuli from the genitourinary tract. Vomiting may be the only symptom of genitourinary tract disease in infants and young children.
    1. Acute pyelonephritis. Vomiting, often projectile and perhaps accompanied by visible peristaltic waves, frequently is the outstanding symptom.
    2. Obstructive anomalies and hydronephrosis. Vomiting frequently occurs in the presence of anomalies of the urinary tract, especially those causing intermittent obstruction.
    3. Acute glomerulonephritis. Vomiting occasionally occurs as a prodrome.
    4. Urinary calculi may at times cause vomiting.
    5. Pregnancy may be a cause of persistent vomiting in adolescent girls.

C. Reflex vomiting due to labyrinthine disturbances
    1. Otitis media with labyrinthitis
    2. Motion sickness: car sickness, sea sickness, air sickness. A familial tendency may be reported.

D. Reflex vomiting due to drugs and poisons. The mucosa of the gastrointestinal tract is directly irritated in most instances, although some drugs also act centrally.

    1. Salicylates

    2. Mustard, ipecac

    3. Digitalis

    4. Vomiting may be an early symptom in children with lead poisoning.

    5. Vomiting is an almost constant symptom of aminophylline toxicity. The vomiting may be intractable and characterized by bloody or coffee-ground vomitus.

E. Heat prostration

F. Hypoadrenalism in young infants with congenital virilizing adrenal hyperplasia may be accompanied by persistent or recurrent vomiting as well as by diarrhea. Visible peristaltic waves may occur. Dehydration may be more severe than would be anticipated from the amount of vomiting or diarrhea. Nausea and vomiting may be early manifestations of Addison's disease in older children.

G. Hypercalcemia. Vomiting, occasionally severe and projectile, may be the initial manifestation in infants with idiopathic hypercalcemia.

H. Neonatal tetany may be accompanied by vomiting, along with convulsive seizures and edema of the hands and feet.

I. Renal insufficiency; uremia

J. Pancreatitis may account for vomiting and abdominal pain in children.

K. Infectious hepatitis. Vomiting may be an early symptom.

L. Reye's syndrome may be characterized early by an upper respiratory infection followed by vomiting, changes in sensorium and behavior.

M. Acidosis. Vomiting may occur in patients in diabetic and other acidotic states.

N. An inborn error of metabolism, especially a disorder characterized by protein intolerance, should be suspected as a cause of persistent vomiting that begins after the institution of feedings in newborn infants. This group includes:

    1. Urea cycle defects characterized by hyperammonemia and lethargy.

    2. Disorders of organic acid metabolism. These patients demonstrate profound lethargy and projectile vomiting accompanied by metabolic acidosis, ketosis, neutropenia and thrombocytopenia.

        a. Methylmalonic acidemia. Other clinical features include hepatomegaly and failure to thrive.

        b. Propionic acidemia. These infants fail to thrive.

        c. Isovaleric acidemia.

        d. Argininemia

Keating, J.P., Feigin, R.D., Tenenbaum, S.M. and Hillman, R.E.: Hyperglycinemia with ketosis due to a defect in isoleucine metabolism: a preliminary report. *Pediatrics* 50:890, 1972.

Snyderman, S.E. et al.: Argininemia. *J. Pediatr.* 90:563, 1977.

    3. Phenylketonuria may cause vomiting in the newborn.

    4. Fructose intolerance (fructosemia) and fructose-1,6-diphosphatase deficiency may be manifested by recurrent nausea, vomiting, diarrhea, failure to thrive, hepatomegaly, malaise and hypoglycemia after ingestion of fructose-containing foods.

Rennert, O.M. and Greer, M.: Hereditary fructosemia. *Neurology 20*:421, 1970.

    5. Hereditary tyrosinemia

III. Central vomiting

  A. Central vomiting due to disease of the central nervous system

      1. Intracranial neoplasms. Vomiting is one of the most common clinical manifestations of an intracranial neoplasm in children. Though vomiting may be accompanied by evidences of increased intracranial pressure, it may occur initially in the absence of such pressure owing to direct involvement of the medullary vomiting center. This may be the case in patients who have a midline tumor of the cerebellum, a tumor involving the fourth ventricle and a pontine or a medullary tumor. *Vomiting in the absence of signs of increased intracranial pressure can be due to an intracranial neoplasm.* Initially, the vomiting often occurs in the morning a short time after awakening and before breakfast. It may be projectile but commonly is not. Nausea often precedes the vomiting but, in many instances, does not. Vomiting is not followed by nausea. Remissions due to spontaneous decompression may occur after the child has been vomiting for several days. Vomiting recurs, however, within a short time. *The presence of an intracranial neoplasm is a serious diagnostic consideration in every child with unexplained vomiting.*

      2. Cerebral edema

        a. Cerebral edema in the newborn infant may be accompanied by vomiting and convulsive seizures during the first two or three days of life.

        b. Traumatic cerebral edema: acute focal edema, acute general edema. Repeated vomiting may occur after a head injury. This need not cause undue concern unless accompanied by alteration in consciousness or neurologic abnormalities.

      3. Intracranial hemorrhage

      4. Subdural hematoma. Vomiting, convulsions and irritability are the cardinal symptoms of this disorder in infants. In approximately 5 per cent of cases, unexplained vomiting is the only symptom. Usually, however, it is accompanied by delay in neuromuscular development, convulsions, macrocephaly, widening of the biparietal diameter, fever and failure to thrive.

      5. Hydrocephalus. Signs and symptoms of increased intracranial pressure owing to acute obstruction of cerebrospinal fluid shunts include vomiting, irritability, lethargy, headache, bulging of the fontanel or rapid increase in head size.

Freeman, J.M. and D'Souza, B.: Obstruction of CSF shunts. *Pediatrics 64*::111, 1979.

      6. Meningitis and meningoencephalitis

      7. Subdural effusions complicating bacterial meningitis

      8. Intracranial abscess

      9. Epilepsy. Rarely, abdominal pain and vomiting may, in themselves, constitute a form of epilepsy. These symptoms may also represent the aura in patients with major seizures.

10. Leigh's disease may be characterized by recurrent vomiting, lethargy and brainstem dysfunction with dysphagia, facial weakness, respiratory irregularity, extraocular palsies and ataxia.
11. Lead poisoning is accompanied by encephalopathy and increased intracranial pressure. Vomiting, often persistent and projectile, is frequent and may be the initial manifestation.
12. Idiopathic hypoglycemia
13. Migraine
14. Salicylism. Vomiting may be the initial manifestation in these children.

B. Central vomiting not due to primary central nervous system disease
  1. Abnormal body metabolites
    a. Uremia
    b. Diabetic acidosis
    c. Hepatic cirrhosis
    d. Chronic acidosis of renal origin may be characterized by recurrent episodes of vomiting.
  2. Acute infections; sepsis or other infections, especially in young infants
  3. Psychogenic vomiting. Vomiting occurs in some children when they are unduly stimulated or excited. Anorexia and vomiting are frequently present in infants and childen when the emotional environment is unpleasant. Some children may gag and vomit if an attempt is made to force them to eat a particular food or foods. Self-induced, recurrent vomiting is sometimes seen in moderately or severely retarded children. Occasionally, vomiting may be related to a school phobia. In this event, vomiting usually occurs before or shortly after breakfast while the child is still at home, or it may occur at school. Vomiting does not occur on Saturday or Sunday.
  4. Cyclic vomiting is characterized by episodes of vomiting that tend to recur two, three or more times a year. These episodes may last for several days. Severe ketosis and, sometimes, acidosis develop. The cause for this syndrome is unknown. These children are often emotionally labile, and a period of cyclic vomiting may be precipitated by some emotional upset. Cyclic vomiting may occur in patients with a diverticulum of the small bowel or recurrent volvulus. This type of vomiting has also been described in children with familial dysautonomia and in those who later experience migraine headaches. Cyclic vomiting has also been considered an autonomic type of epilepsy.

Reinhart, J.B., Evans, S.L. and McFadden, D.L.: Cyclic vomiting in children: seen through the psychiatrist's eye. *Pediatrics 59*:371, 1977.

  5. Anorexia nervosa and bulimia (megaphagia) may be accompanied by self-induced vomiting. Bulimia occurs in both anorexia nervosa and the Kleine-Levin syndrome.

Rich, C.L.: Self-induced vomiting. Psychiatric considerations. *JAMA 239*:2688, 1978.

# ETIOLOGIC CLASSIFICATION OF REGURGITATION

I. "Physiologic" regurgitation, 285
II. Faulty feeding techniques, 285
III. Gastroesophageal reflux, 285
IV. Congenital esophageal obstructions, 286
   A. Esophageal atresia, 286
   B. Stenosis of esophagus, 286
   C. Congenitally short esophagus, 286
   D. Esophageal hiatus hernia, 286
   E. Webbing of esophagus, 287
   F. Cardiospasm, 287
   G. Congenital vascular ring, 287
   H. Duplication of esophagus, 287
V. Acquired esophageal lesions, 287
   A. Esophagitis, 287
     1. Infectious diseases
     2. Ingestion of corrosive agents
     3. Cardiac disease
     4. Chronic pulmonary infections
     5. Esophageal chalasia or hiatus hernia
   B. Strictures, 287
     1. Infectious diseases
     2. Scleroderma
     3. Corrosive agents
     4. Foreign body

   C. Esophageal diverticulum, 287
   D. Traumatic pseudodiverticulum of pharynx, 287
   E. Foreign body, 287
   F. Retroesophageal abscess, 287
     1. Extension of retroesophageal abscess
     2. Esophageal perforation
     3. Foreign bodies
     4. Vertebral tuberculosis
     5. Ulceration from tracheotomy tube
     6. Suppurating mediastinal lymph nodes
VI. Rumination, 288
VII. Pyloric stenosis, 288
VIII. Miscellaneous causes, 288
   A. Dyspnea, 288
   B. Increased intra-abdominal pressure, 288
     1. Ascites
     2. Abdominal cysts
     3. Organ enlargements
     4. Neoplasms
   C. Eventration of diaphragm, 288

# ETIOLOGIC CLASSIFICATION OF VOMITING

I. Mechanical vomiting, 290
   A. Obstructive, 290
     1. Intestinal atresia
     2. Imperforate anus
     3. Meconium ileus
     4. Meconium plug
     5. Intestinal stenosis
     6. Neonatal small left colon syndrome
     7. Malrotation of bowel
     8. Midgut volvulus
     9. Pyloric stenosis
     10. Pylorospasm
     11. Torsion of stomach
     12. Annular pancreas
     13. Diaphragmatic hernia
     14. Duplications of alimentary tract
     15. Incarcerated or strangulated hernias
     16. Intussusception
     17. Adhesive bands
     18. Foreign bodies in the gastrointestinal tract
     19. Paralytic ileus
     20. Intramural hematoma
     21. Hirschsprung's disease
     22. Sigmoid volvulus
     23. Chronic idiopathic pseudoobstruction syndrome

     24. Ascariasis
   B. Nonobstructive, 293
     1. Severe cough
II. Reflex causes, 294
   A. Stimuli from gastrointestinal tract, 294
     1. Swallowing amniotic fluid
     2. Postnasal drip and pharyngeal mucus
     3. Edematous uvula
     4. Gastritis
     5. Spontaneous gastric perforation
     6. Gastrointestinal allergy
     7. Peptic gastric or duodenal ulcer
     8. Enterocolitis
     9. Necrotizing enterocolitis
     10. Celiac disease
     11. Appendicitis
     12. Acute peritonitis
     13. Hemorrhagic diseases
     14. Superior mesenteric artery syndrome
     15. Mesenteric vascular occlusion
   B. Stimuli from genitourinary tract, 295
     1. Acute pyelonephritis
     2. Obstructive anomalies and hydronephrosis
     3. Acute glomerulonephritis
     4. Urinary calculi
     5. Pregnancy

C. Labyrinthine disturbances, 295
  1. Otitis media with labyrinthine disturbances
  2. Motion sickness
D. Drugs and poisons, 295
  1. Salicylates
  2. Mustard, ipecac
  3. Digitalis
  4. Lead poisoning
  5. Aminophylline toxicity
E. Heat prostration, 296
F. Hypoadrenalism, 296
G. Hypercalcemia, 296
H. Neonatal tetany, 296
I. Renal insufficiency, uremia, 296
J. Pancreatitis, 296
K. Infectious hepatitis, 296
L. Reye's syndrome, 296
M. Acidosis, 296
N. Metabolic errors, 296
  1. Urea cycle defects
  2. Disorders of organic acid metabolism
  3. Phenylketonuria
  4. Fructosemia, fructose-1, 6-diphosphatase deficiency

  5. Hereditary tyrosinemia
III. Central vomiting, 297
A. Central nervous system causes, 297
  1. Intracranial neoplasms
  2. Cerebral edema
  3. Intracranial hemorrhage
  4. Subdural hematoma
  5. Hydrocephalus; obstructed shunt
  6. Meningitis and meningoencephalitis
  7. Subdural effusions
  8. Intracranial abscess
  9. Epilepsy
  10. Leigh's disease
  11. Lead poisoning
  12. Idiopathic hypoglycemia
  13. Migraine
  14. Salicylism
B. Other causes, 298
  1. Abnormal body metabolites
  2. Acute infections
  3. Psychogenic vomiting
  4. Cyclic vomiting
  5. Anorexia nervosa, bulimia

---

CHAPTER 32

# DIARRHEA

Diarrhea refers to an increased frequency and water content of the stools owing either to solute malabsorption, fluid secretion or motility disturbance.

Banwell, J.G. et al.: Fluid and electrolyte transport in the small intestine. *Am. J. Clin. Nutr. 23*:1559, 1970.
Jeejeebhoy, K.N.: Symposium on diarrhea. I. Definition and mechanisms of diarrhea. *Can. Med. Assoc. J. 116*:737, 1977.
Phillips, S.F.: Diarrhea: pathogenesis and diagnostic techniques. *Postgrad. Med. 57*:65, 1975.

## ETIOLOGIC CLASSIFICATION OF DIARRHEA BY AGE PERIODS

I. *The newborn infant*
    Diarrhea may begin insidiously with restlessness, irritability, lethargy, refusal of food, vomiting and weight loss preceding a change in the frequency or consistency of the stools. The sudden passage of a large, watery stool may be the initial symptom.
A. Overfeeding may cause loose stools in the premature infant.

B. Viral diarrhea of the newborn may occur in epidemic form. Stools are yellow, liquid and explosive. Etiologic agents in viral diarrhea of the newborn include rotavirus and echovirus types 11, 14 and 18.

C. Necrotizing enterocolitis, which occurs primarily in low-birth-weight infants who have experienced stress such as hypoxia, is characterized by poor feeding, diarrhea, blood in the stools, bilious vomiting, abdominal distention, lethargy and signs of peritonitis. Roentgenographic examination reveals pneumatosis or pneumoperitoneum. The onset is usually in the first five days of life but may not occur until three weeks of age.

Santulli, T.V. et al.: Acute necrotizing enterocolitis in infancy: a review of 64 cases. *Pediatrics* 55:376, 1975.

D. Bacterial diarrhea of the newborn
1. Enteropathogenic, enterotoxigenic and enteroinvasive Escherichia coli. Certain serogroups of Escherichia coli cause sporadic and epidemic outbreaks of diarrheal disease in newborn and older infants. The infection may be subclinical, mild, severe or fulminant. The enterotoxigenic form is most frequently etiologic in infants, causing green, foul-smelling stools with mucus, while in older children the enteroinvasive form produces symptoms that may simulate shigella dysentery. Fever and vomiting may accompany the diarrhea.
2. Salmonella. Stools are green and mucoid and may contain blood. Abdominal distention, vomiting, dehydration, rapid weight loss, fever, stupor and convulsions may occur. Splenomegaly and jaundice may also be noted. Bacteremia, meningitis, peritonitis, pyogenic arthritis, osteomyelitis and pleurisy are possible complications. The course may be mild, severe with sepsis, or prolonged and typhoidal. Salmonella enteritis in the mother may cause infection of the newborn infant during delivery.

E. Parenteral diarrhea refers to the occurrence of loose stools in the presence of extraintestinal infections (e.g., respiratory or urinary tract infections).

F. Dietary factors. Few instances of diarrhea are due to the usual formulas used in the feeding of newborn infants. Cow milk allergy, a rare and frequently overdiagnosed disorder, may become symptomatic in the first weeks of life with colic, loose stools and, perhaps, bright red blood in the stools.

G. Congenital enterokinase deficiency, an extremely rare defect in the intestinal mucosa, causes diarrhea and hypoproteinemia.

Haworth, J.C., Gourley, B., Hadorn, B. and Sumida, C.: Malabsorption and growth failure due to intestinal enterokinase deficiency. *J. Pediatr.* 78:481, 1971.

H. Congenital alkalosis with diarrhea (congenital chloridorrhea), a rare familial disease, is characterized by intractable, watery diarrhea beginning shortly after birth. Extreme alkalosis results from excessive loss of chloride ion in the stools.

McReynolds, E.W., Roy, S., III and Etteldorf, J.N.: Congenital chloride diarrhea. *Am. J. Dis. Child.* 127:566, 1974.

II. *Older infants and children*
A. Infections
1. Parenteral diarrhea. Children may have loose stools at the onset of or during an acute respiratory or urinary tract infection.

2. Acute gastroenteritis syndrome (winter vomiting disease, epidemic nausea and vomiting, viral diarrhea). Next to respiratory disease, acute gastroenteritis is the most common illness in children. About 20 to 30 per cent of episodes of infectious diarrhea has a bacterial etiology. Another 20 to 30 per cent is of undetermined etiology. The remaining 50 per cent has a viral etiology, most commonly the rotavirus. Except for echovirus 11, proof is lacking for the etiologic association of other enteroviruses or adenoviruses in acute gastroenteritis. The acute gastroenteritis syndrome is more common in the winter and occurs in family and community outbreaks. While it affects younger children primarily, it may occur in adults. Diarrhea usually follows nausea and vomiting after a few hours. There may be 2 to 20 watery bowel movements a day. The stools do not contain blood or pus. Abdominal cramps, muscle aching and weakness are often prominent. Fever and dehydration may occur. Duration of the illness is usually one or two days.

Hodes, H.L.: Viral gastroenteritis. *Am. J. Dis. Child. 131*:729, 1977.
Rodriguez, W.J. et al.: Clinical features of acute gastroenteritis associated with human reovirus-like agent in infants and young children. *J. Pediatr. 91*:188, 1977.
Steinhoff, M.C.: Viruses and diarrhea — a review. *Am. J. Dis. Child. 132*:302, 1978.
Tallett, S. et al.: Clinical, laboratory, and epidemiologic features of a viral gastroenteritis in infants and children. *Pediatrics 60*:217, 1977.

3. Infectious hepatitis. Mild diarrhea may occur during the preicteric phase.
4. Bacterial diarrhea. Stool cultures should be obtained and plated immediately.
   a. Staphylococcal food poisoning. Severe vomiting, retching, abdominal pain and diarrhea occur within one to six hours after ingestion of food contaminated with staphylococcal exotoxin. Several members of a family may simultaneously become ill. Stools are watery and may contain blood. Shock and cyanosis may occur in severe cases. Staphylococcal pseudomembranous colitis with explosive diarrhea and a pseudomembrane noted on endoscopy may occur in patients receiving antibiotics.
   b. Salmonella (excluding typhoid fever). Vomiting, abdominal pain, fever and diarrhea with watery, mucoid and sometimes bloody stools may be due to a salmonella enteric infection. Bacteremia with subsequent localization in joints, bones, meninges or soft tissues may occur as a complication. Splenomegaly, jaundice, meningismus, convulsions and stupor may appear. The diagnosis is established by stool and blood cultures.
   c. Typhoid fever. Frequent watery or mucoid stools occur in approximately half the patients with typhoid fever. Very young infants are often asymptomatic except for mild gastroenteritis.
   d. Shigella (bacillary dysentery) usually occurs between 1 and 5 years of age with about 25 per cent occurring under 1 year of age. The onset is abrupt with vomiting, abdominal cramps, high fever, prostration and explosive, odorless, greenish-yellow and watery stools. Within a few hours the stools may contain mucus, pus and streaks of bright red blood. Meningismus, disorientation, coma and convulsions may sug-

gest encephalitis. Bacteremia is relatively infrequent. Bronchitis or pneumonitis may also occur. Diarrhea may continue intermittently for weeks or months. Other members of the family are usually carriers or have active disease. Stool cultures should be obtained on all family members. Since amebae and other intestinal parasites are also frequently present, stools should be examined for ova and parasites.

e. Pseudomonas aeruginosa may also cause severe diarrhea. Colonization or overgrowth of the intestinal tract by Klebsiella pneumoniae or staphylococci, pneumococci or streptococci may cause diarrhea.

f. Enteropathic E. coli may be etiologic in diarrhea in children under two years of age. Symptoms include anorexia and vomiting. The stools have a foul odor and are green, loose and slimy. Usually, there is no history of diarrhea in household contacts.

g. Tularemia may be accompanied by diarrhea, vomiting and abdominal pain.

h. Brucellosis. Diarrhea or bloody stools may occur during the acute phases of this disease.

i. Tuberculous enteritis may have a protracted course with intermittent diarrhea and tenesmus. Blood in the stools is usually microscopic in amount. Tuberculosis of the respiratory tract is usually the site of the primary infection.

j. Non-cholera vibrio infections

Hughes, J.M., Hollis, D.G., Gangarosa, E.J. and Weaver, R.E.: Non-cholera vibrio infections in the United States. *Ann. Int. Med. 88*:602, 1978.

k. Yersinia enterocolitica may cause diarrhea in infants and young children. Usually mild and self-limited, the diarrhea may be severe, with blood in the stools and fever.

l. Campylobacter enteritis may be characterized by diarrhea, abdominal pain and fever. The stools are watery, profuse and foul-smelling.

Rettig, P.J.: Campylobacter infections in human beings. *J. Pediatr. 94*:855, 1979.

m. Altered gastrointestinal flora secondary to the use of broad-spectrum antibiotics may cause chronic diarrhea.

Connor, J.D. and Barrett-Connor, E.: Infectious diarrhea. *Pediatr. Clin. N. Am. 14*:197, 1967.
Cramblett, H.G., Azimi, P. and Haynes, R.E.: The etiology of infectious diarrhea in infancy, with special reference to enteropathogenic E. coli. *Ann. N.Y. Acad. Sci. 176*:80, 1971.
Drachman, R.H.: Acute infectious gastroenteritis. *Pediatr. Clin. N. Am. 21*:711, 1974.
Nelson, J.D. and Haltalin, K.C.: Accuracy of diagnosis of bacterial diarrheal disease by clinical features. *J. Pediatr. 78*:519, 1971.

5. Protozoan diarrhea

a. Amebiasis may be characterized by intermittent episodes of diarrhea with four to six liquid stools a day. The stools may contain only microscopic amounts of blood, mucus and pus. Constipation is often present between episodes of diarrhea. In the severe dysenteric form the stools are at first watery, green and slimy. Nausea, abdominal cramps, tenesmus and fever are also present. Blood-flecked stools and mucus appear within a short time, and as many as 15 to 20 stools may be passed in 24 hours. Chronic amebiasis may simulate ulcerative colitis with blood, mucus and pus intermittently present in the stools. For microscopic examination, the stools must be fluid, freshly passed and warm. They are best obtained by mild saline catharsis, saline enema or aspiration of lesions at the time of proctoscopy. Whenever possible, bloody mucus should be selected for examination. If amebae are found in the patient, all members of the family should have stool examinations. Stool cultures for salmonella or shigella organisms should also be obtained.

    b. Giardia lamblia. The celiac syndrome may be produced by extensive coating of the mucosal surfaces of the duodenum and jejunum by this protozoan. While the cysts may be demonstrable by duodenal aspiration in addition to examination of the stools, the latter is positive in only 30 per cent of cases. Therefore, Giemsa-stained smears of the mucus adhering to intestinal biopsies may be diagnostically useful. Giardiasis is one of the causes of malabsorption in patients with primary immunodeficiency syndromes. In its acute phase, giardiasis may cause explosive, watery, foul-smelling stools with abdominal distention and flatulence.

Ament, M.E.: Diagnosis and treatment of giardiasis. *J. Pediatr. 80*:633, 1972.
Burke, J.A.: Giardiasis in childhood. *Am. J. Dis. Child. 129*:1304, 1975.

    6. Parasitic diarrhea
        a. Nematodes (roundworms)
           (1) Trichuriasis (whipworm disease). Rarely, bloody, mucoid diarrhea may occur.
           (2) Hookworm disease. Unformed, tarry stools may be present in patients with heavy hookworm infestation.
           (3) Strongyloidiasis (threadworm disease). Mucoid diarrhea, at times severe, may be persistent or alternate with constipation.
        b. Platyhelminthes (flatworms)
           (1) Taeniasis (tapeworm infestation). During the early stages mucoid diarrhea is frequent.

Katz, M.: Parasitic infections. *J. Pediatr. 87*:165, 1975.

    7. Fungal diarrhea
        a. Histoplasmosis. Diarrhea is frequent in the disseminated form of this disease. Blood may appear in the stools if ulceration of Peyer's patches occurs.
        b. Candida
  B. Malabsorption syndromes
    1. Celiac disease is due to intolerance to wheat gluten (gluten-induced enteropathy). Vomiting may be the initial manifestation. Intermittent diarrhea may begin at any time from birth to the end of the second year. In an occasional child, symptoms begin later. The stools are often fluid or mushy and vary in color from pale cream to greenish-yellow. Mucus may cause the stools to have a metallic sheen. Occasionally, oily or greasy droplets appear on the surface of a fluid stool. The volume is usually larger than normal and, eventually, the stools have an offensive

odor. One to ten stools a day may be passed during diarrheal episodes that last days, weeks or months. Irritability may be notable during these periods. Remissions are frequent at first, and the stools may be normal or constipated between episodes.

Three-day total stool fat determinations verify the presence of steatorrhea. In celiac disease, the fecal fat output exceeds 5 and frequently 10 gm. a day while the child is receiving an adequate fat intake in a normal diet. In addition to the increase in fecal fat, the laboratory findings most consistently present include low concentrations of serum proteins, serum folate and serum carotene. Serum carotene levels greater than 100 $\mu$g./100 ml. are normal and exclude the possibility of malabsorption. Values between 20 and 50 $\mu$g./100 ml. are suggestive of but not specific for malabsorption. Serum carotene levels less than 20 $\mu$g./100 ml. are seen almost exclusively in malabsorption states. The Sudan III stain for fecal fat may confirm a clinical impression that the stool contains excessive fat but may be falsely negative. Normal stools do not contain Sudan III staining material or only small particles. With a marked increase in stool fat, many fat droplets are noted on microscopic examination.

Goldbloom, R.B., Blake, R.M. and Cameron, D.: Assessment of three methods for measuring intestinal fat absorption in infants and children. *Pediatrics 34*:814, 1964.
Jones, W.O. and Di Sant'Agnese, P.A.: Laboratory aids in the diagnosis of malabsorption in pediatrics. *J. Pediatr. 62*:44, 1963.

Biopsy specimens of the small intestinal mucous membrane, obtained by intubation, demonstrate characteristic mucosal changes. The disorder should respond promptly to a gluten-free diet.

Dermatitis herpetiformis (see page 256) may be accompanied by celiac symptoms and changes in the intestinal mucosa. Tropical sprue may also occur in children.

Ament, M.E.: Malabsorption syndromes in infancy and childhood. Parts I and II. *J. Pediatr. 81*:685, 867, 1972.
Santiago-Borrero, P.J., Maldonado, N. and Horta, E.: Tropical sprue in children. *J. Pediatr. 76*:470, 1970.
Shuster, S., Watson, A.J. and Marks, J.: Coeliac syndrome in dermatitis herpetiformis. *Lancet 1*:1101, 1968.

2. Cystic fibrosis. Early, the clinical manifestations may be chiefly those of a persistent respiratory infection. The stools may be normal at this time. When solid foods are introduced, the stools may become foamy, bulky and foul-smelling. Often, the stools remain formed or soft and are rarely watery. Increased frequency occurs occasionally, but constipation may be present. In infants up to one year of age who present with evidence of malabsorption but no history of respiratory infections, a sweat chloride determination should be obtained. At times, steatorrhea will be the only presenting clinical manifestation.

3. Pancreatic enzyme deficiency may occur independently of cystic fibrosis in a syndrome characterized by steatorrhea, failure to thrive and neutropenia. Complete absence of trypsinogen may also occur.

Shwachman, H., Diamond, L.K., Oski, F.A. and Khaw, K.: The syndrome of pancreatic insufficiency and bone marrow dysfunction. *J. Pediatr. 65*:645, 1964.
Townes, P.L.: Trypsinogen deficiency disease. *J. Pediatr. 66*:275, 1965.

4. Short bowel syndrome due to massive resection of the small bowel may be associated with malabsorption owing to inactivation of the pancreatic enzymes and inability to reabsorb conjugated bile salts.

5. Other causes of steatorrhea include gastrointestinal allergy, absence of bile in the stools, bile salt deficiency, administration of broad-spectrum antibiotics, intestinal stenosis and intestinal malrotation (stasis syndrome). Steatorrhea may be associated with hypoparathyroidism and with Wolman's disease.

Powell, G.K., Jones, L.A. and Richardson, J.: A new syndrome of bile acid deficiency — a possible synthetic defect. *J. Pediatr. 83*:758, 1973.

6. Parasites. Giardiasis is the parasite most commonly associated with malabsorption. Other parasites are Strongyloides stercoralis, Capillaria philippinensis and Coccidia.

7. Abetalipoproteinemia is characterized by steatorrhea, thorny projections on the erythrocytes (acanthocytosis), atypical retinitis pigmentosa, progressive ataxia and virtual absence of beta-lipoprotein. Diarrhea in the first two years of life is usually the initial symptom. Neurologic symptoms occur many years later. A low serum cholesterol level in a young child with the celiac syndrome suggests this disorder. The diagnosis may be established by lipoprotein immunoelectrophoresis.

8. Primary immunodeficiency syndromes may be accompanied by gastrointestinal symptoms such as vomiting, diarrhea, steatorrhea, weight loss and protein-losing enteropathy. Giardiasis may be present in patients with primary B-cell deficiency. Chronic watery diarrhea in patients with T-cell defects is probably due to mucosal structural changes.

Ament, M.E., Ochs, H.D. and Davis, S.D.: Structure and function of the gastrointestinal tract in primary immunodeficiency syndromes. A study of 39 patients. *Medicine 52*:227, 1973.
Gryboski, J.D., Self, T.W., Clemett, A. and Herskovic, T.: Selective immunoglobulin A deficiency and intestinal nodular lymphoid hyperplasia: correction of diarrhea with antibiotics and plasma. *Pediatrics 42*:833, 1968.
Horowitz, S. et al.: Small intestinal disease in T cell deficiency. *J. Pediatr. 85*:457, 1974.

9. Intestinal lymphagiectasis. In addition to chylous ascites and edema, diarrhea may be secondary to malabsorption of fat.

10. Carbohydrate malabsorption. The diarrhea of carbohydrate malabsorption results from the osmotic effects of nonhydrolysed, unabsorbed sugar in the small bowel and from the acid metabolites formed by bacterial fermentation of the sugars in the colon. Stools are watery, frothy, often profuse, acid and frequently accompanied by flatus and excoriation of the perianal skin.

Carbohydrate malabsorption states may be congenital or acquired and related to disaccharides or monosaccharides. The exceedingly rare congenital disorders may cause diarrhea, vomiting and failure to thrive from the first day of life (lactase deficiency and glucose-galactose malabsorption) or after the first month (sucrase-isomaltase deficiency) unless carbohydrates are removed from the diet. Secondary types of carbohydrate malabsorption include lactase deficiency, lactase deficiency with deficiency of other disaccharides or temporary monosaccharide malabsorption.

Secondary lactase deficiency, by far the most common, follows any disorder that damages the epithelium, especially the brush border of the intestinal mucosa. Acute gastroenteritis is the most frequent cause of secondary lactase deficiency, which lasts from a few days to several weeks. If the carbohydrate intolerance persists over three weeks, the infant has usually become intolerant to all monosaccharides. Other disorders that lead to secondary deficiencies include celiac disease, giardiasis, cow milk sensitivity, sensitivity to soy protein isolate, leukemia treated with antimetabolites, protein-calorie malnutrition and gastrointestinal tract surgery in the newborn. Secondary lactase deficiency is especially common following diarrhea in newborn infants. Disaccharidase deficiency also occurs in many children with immunologic disorders.

Carbohydrate malabsorption may be suspected on the basis of the history and the examination of the stool. Screening stool examinations are (1) determination of the stool pH and (2) testing of the stool for reducing substances. In the screening tests, only the liquid portion of the stool uncontaminated by urine should be used. Stools should be collected on a piece of plastic inserted in the diaper and tested promptly. The pH may be determined by a Combistic or pH paper. Normally, the fecal pH is between 7 and 8. In carbohydrate malabsorption, the pH is less than 5.5 to 6, an abnormally low value.

The screening test for sugar in the stool employs the Clinitest reagent. A Clinitest tablet is added to 15 drops of a mixture of 1 part fluid stool to 2 parts of water. The resulting color is then compared to a color chart. Values above 0.5 per cent are abnormal. If sucrose is thought to be the offending sugar, the stool should be hydrolyzed using 1N HCl instead of water for dilution and boiling for 30 seconds to convert the sucrose to glucose and fructose.

In the presence of a suggestive history and positive screening tests, removal of the sugar from the diet should promptly relieve the diarrhea. If more sophisticated diagnostic tests are needed, specific carbohydrate tolerance tests may be used.

Dahlqvist, A.: Disaccharide intolerance. *JAMA 195*:225, 1966.
Dubois, R.S. et al.: Disaccharidase deficiency in children with immunologic deficits. *J. Pediatr. 76*:377, 1970.
Gracey, M. and Burke, V.: Sugar-induced diarrhea in children. *Arch. Dis. Child. 48*:331, 1973.
Lifshitz, F. et al.: Monosaccharide intolerance and hypoglycemia in infants with diarrhea. I. Clinical course of 23 infants. *J. Pediatr. 77*:595, 1970.
Schneider, A.J., Kinter, W. B. and Stirling, C.E.: Glucose-galactose malabsorption. *N. Engl. J. Med. 274*:305, 1966.
Townley, R.R.W.: Disaccharidase deficiency in infancy and childhood. *Pediatrics 38*:127, 1966.

Lactose intolerance differs from congenital lactase deficiency in that the patients as young children usually do not have symptoms but demonstrate milk-induced abdominal cramps and diarrhea as adolescents or adults.

Huang, S-S. and Bayless, T.M.: Lactose intolerance in healthy children. *N. Engl. J. Med. 276*:1283, 1967.

C. Gastrointestinal allergy. In the newborn period, gastrointestinal allergy to cow milk may cause clinical manifestations that range from severe diarrhea and shock to chronic diarrhea with mucus, gross or occult blood in the stools and steatorrhea. Diagnostic criteria include cessation of symptoms with elimination of milk and their recurrence within 48 hours of a rechallenge on 3 occasions. Most patients develop symptoms during the first 6 weeks of life. Tolerance to milk is gradually acquired by 2 to 5 years of age. Some infants are also extremely sensitive to soy protein and develop vomiting and diarrhea after its ingestion. Elimination diets may be helpful diagnostically when gastrointestinal allergy is suspected.

Bahna, S.L. and Heiner, D.C.: Cow's milk allergy: pathogenesis, manifestations, diagnosis and management. *Adv. Pediatr. 25*:1, 1978.
Gryboski, J.D.: Gastrointestinal milk allergy in infants. *Pediatrics 40*:354, 1967.
Mendoza, J., Meyers, J. and Snyder, R.: Soybean sensitivity. *Pediatrics 46*:774, 1970.

D. Antibiotic diarrhea due to alteration of the intestinal flora
E. Endocrine and metabolic diarrhea
   1. Hyperthyroidism
   2. Uremia
   3. Nephrosis. Episodes of nonspecific diarrhea may occur in children with nephrosis.
   4. Cystinosis
   5. Hereditary tyrosinemia
   6. Wolman's disease
   7. Chronic diarrhea with abdominal distention and wasting is the presenting symptom in some patients with a ganglioneuroma or ganglioneuroblastoma. The symptoms may suggest either celiac disease or cystic fibrosis. Bowel movements are foul-smelling, frequent, frothy and loose, watery or greasy. There is a history of weight loss or failure to gain. Lethargy, irritability, excessive perspiration and hypertension may also be noted. Preoperatively, the urinary excretion of norepinephrine, 3-methoxy-r-hydroxy mandelic acid and related metabolites is increased. Complete reversal of symptoms follows removal of the tumor.
   8. The Zollinger-Ellison syndrome is manifested by severe diarrhea, with or without peptic ulcer and marked hyperchlorhydria.
   9. Nonbeta islet cell hyperplasia may be associated with chronic diarrhea.

Grishan, F.K., Soper, R.T., Nassif, E.G. and Younoszai, M.K.: Chronic diarrhea of infancy: nonbeta islet cell hyperplasia. *Pediatrics 64*:46, 1979.

F. Miscellaneous causes of diarrhea
   1. Gastrointestinal hemorrhage (see page 342)
   2. Acute appendicitis with pelvic position of the appendix
   3. Acute peritonitis. Diarrhea may occur early.
   3. Laxatives, cathartics or high sulfate content of well water (over 400 mg. of sulfate per liter) given to infants.

Chien, L., Robertson, H. and Gerrard, J.W.: Infantile gastroenteritis due to water with high sulfate content. *Can. Med. Assoc. J. 99*:102, 1968.

   5. Diffuse familial polyposis of the colon. Loose stools with or without mucus and blood are present in the majority of patients. Polyps may be palpable on rectal examination.

6. Protein-losing enteropathy may be characterized by diarrhea as well as marked hypoproteinemia and edema. Because of this diagnostic possibility, serum protein electrophoresis may be indicated as part of the work-up of patients with chronic diarrhea.
7. Dietetic candies containing sorbitol when eaten in large quantities may cause diarrhea because of the osmotic effect of the sugar.

Gryboski, J.D.: Diarrhea from dietetic candies. *N. Engl. J. Med. 275*:718, 1966.

8. Foreign body in the intestine or rectum.
9. Hirschsprung's disease. Enterocolitis with the acute onset of diarrhea, vomiting, abdominal distention, lethargy, fever and dehydration at two or three weeks of age is a life-threatening complication. Massive dilatation of the colon may occur.
10. Rectal stenosis. Fluid stools may occur around a fecal impaction.
11. Starvation stools may be watery, greenish and mucoid.
12. Ulcerative colitis. Unexplained, intermittent, mucoid diarrhea may precede by weeks or months the appearance of mucus, pus and blood in the stools. The onset may be sudden or insidious. In the latter event, the first symptom is an increased number of bowel movements. At times, rectal bleeding is the initial symptom. When involvement is localized chiefly to the rectum and rectosigmoid, blood, pus and mucus may be noted in the stools. In such cases, the bowel movements may be of normal consistency or even constipated. Blood on the stools in the absence of diarrhea may be the first symptom of ulcerative colitis. In severe ulcerative colitis, the patient has more than six diarrheal stools a day. Anemia may be due to the considerable blood loss experienced and to the inflammation. Fever and weight loss are common. Extraintestinal complications include arthritis, erythema nodosum, pyoderma gangrenosum, aphthous ulcers in the mouth, growth retardation and delayed puberty. Crohn's disease involving the colon is a differential consideration. Abdominal cramps and tenderness may also be present. The sense of urgency and tenesmus may be severe and the patient may be awakened several times a night to have a bowel movement.

Ament, M.E.: Inflammatory disease of the colon: ulcerative colitis and Crohn's colitis. *J. Pediatr. 86*:322, 1975.
Michener, W.M.: Ulcerative colitis in children. *Pediatr. Clin. N. Am. 14*:159, 1967.

13. Crohn's disease (regional enteritis) may be characterized by chronic, persistent diarrhea. Cramping abdominal pain, loss of weight and fever may also be present. Initial symptoms, appearing before diarrhea, may include growth failure, delayed puberty and fever of undetermined origin. Perianal disease with anal fissures and fistulae may also be a presenting finding.
14. Constipation with fecal retention may be accompanied by so-called paradoxical diarrhea, with involuntary passage of liquid stool around the hard fecal mass in the rectum.
15. Pseudomembranous colitis due to staphylococcal enterocolitis is a rare but serious disorder in children. Symptoms and findings include fever, vomiting, diarrhea, distended abdomen, abdominal tenderness, dehydration and possibly shock. A pseudomembrane is noted on endoscopic examination.

Prince, A.S. and Neu, H.C.: Antibiotic-associated pseudomembranous colitis in children. *Pediatr. Clin. N. Am.* 26:261, 1979.

G. Psychogenic diarrhea
   1. Fear or anxiety
   2. Encopresis (see page 320)
   3. Chronic diarrhea in young children may be etiologically related to emotional turmoil and conflict in the family. In such instances, the periods of diarrhea parallel times of increased emotional tension and discord in the family. On admission of the patient to the hospital, this type of chronic or recurrent diarrhea dramatically ceases.
H. Irritable colon syndrome or chronic nonspecific diarrhea is characterized by persistent or recurrent diarrhea in children between the ages of six months and four years. Three to ten stools are passed each day with the early morning stool formed and the others small and containing mucus and vegetable fibers. The cause is unknown. Emotional factors, respiratory tract infections and allergic reactions may be contributory. Stool cultures should be obtained to rule out a salmonella infection.

Davidson, M. and Wasserman, R.: The irritable colon of childhood (chronic nonspecific diarrhea syndrome). *J. Pediatr.* 69:1027, 1966.

## COMPLICATIONS OF ACUTE DIARRHEA

I. Dehydration manifested by:
   A. Visible dryness of the tongue and mucous membranes; stringy oral secretions
   B. Sunken anterior fontanel
   C. Reduced tissue turgor determined by pinching up the skin of the abdominal wall between the thumb and index finger. If the fold persists for several seconds after release, significant dehydration is present. Tissue turgor is also poor in malnourished infants owing to loss of subcutaneous fat.
   D. Weight loss. In acute illnesses, weight loss is chiefly due to dehydration. Fluid loss can be calculated almost directly from the weight loss. For example, a baby who has acutely lost 1 pound has an accumulated fluid deficit of approximately 450 ml.
   E. Fever
   F. Reduced frequency of urination
   G. Dark urine

Finberg, L.: The management of the critically ill child with dehydration secondary to diarrhea. *Pediatrics* 45:1029, 1970.
Weil, W.B., Jr. and Bailie, M.D.: *Fluid and Electrolyte Metabolism in Infants and Children.* New York, Grune and Stratton, 1978.

II. Shock
III. Hypokalemia
IV. Hypernatremia and hyperosmolarity. Hypertonic dehydration usually occurs in infants under the age of one year with gastroenteritis. There is often a history of refusal of fluids for many hours or a few days. Some patients have

received oral electrolyte solutions. An occasional patient has concomitant renal disease. The infant may not appear dehydrated. Tissue turgor may be fair, but the skin often feels doughy or velvety. High fever may be present. Signs of central nervous system dysfunction include unusual irritability or lethargy, hypertonicity, meningismus, convulsions, stupor and coma.

Finberg, L.: Hypernatremic (hypertonic) dehydration in infants. *N. Engl. J. Med. 289*:196, 1973.

  V. Bacteremia. The younger the patient, the greater the hazard of bacteremia.
  VI. Pyogenic arthritis
  VII. Peritonitis
VIII. Pneumonia
  IX. Pyelonephritis
  X. Meningitis
  XI. Encephalopathy
    A. Thrombosis of cortical veins
    B. Hypernatremia
  XII. Phlebothrombosis
    A. Thrombosis of the large cortical veins or dural sinuses in severely dehydrated infants and children may cause convulsive seizures, coma and paresis.
    B. Thrombosis of the renal veins may be followed by sudden enlargement of one or both kidneys, shock, hematuria and azotemia. Symptoms may be minimal, however, and the urinary findings attributed to the primary dehydration. Bilateral renal vein thrombosis may result in the nephrotic syndrome.
    C. Renal artery thrombosis followed by oliguria, anuria, hematuria, albuminuria, casts and azotemia.
  XIII. Perianal excoriation results from maceration and tryptic digestion of the perianal skin. This complication is especially noted in disaccharidase deficiency.
  XIV. Anal prolapse
  XV. Intussusception may occur during the course of severe diarrhea. The diagnosis may be overlooked if the abdominal pain and blood in the stools are attributed to dysentery.

## GENERAL REFERENCES

Gall, D.G. and Hamilton, J.R.: Chronic diarrhea in childhood. *Pediatr. Clin. N. Am. 21*:1001, 1974.
Gryboski, J.D. (ed.): *Gastrointestinal Problems in Infants*. Philadelphia, W. B. Saunders Co., 1975.
Gryboski, J.D.: Chronic diarrhea. *Cur. Prob. Pediatr. 9*:3, 1979.
Poley, J.R.: Chronic diarrhea in infants and children. Parts I and II. *South. Med. J. 66*:1035, 1133, 1973.
Roy, C.C., Silverman, A. and Cozzetto, F.J.: *Pediatric Clinical Gastroenterology*. 2nd ed. St. Louis, C. V. Mosby Co., 1975.

## ETIOLOGIC CLASSIFICATION OF DIARRHEA BY AGE PERIODS

I. The newborn infant, 300
  A. Overfeeding, 300
  B. Viral diarrhea, 301
  C. Necrotizing enterocolitis, 301
  D. Bacterial diarrhea, 301
    1. E. coli
    2. Salmonella
  E. Parenteral diarrhea, 301
  F. Dietary factors, 301
  G. Congenital enterokinase deficiency, 301
  H. Congenital alkalosis with diarrhea, 301
II. Older infants and children, 301
  A. Infections, 301
    1. Parenteral diarrhea
    2. Acute gastroenteritis syndrome
    3. Infectious hepatitis
    4. Bacterial diarrhea
    5. Protozoan diarrhea
    6. Parasitic diarrhea
    7. Fungal diarrhea
  B. Malabsorption syndromes, 304
    1. Celiac disease
    2. Cystic fibrosis
    3. Pancreatic enzyme deficiency
    4. Short bowel syndrome
    5. Other causes of steatorrhea
    6. Parasites
    7. Abetalipoproteinemia
    8. Primary immunodeficiency
    9. Intestinal lymphangiectasis
    10. Carbohydrate malabsorption
  C. Gastrointestinal allergy, 308
  D. Antibiotic diarrhea, 308

  E. Endocrine and metabolic diarrhea, 308
    1. Hyperthyroidism
    2. Uremia
    3. Nephrosis
    4. Cystinosis
    5. Hereditary tyrosinemia
    6. Wolman's disease
    7. Ganglioneuroma or ganglioneuroblastoma
    8. Zollinger-Ellison syndrome
    9. Nonbeta islet cell hyperplasia
  F. Miscellaneous causes, 308
    1. Gastrointestinal hemorrhage
    2. Acute appendicitis
    3. Acute peritonitis
    4. Laxatives, cathartics or high sulfate content of well water
    5. Diffuse familial polyposis of colon
    6. Protein-losing enteropathy
    7. Dietetic candy with sorbitol
    8. Foreign body in intestine or rectum
    9. Hirschsprung's disease
    10. Rectal stenosis
    11. Starvation
    12. Ulcerative colitis
    13. Crohn's disease
    14. Constipation with fecal retention
    15. Pseudomembranous colitis
  G. Psychogenic diarrhea, 310
    1. Fear or anxiety
    2. Encopresis
    3. Familial turmoil or conflict
  H. Irritable colon syndrome, 310

CHAPTER **33**

# CONSTIPATION

Constipation refers to difficulty in defecating. The stools may be normal, large cylindrical masses or hard, dry pellets. The bowel movements are characteristically infrequent; however, a few pellets may be passed several times a day. In the presence of a fecal impaction the stools may become fluid (paradoxical diarrhea). The symptoms of constipation include mild anorexia, tenesmus, straining and abdominal pain. Pain on defecating is frequent. The stools may be streaked with bright red blood as a result of mucosal injury. Anal fissures are common, and anal or rectal prolapse may occur in debilitated patients. Fecal material is often palpable in the lower abdomen as firm, irregular, cylindrical masses that indent on pressure.

## NORMAL STOOLS

*Meconium stools* are greenish-black, odorless, thick and sticky. Four or five are passed each day during the first three to four days of life. Delay in passage of meconium stools in the first day of life may be due to Hirschsprung's disease, intestinal obstruction, meconium plug, hypothyroidism, sepsis with adynamic ileus or maternal addiction.

*Transitional stools* are mixed, greenish-brown, thin and slimy, and may contain milk curds. Four to eight stools are passed per day between the fourth and seventh days of life.

The number of stools passed by normal infants during the first week of life gradually increases to reach a peak usually on the fifth day. A relation exists between the number of stools and the infant's total food intake. During any one day a small number of normal newborns have no bowel movements; on the other hand, a few babies pass as many as 12 to 14 stools. The diagnosis of constipation or diarrhea in this age period, therefore, is not based on the frequency of stools alone but is also based on their nature and on other clinical findings. Since mothers are frequently concerned about the number of stools their babies pass, it is usually well to inform them as to what to expect in the first week of life.

*Milk stools* are passed after the first week of life. *Breast-fed* babies have homogeneous, pasty, mushy (like cream soup), slightly sour-smelling, light yellow stools that cling to or sink into the diaper. One to eight are passed each day, and many babies have a stool after each feeding. The average is two to four a day. Faintly green stools containing a small amount of mucus are seen occasionally. An infant is rarely, if ever, constipated while exclusively on a breast milk diet. Babies fed on *cow milk* have putty-like, firm, pale yellow stools that do not cling to the diaper. One to four are passed each day, with an average of one or two. The presence of tough curds may give the stool a scrambled-egg appearance. Milk stools turn green or brown on exposure to air.

The frequency of stools usually decreases between one and three months of age in both breast- and bottle-fed infants. A few normal babies may then have stools as infrequently as every second or third day. By one year of age the majority of infants have only one stool a day, but individual infants may have more or fewer.

When chopped foods are first added to a baby's diet, they may appear in the stool almost unchanged. Visible mucus is often present in the stools of babies during respiratory infections. A light-colored, seemingly acholic stool may occasionally be passed in normal infants and children, usually in relation to a respiratory infection.

In some children seen because of constipation, the parents report that the stools are so large that they plug up the toilet. This history is not specific for Hirschsprung's disease or pathognomonic for any other etiology.

## PHYSIOLOGY OF DEFECATION

In the first year of life, defecation is primarily a reflex act. Mass peristaltic movements initiated by fecal bulk traverse the entire colon (unless the myenteric plexus is not intact). These movements are influenced by parasympathetic (excitatory) and sympathetic (inhibitory) impulses. When the rectum becomes distended with feces, afferent fibers conduct impulses to the "defecation center" in the second, third and fourth sacral segments of the spinal cord. Motor impulses from this area then cause relaxation of the internal anal sphincter. This sphincter is also subject to parasympathetic inhibition and sympathetic excitation. The afferent impulses that ascend the spinal cord also cause contraction of the voluntary muscles of defecation. Closure of the glottis and contraction of the diaphragmatic and abdominal muscles lead to an increase in the intra-abdominal and intrarectal pressures. Dilatation of the external anal sphincter occurs reflexly. The levator ani muscles contract and lift the anus over the fecal mass.

During the first year of life, each mass peristaltic movement is followed by the passage of a stool, since defecation is not voluntarily inhibited. The defecation reflex normally prevents an excessive accumulation or desiccation of feces. In the second year of life and thereafter, voluntary cortical control of defecation is possible through the willful contraction or relaxation of the external anal sphincter (striated muscle). In older children, the number of stools normally passed a day varies with the child. Most children have one bowel movement a day; some have two a day; still others have a stool every other day or even less frequently without symptoms.

**Bowel Training.** There is a cultural concern with gastrointestinal function. Bowel training is still, at times, compulsively undertaken. Many parents have been conditioned to the concept that it is essential for the child to have one bowel movement a day. A premium is often placed on early cleanliness. These attitudes ignore the natural frequency of the stools and the level of neuromuscular development as an indication for training. Since the passage of bowel movements often becomes a point of coercion and conflict, constipation frequently arises during the training period, especially if upsetting events such as divorce, a move or a mother's return to work occur concurrently.

1. "CATCHING" THE STOOL. After the first few months of life, the majority of babies have stools at fairly predictable times, but a few infants remain totally irregular. If the baby is regular, has an adequate sense of balance and can sit well alone, mothers sometimes attempt "catching" of the stool. Catching does not constitute training of the baby, and defecation continues to be a reflex activity without a voluntary component. The baby does not have the cortical development to understand what is desired of him, does not associate words with the act and does not have the neuromuscular development to inhibit his defecation reflex. At best, catching the stool is an aid for the mother to avoid cleaning diapers. If it is successful, a mother may feel that she has trained the baby. When the baby begins to walk, however, the stools are often passed more irregularly and, therefore, become difficult to catch. Mothers who have prided themselves on early training may then find that all semblance of it has disappeared.

2. CHOICE OF A POTTY. The potty seat should facilitate defecation and prevent fear. This is possible if the following requirements are met: a seat small enough to support the ischial tuberosities, an adequate back and arm rest and a firm foot rest. Although a potty seat that can be placed on the floor would seem the most desirable type, the psychologic advantage of identification by the child with other members of the family has made the use of a potty seat attached to the adult seat seem more advantageous. Because of the fear of falling, the parent should remain with the child if the adult toilet is used. As the child grows older, small stairs to the adult toilet should be available so that he can go to the toilet as he desires.

The potty also should permit an optimal position for defecation. The infant must be able to lean forward with the thighs partially flexed on the abdomen, the feet firmly planted on the floor or a foot rest and the ischial tuberosities adequately supported. This position permits a fulcrum action of the levator ani muscles and places the accessory muscles of defecation at a mechanical advantage.

3. TRAINING TECHNIQUES. The use of the toilet is a habit that need not be "trained into" a child. Bowel control is a complicated function that requires a relatively advanced degree of neuromuscular, social and emotional development. The baby must wish to please his mother by controlling bowel function. He must be aware that a movement is coming, be able to withhold it through cortical inhibition, understand what is expected of him when he is placed on the potty and be able to verbalize his need to defecate in some manner. These capacities develop slowly and cannot be accelerated by external pressure. They are seldom present before the second year of life. Parents often have the erroneous idea, however, that bowel training requires an all-out effort on their part. Actually, little training is necessary. Children in permissive societies learn bowel control by imitation and are often spontaneously trained by the age of two years.

Training can be delayed advantageously until the infant is proficient at walking because until that time bowel movements are apt to be irregular as the new skill is being integrated and because it is difficult for the child to acquire multiple skills simultaneously. Usually, walking has been mastered by 14 to 15 months of age, and training can be started then. If the baby has regular movements, he can be placed on the potty at the expected usual time. If he is irregular, the mother should wait until he grunts or strains or otherwise indicates the coming of the stool. He should not be placed on the potty at a predetermined time and given a suppository to induce a stool. The mother should use the same word for defecation each time. Ten minutes is usually sufficient for a sitting, and a baby may be removed from the potty sooner if he is resistant. Attempts at training may be stopped temporarily if resistance develops, and attempts may be temporarily abandoned when the baby is tired or ill. Lapses in training are frequent throughout the second year and are especially apt to occur during periods of integration of new skills or emotional disturbance.

Brazelton, T.B.: A child-oriented approach to toilet training. *Pediatrics 29*:121, 1962.

4. RESISTANCE TO TRAINING often develops at some point. It usually has an emotional basis and may be managed by a reduced emphasis on the training process. Early in the course of training, an infant may not use his word for defecation until after a movement has occurred. This indicates that the baby is learning to connect the word with the act and is an essential feature of training. It does not represent resistance or cause for discouragement. A baby in the second year may have a bowel movement after he has been removed from the potty and dressed. This sometimes indicates resistance and often correlates with negativism in other aspects of personal-social behavior; on the other hand, it may be interpreted to the mother as an encouraging sign (i.e., that the child has just about mastered this complicated business and will likely soon be successful). This is usually transient and should not become a matter of undue concern. If all goes well, the child usually manages his clothes and goes to the toilet himself by two or three years of age. Lapses, however, may still occur in the third year. The causes for true resistance to training include the following:

a. *Fear.* Resistance to training may be due to fear. The baby may be afraid of the potty because he has had painful stools there. He may have a fear of falling from the adult toilet. Occasionally, he fears the flushing of the toilet after defecation. Because the baby cannot verbalize these fears, they usually appear as resistance to training.

b. *Maternal disgust.* A baby frequently has pride in his stool. He may admire it and even call his mother from another room to see it. Sometimes, he may play with it. In contrast to this, his mother may disgustedly flush the stool down the toilet and react with revulsion when she discovers a stool in his pants or finds him playing with it.

c. *Disturbed mother-child relations.* During training, the infant learns that the passage of his stool on the potty pleases his mother. He also learns that he can withhold or pass it at will. From this time on he can either give up his stools for the approval of his mother or he can withhold them. Punishment, unpleasantness and coercion in bowel training may elicit reactive withholding of the stool and resistance to training.

## ETIOLOGIC CLASSIFICATION OF CONSTIPATION AND INFREQUENT STOOLS

I. Interference with mass peristaltic movements of the colon
  A. Reflex mechanisms of mass peristalsis anatomically intact
    1. Lack of fecal bulk causes an inadequate stimulus to mass peristaltic movements.
      a. Anorexia, underfeeding, vomiting and starvation
      b. Lack of roughage in the diet
        (1) Continued use of pureed foods after 10 to 12 months of age
        (2) Preponderance of highly refined starches in the diet
        (3) High protein diet. Protein is almost completely digested and absorbed, leaving little residue.
      c. Enemas, laxatives and suppositories empty the colon and remove the stimulus to peristalsis for two to three days. Diarrhea is usually followed by infrequent stools for several days.
    2. Hard stools interfere with the effectiveness of mass peristaltic movements.
      a. Cow milk stools
        (1) Substitution of a supplemental bottle of cow milk for one of the breast feedings may cause solidification of the stools and a decrease in frequency.
        (2) Excessive cow milk intake. Occasionally, infants refuse solid foods in the latter half of the first year of life and satisfy their caloric needs by an excessive intake of cow milk — as much as 2 quarts a day. The high calcium content of this diet leads to the formation of calcium caseinate and soaps in the stools. These substances supply bulk but do not stimulate peristalsis.
      c. Desiccated stools
        (1) Dehydration and fever cause dessication of the stools by diminishing intestinal secretions and increasing water absorption from the colon. A transient period of constipation is common during acute febrile illnesses. In hot weather, babies may be constipated if not

offered sufficient water. The stools may be desiccated in patients with infantile renal acidosis, diabetes insipidus or idiopathic hypercalcemia.

    (2) Withholding the stool. The longer a stool is withheld, the more water is reabsorbed in the rectum.

3. Mechanical obstruction blocks the fecal stream and interferes with the progress of a mass peristalic movement. Obstipation or intractable constipation may occur.

    a. Intestinal atresia

    b. Imperforate anus. Constipation may be the presenting complaint in infants with an imperforate anus and rectoperineal fistula.

    c. Meconium ileus

Donnison, A.B., Schwachman, H. and Gross, R.E.: A review of 164 children with meconium ileus seen at the Children's Hospital Medical Center, Boston. *Pediatrics 37*:833, 1966.

    d. Meconium-ileus equivalent (kiotileus) refers to the intestinal obstruction that occasionally occurs in older children with cystic fibrosis. Firm, rubbery masses of stool are palpable on abdominal examination.

    e. An inspissated meconium plug in the lower colon in the newborn infant may cause intestinal obstruction and failure to pass meconium. The signs and symptoms include those of intestinal obstruction with abdominal distention, vomiting that may be bilious and intestinal patterning. Roentgenographic examination, other than being compatible with low intestinal obstruction, does not differentiate meconium ileus, small intestinal atresia or Hirschsprung's disease from the meconium plug syndrome. The barium enema, which reveals a normal-caliber colon, is both diagnostic and often therapeutic. Cystic fibrosis and Hirschsprung's disease are among the disorders associated with the meconium plug syndrome.

Ellis, D.G. and Clatworthy, H.W., Jr.: The meconium plug syndrome revisited. *J. Pediatr. Surg. 1*:54, 1966.

Mikity, V.G., Hodgman, J.E. and Paciulli, J.: Meconium blockage syndrome. *Radiology 88*:740, 1967.

    f. Intestinal stenosis, especially rectosigmoidal and anal

    g. Malrotation of the bowel

    h. Volvulus

    i. Duplication of the alimentary tract, especially of the rectum

    j. Incarcerated hernia

    k. Intussusception

    l. Congenital or acquired adhesive peritoneal bands

4. Paralytic ileus

    a. Peritonitis

    b. Postoperative ileus

    c. Reflux ileus associated with pneumonitis or other acute illness

    d. Severe hypokalemia

B. Anatomically defective reflex mechanisms of mass peristalsis. Aganglionic megacolon or Hirschsprung's disease is due to a segmental absence of parasympathetic ganglion cells in the myenteric plexus. The affected segment usually begins at or near the anus and extends proximally some 5 to 20 cm. Occasionally, the defect may involve the entire colon and part of the ileum. The absence of ganglion cells interferes with normal mass peristalsis and causes a functional obstruction. The bowel above the site of functional obstruction becomes dilated and hypertrophied. In contrast to other types of megacolon, dilatation of the colon almost never extends to the anus in these patients.

Symptoms may begin at birth or the first day of life with delayed passage of meconium and abdominal distention. Most normal infants pass meconium in the first 24 hours. In other instances, evidence of intestinal obstruction does not appear until a few days later. Some newborn infants demonstrate severe obstipation, while others have intermittent episodes of constipation, abdominal distention and vomiting. Hirschsprung's disease is not an uncommon cause of acute intestinal obstruction in the newborn.

Rectal examination reveals a normal anal sphincter, a well-formed anal canal and a small, empty rectal ampulla. That the baby evacuates the colon on rectal examination does not rule out aganglionic megacolon. Roentgenographic examination with a lateral view demonstrates a low intestinal obstruction and a small, air-containing rectum. The diagnosis may be confirmed by barium examination without prior preparation of the colon. With the patient in the oblique or lateral position, a small amount of barium is allowed to run slowly into the rectum. An excessive amount overdistends the rectum and obliterates the diagnostic findings. In patients with aganglionic megacolon, a narrowed, irregular segment of the rectum is visualized. Turbulent and purposeless peristalsis may also appear. The bowel proximal to the narrowed segment, usually at the junction of the rectum and sigmoid, is usually dilated and redundant.

Accurate diagnosis of Hirschsprung's disease may be difficult in newborn infants and during the first several months of life. The barium enema does not always demonstrate the classic findings as seen in older patients, since dilatation and hypertrophy of the proximal colon may not yet have developed. Such infants will have a normal sized colon but may demonstrate delayed evacuation of the barium. X-rays, especially lateral views, should, therefore, be repeated in 24 and 48 hours. Normal infants usually pass the barium in 24 hours, but, in Hirschsprung's disease, the barium is retained and mixed with fecal material. Rectal biopsy is diagnostic in equivocal cases. Not infrequently, these patients have associated anomalies in the urinary tract (e.g., a large, atonic bladder with or without megaloureters). If surgical correction is not performed early, chronic abdominal enlargement gradually develops. Enterocolitis is a major complication of Hirschsprung's disease. Clinical manifestations include massive dilatation of the colon, diarrhea, vomiting, fever, dehydration and lethargy.

Anatomic megacolon is due to a congenital anorectal stenosis or to stricture of the rectum that develops after surgical correction of an imperforate anus. Rarely, intrinsic or extrinsic tumors may cause a megacolon. Anatomic megacolon can be diagnosed by history and by digital examination of the rectum. The onset of symptoms is usually gradual, and the time of onset depends upon the degree of obstruction. A few patients with fecal impaction and soiling have a short area of achalasia proximal to the anus demonstrable by motility studies.

II. Interference with the spinal arc

A. Voluntary inhibition of defecation may cause disappearance of the stimulus to defecate. The stool may then become desiccated and its passage accompanied by pain. This, in turn, may cause further inhibition of defecation.

1. Children may be too busy to take time from their play.
2. The school child may be afraid of being late for school if he stops to defecate. At school, he may be embarrassed to ask permission to leave the room.
3. Hospitalized infants or young children may not be able to make their need to defecate known to the staff.
4. After the age of four years or so, a child may desire privacy when he uses the toilet.
5. Travelling disrupts routines. The child may feel anxious or insecure when away from familiar surroundings, or a toilet may be inaccessible to him. Some children experience difficulty in using a toilet away from home.

B. Excessive use of suppositories, laxatives and enemas. These agents empty the colon so that stools are infrequent for two to three days. This may create the false impression that constipation has recurred or is still present. In patients who receive laxatives over a prolonged period of time, the bowel becomes insensitive to its own physiologic reflexes and dependent on the artificial agents.

C. Spinal cord lesions. Interruption of the spinal cord above the defecation center in the second, third and fourth sacral segments causes a loss of voluntary control. Defecation then reverts to a reflex act with the rectum emptying automatically with each mass peristaltic movement of the colon. Destruction of the cord at the defecation center causes the loss of all rectal sensation and relaxation of the external anal sphincter. This results in incontinence rather than automaticity. Fecal impaction frequently occurs in patients with either type of spinal cord lesion. It is rare for a neurologic lesion to produce fecal incontinence without a disturbance in bladder control.

Rectal continence is sustained through the actions of the internal sphincter, which is under reflex control, and of the striated muscle external sphincter, which is under both reflex and voluntary control. Rectal incontinence occurs only when the somatic innervation of the external sphincter has been impaired. In such instances, a full rectum produces reflex relaxation of the internal sphincter. Without adequate voluntary and reflex action of the external sphincter, incontinence results.

White, J.J. et al.: A physiologic rationale for the management of neurologic rectal incontinence in children. *Pediatrics* 49:888, 1972.

1. Transection of the spinal cord
2. Meningomyelocele
3. Spina bifida occulta associated with myelodysplasia
4. Diastematomyelia is characterized by difficulty in walking. Dribbling of

        urine and fecal incontinence are frequent associated findings. Fecal impaction may occur.

    5. Neoplasms

III. Interference with relaxation of the anal sphincters

    A. Anal fissures are one of the most frequent causes of constipation in early infancy. A bowel movement may not occur for several days, and the stools are apt to be hard and streaked with bright red blood. The infant may be irritable and cry excessively, especially before and after passage of a bowel movement. The majority of fissures can be visualized with the infant in a knee-chest position and the buttocks spread to reveal the mucocutaneous junction of the anus. Early lesions have the appearance of superficial erosions. More advanced lesions are seen as linear or elliptical breaks in the skin. Long-standing fissures are deep and indurated. In the presence of a suggestive history, rectal examination may be performed when a fissure is not visualized. Internal fissures are often visible through the relaxed anal sphincter as the examining finger is withdrawn.

        Fissures involuntarily inhibit defecation by producing spasm of the external anal sphincter. This results in desiccation of the stools. The cycle becomes self-perpetuating since the passage of hard stools traumatizes the mucosa and prevents healing of the fissure. Anal fissures occasionally occur in patients with anal stenosis. They may also occur in older children with pinworms as a result of perianal scratching.

    B. Anal stenosis

      1. Congenital anal stenosis is a common cause of constipation in young infants. Anal fissures are often also present.

      2. Acquired stricture may be a complication of surgery for imperforate anus.

IV. Interference with contraction of the voluntary muscles of defecation

    A. Congenital deficiency or complete absence of the abdominal musculature is characterized by a protuberant and often asymmetrically shaped abdomen. Constipation is always a problem. The bladder may be enlarged, and hydroureter and hydronephrosis are usually present.

    B. Floppy infant syndrome

    C. Cerebral palsy

    D. Poliomyelitis

    E. Guillain-Barré syndrome

    F. Postdiphtheritic paralysis

    G. Rickets may be accompanied by flabby, weak, abdominal musculature.

    H. Anemia may be associated with flabby, weak, hypotonic musculature.

    I. Constipation in infants and children with hypothyroidism is due to hypotonia of the abdominal and intestinal musculature. Constipation may be an early symptom in congenital hypothyroidism.

    J. Infantile botulism may initially cause constipation. Later findings include poor cry, weak suck, dysphagia and loss of head control.

V. Interference with autonomic and cortical control of defecation.

    A. Irritable colon

    B. Encopresis with functional megacolon secondary to chronic constipation is characterized by repeated fecal soiling owing to the involuntary passage of small amounts of feces into the underpants of a child over four years of age in the absence of neurologic or other anatomic factors. Fecal soiling of the underclothing with soft fluid stool is an almost constant finding. The child with encopresis often seems unaware of his odor. Periodically, voluminous stools are passed spontaneously. Rectal examination reveals a large rectal vault packed with feces that may be surprisingly soft in many cases but often firm or hard. Constipation is usually long-standing so that enormous amounts of stool may be found on physical or plain x-ray examination of the abdomen. Some children are found to have only rectal retention with a megarectum rather than a megacolon.

The child who has encopresis without constipation usually has major psychopathology. The severe constipation in children with encopresis may be due to painful defecation secondary to an anal fissure, coercive bowel training, fear of the toilet, or reactive voluntary withholding of bowel movements. The accumulated fecal mass causes distention of the rectum. Sensory receptors in the rectal wall and puborectalis muscle then lead reflexly to relaxation of the internal sphincter. With subsequent relaxation of the levator ani and shortening of the anal canal, the external sphincter relaxes and encopresis occurs.

Colicky abdominal pain is frequent. Abdominal distention is less prominent than with aganglionic megacolon and is usually minimal, even after several years. When emotional factors are prominent, children with encopresis may refuse to use the toilet. Rather, they hold their lower extremities tightly together and strain in an apparent attempt to withhold the stool.

An intravenous pyelogram should be obtained in patients with chronic fecal impaction because secondary hydronephrosis and vesicoureteral reflux are often present.

Bellman, M.: Studies on encopresis. *Acta Pediatr. Scand. Suppl.* 170, 1966.
Levine, M.D. and Bakow, H.: Children with encopresis: a study of treatment outcome. *Pediatrics 58*:845, 1976.

## GENERAL REFERENCES

Davidson, M.: Constipation. In Green, M. and Haggerty, R.J. (eds.): *Ambulatory Pediatrics*. 1st ed. Philadelphia, W. B. Saunders Co., 1968.
Davidson, M., Kugler, M.M. and Bauer, C.H.: Diagnosis and management in children with severe and protracted constipation and obstipation. *J. Pediatr. 62*:261, 1963.
Fitzgerald, J.F.: Constipation. In Green, M. and Haggerty, R.J. (eds.): *Ambulatory Pediatrics II*. Philadelphia, W. B. Saunders Co., 1977, p. 118.
Fitzgerald, J.F.: Encopresis. In Green, M. and Haggerty, R.J. (eds.): *Ambulatory Pediatrics II*. Philadelphia, W. B. Saunders Co., 1977, p. 121.

## ETIOLOGIC CLASSIFICATION OF CONSTIPATION AND INFREQUENT STOOLS

CHAPTER 34

# DYSPHAGIA

Dysphagia may be defined as difficulty in swallowing, characterized variously by choking, return of fluids and food through the nose, hesitation in swallowing, pain during deglutition, retrosternal discomfort and regurgitation with aspiration of food. Cineradiography may be a helpful tool in the study of selected patients, particularly those thought to have a neuromuscular disorder. In other cases, direct endoscopy is indicated.

## ETIOLOGIC CLASSIFICATION OF DYSPHAGIA

I. Anatomic
    A. Congenital malformations
        1. Cleft palate
        2. Macroglossia
        3. Micrognathia
        4. Intrinsic esophageal lesions (e.g., atresia, stenosis, webs). With an H-type tracheoesophageal fistula, severe choking and coughing may follow feeding.
    B. Acquired malformations
        1. Esophageal stenosis may occur postoperatively in infants with esophageal atresia and tracheoesophageal fistula.
        2. Esophagitis secondary to gastroesophageal reflux or hiatus hernia may cause marked dysphagia.

Christie, D.L., O'Grady, L.R. and Mack, D.: Incompetent lower esophageal sphincter and gastroesophageal reflux in recurrent acute pulmonary disease of infancy and childhood. *J. Pediatr. 93*:23, 1978.

3. Esophageal involvement may occur with scleroderma or lupus erythematosus.
4. Alkali burns of the esophagus

Girdany, B.R.: The esophagus in infancy: congenital and acquired diseases. *Radiol. Clin. N. Am. 1*:557, 1963.

C. Encroachment; compression; displacement
   1. Enlarged tonsils
   2. Cardiac enlargement
   3. Vascular ring
   4. Mediastinal tumors
   5. Retropharyngeal abscess
   6. Goiter, Hashimoto's thyroiditis
D. Inflammatory lesions
   1. Herpetic gingivostomatitis
   2. Thrush
   3. Peritonsillar abscess
   4. Pharyngitis
   5. Epiglottitis

II. Neuromuscular
A. Brain damage; intellectual retardation; cerebral palsy. Difficulty in sucking and swallowing may be the first indication of maldevelopment of or damage to the central nervous system. The mother may report that the baby requires more than an hour to take one ounce of milk or that he does not seem to know how to suck or use his tongue.
B. Infants with hypothyroidism may feed poorly and have difficulty in sucking and swallowing.
C. Floppy infant syndrome. Infants with generalized hypotonia may have difficulty in feeding.
D. Pharyngeal paralysis
   1. Evidence of difficulty in swallowing is an early sign of bulbar poliomyelitis.
   2. Postdiphtheritic paralysis; tick paralysis; Guillain-Barré syndrome
   3. Isolated palatal paralysis may become manifest soon after birth with regurgitation of liquids through the nose while feeding.
   4. Botulism produces dysphagia along with constipation, diplopia, photophobia, blurring of vision and generalized weakness occurring 18 to 36 hours after ingestion of the toxin.

Johnson, R.O., Clay, S.A. and Arnon, S.S.: Diagnosis and management of infant botulism. *Am. J. Dis. Child. 133*:586, 1979.

   5. Pseudobulbar or suprabulbar paresis due to involvement of nerve tracts from the cortical motor areas for the lips, palate and tongue to the medullary motor nuclei. Clinical manifestations result from weakness and/or spasticity of the lips, tongue, palate and pharyngeal muscles. A jaw jerk is present.
   6. Congenital absence of cranial nerve nuclei
   7. Möbius's syndrome may cause dysphagia in infants
E. Pharyngeal or cricopharyngeal incoordination

Utian, H.L. and Thomas, R.G.: Cricopharyngeal incoordination in infancy. *Pediatrics* *43*:402, 1969.

    F. Congenital myotonic dystrophy may be characterized by difficulties in sucking and swallowing.

    G. Pontine glioma

    H. The infantile form of Gaucher's disease may be characterized by dysphagia and laryngospasm.

    I. Familial dysautonomia. These patients often have difficulty in swallowing and appear to aspirate food.

    J. Rabies is characterized by spasms of the pharynx and larynx when attempts are made to swallow liquids or solids.

    K. Phenothiazine toxicity

    L. Lesch-Nyhan syndrome may cause athetoid dysphagia.

    M. Myasthenia gravis may be characterized by dysphagia and by difficulty in chewing due to weakness of the jaw muscles. Regurgitation may occur through the nose.

    N. Subacute necrotizing encephalomyelopathy (Leigh's syndrome), which has its onset in infancy, may be characterized by dysphagia as well as other signs of brainstem dysfunction.

III. Psychologic and functional disturbances

    A. Globus hystericus associated with spasm of the upper pharyngeal constrictors is characterized by a "lump" in the throat, difficulty in swallowing and, at times, by retrosternal discomfort.

    B. A type of pseudodysphagia may occur in which a child refuses to chew foods that are chopped and restricts his diet to those that are pureed. Other children hold food in their mouths creating a "chipmunk' appearance with their distended cheeks. If the child is not retarded, this usually reflects problems in the mother-child relationship.

    C. Cardiospasm occasionally occurs in older children and adolescents. Early, dysphagia for solid foods is recurrent and transient. There may be only a brief delay in swallowing. Later, dysphagia is constant and undigested food is regurgitated. The patient may complain of vague discomfort or pressure in the lower substernal region.

IV. Foreign body lodged in the esophagus may cause dysphagia, total inability to swallow and/or pain on swallowing.

 V. Respiratory and cardiac disorders. Infants with dyspnea may have dysphagia because the act of swallowing accentuates the respiratory difficulty. Infants with hypoxia or shortness of breath may appear to have dysphagia since they require a long time to take even small feedings.

    A. Larynx

        1. Congenital laryngeal disorders such as inspiratory laryngeal collapse

        2. Epiglottitis, acute laryngotracheobronchitis

    B. Pulmonary disease

    C. Cardiac disease

## GENERAL REFERENCE

Illingworth, R.S.: Sucking and swallowing difficulties in infancy: diagnostic problem of dysphagia. *Arch. Dis. Child. 44*:655, 1969.

## ETIOLOGIC CLASSIFICATION OF DYSPHAGIA

I. Anatomic, 322
  A. Congenital malformations, 322
    1. Cleft palate
    2. Macroglossia
    3. Micrognathia
    4. Intrinsic esophageal lesions
  B. Acquired malformations, 322
    1. Esophageal stenosis
    2. Esophagitis
    3. Scleroderma or lupus erythematosus
    4. Alkali burns of esophagus
  C. Encroachment; compression; displacement, 323
    1. Enlarged tonsils
    2. Cardiac enlargement
    3. Vascular ring
    4. Mediastinal tumors
    5. Retropharyngeal abscess
    6. Goiter, Hashimoto's thyroiditis
  D. Inflammatory lesions, 323
    1. Herpetic gingivostomatitis
    2. Thrush
    3. Peritonsillar abscess
    4. Pharyngitis
    5. Epiglottitis
II. Neuromuscular, 323
  A. Brain damage, intellectual retardation, cerebral palsy, 323
  B. Hypothyroidism, 323
  C. Floppy infant syndrome, 323
  D. Pharyngeal paralysis, 323

    1. Bulbar poliomyelitis
    2. Postdiphtheritic paralysis, tick paralysis, Guillain-Barré syndrome
    3. Isolated palatal paralysis
    4. Botulism
    5. Pseudobulbar or suprabulbar paresis
    6. Congenital absence of cranial nerve nuclei
    7. Möbius's syndrome
  E. Pharyngeal or cricopharyngeal incoordination, 323
  F. Congenital myotonic dystrophy, 324
  G. Pontine glioma, 324
  H. Gaucher's disease, 324
  I. Familial dysautonomia, 324
  J. Rabies, 324
  K. Phenothiazine toxicity, 324
  L. Lesch-Nyhan syndrome, 324
  M. Myasthenia gravis, 324
  N. Subacute necrotizing encephalomyelopathy, 324
III. Psychologic and functional disturbances, 324
  A. Globus hystericus, 324
  B. Pseudodysphagia, 324
  C. Cardiospasm, 324
IV. Foreign body in esophagus, 324
V. Respiratory and cardiac disorders, 324
  A. Larynx, 324
  B. Pulmonary disease, 324
  C. Cardiac disease, 324

CHAPTER **35**

# ABDOMINAL PAIN

Abdominal pain is one of the most common and yet, at times, one of the most difficult symptoms to evaluate in infants and children. Abdominal pain may be suspected in infants in the presence of screaming or persistent crying, restlessness, irritability, squirming, grunting respirations, flexion of the thighs on the abdomen and refusal to eat.

The clinical classification of abdominal pain presented here is not based on the underlying disturbances or sensory mechanisms that produce this symptom, since these mechanisms are not completely understood.

## ETIOLOGIC CLASSIFICATION OF ABDOMINAL PAIN

I. Intra-abdominal causes
  A. Gastrointestinal tract
    1. Colic is a nonspecific symptom state occurring during the early months of life and characterized by vigorous and prolonged crying, presumably owing to intermittent abdominal pain. The episodes are sudden in onset and, in many cases, begin about the same time each day. The infant appears to be in great pain and is often inconsolable. His face becomes flushed, his abdomen distended, and his extremities drawn up against his body. Often, his crying does not diminish even though he is picked up and rocked.

      The incidence and frequency of colic appear to vary in different social groups and families, with the baby's temperament and with his manner of relieving tension. In some, colic is rarely seen or occurs only occasionally while other infants experience this discomfort almost every evening for two or three months. Many factors may be etiologic. Errors in feeding technique such as excessive air swallowing, improperly sized nipple holes, bottle-propping, failure to burp the infant and the ingestion of an excessive amount of a too-dilute formula are considerations. Underfeeding as well as overfeeding should be investigated. Gastrointestinal allergy may play a role at times. In other instances, colic may reflect tenseness in the mother and the household.

    2. Peptic ulcer in children, usually duodenal rather than gastric, is a relatively rare cause of abdominal pain, which may be periumbilical, epigastric or poorly localized. Although it may be severe and cause the child to cry, usually the pain is described as a persistent stomach ache. Episodes of pain last from a few minutes to hours. Pain is more frequent at night than during the daytime. Pain may occur in the morning before breakfast and before other meals, but there is usually no relation to meals. Pain may be relieved by milk or other food, but it also may become worse for a time after eating. At times, relief occurs after vomiting.

      Peptic ulcers in infants and children are not always accompanied by abdominal pain. In premature and very young infants, vomiting is a more prominent clinical manifestation. Recurrent or cyclic vomiting, with or without nausea, may be the chief symptom in young children. The occurrence of peptic ulcers in children with burns, head injuries, intracranial tumors, infections of the central nervous system, severe stress and steroid therapy is well known. Since hematemesis and melena may occur in children with a peptic ulcer, examination of stools for occult blood is indicated. Demonstration of an actual ulcer crater by x-ray or endoscopy is necessary for diagnosis.

Deckelbaum, R.J., Roy, C.C., Lussier-Lazaroff, J. and Morin, C.L.: Peptic ulcer disease: a clinical study in 73 children. *Can. Med. Assoc. J. 111*:225, 1974.
Rosenlund, M.L. and Koop, C.E.: Duodenal ulcer in childhood. *Pediatrics 45*:283, 1970.

    3. The Zollinger-Ellison syndrome, which consists of peptic ulceration, hypertrophy of gastric mucosa, gastric hypersecretion with increased

acidity and non-beta islet cell tumor of the pancreas, has been reported in children over seven years of age. Presenting complaints include abdominal pain, vomiting, hematemesis and melena. The ulcers usually are duodenal but may occur also in the stomach or jejunum.

Buchta, R.M. and Kaplan, J.M.: Zollinger-Ellison syndrome in a nine-year-old child: a case report and review of this entity in childhood. *Pediatrics* 47:594, 1971.

4. Dietary indiscretion, either overindulgence or the ingestion of foods not easily digested, is a common cause of acute abdominal pain in young children.

5. Appendicitis is the most common cause for abdominal surgery in childhood. While the diagnosis of appendicitis is often not difficult, it may be most challenging. The classic history begins with abdominal pain followed by nausea, vomiting and fever. With these symptoms, appendicitis is always a diagnostic consideration. Initially, the pain may be periumbilical or epigastric. Young children, of course, do not localize their complaint well. After a time, perhaps a few hours, the pain may become localized in the right lower quadrant or in the region of the umbilicus. The pain is rarely severe. It is usually constant but may be colicky or intermittent. If rupture of the appendix occurs, the child may complain less of pain for an hour or two. The pain soon returns, however, with increased intensity. The symptoms associated with abdominal pain and appendicitis in infants and very young children — irritability, restlessness, unexplained crying, refusal of feedings and vomiting — are often overlooked.

Vomiting, with or without nausea, is almost a constant feature in children with appendicitis. The diagnosis is less likely if this symptom is absent. Vomiting may occur once, twice or repeatedly. Younger children seem to vomit more often than those who are older. Fever is usually low grade and, unless a complication occurs, rarely exceeds 38.9° C. (102° F.). Bowel movements are usually normal, or constipation may be present. Diarrhea may occur if the inflamed appendix lies next to the terminal ileum or sigmoid. Diarrhea may also appear in children with early peritonitis. Appendicitis may occur as a complication of measles and in children who have an upper respiratory tract infection, enteritis or rheumatic fever.

The physical findings, discussed on pages 134 and 147, are of great importance in deciding whether or not acute appendicitis is present. If these findings have not developed when the child is first seen, repeated examinations are indicated over a period of a few hours. In this circumstance, it is usually best to hospitalize the patient unless he can be kept under close personal supervision at home.

The place of the white blood cell count, urinalysis and a chest roentgenogram in the diagnostic work-up of these patients is well known. A plain film of the abdomen may demonstrate the presence of a fecalith.

Mesenteric lymphadenopathy due to Yersinia enterocolitica may cause abdominal pain that closely resembles acute appendicitis. When a normal appendix is found in the presence of mesenteric adenitis, a node should be biopsied for culture.

Rowe, M.I.: Diagnosis and treatment: appendicitis in childhood. *Pediatrics 38*:1057, 1966.

6. Intussusception is an especially important diagnostic consideration in infants with abdominal pain. Immediate diagnosis and treatment are imperative if mortality is to be minimized. Brennemann's description of the pain is classic: "The onset is dramatic. Awake or asleep the baby suddenly cries out with a pain that is obviously extreme. He screams, claws, and clambers up on his mother, twists, and squirms, and nothing gives any relief until, almost as suddenly, there is a lull with absence of pain, only to be followed by a similar painful episode. This sudden onset is of great diagnostic value. As in almost no other condition the mother usually states the exact hour at which the pain began. In the course of some hours the pains become less severe, as a rule not enough to cause the child to cry out as before. With each recurrence he merely squirms, throws himself to one side, doubles up, whimpers, moans or sighs. His facies usually becomes so distinctive that it, too, is of diagnostic value. He appears calm, too calm, paying little attention to his surroundings and yet seems preoccupied and apprehensive."

The history of abdominal pain, sudden in onset, lasting several seconds and recurring every 5 to 15 minutes, always means intussusception until that diagnosis is ruled out. In some instances, pain may not be a prominent feature or may be persistent rather than intermittent. Between the paroxysms of pain the child may appear completely normal. Vomiting occurs early in many of these patients. Blood in the stools is usually a relatively late finding. The physical findings in patients with intussusception have been described on page 133. Although the diagnosis can usually be made readily on the basis of the history and physical examination, a barium enema is diagnostic and usually therapeutic. Since diarrhea may occur in patients with intussusception, this possibility should be considered in infants seen with an atypical picture of dysentery.

Chronic intussusception is a rare cause of recurrent pain in childhood. Intermittent vomiting and the passage of small amounts of blood in the stool may occur.

7. Intestinal malrotation may at times be responsible for recurrent abdominal pain. Nausea and vomiting may also be present.

8. Volvulus

9. Intra-abdominal hernia

10. Meckel's diverticulum. Blood in the stools, usually sudden and large in amount, suggests a Meckel's diverticulum. On the other hand, Meckel's diverticulitis may be characterized by abdominal pain, tenderness, vomiting and fever — symptoms indistinguishable from those of appendicitis. The findings, however, usually do not become localized in the right lower quadrant. Meckel's diverticulum may also cause recurrent, somewhat diffuse, periumbilical discomfort.

11. A mesenteric cyst may be responsible for recurrent abdominal pain. Bleeding into the cyst may cause acute, severe pain.

12. Duplications of the intestinal tract may be characterized by intermittent, colicky abdominal pain and vomiting.

13. Intestinal polyps are a rare cause of intermittent abdominal pain and discomfort.
14. With an incarcerated hernia, the infant is irritable, fretful and in severe pain. His respiratory rate is increased. He may refuse his feedings and vomit.
15. Intestinal obstruction, complete or incomplete, is characterized by intermittent, colicky pain. The intensity of the pain varies somewhat with the degree of obstruction.
16. Constipation may cause vague, chronic abdominal pain and discomfort in children.
17. Sigmoid volvulus may simulate some of the symptoms of intussusception, including anorexia, abdominal cramps, tenderness, a palpable mass and rectal bleeding.

Campbell, J.R. and Blank, E.: Sigmoid volvulus in children. *Pediatrics 53*:702, 1974.

18. The diagnostic work-up of children with abdominal pain should include examination of stools for ova and parasites. Pinworms may rarely cause appendicitis.
19. The onset of diarrhea in patients with dysentery may be preceded by abdominal pain, tenderness, vomiting and fever. Usually, the abdominal pain is not severe, and localization does not occur.
20. Abdominal pain and diarrhea with watery, mucoid and sometimes bloody stools may occur in patients with salmonella enteritis.
21. An increase in the frequency of stools, abdominal discomfort and abdominal cramps may be the earliest clinical manifestations of ulcerative colitis. At times, however, abdominal pain is not present.
22. Children with regional enteritis or Crohn's disease may have recurrent episodes of abdominal pain and cramps, anorexia, vomiting, diarrhea, fever and weight loss. The symptoms of acute regional enteritis may closely simulate those of acute appendicitis.

Dubois, R.S., Rothschild, J. and Silverman, A.: The pediatric corner: the varied manifestations of Crohn's disease in children and adolescents. *Am. J. Gastroenterol. 69*:203, 1978.

23. Rarely, colicky abdominal pain may be caused by an allergic response to specific foods. Diarrhea, nausea and vomiting may also occur.
24. Lactose intolerance, a common trait in many population groups during adolescent and adult years, is characterized by bloating, flatulence, abdominal pain, diarrhea and cramps after drinking milk.

Barr, R.G., Levine, M.D. and Watkins, J.B.: Recurrent abdominal pain of childhood due to lactose intolerance. *N. Engl. J. Med. 300*:1449, 1979.
Bayless, T.M., et al.: Lactose and milk intolerance: clinical implications. *N. Engl. J. Med. 292*:1156, 1975.
Committee on Nutrition, American Academy of Pediatrics: The practical significance of lactose intolerance in children. *Pediatrics 62*:240, 1978.

25. Abdominal pain, at times severe, may occur in patients with cystic fibrosis. The cause has been attributed to such factors as steatorrhea with excessive fermentation of intestinal contents, irritability of the descending loop of the duodenum or pancreatitis.
26. Hereditary angioneurotic edema may cause severe recurrent episodes

of abdominal pain due to edema of the bowel wall occurring, at times, in the absence of edema of the skin.

B. Urinary tract

    1. Abdominal pain, especially chronic or recurrent, is often attributable to urinary tract disease. Obstruction of the urinary tract with or without superimposed infection is the most important type of renal disease associated with this symptom. Urologic abdominal pain may be present in the back, the flank or the lower abdomen. Fever, nausea and vomiting may also be present.

    2. Patients with Henoch-Schönlein purpura, hemophilia or other systemic hemorrhagic disease may have colicky renal pain owing to the passage of blood clots down the ureter.

    3. Colicky pain may also be caused by a renal calculus with radiation of the pain along the course of the ureter to the genitalia.

    4. Abdominal pain occasionally occurs as an early manifestation of acute glomerulonephritis.

C. Liver and gallbladder

    1. Infectious hepatitis may be characterized by abdominal discomfort and pain in the right upper quadrant. The possibility of nonicteric hepatitis should be considered in patients who complain of right upper quadrant or epigastric pain.

    2. Cholecystitis, although rare, does occur in childhood. It is characterized by severe abdominal pain, chiefly in the right upper quadrant, and by nausea, vomiting and fever. Tenderness, guarding and a mass may be noted on physical examination. Jaundice may also occur. Cholecystography is indicated.

Andrassy, R.T. et al.: Gallbladder disease in children and adolescents. *Am. J. Surg. 132*:19, 1976.
Pieretti, R., Auldist, A.W. and Stephens, C.A.: Acute cholecystitis in children. *Surg. Gynecol. Obstet. 140*:16, 1975.

    3. Cholelithiasis. Patients with cholelithiasis may have repeated episodes of abdominal pain, chiefly in the right upper quadrant, accompanied by nausea and vomiting, tenderness and muscle guarding. Jaundice is an occasional symptom. In children, this disorder is usually associated with some systemic disorder such as chronic hemolytic anemia, Wilson's disease, cystic fibrosis or metachromatic leukodystrophy.

Ariyan, S., Shessel, F.S. and Pickett, L.K.: Cholecystitis and cholelithiasis masking as abdominal crises in sickle cell disease. *Pediatrics 58*:252, 1976.
Rosenfield, N. et al.: Cholelithiasis and Wilson's disease. *J. Pediatr. 92*:210, 1978.

    4. Passive congestion of the liver

    5. Intrahepatic sinusoidal plugging during a sickle cell crisis may cause fever, jaundice, hepatomegaly, leukocytosis, elevated alkaline phosphatase and acholic stools.

    6. Choledochal cyst or cystic dilatation of the gallbladder may cause abdominal pain. Jaundice of the obstructive type and a palpable mass in the right upper quadrant are also frequently present. The discomfort is usually localized in the right upper part of the abdomen.

    7. Hydrops, or acute distention, of the gallbladder may cause a right upper quadrant mass, severe pain and rigidity of the rectus muscle.

8. Hepatic tumors may cause abdominal discomfort.
9. Chiari's syndrome, or thrombosis of the hepatic veins, is characterized, in part, by upper abdominal pain.

D. Spleen
1. Traumatic rupture of the spleen may cause tenderness and muscle spasm in the left upper quadrant.
2. Splenomegaly produces abdominal discomfort.
3. Congestive splenomegaly may be associated with left upper quadrant pain during episodes of hematemesis.

E. Pancreas
1. Acute pancreatitis is characterized by the abrupt onset of midepigastric or generalized constant abdominal pain, nausea, protracted vomiting, jaundice, fever, and abdominal tenderness most prominent in the epigastrium or around the umbilicus. The patient usually appears acutely ill and may be in shock. Physical examination reveals maximal tenderness in the midepigastric area with muscle guarding and rigidity. The abdomen is distended and has a firm, doughy feel. The child may assume the knee-chest position for relief of pain. Bluish discoloration of the umbilicus or flanks may occur if intra-abdominal hemorrhage has occurred. Pleural effusion may develop in some patients. Daily determination of the serum amylase is indicated when pancreatitis is suspected. Hyperglycemia and hypocalcemia may also occur. Pancreatitis may be associated with mumps, sepsis, blunt or penetrating trauma or mechanical obstruction of the pancreatic ducts by ascaris. Acute pancreatitis may also be induced by drugs such as azathioprine, isoniazid, 6-mercaptopurine, L-asparaginase and steroid therapy. Obstruction of the pancreatic or distal common bile duct, usually owing to a congenital anomaly of the ducts, may be etiologic. Chronic relapsing pancreatitis is characterized by recurrences of pain and upper abdominal discomfort. Pancreatic calcifications, diabetes mellitus and steatorrhea may occur. Recurrent pancreatitis may be hereditary, including familial hyperlipemia, or associated with hyperparathyroidism or cystic fibrosis. Fat necrosis associated with pancreatitis may cause fever, tender subcutaneous nodules, polyarthritis and bone pain.

Fonkalsrud, E.W., Henney, R.P., Riemenschneider, T.A. and Barker, W.F.: Management of pancreatitis in infants and children. *Am. J. Surg. 116*:198, 1968.
Jordan, S.C. and Ament, M.E.: Pancreatitis in children and adolescents. *J. Pediatr. 91*:211, 1977.
Shwachman, H., Lebenthal, E. and Khaw, K.-T.: Recurrent acute pancreatitis in patients with cystic fibrosis with normal pancreatic enzymes. *Pediatrics 55*:86, 1975.
Williams, T.E., Jr., Sherman, N.J. and Clatworthy, H.W., Jr.: Chronic fibrosing pancreatitis in childhood: a cause of recurrent abdominal pain. *Pediatrics 40*:1019, 1967.

2. Congenital fibrosis of the sphincter of Oddi may be associated with abdominal pain.
3. Pseudocyst of the pancreas is characterized by abdominal pain, anorexia, nausea, vomiting, distention and an abdominal mass, usually tender and firm, in the upper abdomen. Ascites, weight loss or fever may also be noted.

Stone, H.H. and Whitehurst, J.O.: Pseudocysts of the pancreas in children. *Am. J. Surg. 114*:448, 1967.

F. Ovaries, uterus
1. Torsion of an ovarian pedicle, cyst or tumor on the right may be accompanied by symptoms indistinguishable from those of acute appendicitis. Torsion of the adnexa is a diagnostic consideration with sudden onset of lower abdominal pain and vomiting, especially if there is a prior history of similar episodes. A pelvic mass can be palpated. Intermittent torsion may cause recurrent symptoms. Rupture of an ovarian follicle at ovulation may cause abdominal pain, the so-called *mittelschmerz*. The episode, characterized by dull but, at times, sharp lower abdominal quadrant pain, occurs two weeks before a menstrual period, usually in older adolescents over 16 years of age. Abdominal and unilateral adnexal tenderness and some muscle guarding may be noted. Pelvic discomfort and cramps may also accompany menstruation.

Ein, S.H., Darte, J.M.M. and Stephens, C.A.: Cystic and solid ovarian tumors in children: a 44-year review. *J. Pediatr. Surg. 5*:148, 1970.
Grosfeld, J.L.: Torsion of normal ovary in the first two years of life. *Am. J. Surg. 117*:726, 1969.
Schultz, L.R., Newton, W.A., Jr. and Clatworthy, H.W., Jr.: Torsion of previously normal tube and ovary in children. *N. Engl. J. Med. 268*:343, 1963.

2. Hematocolpos in adolescent girls may be accompanied by constant or intermittent abdominal pain.
3. Dysmenorrhea is characterized by lower abdominal and back pain accompanied, at times, by headache, nausea and vomiting.

G. Primary streptococcal or pneumococcal peritonitis is rare. Generalized, but usually not severe, abdominal pain is present. Tuberculous peritonitis is usually characterized more by abdominal discomfort than by actual pain. At times, however, the pain may be severe. After rupture of an appendix, the child may complain less of pain for an hour or two. The abdominal pain then becomes generalized, and the child lies very still in an effort to minimize it.

H. Mesenteric lymphadenitis is a diagnosis made essentially by exclusion. With a history of abdominal pain, vomiting and fever, the suspicion of acute appendicitis is always warranted. A period of observation may be required to eliminate or confirm this possibility. If the symptoms do not progress and significant tenderness is absent, appendicitis can eventually be excluded. When appendicitis cannot be ruled out, laparotomy is indicated. If mesenteric adenitis is found with a normal appendix, a node should be cultured for Yersinia enterocolitica. Tuberculosis of the mesenteric lymph nodes may cause chronic abdominal pain.

Blattner, R.J.: Acute mesenteric lymphadenitis. *J. Pediatr. 74*:479, 1969.

I. Iliac adenitis may cause lower abdominal pain, tenderness, fever and leukocytosis.
J. Leukemia and other lymphomas may cause abdominal pain through involvement of mesenteric or retroperitoneal lymph nodes.
K. Mesenteric vein thrombosis
L. Salpingitis and pelvic inflammatory disease is characterized by lower abdominal pain, bilateral adnexal tenderness and tenderness on motion of the

cervix. Acute salpingitis caused by N. gonorrhoeae is accompanied by fever, leukocytosis, elevated sedimentation rate and positive cervical culture for gonorrhea. Gonococcal perihepatitis may accompany acute salpingitis.

Litt, I.F., Edberg, S.C. and Finberg, L.: Gonorrhea in children and adolescents: a current review. *J. Pediatr. 85*:595, 1974.

M. Superior mesenteric artery syndrome is produced by duodenal obstruction proximal to the ligament of Treitz. Symptoms, which are intermittent or constant, include postprandial fullness, abdominal pain and cramps, nausea and vomiting and failure to gain weight. Weight loss and a hyperextension body cast are among precipitating causes.

Hyde, J.S. et al.: Superior mesenteric artery syndrome. *Am. J. Dis. Child. 106*:25, 1963.

II. Extra-abdominal causes
   A. Lungs. Right lower lobe pneumonia with diaphragmatic pleurisy may cause abdominal pain, vomiting and perhaps muscle guarding on the right, somewhat suggestive of appendicitis. A chest roentgenogram may be indicated for differentiation.
   B. Heart
      1. Rheumatic fever. Abdominal pain may be one of the initial symptoms, preceding other manifestations, or may occur later during the course of the disease. Fever, vomiting and leukocytosis may be accompanying findings. Usually, the abdominal pain is diffuse or epigastric. Abdominal tenderness and rigidity may not be present. On the other hand, localizing findings may occur in the right lower quadrant. Differentiation between the abdominal manifestations of rheumatic fever and appendicitis may be difficult or impossible.

Lin, J-S. and Rodriguez-Torres, R.: Appendectomy in children with acute rheumatic fever. *Pediatrics 43*:573, 1969.

      2. Pericarditis may be accompanied by epigastric complaints.

Boles, E.T. and Hosier, D.M.: Abdominal pain in acute myocarditis and pericarditis. *Am. J. Dis. Child. 105*:70, 1963.

      3. Infants with congenital endocardial fibroelastosis may appear to have intermittent episodes of colicky abdominal pain.
   C. Central nervous system and spinal cord
      1. Abdominal epilepsy. Abdominal pain is a common aura of epileptic seizures. Unusually, paroxysmal episodes of abdominal pain may be ascribed to abnormal cerebral discharges. The abdominal pain is severe and colicky, sudden in onset and periumbilical or epigastric in location. Pain lasts only a few minutes and may be followed by postictal sleep. That some clouding of consciousness, disorientation or confusion occurs during the attack is an important diagnostic point. Episodes of abdominal pain may recur several times over a period of a few days. The electroencephalogram is abnormal. These patients may or may not have a history of convulsive seizures. In addition to periodic abdominal pain, epileptic equivalent states may be characterized by nausea, vomiting, headache and fever.

Babb, R.R. and Eckman, P.B.: Abdominal epilepsy. *JAMA 222*:65, 1972.
Douglas, E.F. and White, P.T.: Abdominal epilepsy — a reappraisal. *J. Pediatr. 78*:59, 1971.

2. Brain tumors and other intracranial lesions may rarely be accompanied by abdominal pain.
3. Herpes zoster
4. Tuberculous spondylitis
5. Spinal cord tumors in the dorsolumbar region may cause acute abdominal pain.

D. Blood
1. Abdominal pain may occur in patients with acute hemolytic anemia and during crises with chronic hemolytic anemia.
2. The symptoms and signs of an abdominal crisis in patients with sickle cell anemia may simulate those of an acute surgical abdomen or gallbladder disease with pain, jaundice, leukocytosis and elevation of liver enzymes. Crises occur in 10 per cent of patients with sickle cell anemia. Usually, the pain remains generalized. Splenic thromboses may be accompanied by pain in the left upper quadrant.
3. Abdominal pain may occur in patients with leukemia.
4. Abdominal pain in patients with anaphylactoid or Schönlein-Henoch purpura may occur either before or after the purpura. The pain is often colicky and may be severe. Nausea, vomiting, hematemesis and melena may occur. Gastrointestinal hemorrhage in patients with other types of purpura may also cause abdominal pain.

Byrn, J.R., Fitzgerald, J.F., Northway, J.D., Anand, S.K. and Scott, J.R.: Unusual manifestations of Henoch-Schönlein syndrome. *Am. J. Dis. Child. 130*:1335, 1976.

5. Hemophilia may cause abdominal pain as a result of retroperitoneal hemorrhage.
6. Acute infectious lymphocytosis may be characterized by abdominal pain.

E. Metabolic
1. Lead poisoning may cause colicky abdominal pain and vomiting.
2. Hyperparathyroidism due to a functioning parathyroid adenoma may be characterized by severe abdominal pain, nausea, vomiting, fever, azotemia, stupor and coma.
3. Addison's disease may be characterized by severe abdominal pain, vomiting and diarrhea.
4. Diabetic acidosis may be accompanied by abdominal pain.
5. Hypoglycemia
6. Hyperlipoproteinemia may be characterized by attacks of colicky abdominal pain along with abdominal tenderness, boardlike rigidity, anorexia, fever and, at times, collapse. Duration of the episodes is one to four days.
7. Acute porphyria may cause colicky abdominal pain.
8. Hereditary angioedema may be characterized by recurrent abdominal pain.
9. Familial paroxysmal polyserositis (Mediterranean fever) may be manifested as paroxysmal peritonitis with exquisite abdominal tenderness,

muscle guarding, vomiting, fever and leukocytosis. In some patients, paroxysmal pleuritis may occur independent of, precede, or follow the abdominal attack.

Siegal, S.: Familial paroxysmal polyserositis. Am. J. Med. 36:893, 1964.

F. Miscellaneous
1. Periarteritis nodosa. Abdominal pain, frequently in the right upper quadrant, may be one of the nonspecific symptoms in these patients.
2. Arachnidism, or black widow spider poisoning, is characterized by severe abdominal pain and rigidity of the abdominal wall without localized tenderness.
3. Epidemic myalgia may be characterized by spasmodic abdominal pain, tenderness and muscle spasm.
4. Mesenteric arteritis, a complication occurring 3 to 6 days following surgical correction of coarctation of the aorta, is characterized by hypertension, abdominal pain, tenderness, distention, vomiting, intestinal bleeding, fever and, if untreated, gangrene of the bowel.
5. Ectopic pregnancy may be characterized by amenorrhea, menorrhagia or irregular bleeding, abdominal pain and a tender adnexal mass unaccompanied by fever or a cervical discharge.

III. Recurrent abdominal pain
Recurrent abdominal pain represents a frequent cause for consultation. A nonorganic etiology is suggested when there is a diffuse or changing localization of the complaint, bizarre radiation of pain, a temporal relation to stressful situations, failure of the patient to be awakened at night by the pain and the absence of abdominal tenderness, muscle spasm or distention. The symptom is especially common in children from the age of 8 to 15. Recurrent abdominal pain under the age of 3 to 5 is more likely organic than biosocial. The severity of the pain provides no clue as to its organic or psychogenic etiology.

Since in the case of somatic complaints such as recurrent abdominal pain, the children are usually around 10 or 11 years of age or adolescents, and their parents are around 35 or 45 years of age, the following kinds of personal, developmental, or family problems and stresses are important to touch upon in the history.

A. Separation experiences
1. The death or the anticipated death of an important family member (e.g., a parent, sibling, grandparent or friend)
2. Divorce or anticipated divorce or desertion. An impending divorce may be suspected on the basis of the symptoms presented by the child.
3. Social or vocational commitments that create a separation between parent and child
4. The child's fear of his own death (e.g., a child who has recovered from a critical illness or who has a long-term, life-threatening illness)
5. Alienation or lack of communication between the patient and his family

B. Illness in the family
1. Physical illness (e.g., cancer or myocardial infarction in a parent or the presence of a long-term handicapping condition such as mental retarda-

tion or myelodysplasia in a sibling). Each parent should be asked if he or she is seeing a physician.

2. Frequently, there are somatic complaints in the parents that serve as a "family" model for the complaint (e.g., the mother may have chronic abdominal pain).

3. Psychologic symptoms and disorders (e.g., anxiety, depression, alcoholism or psychosis). One may use here such leading questions as, "Who's the nervous one in your family?" or "Who does the worrying around your house?"

4. Hypochondriasis or parental preoccupation with illness.

C. Marital discord needs to be kept in mind as a possibility.

D. Unsatisfactory parent-child interaction (e.g., over-expectation, over-restriction, unfavorable comparison with a sibling, disappointment in the child).

E. How the child and his family deal with angry feelings. The outward expression of anger is especially difficult for the child whose parent is chronically or seemingly seriously ill.

F. Evidence of depressive reaction in the child (e.g., school underachievement, trouble sleeping, overeating or undereating as well as "feeling blue")

G. Child's ability to get along with peers

H. Child's preparation for sexual development; his sexual concerns

I. School and learning problems

J. Sleeping arrangements that are not appropriate for the child's age

IV. Further questioning to determine etiology

A. Why do the parents come now when the complaint may have been going on a long time?

B. What do the parents and child think is wrong?

C. What does the symptom bring to the child in terms of secondary gain?

D. Is the symptom masking a school phobia?

E. What do the parents and child expect to be done?

F. Does the pain awaken the child at night? Generally, recurrent abdominal pain of a psychologic etiology does not.

With presenting complaints of this kind, one may open the interview with a statement somewhat as follows, "In seeing many children with this symptom, I find that it is sometimes due to physical causes, sometimes due to stresses at this stage of life and sometimes to both. But *pain is pain* no matter what the cause, so it's my practice to look thoroughly at all possibilities, physical, psychologic and . . . whatever."

This opening clarification precludes an impression on the part of the parents or child that the doctor, in a snap decision, has concluded that the symptom is all "in the child's head" or that the child is "making it up." If the parents of a child with abdominal pain ask about this, the doctor may respond with a statement such as, "Well, it's not in his head, it's in his stomach."

Green, M.: A developmental approach to symptoms based on age groups. *Pediatr. Clin. N. Am.* 22:571, 1975.

# ETIOLOGIC CLASSIFICATION OF ABDOMINAL PAIN

I. Intra-abdominal causes, 326
  A. Gastrointestinal tract, 326
      1. Colic
      2. Peptic ulcer
      3. Zollinger-Ellison syndrome
      4. Dietary indiscretion
      5. Appendicitis
      6. Intussusception
      7. Intestinal malrotation
      8. Volvulus
      9. Intra-abdominal hernia
      10. Meckel's diverticulum
      11. Mesenteric cyst
      12. Duplications of the intestinal tract
      13. Intestinal polyps
      14. Incarcerated hernia
      15. Intestinal obstruction
      16. Constipation
      17. Sigmoid volvulus
      18. Parasites
      19. Dysentery
      20. Salmonella enteritis
      21. Ulcerative colitis
      22. Regional enteritis or Crohn's disease
      23. Allergic response to food
      24. Lactose intolerance
      25. Cystic fibrosis
      26. Hereditary angioneurotic edema
  B. Urinary tract, 330
      1. Obstruction
      2. Systemic hemorrhagic disease
      3. Renal calculus
      4. Acute glomerulonephritis
  C. Liver and gallbladder, 330
      1. Infectious hepatitis
      2. Cholecystitis
      3. Cholelithiasis
      4. Passive congestion of the liver
      5. Sickle cell crisis
      6. Choledochal cyst or cystic dilatation of the gallbladder
      7. Hydrops of gallbladder
      8. Hepatic tumors
      9. Chiari's syndrome
  D. Spleen, 331
      1. Traumatic rupture
      2. Splenomegaly
      3. Congestive splenomegaly
  E. Pancreas, 331
      1. Acute pancreatitis
      2. Congenital fibrosis
      3. Pancreatic pseudocyst
  F. Ovaries, uterus, 332
      1. Torsion of ovarian pedicle, cyst or tumor
      2. Hematocolpos
      3. Dysmenorrhea
  G. Primary streptococcal or pneumococcal peritonitis, 332
  H. Mesenteric lymphadenitis, 332
  I. Iliac adenitis, 332
  J. Leukemia and other lymphomas, 332
  K. Mesenteric vein thrombosis, 332
  L. Salpingitis and pelvic inflammatory disease, 332
  M. Superior mesenteric artery syndrome, 333

II. Extra-abdominal causes, 333
  A. Right lower lobe pneumonia with diaphragmatic pleurisy, 333
  B. Heart, 333
      1. Rheumatic fever
      2. Pericarditis
      3. Congenital endocardial fibroelastosis
  C. Central nervous system and spinal cord, 333
      1. Abdominal epilepsy
      2. Brain tumors and other intracranial lesions
      3. Herpes zoster
      4. Tuberculous spondylitis
      5. Spinal cord tumors in the dorsolumbar region
  D. Blood, 334
      1. Acute hemolytic or chronic hemolytic anemia
      2. Sickle cell crisis
      3. Leukemia
      4. Anaphylactoid or Schönlein-Henoch purpura
      5. Hemophilia
      6. Acute infectious lymphocytosis
  E. Metabolic, 334
      1. Lead poisoning
      2. Hyperparathyroidism
      3. Addison's disease
      4. Diabetic acidosis
      5. Hypoglycemia
      6. Hyperlipoproteinemia
      7. Acute porphyria
      8. Hereditary angioedema
      9. Familial paroxysmal polyserositis
  F. Miscellaneous, 335
      1. Periarteritis nodosa
      2. Arachnidism
      3. Epidemic myalgia
      4. Mesenteric arteritis
      5. Ectopic pregnancy

III. Recurrent abdominal pain, 335
  A. Separation experience, 335
      1. Death or anticipated death in family
      2. Divorce or anticipated divorce or desertion
      3. Social or vocational separation of parent and child
      4. Child's fear of his own death
      5. Alienation or lack of communication in family
  B. Illness in family, 335
      1. Physical illness
      2. Parents' complaints as "model" for child
      3. Psychologic symptoms and disorders
      4. Hypochondriasis
  C. Marital discord, 336
  D. Unsatisfactory parent-child interaction, 336
  E. Expression of angry feelings, 336
  F. Depressive reaction in child, 336
  G. Child's interaction with peers, 336
  H. Child's sexual concerns, 336
  I. School and learning problems, 336
  J. Inappropriate sleeping arrangements for child's age, 336

# CHAPTER 36

# ANOREXIA

A complete list of the causes of anorexia would include most of the diseases known to pediatrics. Food intake diminishes during almost every acute or chronic illness, in the presence of anemia, with urea cycle disorders in newborn infants, in such endocrine diseases as hypothyroidism and Addison's disease, in infectious hepatitis, with endocardial fibroelastosis and in vitamin D poisoning, diabetes insipidus, infantile renal acidosis, idiopathic hypercalcemia and lead poisoning. The common cold in infants is usually preceded by the sudden loss of appetite. Anorexia due to organic disease commonly results in a uniform refusal of all foods.

The physiologic mechanisms involved in the regulation of food intake are incompletely understood. *Appetite* refers to a desire for certain foods. Though appetite must have a physiologic basis, it is also determined by cultural patterns and modified by psychologic factors. A gastric factor is probably present, the appetite depending upon whether the tone of the gastric musculature is good or poor. The gastric tone may either be inhibited or increased by stimuli from the cortical and hypothalamic areas of the brain transmitted through the vagus and splanchnic nerves. Anxiety, worry, fear and resentment cause a diminution in appetite even when the gastric tone is high.

*Hunger* is caused primarily by the occurrence of vigorous gastric peristaltic contractions when the stomach is empty. The frequency and intensity of these contractions vary among different persons. Afferent impulses that arise in the gastric mucosa stimulate parasympathetic centers in the brain stem; efferent impulses then pass through the vagus and stimulate the gastric musculature. Non-nutritive as well as nutritive substances placed in the mouth or entering the stomach can cause cessation of peristalsis. When food reaches the duodenum, the enterogastrone that is secreted inhibits gastric contractions. Psychologic factors can stop peristalsis or mask the sensation of hunger.

*Satiety* is reached when the hunger-appetite mechanism has caused a certain amount of food to be ingested. The hypothalamus determines, to some extent, when satiety is reached, but conditioning also plays an important role.

Normally, hunger determines when a person eats, appetite what he eats and satiety how much he eats. Fortunately, well infants and children generally take food at the right time and in the correct amounts if it is offered to them in nurturing environments. Babies also accept solid foods and feed themselves when their neuromuscular progress permits them to do so. Eating should constitute no problem. The physician may need to help parents understand and accept normal feeding patterns of infants and children.

## DEVELOPMENTAL GUIDES TO FEEDING

**Periodicity of Hunger.** Babies have hunger contractions shortly after birth. Within a few days, a rhythmical pattern develops in most babies. Parents can generally tell when hunger occurs, because the infant shows his discomfort at first by restlessness and then by crying — the physiologic indications that a baby is ready to eat.

The frequency of hunger contractions is an individual matter. The interval may be three hours for one baby and four hours for another. The same infant may have a three-hour interval at one time of day and a five-hour period at another, but a similar pattern occurs on successive days. Babies should be fed according to their own individual hunger rhythms since rigidly prescribed feeding schedules ignore the hunger mechanism.

Aldrich and Hewitt studied the individual hunger rhythms in 100 infants permitted a self-regulatory feeding pattern during the first year of life. In the first month after birth, the majority of infants wanted to be fed at a three-hour interval. Ten per cent, however, chose a two-hour schedule. Only two babies had irregular hunger rhythms. Not until the third month did a predominant number of infants want a four-hour schedule. One third of the babies still preferred to be fed every three hours at that time.

Aldrich, C.A. and Hewitt, E.S.: Self-regulatory feeding program for infants. *JAMA 135*:340, 1947.

It is now well recognized that some mothers are not able to interpret their infant's needs accurately; consequently, their infants do not do well on a flexible schedule. Such mothers are more comfortable when they can follow a definite feeding schedule, which the physician can suggest on the basis of his knowledge of hunger patterns. In the majority of instances, however, the self-regulatory program meets the infant's needs and presents no problem to the mother.

**Rooting Reflex.**   When an infant's cheek or the corner of his mouth is stimulated by contact with the breast or nipple, the infant automatically turns toward the stimulus prepared to suck.

**Sucking Reflex.**   The presence of the sucking reflex in term and in most prematures is the neuromotor indication for liquid feedings. Some infants suck vigorously through an entire meal; others may stop several times during a feeding. When sucking stops and the infant falls asleep, the hunger-appetite mechanism has been satisfied.

**Protrusion Reflex.**   As a result of this reflex, solid food placed in the anterior third of the mouth in young infants is reflexly pushed out by the tongue. This reflex does not interfere with nursing, since the nipple empties into the back of the mouth and throat. It may, however, make the early feeding of solid foods difficult. The protrusion reflex normally disappears between the third and fifth months of life, most commonly in the fourth month.

**Appetite Development.**   *Hunger* is the factor that chiefly controls food intake during early infancy. *Appetite,* which may be evident by three months of age, usually does not become important until the latter half of the first year. Before this time, almost any food of liquid consistency is accepted, including soy bean or protein hydrolysate milks. In the third month of life, however, it may be difficult to get a baby to change from a cow milk to a substitute formula. In other instances, this difficulty is not encountered until the eighth or ninth month.

In the latter half of the first year, family dietary patterns, maternal dislike of foods being offered, or unpleasantness associated with the introduction of certain foods are conditioning factors for impaired appetite. By 12 months of age the baby shows definite preferences and dislikes. He takes time to look over the foods offered and selects those he likes. At eight months, he may have seemed too hungry to care at mealtimes.

**Self-Feeding.** The neuromuscular development of a baby normally permits self hand-feeding before a year of age. If a baby is prevented from feeding himself, this ability may be delayed for many weeks or months.

At approximately four months of age, the baby begins to acquire some control of his hands and skill in their use. He recognizes his bottle and may reach out for it. At five to six months, he can put his hands around the bottle and guide it to his lips. By approximately nine to ten months of age, a baby has acquired the ability of prehension, and shortly after this he learns to chew. He can then be encouraged to feed himself a cracker or a cookie. At nine months, an empty cup may be placed on his tray for practice. At ten months, he can begin practicing with a spoon. Because the neuromuscular control needed is not as great, he becomes proficient in the use of a cup before he is skilled in handling a spoon. Shortly after 12 months of age, he can use a cup well. He works with the spoon in earnest between 12 and 14 months but is not really skilled at it until about 18 months.

Self-feeding between 12 and 18 months is apt to be a mixture of spoon-feeding, hand-feeding and cup-glass-feeding. The result is usually messy, but the infant learns by practice. By 18 to 21 months, babies who have been permitted to do so usually feed themselves well.

**Chewing.** Chewing motions usually appear by about the eighth or ninth month and are the neuromuscular indication that lumpy foods can be introduced whether teeth are present or not. The baby may initially resist a change in the consistency of his food. If this is the case, the mother may wait a few days before making another attempt. Some infants, especially children who have been chronically ill or are emotionally upset or retarded, continue to refuse lumpy foods for some time.

**Emotional Development and Feeding.** In addition to being related to an infant's physiologic needs and neuromuscular progress, feeding is also closely entwined with emotional development. Many new types of psychobiologic integration are required in the progressive steps of self-feeding, and these steps may be resisted at one or more points. Feeding is often the first arena for a struggle between parent and child. That is why new foods or techniques are introduced gradually and temporarily stopped if resistance develops. If the general physical care and the emotional environment are favorable, problems in the feeding sphere are usually transient. If not, the feeding problem may persist and become worse. Food is made a point of struggle. When this happens, the important physiologic criteria of the infant's nutritional needs are obscured.

When physiologic and developmental guides to infant feeding are persistently ignored, due to lack of a satisfactory parent-child relationship, psychogenic anorexia may develop. The parent may be unable to supply a healthy, positive stimulus to the infant's development. Evidence of this may be present also in areas other than feeding.

Force has been used in almost every case of psychogenic anorexia. The infant resists force by not eating. Gagging and vomiting may also occur. The parent may attempt to make the baby conform to adult or other inappropriate standards. The child is not given the support he needs to achieve new feeding patterns, and his hunger-appetite mechanism becomes suppressed by anger and frustration.

The history may indicate that the baby may be forced to restrict his self-feeding attempts because they are messy and to be neat before he is able. The baby's food preference may be ignored, and he may be forced to accept foods that are "good for him" or to take additional food even though his hunger-appetite mechanism is functioning normally. Some older infants and young children with psychologic anorexia limit their intake to a certain few foods and refuse or are wary of anything else. This may also be a manifestation of anxiety in young children.

Infants who receive poor physical care seem to have little appetite and often feed poorly, perhaps because they are uncomfortable in the feeding situation and unsatisfied most of the time.

Excessive milk intake in infants may be the result of psychogenic anorexia. The baby clings to his early feeding pattern and refuses solid foods. The milk intake is increased to meet caloric needs, and, eventually, two or more quarts of milk a day may be taken. Because of the lack of iron in this diet, and possible blood loss in the stools due to sensitivity to cow milk, iron deficiency anemia results and further accentuates the anorexia.

Temporary anorexia may occur during teething. Most infants and children also eat less during hot weather.

It is sometimes stated that "physiologic anorexia" occurs uniformly in the second year of life, owing to the deceleration of growth that occurs at this time. Current experience does not seem to confirm this. The total amount of food taken by a baby in the second year is greater than in the first year.

Psychogenic anorexia in the preschool and school age child usually represents a continuation of the feeding difficulties present during infancy. By this time, the problem is difficult to treat. Even with guidance, it may persist for weeks or months. There may be a history of delayed self-feeding or chewing, chewing but not swallowing solid foods, gagging and choking, coaxing and cajoling, and family scenes centering about the child's refusal to eat. Anorexia may be used as a means of gaining attention, as a manifestation of general negativism or as a symptom of some other disturbance in parent-child relations.

Anorexia may be highly selective in these children. Fussiness about foods is often prominent. Milk may be taken from a cup, but not a glass. A child may insist on hamburgers, soda pop and ice cream. He eats these with relish and refuses to touch other foods. The child may drink large volumes of milk to meet his nutritional and caloric needs, but refuse most solid foods.

Children with psychogenic anorexia are often thin, and their body measurements frequently fall in the lower percentiles. At times, however, a mother may complain that her child has anorexia and is underweight when he is actually well nourished or obese. The family dietary pattern in these instances may tend toward an excessive intake of food. The child in attempting to follow his own hunger-appetite mechanism does not conform.

*Anorexia nervosa* is the most serious of all feeding disturbances. The hunger-appetite mechanism may be completely suppressed. Loss of weight and malnutrition may be severe, exceeding 20 per cent or more of body weight, and death may occur. Menstruation either ceases or does not begin. Anorexia nervosa occurs most frequently in preadolescent and adolescent girls, usually from middle class families, although it may also develop in boys. The refusal to eat or rigorous dieting may begin after a friend or relative has expressed concern about the child's becoming obese.

Because of a distorted body image, the child does not see herself as too thin even after large losses of weight. The patient strongly resists gaining weight and may be very manipulative. One may elicit a history of strenuous exercise, secret dieting or use of laxatives. At other times, there is a history of overeating followed, at times, by self-induced vomiting. Many of these children are almost constantly active, seemingly without fatigue.

Anorexia nervosa is not a specific clinical entity but is associated with a number of personality disturbances, environmental situations, parental attitudes and with varying degrees of severity. The families are often overprotective and closely knit. Problems other than the one related to food are initially denied. Some patients are severely emotionally disturbed, i.e., prepsychotic or psychotic, others are depressed, while the symptom in still others is reactive to a disturbing situation.

Bruch, H.: *Eating Disorders: Obesity, Anorexia Nervosa and the Person Within.* New York, Basic Books, 1973.

Minuchin, S., Rosman, B.L., Baker, L. and Liebman, R.: *Psychosomatic Families; Anorexia Nervosa in Context.* Cambridge, Harvard University Press, 1978.

*Pica,* the eating of non-nutritious substances such as dirt, clay, paint and coal, may predispose to lead poisoning or visceral larva migrans. Persistent pica is usually due to insufficient maternal supervision and availability.

Zinkham, W.H.: Visceral larva migrans. *Am. J. Dis. Child. 132*:627, 1978.

CHAPTER 37

# RECTAL BLEEDING

*Melena* refers to the passage of black tarry stools due to bleeding presumably above the ileocecal valve. *Hematochezia* refers to the passage of brick-red or red-brown colored blood from the distal small bowel or proximal colon. Bleeding from the anorectum appears as bright red blood on the outside of the stool, on toilet paper or in the toilet bowl water. The presence of blood may be confirmed by the stool guaiac test. With confirmed rectal bleeding, sigmoidoscopy, barium enema and angiography may be selectively indicated in addition to the usual physical, rectal and laboratory examinations. The passage of a nasogastric tube to determine the presence or absence of blood in the stomach may help localize the site of bleeding. Blood present in the gastric aspirate may arise from gastritis, esophageal varices, hiatus hernia or a gastric ulcer. If no blood is aspirated from the stomach, the site of hemorrhage is likely distal to the ligament of Treitz.

Endoscopy is helpful in the diagnosis of esophagitis, varices, gastritis, gastric ulcers, polyps, ulcerative colitis, granulomatous colitis and other gastrointestinal lesions.

Selective angiography of the mesenteric vessels may be diagnostically helpful with severe gastrointestinal hemorrhage. It may be an important first step in localizing the site of intestinal hemorrhage due to a stress ulcer, identifying a Meckel's diverticulum or determining the cause of hematobilia. If this study is inconclusive, barium studies can then be conducted. Mesenteric angiography may also be indicated with a history of recurrent gastrointestinal bleeding or chronic blood loss unexplained by previous barium studies.

## ETIOLOGIC CLASSIFICATION OF RECTAL BLEEDING

I. During the first day of life grossly bloody stools may be due to the swallowing of over 30 ml. of maternal blood. The Apt test may be used to demonstrate whether the blood is of maternal or infant origin.

   One part of stool is mixed with five to ten parts water. The stool must be red and grossly bloody since in a tarry stool the oxyhemoglobin has already been changed to hematin. There must be a pink supernatant solution; otherwise, the subsequent color change will not be seen. This mixture is then centrifuged at 2000 r.p.m. for 1 to 2 minutes, and the pink hemoglobin solution is decanted off. One part of 0.25-normal sodium hydroxide solution is then mixed with 5 parts of the hemoglobin solution. In the presence of adult hemoglobin, the solution will change to a yellow-brown color within two minutes; in the presence of fetal hemoglobin, which is alkali-resistant, the solution remains pink.

II. Esophageal varices secondary to portal hypertension. Varices can be visualized on endoscopy, or at times, with careful x-ray examination. The cause of portal hypertension may be demonstrated by mesenteric arteriography or preoperative percutaneous splenoportography.

III. Peptic ulcer. Stress ulcers in the stomach or duodenum due to a central nervous system disorder, burn or anoxia may cause marked blood loss. The Zollinger-Ellison syndrome may cause gastrointestinal hemorrhage.

Abramson, D.J.: Curling's ulcer in childhood: review of the literature and report of five cases. *Surgery 55*:321, 1964.
Stevens, H., Gwin, G.H., and Gilbert, E.F.: Gastrointestinal ulceration and central nervous system lesions. *Am. J. Dis. Child. 106*:613, 1963.

IV. Duplication of the bowel.

V. Intussusception. While the passage of blood mixed with feces or a small amount of mucus (red currant jelly stool) occurs in the first 24 hours of this disease in about half of the patients, it is not essential for early diagnosis. Chronic recurrent sigmoid intussusception, reported in children with chronic constipation, is characterized by small amounts of bright red blood in the stools.

VI. Volvulus in the newborn, usually associated with malrotation of the bowel, may be characterized by vomiting, abdominal distention, an abdominal mass and bloody stools. In the newborn infant, this clinical presentation should more strongly suggest a volvulus than an intussusception.

VII. Intestinal gangrene, which may be secondary to volvulus or a compromised blood supply, may cause massive gastrointestinal hemorrhage in infancy. Clinical findings may include pain, abdominal distention, vomiting and shock. Barium examinations are contraindicated. Preoperative mesenteric arteriography may be helpful.

VIII. Meckel's diverticulum is often characterized by the sudden, massive and painless passage of blood, either melena or hematochezia, in infants and young children. In the latter event, the blood may be brick or bright red and clotted. A technetium scan may help localize the bleeding site.

IX. Intestinal polyps in the colon or rectum are frequent causes of hematochezia in children. Instead of a copious passage of blood, there is intermittent and recurrent spotting, blood-stained mucus or streaks of bright red blood in the stool. An air contrast study of the colon may be diagnostic. Sigmoidoscopy is always indicated. Most polyps are of the juvenile retention type. A few represent familial adenomatous polyposis of the colon, Gardner's syndrome, generalized juvenile gastrointestinal polyposis or Peutz-Jegher's syndrome.

Sachatello, C.R., Pickren, J.W., and Grace, J.T., Jr.: Generalized juvenile gastrointestinal polyposis. *Gastroenterology 58*:699, 1970.

X. Anal fissure is the most common cause of blood on the stools in young infants.

XI. Rectal prolapse may cause blood on the stools.

XII. Amebic dysentery may cause a bloody, mucoid rectal discharge.

XIII. Bacillary dysentery may present with a bloody mucoid stool.

XIV. Hookworm and whipworm disease (trichuriasis) and other intestinal parasites may cause blood in the stools.

XV. Rectal bleeding along with loose stools and mucus may occur in young infants allergic to cow milk. The blood, which is bright red, may be copious in amount or mixed in with the stool as tiny clots. Colicky abdominal pain is another prominent manifestation.

XVI. Whole cow milk may cause chronic occult gastrointestinal blood loss in infants under 18 months of age with resultant iron deficiency anemia.

XVII. Necrotizing enterocolitis in the newborn is often characterized by the passage of bloody mucus in addition to other symptoms.

XVIII. Ulcerative colitis may be characterized at its onset by rectal bleeding without diarrhea, especially when the disease is limited to the rectosigmoid. Blood may be mixed with pus and mucus.

XIX. Foreign bodies and trauma may cause rectal bleeding.

XX. Hemangioma involving the bowel wall.

XXI. Gastrointestinal neurofibromatosis may cause chronic blood loss.

XXII. Malignancies involving the bowel wall.

XXIII. Systemic hemorrhagic diseases, including Henoch's purpura. Melena is often a clinical manifestation in hemorrhagic disease of the newborn. Other congenital or acquired deficiency of coagulation factors or platelets are less common causes of gastrointestinal hemorrhage.

XXIV. Traumatic hematobilia in which bleeding occurs into the biliary tract after blunt or penetrating abdominal trauma is characterized by colicky right upper quadrant abdominal pain, at times radiating to the shoulder, followed by hematemesis with relief of the pain. A right upper quadrant mass and obstructive jaundice may occur. While gastrointestinal hemorrhage may occur within hours, it may be postponed until weeks or months after the injury. Abdominal angiography permits preoperative diagnosis by demonstration of a traumatic aneurysm of the hepatic artery.

Hawes, D.R., Franken, E.A., Jr., Fitzgerald, J.F. and Battersby, J.S.: Traumatic hematobilia. Angiographic diagnosis. *Am. J. Dis. Child.* *125*:130, 1973.

XXV. A "red diaper" syndrome in which red pigmentation of soiled diapers occurs after storage in the diaper receptacle for 24 to 36 hours is due to Serratia marcescens in the stools.

XXVI. Multiple intestinal telangiectasis associated with recurrent melena has been reported in a few patients with Turner's syndrome.

XXVII. In some instances, the cause of rectal bleeding, even when massive, remains undetermined even after extensive investigation, especially in the newborn infant. Although much blood may be lost, the bleeding stops spontaneously in most infants. Laparotomy is rarely either of diagnostic or therapeutic help. X-ray studies are seldom indicated during the period of acute hemorrhage.

Sherman, N.J. and Clatworthy, H.W.: Gastrointestinal bleeding in neonates: a study of 94 cases. *Surgery* *62*:614, 1967.

## GENERAL REFERENCES

Collins, R.E.C.: Some problems of gastrointestinal bleeding in children. *Arch. Dis. Child.* *46*:110, 1971.

Franken, E.A., Jr.: Gastrointestinal bleeding in infants and children. Radiologic investigation. *JAMA* *229*:1339, 1974.

Ternberg, J.L. and Koehler, P.R.: The use of arteriography in the diagnosis of the origin of acute gastrointestinal hemorrhage in children. *Surgery* *63*:686, 1968.

---

## ETIOLOGIC CLASSIFICATION OF RECTAL BLEEDING

# CHAPTER 38

# JAUNDICE

## CLINICAL CONSIDERATIONS

Jaundice refers to a yellowish discoloration of the sclera, mucous membranes and skin owing to an excess of bilirubin in the blood. Tears, nasal secretions, saliva and cerebrospinal fluid may also be stained. The level of serum bilirubin at which clinical jaundice appears varies in different age groups. Jaundice is evident in most newborn infants with a serum bilirubin concentration of 5 to 7 mg./dl., whereas jaundice appears in older persons when the serum bilirubin level reaches about 2 mg./dl.

Strong natural light is optimal for the clinical detection of jaundice, and minimal jaundice may be missed in a darkened room. If artificial light is used, only white fluorescent light permits early detection. Jaundice usually is evident in the sclerae or in the mucous membrane of the hard palate before it is visible in the skin. Indeed, these may be the only sites in which jaundice can be detected in darkly pigmented patients. Since the clinical detection of jaundice in newborn infants is unreliable, measurements of serum bilirubin levels are indicated when hyperbilirubinemia is suspected.

The exact shade of jaundice is of little diagnostic importance. In jaundice of long duration, the tissues are apt to have a greenish appearance, which is due to the oxidation of bilirubin to biliverdin. Pruritus rarely accompanies jaundice in children but occasionally is a significant problem with obstructive jaundice.

Carotenemia, a common cause of skin pigmentation in infants, which is the result of a large intake of carotene-containing foods, is to be differentiated from jaundice. The yellow discoloration of the skin with carotenemia does not involve the sclerae and is most evident in the nasolabial folds and on the palms and soles.

## BILE PIGMENT METABOLISM

The initial steps in the transformation of hemoglobin to bilirubin occurs in the reticuloendothelial cells of the bone marrow, the spleen and the liver. The first step is the formation of water-insoluble free bilirubin. Bilirubin at this stage is transported in the plasma attached to protein, chiefly albumin. Bilirubin can be displaced from this albumin binding by several drugs (sulfonamides, aspirin, salicylate, oxacillin, cephalothin), metabolic states (hypoxia, acidosis, hypoglycemia, hypothermia, hypoproteinemia) or a high concentration of free fatty acids (secondary to use of soy bean fat emulsions such as Intralipid). The liver normally conjugates free bilirubin to form water-soluble bilirubin glucoronide, which is excreted in the bile. Unconjugated and conjugated bilirubin are roughly synonymous with indirect- and direct-reacting bilirubin, respectively. The conversion of bilirubin to water-soluble glucuronide apparently occurs in the hepatic parenchymal

346

cells. Glucoronyl transferase, the enzyme that catalyzes this reaction, is relatively deficient in newborn infants, especially premature ones, and in patients with familial nonhemolytic jaundice (Crigler-Najjar syndrome). This deficiency leads to an elevated serum level of unconjugated bilirubin.

Bilirubin is excreted into the bile capillaries and the intestinal tract as a sodium salt. Under abnormal circumstances, sodium bilirubinate may regurgitate into the blood stream, where it probably circulates as a readily dissociable complex with albumin. This compound readily passes through the glomeruli.

In the newborn infant, some of the conjugated bilirubin is converted to its unconjugated form, reabsorbed into the enterohepatic circulation and presented to the liver for reprocessing.

Fleischner, G. and Arias, I.M.: Recent advances in bilirubin formation, transport, metabolism and excretion. *Am. J. Med. 49*:576, 1970.

The stools of young infants frequently contain no urobilinogen, the biliary pigments being excreted unchanged as sodium bilirubinate for a variable period of days or weeks after birth. This is presumably due to an absence or diminished number of intestinal bacteria capable of transforming bilirubin to urobilinogen. Similar alterations in flora may occur at any age during diarrhea or after the oral administration of broad-spectrum antibiotics.

In older infants and children, as a result of bacterial action in the intestine, sodium bilirubinate is first reduced to two colorless substances, mesobilirubinogen and stercobilinogen, which collectively are designated as urobilinogen. Urobilinogen is then rapidly oxidized to two orange-yellow pigments designated as urobilin.

The stools of young infants are often green during episodes of diarrhea. Green-colored stools may be present in some normal breast-fed infants. These changes are apparently due to the direct oxidation of bilirubin to green biliverdin instead of the usual bacterial reduction to urobilinogen.

## THE HEPATIC LOBULE

As blood traverses the sinusoids to the central vein, unconjugated or partially conjugated bilirubin and urobilinogen are removed by either the parenchymal or Kupffer cells. The ampulla and primary bile canaliculus through which bile enters the biliary system are particularly vulnerable structures that may become obstructed by surrounding edema or increased connective tissue in liver disease, and by inspissated bile.

Lymph vessels play an important role in regurgitation jaundice, and at least a part of the regurgitated bilirubin reaches the systemic circulation through these channels.

## PHYSIOLOGIC CLASSIFICATION OF JAUNDICE

Two types of jaundice, retention and regurgitation, can be distinguished. Retention jaundice results from failure of the liver cells to convert bilirubin to bilirubin glucuronide at a rate that will prevent accumulation of the unconjugated pigment in the blood. Bile is not present in the urine. Regurgitation jaundice results from the return of bilirubin to the blood stream after its conversion to bilirubin glucuronide. Bile is present in the urine.

**Pathogenesis of Retention Jaundice.** Retention jaundice may occur in the presence of excessive hemolysis and/or pigment production, impaired liver uptake or defective conjugation.

When the rate of destruction of red blood cells is accelerated in hemolytic anemia, increased quantities of bilirubin reach the hepatic cells for processing. Normally, the capacity of the liver for bilirubin excretion is great; however, in the presence of a hemolytic anemia, hepatic cellular function may be impaired. Because of the resultant limited conversion and excretion of unconjugated bilirubin, a portion of the pigment is retained in the blood.

The increased amount of sodium bilirubinate that enters the intestine causes increased fecal excretion of urobilinogen in older infants and children. The intestinal reabsorption of urobilinogen is also increased. In the presence of impaired liver function, however, the excretion of urobilinogen by the liver is diminished. As a result, an increased amount of urobilinogen may pass into the systemic circulation and appear in the urine. Bile is not present in the urine even though the serum levels of bilirubin may be increased.

Complete or partial intrahepatic biliary obstruction may appear during the course of a severe hemolytic anemia, especially in infants. The exact cause of this obstruction is not known. Hypoxic or toxic damage to the ampullae and bile canaliculi may permit leakage of conjugated bilirubin and water while other components of the bile, unable to escape, may remain within the lumen and form obstructing bile thrombi. When intrahepatic obstruction occurs, the findings of regurgitation jaundice are added to those of retention jaundice.

In patients with nonhemolytic retention jaundice, bilirubin, though formed in usual amounts, is not processed at a normal rate by the impaired Kupffer cell–liver cell mechanism. As a result, unconjugated bilirubin accumulates in the blood. Bile does not appear in the urine. Hepatic immaturity in the newborn (physiologic jaundice of the newborn), hereditary hepatic dysfunction (familial nonhemolytic jaundice) and acquired hepatocellular disease are associated with this type of jaundice. In other instances, hypoxia associated with neonatal respiratory distress may impede the partial conjugation of bile to its monoglucuronide form.

**Pathogenesis of Regurgitation Jaundice.** Regurgitation jaundice may occur secondary to necrosis of liver cells or obstruction of the bile ducts.

In hepatocellular disease, necrosis of hepatic cord cells disrupts the continuity of the bile capillaries. Bilirubin glucoronide can then regurgitate into the tissue space that surrounds the hepatic cords or into the sinusoids. Thus, regurgitated bilirubin passes into the systemic circulation indirectly by lymphatic absorption from the tissue spaces or directly through the sinusoidal circulation. Bile is present in the urine. Fecal urobilinogen absorbed from the intestine is not readily excreted by the Kupffer cell–liver cell mechanism, and urobilinogenuria occurs.

With advancing hepatocellular disease and further functional impairment of hepatic cells, the findings of retention jaundice are added to those of regurgitation. Bilirubinuria continues or is augmented. Urobilinogenuria is pronounced.

In the presence of severe hepatocellular disease, leakage of bile or obstruction of the ampullae and primary bile canaliculi may cause complete cessation of the outflow of bile. The stools become acholic. Urobilinogenuria also disappears. Prompt-reacting bilirubin rises in the serum while the retention of unconjugated bilirubin continues. Bilirubinuria reaches its maximum level during this phase.

During recovery and with relief of the intrahepatic obstruction, there is a sudden influx of bilirubin into the stool with a corresponding rise in the concentration of fecal urobilinogen. The prompt-reacting bilirubin in the serum falls, and bilirubinuria gradually subsides. As urobilinogen absorption from the intestine occurs again, urobilinogenuria temporarily reaches high levels.

In hepatocanalicular jaundice, injury to the epithelium of the ampulla and primary bile canaliculus may permit extravasation of fluid and sodium bilirubinate into the surrounding tissues. Absorption then occurs through the lymphatics. Obstructing bile thrombi may or may not form from the concentrated solid material that remains behind in the lumen. The ampulla and bile canaliculus may also be subjected to external compression as a result of edema or fibrous proliferation in the surrounding tissues. Laboratory findings in hepatocanalicular disease include acholic stools, absence of urobilinogenuria, elevation of the prompt-reacting bilirubin in the serum and the presence of bile in the urine.

With complete obstruction, the backflow of bile caused by the presence of obstruction hypothetically results in overdistention and disruption of the bile capillaries. Bilirubin glucuronide then regurgitates into the tissue spaces and into the sinusoidal blood. The stools are acholic. Bile is present in the urine. The elevation of serum bilirubin is primarily due to prompt-reacting bilirubin. When obstruction is prolonged, total serum bilirubin may rise far above the value for prompt-reacting bilirubin owing to the occurrence of hepatocellular damage and retention in addition to regurgitation. Laboratory tests of hepatocellular function usually do not become abnormal until obstructive disease has existed for a number of days.

The mechanism of jaundice in incomplete obstruction is the same as that already described. Laboratory findings are also identical except that the stools are not completely acholic.

Schmid, R.: Bilirubin metabolism in man. *N. Engl. J. Med. 287*:703, 1972.

## ETIOLOGIC CLASSIFICATION OF JAUNDICE

I. Retention jaundice
   A. Hemolytic. Not all patients with hemolytic anemia become jaundiced; nevertheless, excessive hemolysis is a frequent cause.
      1. The appearance of jaundice in the first 24 to 48 hours of life or intense icterus at any time in the early neonatal period raises the possibility of hemolytic disease of the newborn owing to maternal-infant blood group incompatibility. The possibility of Rh sensitization should, of course, have been determined by examination of maternal blood for antibodies during the thirty-fourth week of gestation. Detection of antibodies at this time indicates that hemolytic disease may occur in the newborn infant. The diagnosis of ABO incompatibility cannot be made prenatally. Early diagnosis here depends upon prompt detection of jaundice in the nursery. Blanching of the skin on the forehead by finger pressure helps make the icterus evident. Jaundice is noted first on the face, then on the chest and abdomen, and finally on the extremities.

      Jaundice is not present at birth. Infants with ABO incompatibility usually are not clinically ill or pale. Rh-sensitized infants with active hemolysis at birth may demonstrate hepatomegaly, splenomegaly, pallor, petechiae and edema.

Laboratory examinations indicated in infants of Rh-sensitized mothers include serum bilirubin, hemoglobin and Rh type. If the infant is Rh-positive and the mother's serum has anti-Rh antibodies, the diagnosis of erythroblastosis is established. The direct Coombs test is almost always positive in infants with Rh sensitization and is a further confirmatory finding. A negative Coombs test does not exclude this possibility. The serum bilirubin should be followed at 6- to 12-hour intervals.

ABO incompatibility occurs in first-born infants about as often as in those born later. The criteria for a presumptive diagnosis of ABO hemolytic disease are jaundice in the first 24 hours of life, serum bilirubin values of 10 mg./dl. or higher in the first 24 hours of life and an maternal-infant ABO blood group incompatibility in the presence of a negative Coombs test. The hemoglobin may not be significantly reduced. Although other procedures, such as examination of the infant's serum for incompatible anti-A or anti-B antibodies, may be performed, they are not essential for the decision as to therapy. Spherocytosis and reticulocytosis are often severe in infants with ABO incompatibility.

Hemolytic disease of the newborn may be due to other blood group incompatibilities (e.g., Kell, MNS, Kidd, and Duffy). The maternal serum may be examined for blood group antibodies other than anti-A or anti-B.

In severely affected infants, the stools may become acholic, and bile may appear in the urine between the sixth and twelfth days of life as a result of intrahepatic obstruction. In infants treated with exchange transfusions, jaundice rarely persists past the first week of life and never past the tenth day. Jaundice of longer duration with elevation of both direct and indirect bilirubin has been termed the inspissated bile syndrome. The cause is unknown. In infants treated with exchange transfusion, the peak level of serum bilirubin is usually reached on the second day of life.

Naiman, J.L.: Current management of hemolytic disease of the newborn infant. *J. Pediatr.* *80*:1049, 1972.

2. Erythrocyte abnormalities
   a. Spherocytosis
   b. Elliptocytosis
   c. Stomatocytosis
   d. Pycnocytosis
3. Erythrocyte enzyme deficiencies
   a. Glucose-1-phosphate
   b. Pyruvic kinase
4. Alpha-thalassemia
5. The administration of large doses (10 mg. or more) of water-soluble analogues of vitamin K to newborn infants, especially prematures, may cause a marked drop in the reduced glutathione content of red cells, hemolytic anemia, hyperbilirubinemia and kernicterus.

B. Nonhemolytic
1. Physiologic jaundice of the newborn due to hepatic immaturity appears commonly in newborn infants between the second and fifth day of life. Jaundice in the first 24 hours of life in the term infant or the first 48 hours in the premature should never be considered physiologic. Physiologic jaundice usually disappears by the fifth to eighth day except in the premature, when it may persist into the second week of life. Jaundice may also persist in infants of diabetic mothers. Physiologic jaundice is of greater intensity and duration in premature than in full-term infants.

   The peak of the bilirubin rise usually occurs on the second to third day in full-term infants and on the fourth to sixth day in prematures. The serum bilirubin level in full-term infants with physiologic jaundice generally is less than 7 mg./dl. and rarely exceeds 10 mg./dl. Values over 12 mg./dl. in term infants should be regarded as pathologic. The level of direct-reacting bilirubin should not be more than 1.5 mg./dl. The total serum bilirubin level should not increase more than 5 mg./dl./day. Bilirubin values in premature infants may rise as high as 15 to 20 mg./dl. or may exceed 20 mg. at the peak even in the absence of maternal-infant blood group incompatibility. The upper limit of normal for serum bilirubin in premature infants is not known. Levels above 15 mg./dl. probably represent an indication for investigation.

   The rate of destruction of red blood cells in the first ten days of life is three times greater than in the adult. Jaundice would not occur, however, even with this degree of pigment production if hepatic function were mature. Physiologic jaundice is thought to be due, in part, to a deficiency of glucuronyl transferase. The resultant limitation of hepatic excretion of bilirubin leads to an accumulation of the indirect fraction in the blood. The premature infant can excrete bilirubin at the rate of only 1 to 2 per cent of the normal adult capacity. Maturation of the glucuronide conjugating system during the first days of life is thought to lead to disappearance of the jaundice with the variable rate of maturation accounting for the intensity and duration of this symptom. The enterohepatic circulation of bilirubin from the newborn intestinal tract back to the liver may contribute to physiologic jaundice of the newborn. Hypoxia, hyaline membrane disease, hypoglycemia, acidosis, hypothermia and hypoproteinemia may be associated with hyperbilirubinemia and predispose to kernicterus at lower bilirubin levels.

Poland, R.L. and Odell, G.B.: Physiologic jaundice: the enterohepatic circulation of bilirubin. N. Engl. J. Med. 284:1, 1971.

2. Unconjugated "physiologic" hyperbilirubinemia may persist for weeks in congenital hypothyroidism owing to delayed maturation of hepatic glucuronyl transferase.
3. Drugs such as novobiocin and chloramphenicol and vitamin K analogues decrease conjugation because of competition for glucuronyl transferase.
4. Neonatal jaundice associated with breast-feeding may appear between

the sixth and eighth days of life. The serum unconjugated bilirubin may reach 15 to 25 mg./dl. in the second and third weeks of life. The jaundice persists for several weeks unless breast-feeding is discontinued. Pregnane-3$\alpha$, 20$\beta$-diol, an inhibitor of glucuronyl transferase, is present in the mother's milk.

Gartner, L.M. and Arias, I.M.: Studies of prolonged neonatal jaundice in the breast-fed infant. *J. Pediatr. 68*:54, 1966.

5. The Lucey-Driscoll syndrome (transient familial hyperbilirubinemia), due to a potent inhibitor of bilirubin glucuronyl transferase in maternal and infant serum, is characterized by severe, transient unconjugated hyperbilirubinemia.

Arias, I.M., Wolfson, J., Lucey, J.F. and McKay, R.J., Jr.: Transient familial neonatal hyperbilirubinemia. *J. Clin. Invest. 44*:1442, 1965.

6. Hereditary hepatic dysfunction (congenital familial nonhemolytic jaundice; the Crigler-Najjar syndrome) is a congenital, familial, nonhemolytic type of jaundice that may be characterized, in part, by kernicterus. The infant is persistently jaundiced from a few days after birth. The patient is unable to conjugate bilirubin because of a congenital absence (type I) or partial deficiency (type II) of the glucuronyl transferase system. The indirect serum bilirubin level in type I is constantly elevated, commonly over 20 mg./dl. Rigidity, athetosis and an expressionless facies may appear between two weeks and three months of age. Some patients do not develop kernicterus, and neurologic findings may not appear for many years. The type II Crigler-Najjar syndrome is characterized by an unconjugated serum bilirubin concentration that ranges from normal to 22 mg./dl. Kernicterus is unusual in this form of the disorder. Phenobarbital administration reduces the serum bilirubin concentration in adults with the type II disorder.

Arias, I.M. et al.: Chronic non-hemolytic unconjugated hyperbilirubinemia with glucuronyl transferase deficiency: clinical, biochemical, pharmacologic and genetic evidence of heterogeneity. *Am. J. Med. 47*:395, 1969.

7. Gilbert's syndrome (constitutional hepatic dysfunction) is characterized by a persistent slight elevation (under 6 mg./dl., but, at times, as high as 12 mg./dl.) of the unconjugated bilirubin level in patients with otherwise normal liver function tests and absence of overt hemolysis. Jaundice is frequently not present.

Berk, P.B., Bloomer, J.R., Howe, R. B. and Berlin, N.I.: Constitutional hepatic dysfunction (Gilbert's syndrome). *Am. J. Med. 49*:296, 1970.

8. Hepatocellular disease. (See discussion under regurgitation jaundice.)
9. Maternal-fetal or fetal-fetal transfusion
10. Hyperviscosity syndrome of the newborn
11. Massive internal hemorrhage (cephalohematoma, subdural hematoma, subcapsular liver hemorrhage) may rarely cause jaundice in the newborn.
12. Pyloric stenosis, duodenal atresia or annular pancreas may be associated with unconjugated hyperbilirubinemia, perhaps due to increased enterohepatic circulation of bilirubin.

13. The use of excessive concentrations of a phenolic disinfectant detergent may cause neonatal hyperbilirubinemia.

Wysowski, D.K. et al.: Epidemic neonatal hyperbilirubinemia and use of a phenolic disinfectant detergent. *Pediatrics 61*:165, 1978.

II. Regurgitation jaundice
  A. Hepatocellular
    1. Viral
      a. Infectious hepatitis (hepatitis A) may occur at any age in epidemic or sporadic incidence. It is, however, extremely rare in the newborn. Prodromal symptoms in older children include anorexia, fatigue, headache, nausea, vomiting, fever, hepatomegaly and right upper quadrant pain. These are variations in the severity of this disease: hepatitis without jaundice, mild hepatitis with jaundice followed by recovery in six to eight weeks, fatal hepatitis simulating acute or subacute yellow atrophy, and chronic hepatitis.

        During the preicteric phase, urine urobilinogen, serum bilirubin and serum transaminase are the most helpful laboratory tests in establishing the presence of hepatocellular disease. During the icteric phase, severe hepatocellular damage is reflected by a decrease in the serum albumin and a rise in the serum bilirubin.

      b. Serum hepatitis (hepatitis B). Serum hepatitis is transmitted through the infusion of blood contaminated with the virus. Neonatal hepatitis may occur in some infants whose mothers have acute hepatitis B prenatally or in the first two months postpartum.

Gerety, R.J. and Schweitzer, I.L.: Viral hepatitis type B during pregnancy, the neonatal period, and infancy. *J. Pediatr. 90*:368, 1977.
Krugman, S. et al.: Viral hepatitis, type B. Studies on natural history and prevention re-examined. *N. Engl. J. Med. 300*:101, 1979.

      c. Chronic active (aggressive) hepatitis occurs predominantly in girls above ten years of age. The onset may be abrupt, resembling acute infectious hepatitis, but more commonly is insidious with some of the following symptoms: progressive jaundice, anorexia, fatigue, abdominal pain, arthralgia, fever and epistaxis. Spider nevi may be present early. There may be recurrent episodes of jaundice, fatigue, pleural pain and colitis. Endocrine changes include acne, amenorrhea, hirsutism, striae, giant hives, erythema multiforme, from that caused by infectious hepatitis occurs in 10 to 15 per cent and splenomegaly are additional findings. The serum bilirubin is usually 5 to 10 mg./dl. The SGOT usually does not exceed 500 units/ml. Hyperglobulinemia is also present.

Maddrey, W.C. and Cohen, S.A.: Acute and chronic hepatitis in adolescents. *Med. Cl. N. Am. 59*:1453, 1975.
Mistilis, S.P. and Blackburn, C.R.B.: Active chronic hepatitis. *Am. J. Med. 48*:484, 1970.

      d. Infectious mononucleosis. Hepatocellular damage indistinguishable from that caused by infectious hepatitis occurs in 10 to 15 per cent of patients with infectious mononucleosis. Differentiation is made on the basis of the peripheral blood smear and the heterophile agglutination test.

    e. Acute and subacute yellow atrophy. (See discussion of infectious hepatitis and of the chemical causes of jaundice.)

    f. Cytomegalovirus may cause hepatitis, pneumonitis, nephrosis, enteritis or meningoencephalitis in young infants. The clinical manifestations of jaundice in the first 24 hours of life, hepatosplenomegaly, petechiae and erythroblastemia may require differentiation from erythroblastosis fetalis and sepsis.

    g. Congenital rubella is characterized by regurgitative jaundice during the first few days of life. Other findings may include thrombocytopenic purpura, failure to thrive, cataracts, microcephaly, deafness and congenital heart disease.

    h. The virus of herpes simplex may cause hepatitis in both newborn and older infants.

2. Spirochetal

    a. Congenital syphilis: syphilitic hepatitis and late-developing syphilitic cirrhosis

    b. Canicola fever (Leptospira canicola); Weil's disease (Leptospira icterohaemorrhagiae). Jaundice occurs in about 50 per cent of patients with Weil's disease and in 15 per cent of those with other forms of leptospirosis.

3. Bacterial

    a. Sepsis. Severe or overwhelming infection is frequently accompanied by jaundice due to hemolysis and/or hepatitis, especially in newborn and young infants. Salmonellosis may produce hepatitis in infants. Brucellosis may cause a mild hepatitis in older children. A severe urinary tract infection may be a cause of jaundice in young infants and, occasionally, in an older child. Blood and urine cultures should be obtained.

Bernstein, J. and Brown, A.K.: Sepsis and jaundice in early infancy. *Pediatrics* 29:873, 1962.

Hamilton, J.R. and Sass-Kortsak, A.: Jaundice associated with severe bacterial infection in young infants. *J. Pediatr.* 63:121, 1963.

Navey, Y. and Friedman, A.: Urinary tract infection presenting with jaundice. *Pediatrics* 62:524, 1978.

Rooney, J.C., Hill, D.J. and Danks, D.M.: Jaundice associated with bacterial infection in the newborn. *Am. J. Dis. Child.* 122:39, 1971.

4. Protozoan

    a. Congenital toxoplasmosis may cause neonatal jaundice, hyperpyrexia, hepatosplenomegaly and purpura.

    b. Amebiasis may rarely produce jaundice as the result of a large solitary abscess or a diffuse amebic hepatitis.

5. Chemical. Any of the following agents may be responsible for hepatocellular damage. Acute poisoning may cause acute yellow atrophy while chronic intoxication may produce cirrhosis.

    a. Chloroform

    b. Carbon tetrachloride

    c. Arsenicals

    d. Gold

    e. Phosphorus

f. Nitrobenzene and its derivatives

g. Almost any drug may cause hepatocellular damage.

6. Mushroom poisoning

7. Cirrhosis

a. Syphilitic, congenital

b. Laennec's cirrhosis leads to anorexia, weight loss, nausea, vomiting, abdominal pain, enlargement of the abdomen, edema of the lower extremities, hematemesis, other hemorrhagic tendencies and jaundice. Acholic stools may appear in some patients. Symptoms are often insidious and may predate jaundice by some time.

8. Inborn errors of metabolism

a. Wilson's disease may first present as hepatic disease without neurologic or ophthalmologic findings. Adolescents with chronic active hepatitis, portal hypertension or cirrhosis should have a serum ceruloplasmin determination and a slit lamp examination for Kayser-Fleischer rings. Fulminant hepatitis may suddenly occur with jaundice, ascites and hepatic failure.

Werlin, S.L., Grand, R.J., Perman, J.A. and Watkins, J.B.: Diagnostic dilemmas of Wilson's disease: diagnosis and treatment. *Pediatrics* 62:47, 1978.

b. Galactosemia is characterized by the accumulation of galactose-1-phosphate and other metabolic products that presumably have a toxic effect on the liver. If the baby is receiving a galactose-containing formula, jaundice usually appears during the first or second week of life along with hepatomegaly, feeding difficulties, vomiting, diarrhea and failure to thrive. Cataracts may develop later. Both the one-minute and the total serum bilirubin values are elevated. Albuminuria and galactosuria are present. Since galactose reduces Benedict's solution, there will be a positive Clinitest reaction but a negative reaction to a glucose oxidase dipstick (Clinistix) if the infant is receiving galactose in the formula. The diagnosis is established by galactose-1-phosphate uridyl transferase assay in erythrocytes. The clinical status improves and the jaundice promptly disappears on a lactose-free diet.

c. Hereditary fructose intolerance may rarely cause jaundice and a reducing substance in the urine if the infant is receiving fructose.

d. Hereditary tyrosinemia may cause conjugated hyperbilirubinemia. Other symptoms include vomiting, diarrhea, failure to thrive, rickets and hypoglycemia.

B. Hepatocanalicular. Damage to the ampullae and the primary bile canaliculi may occur in such widely dissimilar diseases as erythroblastosis fetalis or Laennec's cirrhosis. Such pathology during the course of infectious hepatitis may lead to chronicity of the disease. The injured ductal epithelium allows leakage of fluid and sodium bilirubinate followed by concentration of the remaining solids within the lumen. The resulting intraluminal bile thrombi may introduce a secondary obstructive factor. Fibrosis or edema may also cause external obstruction of the ampullae or primary canaliculi. In patients with hepatocanalicular disease, the laboratory findings are those of biliary obstruction. Cholestatic hepatitis is a chronic form of hepatitis characterized by pruritus and laboratory evidences of intrahepatic bile stasis such as bile in the urine and elevation of the direct serum bilirubin and alkaline phosphatase.

C. Obstructive

1. Congenital

a. Congenital atresia of the extrahepatic bile ducts. Since the onset of icterus in this disorder often coincides with that of physiologic jaundice, biliary atresia is frequently not suspected until the infant is about three weeks of age. The stools are acholic, but they frequently have a pale yellow appearance caused by an outer pigmented ring of stained intestinal secretions and epithelial cells. Because of the rapidity of the development of cirrhosis in infants with atresia of the extrahepatic biliary tree, the cause of obstructive jaundice in the newborn should optimally be established during the first and not later than the second month of life. Although so-called classic histologic and laboratory findings have been described in biliary atresia, there are many exceptions to this pattern (e.g., urobilinogen may be found in the stools or urine, there may be a history of normally pigmented stools, jaundice may have been persistent from the early days of life, the serum bilirubin rather than continuing to rise may actually fall, and the jaundice may appear to lessen.) Differentiation between biliary atresia and other causes of neonatal cholestatic jaundice requires an [131]I rose bengal excretion test, a percutaneous liver biopsy and an operative cholangiogram.

b. Abnormalities in the development of hepatic bile ducts with or without an associated extrahepatic atresia have variously been termed hypoplasia of intrahepatic bile ducts, paucity of intrahepatic bile ducts and intrahepatic biliary atresia. This group of lesions, largely congenital or, in some cases, thought to be acquired, is not well understood. Diagnosis is possible only by biopsy. Usually, the findings are identical with those of congenital atresia of the major bile ducts. Occasionally, however, the intrahepatic ducts are not completely atretic. In this event, some bilirubin may be excreted into the intestinal tract.

An association between hypoplasia of the intrahepatic ducts and a characteristic facies has been described with a prominent forehead, deeply set eyes, mild hypertelorism, a straight nose and a small, pointed chin. A murmur consistent with pulmonary stenosis or pulmonary artery hypoplasia, vertebral arch defects and growth retardation are other findings.

Alagille, D., Odievre, M., Gautier, M. and Dommergues, J.P.: Hepatic ductular hypoplasia associated with characteristic facies, vertebral malformations, retarded physical, mental, and sexual development, and cardiac murmurs. *J. Pediatr.* 86:63, 1975.

c. The term "inspissated bile syndrome" has been applied to a group of infants who have prolonged obstructive jaundice associated with erythroblastosis fetalis characterized by persistence of jaundice over three weeks, a rise in both direct and indirect bilirubin, maternal-infant blood group incompatibility and the presence of other clinical manifestations of hemolytic disease of the newborn. Rarely, an infant with maternal-infant blood group incompatibility shows elevation of the cord blood direct bilirubin level and evidence of biliary obstruction.

d. Fibrocystic disease may cause obstructive jaundice.

e. "Neonatal hepatitis," or neonatal jaundice with giant cell transformation of the hepatic parenchyma, are terms applied to a clinical and histologic pattern associated with cholestasis and obstructive jaundice in the newborn. Jaundice begins in the early weeks of life and, along with dark urine and acholic stools, may persist for months. Moderate hepatomegaly and splenomegaly are commonly found. The exact etiology is not known. Histologic examination demonstrates replacement of normal parenchyma by multinucleated giant liver cells, lack of intercellular bile canaliculi and absence of bile from efferent bile passages. Differentiation from congenital atresia of the extrahepatic biliary tree may not be possible on the basis of clinical history and physical examination. [131]I rose bengal excretion test may help in the evaluation of biliary obstruction with less than 10 per cent excretion of rose bengal in the stool. Percutaneous liver biopsy may also provide important diagnostic information. Operative cholangiograms may offer the only means for definitive diagnosis. Giant cell transformation of the liver cells has also been described in infants with hemolytic disease of the newborn, congenital spherocytosis, herpes simplex hepatitis and cytomegalovirus disease.

Brough, A.J. and Bernstein, J.: Liver biopsy in the diagnosis of infantile obstructive jaundice. *Pediatrics 43*:519, 1969.

f. Alpha$_1$-antitrypsin deficiency may account for a highly variable clinical picture. Prolonged obstructive jaundice may begin in the first ten weeks of life — occasionally, the first day, with acholic stools, dark urine and hepatomegaly. Some infants demonstrate only abnormal liver function tests while others have no evidence of liver disease. Cirrhosis and portal hypertension may develop.

Andres, J. et al.: Alpha$_1$-fetoprotein in neonatal hepatobiliary disease. *J. Pediatr. 91*:217, 1977.
Odievre, M. et al.: Alpha$_1$-antitrypsin deficiency and liver disease in children: phenotypes, manifestations, and prognosis. *Pediatrics 57*:226, 1976.
Sveger, T.: Alpha$_1$-antitrypsin deficiency in early childhood. *Pediatrics 62*:22, 1978.

g. Parenteral alimentation in infants may be complicated by conjugated hyperbilirubinemia, elevation of both serum transaminase and alkaline phosphatase and hyperammonemia.

Bernstein, J., Chang, C.H., Brough, A.J. and Heidelberger, K.P.: Conjugated hyperbilirubinemia in infancy associated with parenteral alimentation. *J. Pediatr. 90*:361, 1977.
Vain, N.E. and Bedros, A.A.: Liver disease in infants receiving total parenteral nutrition. *Pediatrics 63*:110, 1979.

h. Glycogenosis types III and IV may cause jaundice in young infants.

i. Benign recurrent cholestasis, which begins in childhood or early adulthood, is characterized by intermittent periods of cholestasis that may last one to six months.

Heathcote, J., Deodhar, K.P., Scheuer, P.F. and Sherlock, S.: Intrahepatic cholestasis in childhood. *N. Engl. J. Med. 295*:801, 1976.
Ruymann, F.B., Takeuchi, A. and Boyce, H.W.: Idiopathic recurrent cholestasis. *Pediatrics 45*:812, 1970.
Stark, H.: Benign recurrent cholestasis in a child. *Pediatrics 41*:636, 1968.
Watson, G.H. and Miller, V.: Arteriohepatic dysplasia: familial pulmonary arterial stenosis with neonatal liver disease. *Arch. Dis. Child. 48*:459, 1973.

j. Byler disease, a fatal familial intrahepatic cholestasis in an Amish kindred, is characterized by jaundice with intermittent exacerbations, hepatosplenomegaly, steatorrhea, failure to thrive and dwarfing. Gastrointestinal symptoms in the form of loose, foul-smelling stools antedate the onset of jaundice by one to eight months.

Clayton, R.J., Iber, F.L., Ruebner, B.H. and McKusick, V.A.: Byler disease. *Am. J. Dis. Child. 117*:112, 1969.

k. Congenital cystic dilatation of the common bile duct (choledochal cyst) in young infants may cause obstructive jaundice with jaundice and acholic stools simulating biliary atresia. In older infants and children, abdominal pain, a palpable mass in the right hypochondrium and obstructive jaundice constitute other findings. These may occur singly or together. They are usually intermittent but occasionally persistent. Fever occurs if cholangitis develops. Portal hypertension may ensue. An upper gastrointestinal series may show displacement of the duodenum to the left and anteriorly. Cholangiograms are diagnostically helpful.

Harris, V.J. and Kahler, J.: Choledochal cyst: delayed diagnosis in a jaundiced infant. *Pediatrics 62*:235, 1978.

l. The common bile duct may be obstructed by a bile plug. Surgical exploration and transcholecystic cholangiography establish the diagnosis.

Bernstein, J., Braylan, R. and Brough, A.J.: Bile plug syndrome: a correctable cause of obstructive jaundice in infants. *Pediatrics 43*:273, 1969.

m. The Dubin-Johnson syndrome, characterized by chronic or intermittent jaundice that fluctuates in intensity, may be evident in the neonatal period or appear in childhood. The serum bilirubin, which may range from 2 to 20 mg./dl., is comprised of 25 to 75 per cent direct-reacting bilirubin. Patients may be either asymptomatic or report vague abdominal pain, fatigue, anorexia, vomiting, diarrhea, dark urine and pale stools. The liver may be enlarged and tender. Bile and urobilinogen are found in the urine. Direct and total serum bilirubin concentrations are elevated. Liver biopsy demonstrates lipofuscin pigment in the liver cells.

n. Rotor's syndrome, a familial disorder, is similar to the Dubin-Johnson syndrome except for absence of the abnormal pigment.

Arias, I.M.: Chronic familial nonhemolytic anemia with conjugated bilirubin in the serum. *Gastroent. 43*:588, 1962.

Dubin, I.N.: Rotor's syndrome and chronic idiopathic jaundice. *Arch. Int. Med. 110*:823, 1962.

2. Biliary cirrhosis
    a. Obstructive biliary cirrhosis
    b. Congenital acholangic biliary cirrhosis
    c. Fibroxanthomatous biliary cirrhosis
    d. Biliary cirrhosis associated with cystic fibrosis
3. Cholelithiasis is a rare cause of jaundice in children. The prevalence of gallstones in patients with sickle cell disease ranges from 5 to 35 per cent. Differentiation between abdominal crises, cholecystitis and cholelithiasis may be difficult. Cholecystograms are indicated in the older child with sickle cell anemia who is seen because of abdominal pain.

Ariyan, S., Shessel, F.S. and Pickett, L.K.: Cholecystitis and cholelithiasis masking as abdominal crises in sickle cell disease. *Pediatrics 58*:252, 1976.

4. Neoplasms of the liver and bile ducts may cause jaundice through obstruction of the common hepatic or bile duct. This is extremely rare in childhood.
    a. Primary neoplasms
        (1) Adenomas may originate from parenchymal liver cells or bile duct epithelium. Cystic adenomas of bile duct epithelium may occur. "Hamartomas" comprise a disorganized mass of liver cells, bile ducts and blood vessels.
        (2) Multiple small cysts may rise from the bile ducts. Patients with polycystic kidneys also have hepatic cysts or hepatic fibrosis. Occasionally, large solitary cysts of unknown origin occur.
        (3) Hemangiomas, endotheliomas, hemangioendotheliomas, fibromas, teratomas, carcinomas and sarcomas are other primary hepatic neoplasms.
        (4) Hodgkin's disease
    b. Metastatic neoplasms: neuroblastoma
5. Inflammatory lesions
    a. Abscess: bacterial; amebic
    b. Tuberculoma
6. Parasites
    a. Amebiasis may cause cholecystitis, hepatitis or an obstructing liver abscess.
    b. Ascaris rarely obstructs the common duct.
    c. Echinococcus
7. Obstruction of extrahepatic bile ducts
    a. Peritoneal adhesions
    b. Leukemia may produce obstruction by enlargement of the lymph nodes at the porta hepatis.
    c. Hodgkin's disease
    d. Post-traumatic
8. Chlorpromazine, trimethoprim-sulfamethoxazole and other drugs may rarely cause jaundice in children because of cholestatic hepatitis.

## GENERAL REFERENCES

Andres, J.M., Mathis, R.K. and Waker, W.A.: Liver disease in infants. Part I: Developmental hepatology and mechanisms of liver dysfunction. *J. Pediatr. 90*:686, 1977.

Mathis, R.K., Andres, J.M. and Walker, W.A.: Liver disease in children. Part II. Hepatic disease states. *J. Pediatr. 90*:864, 1977.

Odell, G.B.: Neonatal jaundice. *In* Popper, H. and Schaffner. F., (eds.): *Progress in Liver Disease.* New York, Grune and Stratton, 1976, p. 457.

Ostrow, J.D.: Jaundice in older children and adults. *JAMA 234*:522, 1975.

Sass-Kortsak, A.: Management of young infants presenting with direct-reacting hyperbilirubinemia. *Pediatr. Clin. N. Am. 21*:777, 1974.

Thaler, M.M.: Neonatal hyperbilirubinemia. *Semin. Hematol. 9*:107, 1972.

## ETIOLOGIC CLASSIFICATION OF JAUNDICE

I. Retention jaundice, 349
  A. Hemolytic, 349
    1. Maternal-infant blood group incompatibility
    2. Erythrocyte abnormalities
    3. Erythrocyte enzyme deficiencies
    4. Alpha-thalassemia
    5. Vitamin K overdose
  B. Nonhemolytic, 351
    1. Hepatic immaturity
    2. Hypothyroidism
    3. Drugs
    4. Breast-feeding
    5. Lucey-Driscoll syndrome
    6. Hereditary hepatic dysfunction
    7. Gilbert's syndrome
    8. Hepatocellular disease
    9. Maternal-fetal or fetal-fetal transfusion
    10. Hyperviscosity syndrome
    11. Massive internal hemorrhage
    12. Pyloric stenosis, duodenal atresia or annular pancreas
    13. Excessive phenolic disinfectant detergent

II. Regurgitation jaundice, 353
  A. Hepatocellular, 353
    1. Viral
    2. Spirochetal
    3. Bacterial
    4. Protozoan
    5. Chemical
    6. Mushroom poisoning
    7. Cirrhosis
    8. Inborn errors of metabolism
  B. Hepatocanalicular, 355
  C. Obstructive, 356
    1. Congenital
    2. Biliary cirrhosis
    3. Cholelithiasis
    4. Neoplasms
    5. Inflammatory lesions
    6. Parasitic infection
    7. Obstruction of extrahepatic bile ducts
    8. Drugs

# CHAPTER 39

# FAILURE TO GAIN: FAILURE TO THRIVE: WEIGHT LOSS

## PATTERNS OF WEIGHT GAIN

The greatest gain in weight during fetal development occurs just before birth, owing to the deposition of subcutaneous fat during the last trimester. A physiologic weight loss may occur three to four days after birth. Usually, the birth weight is regained by the tenth to the fourteenth day. Premature infants may experience a relatively larger physiologic weight loss and may require somewhat longer to regain their birth weight.

Weight gain during early infancy is relatively rapid, amounting to 5 or 6 and sometimes up to 10 ounces a week. In the latter half of the first year the gain is slower, 3 to 5 ounces a week. During the first year of life infants should demonstrate a steady weight gain. Failure to do so calls for a careful investigation. During infancy, regular weight gain and growth in length are perhaps the best indicators of normal nutrition and health. *As a general rule, if an infant fails to gain on a formula that is quantitatively and qualitatively correct, there is something wrong with the infant or the feeding situation and not with the formula.* Alterations in the formula or changing to other preparations will usually not correct this problem.

The caloric requirement of the infant depends upon his basal metabolic rate, the rapidity of growth, the degree of activity, the amount of nonutilized food that is lost in the excreta and the specific dynamic action of food. Since adipose tissue is not as active metabolically as other tissue, a malnourished infant with little or no subcutaneous fat has a higher level of metabolism relative to his weight than a normal infant of the same age or weight. Thus, the caloric requirement of the undernourished child per unit of body weight is greater than that of the well-nourished infant. This requirement is also increased in malnourished infants because of the active anabolic processes that occur during recovery. Significant differences in activity among infants and children also account for variability in food requirements. The allowance for activity is much greater in active, kicking, tense infants than in placid, somnolent babies. Crying may raise metabolic requirements 100 per cent or more above the basal metabolic level.

In the presence of diarrhea or impaired absorption, fecal loss of food may be as great as 30 to 40 per cent. Fever causes a significant increase in the total energy requirement. Each degree Fahrenheit elevation in the body temperature increases caloric needs by about 7 per cent. In the first few days of life, the total caloric requirement is about 80 calories per kilogram per day. During the first year of life a normal infant requires 100 to 120 calories per kilogram of body weight. This requirement decreases about 10 Kcal./kg. during each succeeding 3-year period.

These figures are merely an approximation; the exact requirement varies from one infant to another. Though these considerations are important in feeding, the best demonstration of caloric adequacy is regular gain in weight. The basal metabolism of the premature infant is relatively less than that of the more mature infant, and as noted earlier, heat production due to muscular activity is relatively less. The rate of growth, however, is much greater.

During the second year of life, the rate of weight gain continues to diminish, the infant gaining 2½ ounces a week. Instead of a steady weight gain each week, the weight may remain constant for two or three weeks at a time. This pattern of periodic rather than constant weight gain becomes more pronounced in older children. From the age of two to five years, the increments in weight are less than at any other time in childhood. The average yearly gain in weight then is 4 to 5 pounds. After the age of five, the increments in weight begin to increase in contrast to the increments in height, which continue to decrease. An acceleration in the increments in weight occurs during the prepuberal years, girls showing this weight acceleration about two years before boys. These different patterns for weight and height increments cause the prepubertal child to appear more stocky than the preschool child.

## ETIOLOGIC CLASSIFICATION OF FAILURE TO THRIVE OR LOSS OF WEIGHT

I. Qualitative or quantitative inadequacy of food intake
   A. Economic privation, starvation
      1. Marasmus due to inadequate caloric intake
      2. Chronic protein malnutrition, kwashiorkor
   B. Anorexia due to organic or psychologic factors
   C. Feeding difficulties due to organic factors
      1. Congenital anomalies such as glossoptosis or cleft palate
      2. Dyspnea causes difficulty in feeding.
      3. Infants and children who are developmentally retarded may feed poorly and therefore fail to thrive.
   D. Calorically inadequate formula. Breast-fed babies may fail to gain adequately because of an inadequate supply of breast milk. Although some infants will appear hungry, others will not cry excessively.
   E. Child neglect with the infant not fed adequately
II. Defects in assimilation of food
   A. Inadequate digestion
      1. Cystic fibrosis. Failure to gain in spite of hunger and a large food intake is an early symptom of this disease.

Shwachman, H., Redmond, A. and Khaw, K-T.: Studies in cystic fibrosis. Report of 130 patients diagnosed under 3 months of age over a 20-year period. *Pediatrics* 46:335, 1970.

      2. The syndrome of pancreatic insufficiency, failure to thrive and neutropenia.
   B. Inadequate absorption
      1. Celiac syndrome (see page 304)
         a. Gluten-induced enteropathy. Failure to thrive is not an early symptom in patients with celiac disease. Vomiting and perhaps diarrhea may occur first, followed by irregular weight gain. Loss of weight

does, of course, become a prominent manifestation in children with untreated celiac disease. Some patients with celiac disease do not have diarrhea but present with failure to thrive and constipation.

McNicholl, B. and Egan-Mitchel, B.: Infancy celiac disease without diarrhea. *Pediatrics* 49:85, 1972.

    b. Giardiasis
    c. Gastrointestinal allergy
    d. Tuberculosis of mesenteric nodes
    e. Biliary atresia
  C. Systemic infections may interfere with normal assimilation. Congenital infections (e.g., rubella) may cause failure to thrive.

Michaels, R.H. and Kenny, F.M.: Postnatal growth retardation in congenital rubella. *Pediatrics* 43:251, 1969.

  D. Protein-losing gastroenteropathy
  E. Hirschsprung's disease
III. Loss of food substances
  A. Vomiting (consult discussion of this symptom in Chapter 31)
  B. Diarrhea (consult discussion of this symptom in Chapter 32)
IV. Failure of utilization or increased metabolism
  A. Excessive crying or activity; restlessness
  B. Prolonged fever
  C. Repeated acute or chronic infections.
    1. Prenatal viral infection or neonatal bacterial sepsis

Hanshaw, J.B. and Dudgeon, J.A.: *Viral Diseases of the Fetus and Newborn.* W. B. Saunders Co., Philadelphia, 1978.

    2. Repeated respiratory infections
    3. Tuberculosis
    4. Intestinal parasites
    5. Histoplasmosis
    6. Urinary tract infections
    7. Sepsis in newborn infants, especially prematures, may be primarily characterized by failure to thrive. Poor feeding, loss of vigor, regurgitation and irritability may be associated symptoms.
  D. The possibility of a malignancy should always be kept in mind with a history of weight loss or unexplained listlessness.
  E. Cardiac disorders. Failure to gain may be the first indication of cardiac disease in infants. As long as an infant with congenital heart disease gains weight normally, his arterial oxygen saturation has not been reduced to a critical level. Failure to gain may be an early symptom of endocardial fibroelastosis and of impending congestive heart failure, especially in infants with ventricular septal defects. Difficulty in feeding due to dyspnea and cough and resultant poor weight gain may be the first manifestations of cardiac failure.

    In addition to appraisal of the heart, determination of the blood pressure is important in infants who are not thriving. Early symptoms in infants with coarctation of the aorta may be anorexia, vomiting, tiring during feedings and failure to gain weight adequately. Older children with pheochromocytomas sometimes present a picture of cachexia.

F. Chronic pulmonary disease; hypoxia. A roentgenogram of the chest is indicated in infants who fail to thrive. Occasionally, unsuspected chronic pneumonitis will be found.

G. Renal disease
   1. Chronic renal insufficiency leading to metabolic acidosis
   2. Renal tubular acidosis (RTA) (idiopathic renal acidosis, hyperchloremic acidosis with nephrocalcinosis) is characterized by a hyperchloremic acidosis. The distal form of RTA (type I) is characterized by urine with a pH greater than 6 regardless of degree of acidosis. The proximal form (type II) demonstrates normal acidification of the urine with a pH less than 5. Type I renal acidosis may be characterized by vomiting, anorexia, constipation, polyuria, polydipsia, dehydration, hypotonia and failure to gain weight between the fourth and sixth months of life. Type II RTA demonstrates growth failure and vomiting but the infants are otherwise asymptomatic. In older children, renal tubular acidosis is characterized by understature, rickets, polyuria, polydipsia and nephrocalcinosis.

Nash, M.A., Torrando, A.D., Griefer, I., Spitzer, A. and Edelmann, C.M., Jr.: Renal tubular acidosis in infants and children. *J. Pediatr. 80*:738, 1972.

   3. Other types of renal disease such as chronic pyelonephritis, chronic glomerulonephritis, hydronephrosis or polycystic disease of the kidneys may lead to failure to thrive. Failure to gain and grow is probably the most common presenting complaint in infants with serious anomalies of the urinary tract.

H. Idiopathic hypercalcemia of infancy is characterized biochemically by hypercalcemia and clinically by anorexia, vomiting, constipation, failure to thrive, irritability, thirst, fever, hypotonia and muscle weakness. The transient mild form begins between three and seven months of age. The severe form, which begins earlier, is associated with hypertension, mental retardation, azotemia, thirst and polyuria. A characteristic elfin face (Williams elfin facies) occurs in the severe form: full, pouting cheeks, large mouth, prominent upper lip, flat bridge, turned-up nose, hypertelorism and epicanthal folds. The facies may not, however, be sufficiently characteristic to suggest the disorder. Idiopathic hypercalcemia with failure to thrive may be clinically indistinguishable from infantile renal acidosis. Hereditary parathyroid hyperplasia with hypercalcemia may also cause failure to thrive.

Fraser, D., Kidd, B.S.L., Kooh, S.W. and Paunier, L.: A new look at infantile hypercalcemia. *Pediatr. Clin. N. Am. 13*:503, 1966.
Goldbloom, R.B., Gillis, D.A. and Prasad, M.: Hereditary parathyroid hyperplasia: a surgical emergency of early infancy. *Pediatrics 49*:514, 1972.

I. Hepatic insufficiency
J. Bartter's syndrome causes severe failure to thrive in the early months of life. Clinical manifestations include vomiting, constipation, hypokalemia, hypochloremia and, at times, hypomagnesemia.

Simopoulos, A.P. and Bartter, F.C.: Growth characteristics and factors influencing growth in Bartter's syndrome. *J. Pediatr. 81*:56, 1972.

K. Chronic anemia

L. Endocrine disorders
  1. Hyperthyroidism. Although these patients commonly have a large food intake, they may lose weight.
  2. Hypothyroidism. Infants and children with hypothyroidism do not thrive well, in part due to difficulty in sucking and swallowing and to lethargy. Failure to thrive may be the first symptom of congenital hypothyroidism.
  3. Diabetes. Failure to gain weight or rapid loss of weight may be early manifestations of this disease.
M. Storage diseases
  1. Glycogenosis
  2. Infantile Gaucher's disease is characterized by physical and mental retardation, splenomegaly, hepatomegaly and neurologic symptoms. Niemann-Pick disease in infants is characterized by physical and intellectual retardation. Massive hepatosplenomegaly is also present.
  3. Wolman's disease is characterized by failure to thrive, steatorrhea, hepatosplenomegaly and calcified adrenals.
N. Inborn errors of metabolism may present with poor feeding, lethargy and failure to thrive.
  1. Galactosemia. Infants with this disorder may demonstrate jaundice during the neonatal period. Failure to thrive is an early symptom, accompanied, at times, by vomiting and diarrhea. The liver becomes enlarged. Galactosemia and albuminuria occur. Cataracts and mental retardation may develop if the disease is unrecognized for some time. Urine may be screened easily for galactose by finding a positive Clinitest reaction in the presence of a negative Testape or Clinistix test. Definitive methods may then be used to determine the presence of galactose. The diagnosis is confirmed by assay of galactose-1-phosphate uridyl transferase activity in erythrocytes.
  2. The de Toni-Fanconi syndrome is characterized by hypophosphatemia, renal hyperaminoaciduria, organic aciduria and renal glycosuria. Hyperchloremic acidosis, hypokalemia, polyuria and albuminuria may be associated findings. Cystinosis, a recessive disorder, is the most common cause of the Fanconi syndrome. A number of other etiologies, such as heavy metal poisoning, may account for damage to the renal tubules. Failure to thrive is an early finding in these infants, along with polydipsia, lassitude and muscle weakness. Older children demonstrate understature, resistant rickets and, occasionally, photophobia. The diagnosis of cystinosis may be established by slit lamp examination of the cornea or study of the bone marrow.

Schneider, J.A., Wong, V. and Seegmiller, J.E.: The early diagnosis of cystinosis. *J. Pediatr.* 74:114, 1969.

  3. Kinky hair disease
  4. Hypophosphatasia. Failure to thrive may occur in the first six months of life in these patients along with anorexia, irritability, vomiting, fever and convulsions.
  5. Hereditary fructose intolerance. With young children, clinical manifestations include failure to thrive, persistent vomiting, hypoglycemia and hepatosplenomegaly.

6. Homocystinuria
7. Hereditary tyrosinemia
8. Almost all of the other inborn errors of metabolism are characterized by failure to thrive if the baby does not die in the immediate newborn period. Often, symptoms and findings include jaundice, hepatomegaly, intractable metabolic acidosis, ketosis, dehydration, anorexia, lethargy, vomiting, diarrhea, convulsions, coma, unusual urine odor, abnormal hair, unusual facies and macroglossia. The specific diagnosis depends on studies such as urine for metabolic genetic screening, including examination for organic acids.

Aleck, K.A. and Shapiro, L.J.: Genetic-metabolic considerations in the sick neonate. *Pediatr. Clin. N. Am. 25*:431, 1978.
Burton, B.K. and Nadler, H.L.: Clinical diagnosis of the inborn errors of metabolism in the neonatal period. *Pediatrics 61*:398, 1978.
Nyhan, W.L.: Approach to the diagnosis of overwhelming metabolic disease in early infancy. *Cur. Prob. Pediatr.* 7:3 (Apr.) 1977.
O'Brien, D. and Goodman, S.I.: The critically ill child: acute metabolic disease in infancy and early childhood. *Pediatrics 46*:620, 1970.
Scriver, C. and Rosenberg, L.E.: *Amino Acid Metabolism and its Disorders*. Philadelphia, W. B. Saunders Co., 1973.

O. Miscellaneous
1. Vitamin A poisoning. Anorexia and malnutrition are part of the clinical manifestations of this disease process.
2. Progressive diaphyseal dysplasia. Children with this syndrome do not thrive. They have muscular weakness, a waddling gait and characteristic diaphyseal changes on roentgenographic examination of the long bones.
3. Chondrodysplasia punctata. Most of these patients fail to thrive, and death frequently occurs in the first year of life. Some, however, develop normally. The tip of the nose is flattened and the nasal bridge depressed.

Sheffield, L.J., Danks, D.M., Mayne, U. and Hutchinson, L.A.: Chrondrodysplasia punctata—23 cases of a mild and relatively common variety. *J. Pediatr.* 89:916, 1976.

4. Leprechaunism (Donohue's syndrome) is characterized by failure to thrive; an elfin facies with large, low-set ears; flat nasal bridge; thickened lips; micrognathia; facial hirsutism; and prominence of the clitoris.

Summitt, R.L. and Favara, B.E.: Leprechaunism (Donohue's syndrome): a case report. *J. Pediatr.* 74:601, 1969.

5. Fetal alcohol syndrome is characterized by failure to thrive; central nervous system dysfunction with microcephaly and mental retardation; facial anomalies including short palpebral fissures; short, upturned nose with hypoplastic philtrum; thinned upper vermilion border of the lip; and retrognathia.

Clarren, S.K. and Smith, D.W.: The fetal alcohol syndrome. *N. Engl. J. Med. 298*:1063, 1978.

6. Fetal anticonvulsant syndromes

Smith, D.W.: Teratogenicity of anticonvulsant medications. *Am. J. Dis. Child. 131*:1337, 1977.

V. Neurologic and psychologic
A. Lack of individual care and deficient environmental stimulation may contribute to poor physical growth during infancy.

B. Infants with cerebral damage, mental retardation or cerebral palsy often do not thrive. Although children who demonstrate excessive muscular activity may have caloric needs considerably above the average, because of feeding difficulties their caloric intake is often less than that of normal children.

C. Subdural hematoma should be considered in all infants who fail to thrive. Convulsions, vomiting and irritability are common associated symptoms.

D. Diencephalic syndrome due to intracranial neoplasms in the region of the hypothalamus and third ventricle in infants and children under two years of age is characterized by a paradoxical alertness, euphoria and hyperactivity in the presence of emaciation. The appetite is normal or increased. Vomiting may occur irregularly. Pallor, nystagmus and tremor may not be noted. The usual signs of intracranial hypertension are absent early.

DeSousa, A.L., Kalsbeck, J.E., Mealey, J., Jr. and Fitzgerald, J.: Diencephalic syndrome and its relation to opticochiasmatic glioma: review of twelve cases. *Neurosurgery* 4:207, 1979.

E. Leigh's syndrome or subacute necrotizing encephalomyelopathy begins in infancy with failure to thrive, recurrent vomiting, dysphagia, ptosis, rolling eye movements, extraocular palsies, irregular, rapid and sighing respirations, sobbing, ataxia, hypotonia and developmental regression.

Burr, I.M., Slonim, A.E., Danish, R.K., Godoth, N. and Butler, I.J.: Diencephalic syndrome revisited. *J. Pediatr.* 88:439, 1976.
Hirschman, G.H. and Chan, J.C.M.: Complex acid-base disorders in subacute necrotizing encephalomyelopathy (Leigh's syndrome). *Pediatrics* 61:278, 1978.

F. Infants whose failure to thrive is associated with maternal deprivation may have an inadequate caloric intake either because they are not offered sufficient food or because they do not eat what is offered. Parenting disorders are discussed further on page 529.

Fischhoff, J., Whitten, C.F. and Pettit, M.G.: A psychiatric study of mothers of infants with growth failure secondary to maternal deprivation. *J. Pediatr.* 79:209, 1971.
Leonard, M.F., Rhymes, J.P. and Solnit, A.J.: Failure to thrive in infants. *Am. J. Dis. Child.* 111:660, 1966.
Whitten, C.F., Pettit, M.G. and Fischhoff, J.: Evidence that growth failure from maternal deprivation is secondary to undereating. *JAMA 209*:1675, 1969.

## GENERAL APPROACH TO FAILURE TO THRIVE

The pediatric interview and the physical examination are of pre-eminent importance in the initial appraisal of failure to thrive. If the initial impression suggests a psychosocial etiology, a period of observation in the hospital with a normal diet and developmentally appropriate nursing care will soon be confirmatory; that is, the baby will gain weight and develop rapidly. Most babies with failure to thrive are in this group. If there is diagnostic uncertainty, selected laboratory procedures may be obtained including CBC, urinalysis, serum electrolytes, calcium, BUN, creatinine and $T_4$ and $T_3$. Other studies (e.g., urine for genetic screening, bone age, skull films, sweat chloride, carotene) may be obtained as appears clinically appropriate.

### GENERAL REFERENCE

Sills, R.H.: Failure to thrive. The role of clinical and laboratory evaluation. *Am. J. Dis. Child.* 132:967, 1978.

# ETIOLOGIC CLASSIFICATION OF FAILURE TO THRIVE OR LOSS OF WEIGHT

I. Qualitative or quantitative inadequacy of food intake, 362
   A. Economic privation, starvation, 362
      1. Marasmus
      2. Chronic protein malnutrition (kwashiorkor)
   B. Anorexia, 362
   C. Feeding difficulties from organic factors, 362
      1. Congenital anomalies
      2. Dyspnea
      3. Developmental retardation
   D. Calorically inadequate formula, 362
   E. Child neglect, 362
II. Defects in assimilation of food, 362
   A. Inadequate digestion, 362
      1. Cystic fibrosis
      2. Syndrome of pancreatic insufficiency, failure to thrive and neutropenia
   B. Inadequate absorption, 362
      1. Celiac syndrome
   C. Systemic infections, 363
   D. Protein-losing gastroenteropathy, 363
   E. Hirschsprung's disease, 363
III. Loss of food substances, 363
   A. Vomiting, 363
   B. Diarrhea, 363
IV. Failure of utilization or increased metabolism, 363
   A. Excessive crying or activity; restlessness, 363
   B. Prolonged fever, 363
   C. Repeated acute or chronic infections, 363
      1. Prenatal viral infection or neonatal bacterial sepsis
      2. Repeated respiratory infections
      3. Tuberculosis
      4. Intestinal parasites
      5. Histoplasmosis
      6. Urinary tract infections
      7. Sepsis
   D. Malignancy, 363
   E. Cardiac disorders, 363
   F. Chronic pulmonary disease; hypoxia, 364

G. Renal disease, 364
   1. Chronic renal insufficiency leading to metabolic acidosis
   2. Renal tubular acidosis
   3. Chronic pyelonephritis, chronic glomerulonephritis, hydronephrosis, polycystic disease of kidneys
H. Idiopathic hypercalcemia of infancy, 364
I. Hepatic insufficiency, 364
J. Bartter's syndrome, 364
K. Chronic anemia, 364
L. Endocrine disorders, 365
   1. Hyperthyroidism
   2. Hypothyroidism
   3. Diabetes
M. Storage diseases, 365
   1. Glycogenosis
   2. Infantile Gaucher's disease
   3. Wolman's disease
N. Inborn errors of metabolism, 365
   1. Galactosemia
   2. de Toni-Fanconi syndrome
   3. Kinky hair disease
   4. Hypophosphatasia
   5. Hereditary fructose intolerance
   6. Homocystinuria
   7. Hereditary tyrosinemia
   8. Other metabolic disorders
O. Miscellaneous, 366
   1. Vitamin A poisoning
   2. Progressive diaphyseal dysplasia
   3. Chondrodysplasia punctata
   4. Leprechaunism
   5. Fetal alcohol syndrome
   6. Fetal anticonvulsant syndromes
V. Neurologic and psychologic, 366
   A. Poor care and environmental stimulation, 366
   B. Cerebral damage, mental retardation, cerebral palsy, 367
   C. Subdural hematoma, 367
   D. Diencephalic syndrome, 367
   E. Leigh's syndrome, 367
   F. Parenting disorders, 367

# CHAPTER 40

# UNDERSTATURE

The chief feature that sets infants and children apart from adults is the dynamic nature of their growth and development. Since growth in height and weight are sensitive reflections of the health of a child, an understanding of these processes is necessary for a proper appraisal of the pediatric patient. The periodic assessment of infants and children permits the early detection of growth deficiencies and pathologic processes, both organic and psychologic, and the prompt institution of preventive and corrective measures. Growth in a child is almost synonymous with health.

In recent years, studies of growth and development have become increasingly detailed, and a number of methods have been developed to assist the physician in the evaluation of the adequacy of these processes. All methods are projected on the premise that growth progresses in a regular, orderly sequence from infancy to maturity. The speed of development and the final proportions achieved vary from child to child, but the pattern for all is similar and, within limits, predictable.

The best approach is a long-term one in which the child is evaluated in terms of his own velocity or rate of growth. The pattern of development for an individual child may be determined by observation over a period of time. Though all suggested techniques of growth assessment involve making some comparison of the individual to his age group, the criterion for the practical clinical importance of any method is how well it permits assessment of the individual in terms of his own potentiality.

## MEASUREMENTS OF PHYSICAL GROWTH

A few selected measurements should be routinely obtained. In infants, these include weight, head circumference and length. In older children, these are the height and weight. Unless these measurements are made accurately, they are obviously of no value. The same technique of measurement should be used each time.

**Technique of Measurements.** For the measurement of head circumference, a nonstretchable measuring tape is passed over the most prominent part of the occiput and above the supraorbital ridges. The total length is more readily and accurately obtained in children up to three years of age in the recumbent position. In young infants, it is, of course, difficult to obtain an entirely accurate measurement of body length unless special measuring devices (neonatomer or infantomer) are used with the help of an assistant. Balance scales of the beam type should be used for the determination of body weight.

Percentile curves, developed by the National Center for Health Statistics and based on large and representative samples of children, for length or height, weight and head circumference are included as an appendix (p. 585). Curves are available for two age groups—birth to 36 months and 2 to 18 years—with separate curves for boys and for girls. For the younger child, there are percentile curves for body weight for age, length for age, body weight for length and head circumference for age. In the older age group, curves are available for height for age and weight for age. In addition, weight for height curves are available for prepubescent boys and girls.

The curves represent the fifth, tenth, twenty-fifth, seventy-fifth, ninetieth and ninety-fifth percentiles. For the young child, the weights are taken with the child nude while in the older child they include a light examination garment. The length curves for the young children (birth to 36 months) are based on recumbent length without shoes. Height in the older children reflects stature in stocking feet.

The body measurements should be evaluated according to their percentile ranking. These rankings should then be compared to each other to determine whether they fall more or less within the same percentile group. Comparison of these percentile rankings with those of previous examinations should be made in order to detect any significant acceleration or deceleration in the rate of growth.

National Center for Health Statistics: NCHS Growth Charts, 1976. Monthly Vital Statistics Report, Vol. 25, No. 3, Supp. (HRA) 76-1120. Rockville, Maryland, Health Resources Administration, 1976.

National Center for Health Statistics: NCHS Growth Charts, 1976. Vital and Health Statistic, Series 11. Rockville, Maryland, Health Resources Administration, 1976.

Owen, G. M.: The assessment and recording of measurements of growth of children: report of a small conference. *Pediatrics* 51:461, 1973.

## OSSEOUS DEVELOPMENT

Investigation of osseous development may be helpful in the clinical evaluation of a child's growth progress. This assessment is based on the time when ossification centers appear and epiphyseal-diaphyseal union occurs. In newborn infants, roentgenograms of the knee or ankle and foot are informative. In later infancy and in childhood, a roentgenogram of the wrist and hand is usually adequate for appraisal of bone age.

The ossification centers usually present at birth in full-term infants are those of the distal end of the femur, the proximal end of the tibia, the head of the humerus, the calcaneus, the talus and the cuboid. Usually, the carpal centers are not present at birth but appear by about two months of age. Two carpal centers are present at one year of age, and, in general, one additional carpal center appears each year, so that seven are present at six years of age. During the third year of life, the metacarpal and phalangeal epiphyseal centers are demonstrable radiologically. The distal radial epiphysis is usually present by the first year, and the distal ulnar epiphysis appears in most girls between the ages of six and eight years and in the majority of boys between seven and ten years of age.

In general, the ossification centers appear in a definite sequence. As with other aspects of growth and development, there is a range of individual variation, less in infants and greater in adolescents. Skeletal development in girls is advanced over that of boys, slightly so at birth, but by as much as two years at puberty. A sesamoid bone appears at the distal end of the first metacarpal in girls one or two years before the menarche.

Osseous development is or may be retarded in the presence of hypopituitarism, hypothyroidism, malnutrition, constitutional dwarfism, chronic disease, severe illness, male hypogonadism and delayed adolescence. Osseous development is accelerated in sexual precocity and, frequently, in patients with obesity. Percentile tables for the appearance of ossification centers are included in the atlas by Greulich and Pyle.

Greulich, W.W. and Pyle, S.I.: Radiographic Atlas of Skeletal Development of the Hand and Wrist. 2nd ed. Stanford, Stanford University Press, 1959.

## GROWTH PATTERNS

Understature or growth retardation is a problem frequently encountered in pediatric practice. A child may be considered understatured when his length or height is three or more standard deviations below the mean for age or the velocity or the rate of his growth is below that expected for his chronologic age. If the child is being seen for the first time, his height may be compared to that of others by reference to a percentile growth chart. It is helpful to have a long-term record of the child's growth, including birth length and weight, to determine whether the present growth status is the result of a constant growth pattern or whether at some point in the past the child began to experience growth failure. The ninety-seventh and the third percentiles represent approximately two standard deviations above and below the mean. The height age of a child is the chronologic age at which his height would equal the fiftieth percentile.

The rate of growth in length is best depicted on height velocity curves, on which increments in height in inches or centimeters per year are plotted against chronologic age.

Tanner, J.M. and Whitehouse, R.H.: Longitudinal standards for height, weight, height velocity and stages of puberty. *Arch. Dis. Child. 51*:170, 1976.

The general growth pattern is characterized in late fetal life and early infancy by phases of rapid growth. Growth then decelerates in rate until adolescence, at which time another growth spurt occurs. Growth in height is finally terminated by epiphyseal closure.

The fiftieth percentile for length at birth is 50 cm. (20 in.). This increases to about 66 cm. (26 in.) at 6 months for girls and 68 cm. (27 in.) for boys; 74 cm. (29 in.) for girls and 76 cm. (30 in.) for boys at one year; 86 to 87 cm. (34 in.) at 2 years of age.

During the preschool period, growth in height decelerates, occurring at the rate of 6 to 8 cm. (2 to 4 in.) a year. Growth does not occur at a constant rate throughout the year but is greater at certain times than at others. This deceleration in rate of growth in height continues during the school age period, with annual increments of about 5 cm. (2 in.). Because the increments in weight are increasing during this time, the child's physique is more stocky than in the preschool period.

Although there is great variability, perhaps due to constitutional differences, among children in the time of onset, magnitude and duration of the adolescent spurt of growth, sufficient constancy and predictability exist to permit generalization. Regardless of the chronologic age at which the acceleration in height and weight begins, all children follow the same general pattern. The adolescent growth spurt occurs about two years earlier in girls than in boys. The annual increment in stature reflects this growth acceleration between the ages of 9 and 12 years in the girl and 11 and 14 years in the boy; thus, between the ages of 11 and 13, girls may be taller than boys of the same age. Children of either sex, however, may experience an early spurt in growth and reach their maximal rate of growth in about one year. Others demonstrate a late and more moderate pattern. Because of early deceleration in their rate of growth, children who mature early may be smaller when growth in height has ceased than those whose maximal rate of growth occurs late. Some children will have completed this adolescent growth phase before others of the same chronologic age have begun. Boys who mature early may attain maximal growth before girls who mature slowly. The period of maximal growth and that of sexual maturation are closely related temporally. Girls usually experience their greatest acceleration in height a year or two before the menarche. Those who experience their maximal growth early usually have an early menarche.

Children who have a delayed adolescence as part of their constitutionally delayed growth and physical maturation constitute a significant proportion of those seen with the complaint of short stature. Usually, these children have been relatively small throughout childhood and have a concomitant retardation in sexual development, skeletal maturation and muscular development. Clinical differentiation may not be possible among delayed adolescence, hypopituitarism and primordial or constitutional dwarfism as causes for understature before sexual, somatic and skeletal growth have occurred at adolescence. Delayed adolescence is, of course, much more common.

## SKELETAL PROPORTIONS

The relation of the body length from the crown to the symphysis pubis (upper segment) and from the symphysis to the sole (lower segment) is of a diagnostic value. The measurement is obtained by subtracting the value of the symphysis-to-sole measurement from the total height. The normal value of this ratio ranges from 1.8 at birth to about 1.0 at 9 years of age and 0.9 at age 18. Normal ratios are found in children with delayed adolescence, hypopituitarism (proportions of a child of the same size), and primordial dwarfism (proportions of an individual of the same age with normal height). Patients with sexual precocity and progeria demonstrate an advanced ratio. The ratio remains relatively high in young children with hypothyroidism, chondrodystrophy and Turner's syndrome and is relatively low in patients with Hurler's syndrome, Morquio's disease and in some patients with hypogonadism.

## FACTORS AFFECTING STATURAL GROWTH

Growth in height requires the capacity of skeletal and other tissues to respond to appropriate hormonal stimuli, the presence of anabolic hormones, adequate nutrition for maintenance of a positive nitrogen balance and properly functioning assimilative and metabolic processes for the utilization of nutritional substances.

Growth retardation occurs during many acute and chronic illnesses in childhood. Compensatory mechanisms permit growth to regain its intrinsic or constitutional pattern after recovery. Apart from the obvious effects of anorexia and fever, the deceleration or arrest of growth that occurs during infections is unexplained.

Inadequate nutrition leads to diminished cartilaginous growth and osteoblastic activity. Insufficient protein intake with resultant negative nitrogen balance interferes with deposition of organic matrix in bone.

Heredity is a main determinant of the pattern and rate of linear growth, probably through conditioning the intrinsic growth potentialities of skeletal and other tissue and their response to growth stimuli. The influence of heredity in any child is difficult to assess, and understature should not be too readily ascribed to "heredity" without due consideration of other possible causes.

Pituitary growth hormone exerts its chief effect on linear growth through stimulation of somatomedin production. Though an isolated growth hormone deficiency may occur, other pituitary hormones may also be lacking.

Deficiency or absence of the thyroid hormone leads to retardation of growth and maturation. Diminution in cellular metabolism, impairment of cardiovascular function and anorexia all contribute to growth retardation. Chondrogenesis and osteogenesis are retarded.

Estrogens in themselves apparently contribute little to statural growth.

Androgenic hormones facilitate protein anabolism and nitrogen retention. Testicular androgen probably accounts for the spurt of growth in boys at adolescence, the appearance of secondary sexual characteristics and muscular development. The function of adrenal androgen as a complementary growth hormone during adolescence is not completely proved.

## ETIOLOGIC CLASSIFICATION OF UNDERSTATURE

I. Skeletal
   A. Constitutional disease of bones (see p. 196)
   B. Osteogenesis imperfecta
   C. Congenital and acquired defects of the spine
      1. Multiple hemivertebrae; Klippel-Feil syndrome
      2. Tuberculosis
      3. Cushing's syndrome
      4. Kyphosis, scoliosis
      5. Primary hyperparathyroidism with collapse of vertebrae
II. Nutritional. Chronic malnutrition causes growth failure (see Chapter 39).
III. Systemic disorders
   A. Glycogenosis
   B. Cystinosis
   C. Galactosemia
   D. Congenital heart disease

Suoninen, P.: Physical growth of children with congenital heart disease. *Acta Paediatr. Scand.* (suppl.) *225*:1, 1971.

   E. Chronic renal disease is a diagnostic possibility in children who demonstrate understature. Poor nutrition, chronic acidosis, osteodystrophy, diminished somatomedin and anemia may occur. Intravenous pyelography may be indicated in some instances. Determinations of the serum creatinine, electrolytes and urinary pH are indicated in patients with possible renal tubular acidosis.

Lewy, J.E. and New, M.I.: Growth in children in renal failure. *Am. J. Med. 58*:65, 1975.
Stickler, G.B.: Growth failure in renal disease. *Pediatr. Clin. N. Am. 23*:885, 1976.

   F. Chronic pulmonary disease, including cystic fibrosis and severe asthma
   G. Chronic hemolytic and other anemias such as sickle cell anemia
   H. Lipoid storage diseases: xanthomatosis, Niemann-Pick disease, Gaucher's disease

    I. Bartter's syndrome
    J. Mucopolysaccharidoses
    K. Rickets
    L. Infections, including intrauterine infections
    M. Gastrointestinal disease
       1. Regional enteritis (Crohn's disease). Growth retardation may precede by years gastrointestinal signs and symptoms.

Homer, D.R., Grand, R.J. and Colodny, A.H.: Growth, course, and prognosis after surgery for Crohn's disease in children and adolescents. *Pediatrics 59*:717, 1977.

Sobel, E.H., Silverman, F.N. and Lee, C.M., Jr.: Chronic regional enteritis and growth retardation. *Am. J. Dis. Child. 103*:569, 1962.

       2. Ulcerative colitis

Berger, M., Gribetz, D. and Korelitz, B.I.: Growth retardation in children with ulcerative colitis: the effect of medical and surgical therapy. *Pediatrics 55*:459, 1975.

       3. Malabsorption syndromes
       4. Hepatic insufficiency

  IV. Constitutional delayed or slow growth and physical maturation is the etiology in most children, usually boys, seen because of short stature. Slow growth is usually first noted in these children at school age. Growth in height is at the rate of 1.5 to 2 in. (4 to 5 cm.) each year. The height age is equal to a chronologic age that is two to four years younger, but normal adult height is eventually attained. The bone age and dental age are usually similarly retarded. Puberty is delayed until 14 or 15 years of age. A similar history is often obtained in other members of the family.

Prader, A.: Delayed adolescence. *Clin. Endocrinol. Metab. 4*:143, 1975.

  V. Genetic factors
    A. Familial growth patterns (see p. 376)
    B. Chromosomal abnormalities
       1. Trisomy 21
       2. Trisomy 18
       3. Trisomy 13
       4. Turner's syndrome. These children demonstrate moderate understature with 1.5 to 2 in. (4–5 cm.) of growth each year and a mean ultimate height of 140 to 145 cm. Growth is noted to be relatively slow early in childhood. The lower extremities are markedly shortened. A sex chromatin buccal smear is indicated in all phenotypic females seen with short stature since they may not present the classical clinical picture of Turner's syndrome. If clinical manifestations of Turner's syndrome are present, karyotype analysis is indicated even if Barr bodies are present.

Leao, J., Voorhess, M.L., Schlegel, R.J. and Gardner, L.I.: XX/XO mosaicism in nine preadolescent girls. Short stature as presenting complaint. *Pediatrics 38*:972, 1966.

McDonough, P.G.: Gonadal dysgenesis and its variants. *Pediatr. Clin. N. Am. 19*:631, 1972.

Newfeld, N.D., Lippe, B.M. and Kaplan, S.A.: Disproportionate growth of the lower extremities. A major determinant of short stature in Turner's syndrome. *Am. J. Dis. Child. 132*:296, 1978.

5. Chromosome deletion syndromes
    a. Cri-du-chat syndrome
    b. Wolf's syndrome
    c. Deletion of long arm of chromosome 18 or 21

VI. Central nervous system
   A. Mental retardation

Mosier, H.D., Jr., Grossman, H.J. and Dingman, H.F.: Physical growth in mental defectives. *Pediatrics 36*:465, 1965.

   B. Craniopharyngiomas cause hypopituitarism.
   C. Gliomas of the optic chiasm
   D. Pineal tumor
   E. Xanthomatosis with involvement of the hypothalamic area may cause hypopituitarism.

VII. Endocrine. The velocity of a child's growth is an important consideration in deciding whether to include an endocrine disorder in the differential diagnosis of short stature. In the presence of a normal growth rate, i.e., at least 1.5 in. or 4 cm. each year, an endocrine etiology for short stature is unlikely. Since dental and osseous development are usually retarded in the presence of an endocrine disorder, normal dental development or normal bone age makes an endocrine cause less likely.

Raiti, S.: Endocrine causes of short stature. *Postgrad. Med. 62*:81, 1977.

   A. Hypopituitarism may be due to developmental, genetic or acquired defects in the production or action of growth hormone involving the hypothalamus, pituitary, somatomedin or cartilage and bone. The deficiency in human growth hormone secretion may be isolated or accompanied by one or more of the other pituitary trophic hormones. Acquired growth hormone insufficiency may be due to birth trauma, hypothalamic gliomas, intrasellar and suprasellar tumors, histiocytosis, trauma and tuberculosis.

   Growth retardation in isolated human growth hormone deficiency (IGHD) may be initially noted in the first year of life or during early childhood. After this time, growth is slow—less than 4 to 5 cm. annually. Differentiation between understature due to hypopituitarism and that attributable to constitutional factors is difficult in childhood unless a lesion involving the pituitary area is demonstrable. Pituitary dwarfs have normal or almost normal body proportions and immature, round, full "doll-like" facial features, including delayed development of the nasoorbital bridge. Obesity often involves the trunk and buttocks. Delay in dentition may not be noted until eruption of the permanent teeth. The bone age is retarded. In type I IGHD, inherited on an autosomal recessive basis, the patient has a high-pitched voice and develops wrinkled skin during adulthood. Type II IGHD, inherited as an autosomal dominant trait, does not have the voice or skin changes. Spontaneous hypoglycemia may be an accompanying problem in type I IGHD. With multitrophic pituitary hormone deficiency, evidence of thyroid or adrenal insufficiency may occasionally be present. Secondary sexual development may be delayed or absent. The diagnosis of hypopituitarism requires a minimum of two definitive stimulation tests of plasma growth hormone. Some slow-growing children thought to have delayed adolescence or constitutional short stature respond to stimulation tests in a borderline or low normal fashion. Because of the possibility that an intracranial lesion is present in these patients, examination of the visual fields and the fundi is indicated. Roentgenographic examination of the skull should also be performed.

Laron's dwarfism, an autosomal recessive syndrome noted in the first year of life, is characterized by marked dwarfism, truncal obesity, partial anodontia, saddle nose, "setting-sun" eye sign, high-pitched voice, frontal bossing and small genitalia. There is a high circulating level of immunoreactive growth hormone but failure to produce somatomedin in response to growth hormone administration. Spontaneous hypogylcemic episodes occur during infancy.

Decreased somatomedin levels occur in chronic protein calorie deficiency (kwashiorkor) and in chronic renal failure, chronic liver disease and long-term administration of corticosteroids.

Brasel, J.A., Wright, J.C., Wilkins, L. and Blizzard, R.M.: An evaluation of seventy-five patients with hypopituitarism beginning in childhood. *Am. J. Med. 38*:484, 1965.
Elders, M.J. et al.: Laron's dwarfism: studies on the nature of the defect. *J. Pediatr. 83*:253, 1973.

    B. Hypothyroidism. Growth arrest or marked slowing may be the chief or only clinical manifestation of hypothyroidism acquired after age two. The $T_4$ level should be determined with the thyroid stimulating hormone (TSH) obtained if hypothyroidism is present.
    C. Some types of sexual precocity and virilism with premature epiphyseal fusion
    D. Hypoadrenocorticism. With adequate replacement therapy, the growth of these children is normal.
    E. Cushing's syndrome is characterized by cessation of growth.
    F. Poorly controlled diabetes (Mauriac syndrome)

Mandell, F. and Berenberg, W.: The Mauriac syndrome. *Am. J. Dis. Child. 127*:900, 1974.

    G. Pseudohypoparathyroidism
    H. Hyperparathyroidism
VIII. Constitutional
    A. Familial short stature, a common cause of referral for short stature, occurs in children whose parents and other relatives are also short, usually less than 5 feet or 152 cm. tall. The height of the parents, grandparents and siblings should be determined. While they may be large at the time of birth due to maternal factors, infants destined on the basis of their genetic heritage to be constitutionally short decelerate to a lower growth channel in the period between two to six months and three years of age, after which the rate of growth is normal for their age.

The work-up of children who demonstrate this pattern of deceleration or whose length is two or more standard deviations below the mean should include, in addition to the history and physical, bone age determination, lateral skull x-ray, serum thyroxine level, BUN, creatinine, serum electrolytes and a urinalysis.

Horner, J.M., Thorsson, A.V. and Hintz, R.L.: Growth deceleration patterns in children with constitutional short stature: an aid to diagnosis. *Pediatrics 62*:529, 1978.
Smith, D.W. et al.: Shifting linear growth during infancy: illustration of genetic factors in growth from fetal life through infancy. *J. Pediatr. 89*:225, 1976.

B. Primordial dwarfism is characteristically, but not always, present at birth. Growth is normal except for its slow rate and the small stature finally attained. Most constitutionally understatured children demonstrate retarded bone age in infancy and early childhood but normal skeletal maturation by adolescence.

C. The term "intrauterine dwarf" or low-birth-weight infant is sometimes applied to full-term infants who weigh 2500 gm. or less at birth and who continue to grow at a slow rate. Genetic or prenatal environmental factors (e.g., placental insufficiency, intrauterine infections, maternal toxemia, smoking or alcohol ingestion), may be etiologic. Mental retardation may or may not be present.

Cruise, M.O.: A longitudinal study of the growth of low birth weight infants. I. Velocity and distance growth, birth to 3 years. *Pediatrics 51*:620, 1973.
Tanner, J.M. and Whitehouse, R.H.: Height and weight charts from birth to 5 years allowing for length of gestation: for use in infant welfare clinics. *Arch. Dis. Child. 48*:786, 1973.

D. Seckel's syndrome (bird-headed dwarfism) is characterized by a small head, narrow face, prominent beaklike nose and low-set ears.

McKusick, V.A. et al.: Seckel's bird-headed dwarfism. *N. Engl. J. Med. 277*:279, 1967.

E. Progeria. Dwarfism in these children usually occurs by about one year of age.

F. Cockayne's syndrome is characterized by dwarfism appearing in the second year, retinitis pigmentosa, optic atrophy, mental retardation, kyphosis, photosensitivity, an aged appearance and intracranial calcification.

Fujimoto, W.Y., Green, M.L. and Seegmiller, E.J.: Cockayne's syndrome. *J. Pediatr. 75*:881, 1969.

G. Pycnodysostosis is a genetic disorder of bone associated with dwarfism, osteopetrosis, partial aplasia of the terminal phalanges with a widened, drumstick appearance of the fingers and toes; persistence of fontanels and cranial sutures; frontal bossing; persistence of deciduous teeth; and a parrot-like nose.

Sepano, H.D., Gorlin, R.J. and Anderson, V.E.: Pycnodysostosis. *Am. J. Dis. Child. 116*:70, 1968.

H. de Lange's syndrome is characterized by severe mental retardation; microbrachycephaly; small nose with upturned nostrils; simian creases; flexion contracture of elbows; hypertrichosis; low hairline; heavy, confluent eyebrows; wide, thin upper lip; micrognathia; anomalies of the extremities and digits with proximally placed thumb.

Ptacek, L.J. et al.: The Cornelia de Lange syndrome. *J. Pediatr. 63*:1000, 1963.

I. Russell-Silver syndrome is characterized by short stature, unusually large anterior fontanel, enlargement of the head, triangular facies, underdeveloped muscle mass and hemihypertrophy.

Tanner, J.M., Lejarraga, H. and Cameron, N.: The natural history of the Silver-Russell syndrome: a longitudinal study of thirty-nine cases. *Pediatr. Res. 9*:611, 1975.

J. Marchesani's syndrome is characterized by small stature, myopia, spherical lens and brachydactyly.

K. Laurence-Moon-Biedl syndrome consists of retinitis pigmentosa, obesity, polydactyly and hypogonadism.

L. Leprechaunism (Donohue's syndrome) is characterized by retarded growth; peculiar facies with large ears; wide eyes and sunken cheeks; and prominence of the nipples, areolae, clitoris and labia minora.

Kallo, A., Lakatos, I. and Szijarto, L.: Leprechaunism (Donohue's syndrome). *J. Pediatr. 66*:372, 1965.

M. Pseudo-pseudohypoparathyroidism is the term applied to patients whose physical appearance suggests the diagnosis of pseudohypoparathyroidism but who have no aberration in calcium–phosphorus metabolism.

N. Congenital telangiectatic erythema of the face (Bloom's syndrome) is associated with dwarfism, sensitivity to sunlight and an increased incidence of leukemia.

Bloom, D.: The syndrome of congenital telangiectatic erythema and stunted growth. *J. Pediatr. 68*:103, 1966.

O. The Rothmund-Thomson syndrome is characterized by short stature; telangiectasia and pigmentation involving the skin of the face, buttocks and extremities in the first three to six months of life; alopecia; cataracts; and hypogonadism.

P. The Williams syndrome is characterized by retardation in growth, elfin facies, mental retardation, congenital heart disease (e.g., supravalvular aortic stenosis) and, in some cases, infantile hypercalcemia.

Jones, K.L. and Smith, D.W.: The Williams elfin facies syndrome: a new perspective. *J. Pediatr. 86*:718, 1975.

Q. The Dubowitz syndrome is characterized by mental retardation, mild microcephaly, eczema and small stature.

IX. Psychosocial dwarfism is caused by emotional deprivation. A history of bizarre polyphagia and polydipsia is uniformly present. Patients eat "two or three times" as much as their siblings, feed from garbage cans and drink water from toilet bowls and other unusual sources. Recovery occurs in the hospital.

Powell, G.F., Brasel, J.A. and Blizzard, R.M.: Emotional deprivation and growth retardation simulating idiopathic hypopituitarism. I and II. *N. Engl. J. Med. 276*:1271, 1279, 1967.

## GENERAL REFERENCES

Felson, B. (ed.): Dwarfs and other little people. *Semin. Roentgenol. 8*:133, 1973.

Frasier, S.D.: Growth disorders in children. *Pediatr. Clin. N. Am. 26*:1, 1979.

Gotlin, R.W. and Mace, J.W.: Diagnosis and management of short stature in childhood and adolescence. Part I. *Cur. Prob. Pediatr. 2*:3 (Feb.) 1972.

Rimoin, D.L. and Horton, W.A.: Short stature, Parts I and II. *J. Pediatr. 92*:523, 697, 1978.

Root, A.W., Bongiovanni, A.M. and Eberlein, W.R.: Diagnosis and management of growth retardation with special reference to the problem of hypopituitarism. *J. Pediatr. 78*:737, 1971.

Smith, D.W.: Compendium on shortness of stature. *J. Pediatr. 70:*463, 1967.
Smith, D.W.: *Growth and Its Disorders.* Philadelphia, W. B. Saunders Co., 1977.
Wilkins, L.: *The Diagnosis and Treatment of Endocrine Disorders in Childhood and Adolescence.* 3rd ed. Springfield, Charles C Thomas, 1965.

## ETIOLOGIC CLASSIFICATION OF UNDERSTATURE

I. Skeletal, 373
 A. Constitutional diseases of bone, 373
 B. Osteogenesis imperfecta, 373
 C. Congenital and acquired defects of spine, 373
  1. Multiple hemivertebrae; Klippel-Feil syndrome
  2. Tuberculosis
  3. Cushing's syndrome
  4. Kyphosis, scoliosis
  5. Vertebral collapse
II. Nutritional, 373
III. Systemic disorders, 373
 A. Glycogenosis, 373
 B. Cystinosis, 373
 C. Galactosemia, 373
 D. Congenital heart disease, 373
 E. Chronic renal disease, 373
 F. Chronic pulmonary disease, 373
 G. Chronic hemolytic and other anemias, 373
 H. Lipoid storage diseases, 373
 I. Bartter's syndrome, 374
 J. Mucopolysaccharidoses, 374
 K. Rickets, 374
 L. Infections, 374
 M. Gastrointestinal disease, 374
  1. Regional enteritis (Crohn's disease)
  2. Ulcerative colitis
  3. Malabsorption syndromes
  4. Hepatic insufficiency
IV. Constitutional delayed or slow growth, 374
V. Genetic factors, 374
 A. Familial growth patterns, 374
 B. Chromosomal abnormalities, 374
  1. Trisomy 21
  2. Trisomy 18
  3. Trisomy 13
  4. Turner's syndrome
  5. Chromosome deletion syndromes

VI. Central nervous system, 375
 A. Mental retardation, 375
 B. Craniopharyngiomas, 375
 C. Gliomas of optic chiasm, 375
 D. Pineal tumor, 375
 E. Xanthomatosis, 375
VII. Endocrine, 375
 A. Hypopituitarism, 375
 B. Hypothyroidism, 376
 C. Sexual precocity and virilism, 376
 D. Hypoadrenocorticism, 376
 E. Cushing's syndrome, 376
 F. Poorly controlled diabetes, 376
 G. Pseudohypoparathyroidism, 376
 H. Hyperparathyroidism, 376
VIII. Constitutional, 376
 A. Familial short stature, 376
 B. Primordial dwarfism, 377
 C. "Intrauterine dwarf," 377
 D. Seckel's syndrome (bird-headed dwarfism), 377
 E. Progeria, 377
 F. Cockayne's syndrome, 377
 G. Pycnodysostosis, 377
 H. de Lange's syndrome, 377
 I. Russell-Silver syndrome, 377
 J. Marchesani's syndrome, 378
 K. Laurence-Moon-Biedl syndrome, 378
 L. Leprechaunism, 378
 M. Pseudo-pseudohypoparathyroidism, 378
 N. Congenital telangiectatic erythema of face, 378
 O. Rothmund-Thomson syndrome, 378
 P. Williams syndrome, 378
 Q. Dubowitz syndrome, 378
IX. Psychosocial dwarfism, 378

# CHAPTER 41

# GIGANTISM, OVERSTATURE

I. Constitutional tall stature generally presents no problem to boys but may be a concern to those 2.3 per cent of girls whose height of two standard deviations above the mean characterizes them as "excessively" tall.

Crawford, J.D.: Treatment of tall girls with estrogen. *Pediatrics 62*:1189, 1978.
Gardner, L.I.: The child with "excessive" height predication. A clinical dilemma. *Am. J. Dis. Child. 129*:17, 1975.
Wettenhall, H.N.B., Cahill, C. and Roche, A.F.: Tall girls: a survey of 15 years of management and treatment. *J. Pediatr. 86*:602, 1975.

II. Acromegalic gigantism is extremely rare in children.

Saxena, K.M. and Crawford, J.D.: Acromegalic gigantism in an adolescent girl. *J. Pediatr. 62*:660, 1963.

III. Sexual precocity or virilization may cause temporary overstature.

IV. Gigantism may rarely occur in patients with a primary deficiency of pituitary gonadotropic or gonadal hormone. Such children, however, usually do not demonstrate unusual overstature. Delay in epiphyseal fusion results in disproportionately long extremities and span.

V. Cerebral gigantism is characterized by gigantism, prominent forehead, high-arched palate, hypertelorism, dolichocephaly, mental retardation (in about 80 per cent), large hands and feet, pointed chin, accelerated bone age, poor fine motor control and premature eruption of teeth. Large at birth, these children grow most rapidly in the first four years of life.

Sotos, J.F., Cutler, E.A. and Dodge, P.: Cerebral gigantism. *Am. J. Dis. Child. 131*:625, 1977.

VI. Patients with Marfan's syndrome are relatively tall.

Pyeritz, R.E. and McKusick, V.A.: The Marfan syndrome. *N. Engl. J. Med. 300*:772, 1979.

VII. Hyperthyroidism may be characterized by acceleration in growth, but the ultimate height of affected children is normal.

VIII. Macrosomia with a birth weight over 10 pounds may occur in babies born to diabetic or prediabetic mothers. Cardiac enlargement, hepatomegaly, normoblastemia, lethargy, a weak cry, respiratory distress and a plethoric, ruddy or cyanotic round face ("tomato face") are characteristic findings. Brawny, generalized, nonpitting edema may be present.

IX. Beckwith-Wiedemann syndrome, characterized in part by omphalocele and macroglossia, is a cause of neonatal gigantism. The bone age may be advanced.

X. Congenital lipodystrophy, a disorder characterized by generalized loss of subcutaneous fat, insulin-resistant diabetes and hepatomegaly, is characterized by accelerated growth and bone age. The hands and feet age are enlarged.

XI. Congenital hemihypertrophy is accompanied by an increased risk of Wilms' tumor, adrenocortical carcinoma, hepatoblastoma or focal nodular hyperplasia of the liver.

CHAPTER **42**

# SYMPTOMS RELATED TO SEXUAL DEVELOPMENT

## NORMAL DEVELOPMENT

The rate of growth of the primary sex organs during most of infancy and childhood is extremely slow. Growth of the ovaries is minimal before the age of eight years. Acceleration of growth then occurs and is especially rapid between 17 and 20 years of age. No significant increase in the size of the uterus occurs until the preadolescent period. In early life, the uterus is olive- or almond-sized. The cervix constitutes two thirds of the length of the uterus, and the corpus accounts for the remaining third. Because the corpus grows relatively more rapidly than the cervix after the age of six years, these relations become reversed. During adolescence, the uterus nearly doubles in length. Little growth of the testis occurs before 11 years of age. Growth is rapid between the ages of 12 and 16 years. The enlargement is chiefly caused by tubular growth rather than by an increase in the interstitial cells. The sex organs undergo 90 per cent of their final growth during adolescence.

The Tanner criteria should be used in assessing sexual maturation. These are included on page 106 (breasts) and page 153 (genitalia). The time of onset and the chronologic progress of sexual maturation differ not only between boys and girls but also between children of the same sex. In general, however, sexual growth follows a definite pattern. It is to be recognized, of course, that an orderly sequence does not always occur. Variations in timing and sequence are probably due to constitutional endocrine patterns.

In some children, sexual maturation occurs at an early age, in others at an average age, and in still others relatively late. In children who mature early sexually, the period of maximal growth occurs early and over a short time. Osseous development is relatively advanced. The converse may be true in children who mature late. A small number of normal children may demonstrate an especially early sexual maturation, in girls from eight to nine years of age and in boys from nine to ten years. Although sexual development at these early ages may be within normal limits, the possibility of abnormal sexual precocity must be considered. These children should, therefore, be observed over time for disease in the central nervous system, gonads or adrenals. At the other extreme, the onset of adolescence may not occur until 16 or 17 years of age. In these instances, the possibility of sexual infantilism is to be considered as well as that of a normal but delayed adolescence. Long-term observation may also be informative here.

At puberty, the luteinizing hormone-releasing factor or hormone is produced in increased amounts from the so-called hypothalamic *gonadostat*, which, at that time, becomes less sensitive to the negative feedback effects of circulating testosterone or estrogen. Before the onset of puberty, small amounts of these gonadal hormones suppress the hypothalamic–pituitary–gonadal axis. With the resetting of the gonadostat at puberty, follicle-stimulating hormone (FSH) and luteinizing hormone (LH) secretion rapidly increase.

In the girl, follicle-stimulating hormone promotes the growth of graafian follicles and prepares the ovary for the secretion of estrogen in response to the luteinizing hormone. The luteinizing hormone causes ovulation and the formation of a corpus luteum, which elaborates progesterone. When failure of sexual maturation is due to hypothalamic or pituitary dysfunction, the excretion of gonadotropins is decreased. The excretion is relatively increased in girls with gonadal deficiency such as in Turner's syndrome since the production of gonadotropins is not inhibited by the negative feedback produced by circulating estrogen that is absent in these patients.

In the male, the luteinizing hormone (interstitial cell-stimulating hormone) promotes the development of the interstitial or Leydig cells and the production of testicular androgen. Androgen, in turn, inhibits the production of LH in the male. The follicle-stimulating hormone leads to the development of the seminiferous tubules and spermatogenesis. As in the female, the excretion of follicle-stimulating hormone is decreased in patients who have pituitary or hypothalamic disorders. Although often increased, the excretion of follicle-stimulating hormone may be normal or low in patients with testicular tubular deficiency.

The ovarian hormones consist of estrogen and progesterone. Produced by the theca cells of the graafian follicles in response to follicle-stimulating and luteinizing hormones, estrogen produces such female secondary sexual characteristics as development of the breasts, labia minora, uterus, ovaries, fallopian tubes, vaginal cornification, increased acidity and skeletal growth and maturation. Progesterone, produced by the corpus luteum after ovulation, is responsible for the secretory endometrial phase.

A vaginal smear may be examined for cornified epithelial cells as a readily available test for estrogen excretion. Estrogen excretion is increased in patients with granulosa cell tumor of the ovary, some adrenocortical carcinomas and hyperplasias, chorionepithelioma and during pregnancy. The excretion is diminished in girls with sexual infantilism due to hypopituitarism or ovarian deficiency.

In the male, androgenic hormones are produced by both the adrenal cortex (about two thirds) and the testes (about one third); in the female, by the adrenals and possibly by the ovaries. Testicular androgen, secreted by the interstitial or Leydig cells in response to the luteinizing hormone, begins to appear between the ages of 11 and 14 years.

The androgenic hormones account for adolescent physical growth and muscular development. In girls, the primary and secondary sexual characteristics that result from androgenic stimulation at puberty include growth of the labia majora and the clitoris, the appearance of axillary and pubic hair and the occurrence of seborrhea and acne. If there is a deficiency of adrenal androgen, sexual hair does not appear in the female. In the male, androgens account for the growth of the testes, scrotum, penis, prostate and seminal vesicles; the appearance of pubic, axillary and facial hair; increased sebaceous secretion; and laryngeal enlargement with voice change.

The excretory end-products of both testicular and adrenocortical androgens, known as the urinary 17-ketosteroids, are diminished in patients with hypopituitarism, severe nutritional deprivation, Addison's disease, and, to some extent, Klinefelter's syndrome. Increased excretion occurs in patients with adrenocortical tumors or hyperplasia and testicular interstitial cell tumors. In patients with sexual precocity of the complete type, the values are increased to those normal for adolescents or adults. Administration of cortisone causes a diminution in the excretion of urinary 17-ketosteroids in patients with congenital adrenal hyperplasia but has no significant effect in the presence of an adrenal tumor.

Recent evidence demonstrates that in the first six months of life, especially in boys, the hypothalamic–pituitary–gonadal axis is active as shown by increased levels of FSH, LH, testosterone and estrogen. At the age of approximately seven years in girls and eight years in boys, there is a substantial increase in adrenal androgens due to maturation of the androgenic zone of the adrenal cortex.

## MENSTRUATION

The menarche occurs, on the average, during the twelfth year. The normal range for this event is between 9 and 16 years with the time strongly influenced by genetic factors. Most girls experience their maximal growth just before the menarche. Rapid deceleration in growth then occurs. In general, acceleration and deceleration in height and weight are greater in girls who menstruate early than in those who do so late.

Estrogen leads to endometrial proliferation during the first phase of the menstrual cycle. Ovulation and corpus luteum formation occur about the fourteenth day of the cycle. Progesterone, produced by the corpus luteum, acts synergistically with estrogen to initiate the secretory phase and to terminate the proliferative phase of the premenstrual endometrium. The concentration of progesterone is diminished during the latter part of the secretory phase, owing to deterioration of the corpus luteum. Menstruation with loss of the epithelium then occurs about the twenty-eighth day.

Menstruation does not necessarily indicate that ovulation has taken place. Anovulatory periods may continue for a few years after the menarche. Irregularities in amount, scanty or excessive, and duration or interval of menstruation are common in adolescent girls and regularity may not be achieved for some two years. Two or more years after the menarche, a positive feedback mechanism becomes established through which the rise in circulating estrogen produced in the maturing ovarian follicle stimulates the increased secretion of gonadotropins, especially luteinizing hormone.

## AMENORRHEA

The physician may be consulted either because menstruation has not begun (primary amenorrhea) or has ceased to occur. Secondary amenorrhea is the term applied when no menstrual period has occurred for three to six months after a regular cycle had been established.

Primary amenorrhea may be considered to be present if the menarche has not occurred by the sixteenth year. If not due to one of the causes of sexual infantilism noted below, amenorrhea may be associated with such disorders as congenital anomalies of the genital tract, imperforate hymen, regional enteritis, cystic fibrosis, chronic renal disease and congenital heart disease. Persistent galactorrhea and amenorrhea are frequently associated with hypothalamic disorders. Hyperprolactinemia may be present.

Brown, D.M.: Multiple hypothalamic-pituitary abnormalities in an adolescent girl with galactorrhea. *J. Pediatr. 91*:901, 1977.

A number of causes may lead to secondary amenorrhea, including acute weight loss due to voluntary food restriction, psychologic stresses, emotional problems, chronic infections and pregnancy. The Stein-Leventhal or polycystic ovary syndrome, rare under the age of 15, is characterized by amenorrhea or oligomenorrhea alternating with excessive bleeding, hirsutism, sterility, obesity and enlarged ovaries. Post-pill amenorrhea may occur in adolescents who take oral contraceptives before establishment of the normal hypothalamic rhythm.

Grodin, J.M.: Secondary amenorrhea in the adolescent. *Pediatr. Clin. N. Am. 19*:619, 1972.

Vigersky, R.A., Andersen, A.E., Thompson, R.H. and Loriaux, D.L.: Hypothalamic dysfunction in secondary amenorrhea associated with simple weight loss. *New Engl. J. Med. 297*:1141, 1977.

Wentz, A.C.: Oligomenorrhea and secondary amenorrhea in the adolescent. *Med. Clin. N. Am. 59*:1385, 1975.

## DYSFUNCTIONAL BLEEDING

Dysfunctional bleeding is present in adolescent girls when the menstrual period lasts longer than seven days (menorrhagia), when the amount of menstrual bleeding is excessive or when menstruation is frequent (metrorrhagia). In most cases, the dysfunctional bleeding is due to anovulatory cycles or absence of the preovulatory rise in luteinizing hormone so that there is minimal or no progesterone effect on the endometrium. Irregular, excessive or prolonged menstrual flow results. Other causes of dysfunctional bleeding include a granulosa cell tumor, the Stein-Leventhal syndrome, systemic hemorrhagic states such as idiopathic thrombocytopenic purpura or von Willebrand's disease, severe hepatic disease, carcinoma of the cervix, clear cell tumors of the genital tract, vaginal foreign body or hypothyroidism.

## DYSMENORRHEA

Dysmenorrhea is characterized by lower abdominal cramping or severe pain during the menstrual period. Nausea, vomiting and diarrhea may also occur. Menstruation may not be accompanied by pain until 4 to 18 months after the menarche since cramps often do not occur before the onset of ovulation. Occasionally, this complaint is attributable to a pelvic lesion, and a gynecologic examination is indicated. In most cases, the cause of dysmenorrhea is unknown. Prostaglandins may play an etiologic role as may psychologic factors.

## SEXUAL PRECOCITY

The lower limits for the onset of adolescence are eight years of age in girls and nine and one-half years in boys. Development of secondary sexual characteristics before this time warrants investigation. Sexual precocity may be isosexual, the result of increased androgen production in the male or of estrogen in the female, or heterosexual, with virilization of the female or feminization of the male. In complete or true precocious puberty, sexual development simulates that which occurs at adolescence, with development of the gonads leading to spermatogenesis in the male and ovulation in the female. Rarely, a patient with true sexual precocity may not demonstrate complete precocity.

In patients with incomplete precocity or pseudoprecocity, the uninvolved testis or ovary remains infantile in size and function. Although primary and secondary sexual characteristics develop, spermatogenesis and ovulation do not. Patients with heterosexual precocity and those with isosexual precocity due to gonadal or adrenal lesions have incomplete precocity. In general, the androgen and estrogen levels in true or complete sexual precocity are normal for the patient's physiologic age. In the incomplete form, these values are usually excessive. Emotional development, intellectual progression and dentition in sexually precocious children correspond more to chronologic than physiologic age.

## ETIOLOGIC CLASSIFICATION OF SEXUAL PRECOCITY

I. Isosexual male precocity
   A. Physiologic or constitutional idiopathic precocity is the most frequent type of isosexual precocity, accounting for 60 to 70 per cent of instances in boys. The mechanism responsible for the onset of adolescence and release of the pituitary gonadotropins becomes activated at an unusually early age, perhaps owing to constitutional or genetic factors. Early pubescence may represent a familial pattern. Normal pubertal growth of the genitalia occurs, secondary sexual characteristics appear, spermatozoa are produced and normal adult stature is attained. The excretion of sex hormones reaches normal adolescent values. Although initial investigation may reveal no evidence of cerebral, adrenal or testicular disease, periodic re-examinations are indicated.
   B. Central nervous system lesions lead to premature secretion of pituitary gonadotropins and to true sexual precocity with a normal pattern of growth of the primary sex organs, the appearance of secondary sexual characteristics and the occurrence of spermatogenesis. Early diagnosis may be difficult because the lesion is often very small, slow-growing and otherwise asymptomatic.
      1. Brain tumors may lead to sexual precocity through direct or indirect involvement of the hypothalamus and floor of the third ventricle. These tumors include hamartomas, gliomas, astrocytomas, ependymomas and cysts. Pineal tumors may cause sexual precocity in boys. Obstruction to the third ventricle leads to internal hydrocephalus.
      2. Postencephalitic and postmeningitic sequelae

    3. Congenital defects of the hypothalamus

    4. Tuberous sclerosis

    5. Tuberculoma involving the hypothalamus

    6. McCune-Albright syndrome characterized by bone lesions and cafe-au-lait spots

C. Gonadal tumors cause incomplete sexual precocity. The uninvolved testis remains infantile in size, and spermatozoa are not prematurely produced. Secondary sexual characteristics may appear.

    1. Interstitial or Leydig cell tumor of the testis is an extremely rare lesion that presents either as a firm, hard nodule in an enlarged testis or as a generalized enlargement of the involved testis. The excretion of 17-ketosteroids is increased. Adrenal "rest" cells present in the testes in patients with congenital virilizing adrenal hyperplasia may cause palpable testicular masses, which can be mistaken for an interstitial cell tumor. Administration of cortisone causes regression of the masses and a fall in 17-ketosteroid output in the former but not the latter.

    2. Teratoma of the testis has caused sexual precocity in one case.

D. Hypothyroidism may unusually cause precocious puberty.

Hemady, Z.S., Siler-Khodr, T.M. and Najjar, S.: Precocious puberty in juvenile hypothyroidism. *J. Pediatr. 92*:55, 1978.

E. Adrenal lesions cause incomplete sexual precocity. The testes remain infantile in size, unless they contain aberrant adrenal tissue, and premature spermatogenesis does not occur. Usually, the excretion of 17-ketosteroids is increased. Absence of such elevation does not exclude a virilizing adrenal tumor.

    1. Adrenocortical virilizing hyperplasia. The clinical characteristics of untreated congenital virilizing adrenal hyperplasia in the male include early enlargement of the penis and prostate; appearance of pubic and axillary hair; acne; rapid somatic growth; unusual muscular development; advanced bone age with early epiphyseal fusion; and deepening of the voice. Although the genitalia may appear large at birth, they may not increase in size noticeably until two or three years of age. Adrenocortical hyperplasia may also occur in the siblings of these patients.

    2. Adrenocortical tumor. The excretion of 17-ketosteroids in these patients does not decrease in response to the administration of cortisone as in patients with congenital adrenocortical hyperplasia. A large output of dehydroisoandrosterone or other 3-$\beta$-hydroxyketosteroids suggests an adrenal neoplasm.

F. Chorionic gonadotropin-producing tumors. True isosexual precocity has been described in boys with a sacrococcygeal teratoma, hepatoblastoma, intracranial teratoma, retroperitoneal carcinoma and thoracic polyembryoma.

Danon, M. et al.: Sexual precocity in a male due to thoracic polyembroma. *J. Pediatr. 92*:51, 1978.

Hung, U. et al.: Precocious puberty in a boy with hepatoma and circulating gonadotropin. *J. Pediatr. 63*:895, 1963.

II. Isosexual female precocity

A. Physiologic, constitutional, idiopathic precocity. Eighty-five to ninety per cent of girls with sexual precocity may be placed in this category. Sexual precocity is complete, with normal maturation of the ovaries, ovulatory menstrual cycles and excretion of sex hormones at levels that are normal for the girl's physiologic rather than chronologic age.

B. Central nervous system lesions cause complete sexual precocity.
   1. With the exception of pineal tumors, intracranial lesions that cause isosexual precocity in the male may also lead to sexual precocity in the female.
   2. The McCune-Albright syndrome, or polyostotic fibrous dysplasia, is characterized by skin pigmentation and sexual precocity.
   3. Silver's syndrome consists of sexual precocity, hemihypertrophy, short stature and elevated gonadotropins.

Silver, H.K.: Asymmetry, short stature and variations in sexual development: a syndrome of congenital malformations. *Am. J. Dis. Child. 107*:495, 1964.

C. Gonadal tumors. Sexual precocity due to gonadal causes is not accompanied by ovulation. There is premature growth and development of those primary secondary sexual characteristics that are influenced by estrogen secretion.
   1. Granulosa cell tumor leads to the development of primary and secondary sexual characteristics. The sexual hair and the advanced physical growth are probably due to adrenocortical activity, perhaps effected by the action of estrogen on the pituitary. The bone age may be also advanced. A whitish vaginal discharge, at times periodic, may be the first clinical manifestation. Vaginal bleeding, which occurs later, may be regular enough to resemble irregular, scanty or profuse menstrual cycles. Vaginal bleeding may occur before, concomitantly with or after the development of other sexual characteristics. Estrogen excretion is increased. An abdominal or pelvic mass may be present.
   2. Follicle cysts
   3. Luteal cyst (possibly)
   4. Teratoma
   5. Chorionepithelioma
D. Medicational precocity. Pseudoprecocious puberty may result from the accidental ingestion of stilbestrol. The areolae and nipples in such instances are deeply pigmented.
E. Hypothyroidism may be accompanied by a syndrome characterized by precocious menstruation, galactorrhea, absence of pubic hair and enlargement of the sella turcica in the presence of retarded skeletal age. These findings disappear after thyroid therapy.

Jenkins, M.E.: Precocious menstruation in hypothyroidism. *Am. J. Dis. Child. 109*:252, 1965.

## DIAGNOSTIC APPROACH TO ISOSEXUAL PRECOCITY

I. History and physical examination
   A. History and physical findings of precocious sexual development with the appearance of secondary sexual characteristics, enlargement of primary

sexual organs and acceleration of physical and osseous development. In girls, the possibility of accidental ingestion of estrogen should be investigated.

B. Symptoms of intracranial lesions: headache, vomiting, visual disturbances, changes in behavior, polydipsia, polyphagia or obesity.

C. Signs of intracranial lesions: papilledema, optic atrophy, defects in the visual fields and enlargement of the head. The signs of a pineal neoplasm may include strabismus, Argyll Robertson pupils and inability to look upward.

D. Other aspects of the physical examination may include abdominal and rectal examination for the presence of an ovarian tumor; examination of the testes for physiologic or pathologic enlargement; and inspection of the skin for the pigmentation seen in patients with the McCune-Albright syndrome.

II. Roentgenographic examinations to be considered

  A. Skull

    1. Calcification of tumor masses. Calcification of the pineal gland may occur normally in a small number of children.

    2. Spreading of sutures

    3. Computerized axial tomography

  B. Bone age

  C. Skeletal roentgenograms for polyostotic fibrous dysplasia

  D. Intravenous pyelogram for evidence of renal displacement by adrenal mass

III. Hormone determinations. Adolescent hormone levels (gonadotropin, estrogen and 17-ketosteroids) are found in patients with complete precocity with excessive values noted in patients with incomplete precocity.

IV. Surgical exploration if the patient is thought to have a neoplasm of the gonads or adrenals. Testicular biopsy may be helpful in differentiating between true sexual precocity and that due to adrenal lesions. Development of interstitial cells occurs in the former but not the latter.

## ETIOLOGIC CLASSIFICATION OF INTERSEXUAL DEVELOPMENT

I. Female

  A. Female pseudohermaphroditism due to congenital virilizing adrenal hyperplasia is transmitted as an autosomal recessive trait. In these sex chromatin-positive infants, the uterus, fallopian tubes and vagina develop as in other females; however, varying degrees of masculinization of the external genitalia are noted. The phallus, which is enlarged at birth, often resembles a penis with hypospadias and chordee. Fusion of the labioscrotal folds ranges from none or minimal with separate urethral and vaginal orifices to the more common situation in which the fusion extends anteriorly and the urethra and vagina open into a urogenital sinus. A penile urethra occurs in a few cases. When diagnosis and treatment have not been established in infancy, there may be an early appearance of sexual and body hair, acne and deepening of the voice. Physical, osseous and muscular growth is also accelerated. Since epiphyseal fusion occurs early, these children ultimately are relatively understatured.

Almost all instances of this syndrome are due to deficiency of the 21-hydroxylase enzyme. In about one third of these children, aldosterone deficiency occurs with a resultant salt-losing tendency. Dehydration, vomiting, perhaps diarrhea, and circulatory collapse may occur. Hypertension has been reported in a few patients as a result of increased production of 11-deoxycorticosteroids.

Differentiation between female pseudohermaphroditism due to congenital virilizing adrenal hyperplasia and that of nonadrenal etiology should be made promptly. This cannot be done on the basis of the physical examination but depends on determination of the urinary excretion of 17-ketosteroids and pregnanetriol. Early in life, the normal value for urinary 17-ketosteroid excretion may be as high as 2.5 mg. per 24 hours, but after 2 weeks it is under 0.5 mg. per day. Usually, values of 2 to 5 mg. per 24 hours are found in patients with congenital virilizing adrenal hyperplasia. When the 17-ketosteroid value is in the nondiagnostic range (less than 2 mg. per 24 hours), demonstration of urinary pregnanetriol offers confirmation. Cortisone causes a diminution in the production of adrenal androgen and in the excretion of 17-ketosteroids.

B. Nonadrenal female pseudohermaphroditism. Partial embryonic masculinization of the external genitalia may occur in female infants whose mothers received synthetic progestogens during pregnancy. Enlargement of the phallus and varying degrees of fusion of the labioscrotal folds may be produced. Differentiation from congenital virilizing adrenal hyperplasia is made by the absence of increased excretion of urinary 17-ketosteroids and failure of progressive virilization. The buccal smear demonstrates a female chromatin pattern. When masculinization has been substantial, differentiation from true hermaphroditism may not be possible without an exploratory laparotomy. Such exploration is not necessary with a history that the mother received androgens or synthetic oral progestogens during the early months of pregnancy. In other cases, there is as yet no clear explanation for the occurrence of nonadrenal female pseudohermaphroditism.

C. Adrenal tumors. Postnatal virilization during the first decade of life is usually due to an adrenal tumor. After the age of 10 or 12 years, virilization may be attributable either to a tumor or to adrenocortical hyperplasia.

D. Postnatal adrenal hyperplasia.

E. Arrhenoblastomas have not been reported before the age of 15 years.

II. Male

Much progress has been made in the understanding of male pseudohermaphroditism in recent years, but the subject remains complex. These patients have testes and a portion or all of the müllerian (female) duct system. The external genitalia may resemble those of either female or male, or may be ambiguous. The anatomic features vary widely. Except for the presence of testes, some of these children may resemble those with female pseudohermaphroditism due to congenital virilizing adrenal hyperplasia. The scrotum may be cleft and resemble labia. Other physical findings may include microphallus, undescended testes, hypospadias and partial vaginal orifice. Acceleration of physical development and bone age do not occur. The excretion of 17-ketosteroids is not increased. The secondary sexual characteristics that appear at puberty may be either male or female. Gynecomastia is common.

A. Male pseudohermaphroditism may result from a defect, inherited as an autosomal recessive trait, in one of the five enzymatic reactions in testosterone biosynthesis from cholesterol.

B. Testicular feminization syndrome, an X-linked recessive trait and due to a defect in androgen actions, occurs in phenotypic females. Testes, which are present bilaterally, may appear as inguinal or labial masses. At puberty, breast development occurs but pubic and axillary hair are absent or scant. Menstruation does not occur, and the uterus and cervix are absent. These patients have a 46XY karyotype.

Crawford, J.D.: Syndromes of testicular feminization. *Clin. Pediatr. 9*:165, 1970.

C. Persistent müllerian duct syndrome (hernia uteri inguinali), due to a recessive trait, is characterized by female internal genitalia in otherwise normal-appearing males.

Brook, C.G.D. et al.: Familial occurrence of persistent müllerian structures in otherwise normal men. *Br. Med. J. 1*:771, 1973.

D. Mixed gonadal dysgenesis is characterized by a streak gonad on one side and a testis on the other. The patient is chromatin negative, and the karyotype is 45XO/46XX. The external genitalia are usually ambiguous. Secondary sex characteristics do not appear. Gynecomastia is frequent.

E. Genetically, the disorders of incomplete male pseudohermaphroditism can be categorized into two groups. Type I, inherited as an X-linked recessive trait resulting from a single mutant, is variably expressed along a spectrum extending from nearly complete failure of virilization to almost complete masculinization. Included in this group are the syndromes described by these investigators: Lubs (which resembles testicular feminization in some respects), Reifenstein (with perineoscrotal hypospadias), Gilbert-Dreyfus, and Rosewater.

Wilson, J.D. et al.: Familial incomplete pseudohermaphroditism, type 1. *N. Engl. J. Med. 290*:1097, 1974.

Type II, inherited as an autosomal recessive trait and due to testicular 17-ketosteroid reductase deficiency, has been termed pseudovaginal perineoscrotal hypospadias. This disorder resembles Reifenstein's syndrome except that gynecomastia does not develop.

Givens, J.R. et al.: Familial male pseudohermaphroditism without gynecomastia due to deficient testicular 17-ketosteroid reductase activity. *N. Engl. J. Med. 291*:938, 1974.

Grumbach, M.M. and Van Wyk, J.J.: Disorders of sex differentiation. *In* Williams, R.H. (ed.): *Textbook of Endocrinology,* 5th ed. Philadelphia, W. B. Saunders, 1974, pp. 423–501.

Imperato-McGinley, J. and Peterson, R.E.: Male pseudohermaphroditism: the complexities of male phenotypic development. *Am. J. Med. 61*:251, 1976.

Opitz, J.M., Simpson, J.L. and Sarto, G.E.: Pseudovaginal perineoscrotal hypospadias. *Clin. Genet. 3*:1, 1972.

Park, I.J., Aimakhu, V.E., and Jones, H.W., Jr.: An etiologic and pathogenetic classification of male hermaphroditism. *Am. J. Obstet. Gynecol. 123*:505, 1973.

III. True hermaphroditism

The external genitalia in these children may appear ambisexual. Both gonads are usually intra-abdominal. Hypospadias and cryptorchidism are diagnostic clues. In adolescence, gynecomastia is common in true hermaphrodites, and the majority of these patients menstruate. Most are chromatin positive, but some are mosaics.

A. The patient may have one ovary and one testis.

B. The patient may have one ovo-testis.

C. The patient may have an ovary and a testis on one side and either an ovary or a testis on the other.

## DIAGNOSTIC APPROACH TO INTERSEXUAL DEVELOPMENT

The psychologic and psychosocial orientation of patients with hermaphroditism corresponds to the gender of their rearing rather than to anatomic or hormonal considerations. A rational decision needs, therefore, to be made as to the child's sex of rearing within a few days after birth. In this decision, the child's functional genital anatomy is a major determinant. A careful diagnostic appraisal is indicated in infants with clearly ambiguous external genitalia, with either hypospadias or testes that cannot be palpated, and those with female external genitalia but with palpable masses in the labia or inguinal regions. Anatomic studies, including surgical exploration and biopsy of the gonads, may be indicated in infants shown not to have congenital virilizing adrenal hyperplasia.

I. Physical examination directed toward the establishment of anatomic relations and structure through inspection of the external genitalia; abdominal palpation; palpation of the inguinal region, labia or scrotum; and rectal examination. The orifice at the base of the phallus should be examined to determine whether it represents an urethral meatus or an urogenital sinus and whether a communication is present between the urethra and the vagina. Urethroscopic examination may be necessary to demonstrate the vagina and cervix.

II. Determination of the sex chromosomal pattern (number of cells with Barr bodies, number of such sex chromatin bodies per nucleus and size of bodies) using buccal mucosal smears may be a helpful screening device in the study of abnormalities of sexual differentiation. The number of Barr bodies is generally one less than the number of X chromosomes. A buccal smear with suitable controls should be obtained on all apparent male infants with bilateral cryptorchidism.

Weldon, V.V., Blizzard, R.M. and Migeon, C.J.: Newborn girls misdiagnosed as bilateral cryptorchid males. *N. Engl. J. Med. 274*:829, 1966.

In patients with abnormal sexual differentiation, a chromatin-positive pattern restricts diagnostic considerations to either female pseudohermaphroditism or true hermaphroditism. A chromatin-negative pattern is consistent with male pseudohermaphroditism, true hermaphroditism, rudimentary testes or gonadal dysplasia with Leydig cells.

III. Roentgenographic studies

A. A vaginogram may be attempted.

B. Calcification in an adrenal tumor or other neoplasm may be demonstrated.

C. An intravenous pyelogram may show displacement of the kidney downward and anteriorly by an adrenal tumor.

IV. The excretion of the 17-ketosteroids is abnormally increased in patients with adrenocortical hyperplasia or tumor. The excretion of large amounts, over 50 mg. a day, of the 17-ketosteroids is presumptive but not absolute evidence that a tumor is present. An increase in the 3-$\beta$-hydroxy 17-ketosteroids has a similar connotation. The finding of increased amounts of dehydroisoandrosterone in the urine is suggestive evidence for an adrenal tumor. Patients with congenital or postnatal adrenal hyperplasia demonstrate a significant reduction in 17-ketosteroid excretion within seven to ten days after the initiation of cortisone treatment. A similar sustained fall is not seen with an adrenal tumor.

In other types of intersex, elevated levels of androgen or estrogen do not occur before puberty.

V. Surgical exploration and possibly gonadal biopsy may be necessary for diagnosis.

Lippe, B.M.: Ambiguous genitalia and pseudohermaphroditism. *Pediatr. Clin. N. Amer.* 26:91, 1979.

## DELAYED SEXUAL MATURATION; SEXUAL INFANTILISM

In general, evidence of sexual development should appear in girls by the age of 15 or 16 years and in boys by 16 to 17 years of age. This permits a distinction to be made between a late onset of normal adolescence and true sexual infantilism. Constitutional delay in sexual development, more common in boys than girls, is accompanied by short stature (page 373), normal velocity of growth and bone age commensurate with height age. The adolescent growth spurt is delayed. Malnutrition due to anorexia nervosa or inflammatory bowel disease may cause delay in sexual development.

## ETIOLOGIC CLASSIFICATION OF DELAYED SEXUAL MATURATION; SEXUAL INFANTILISM

I. Central
   A. The exact clinical picture in patients with sexual infantilism due to hypopituitarism (panhypopituitarism, partial pituitary insufficiency; deficiency of pituitary gonadotropins) is determined by whether the deficiency is limited to the pituitary gonadotropins or whether other tropic hormones are involved; thus, sexual hair appears, though perhaps in diminished amount, in patients with normal adrenocorticotropic activity. The excretion of 17-ketosteroids is only moderately decreased or corresponds to what would be normal for the female. Abnormalities of the hypothalamic pituitary axis are characterized by low serum gonadotropin concentrations. Serum and urinary levels of luteinizing hormone and follicle-stimulating hormone may be determined by radioimmunoassay.

   Varying degrees of failure of sexual development may occur. In the male, the testes may show some development, although they do not reach normal mature size. Usually, there is lack of spermatogenesis in the male and amenorrhea or irregular and scanty menstruation in the female. Excretion of follicle-stimulating hormone is decreased or absent. If other tropic hormones are deficient, growth retardation, absence of sexual hair and hypoglycemia may be noted.

B. Involvement of the hypothalamus may lead to a diminished secretion of pituitary gonadotropins.

    1. Failure of sexual development may be due to suprasellar cysts, gliomas, craniopharyngiomas or other intracranial tumors that involve the hypothalamus. Hypothalamic involvement may also occur with trauma, encephalitis or sarcoidosis.

    2. Laurence-Moon-Biedl syndrome. The sexual infantilism in these patients is probably due to a congenital, genetically determined hypothalamic defect.

    3. Kallmann's syndrome. In addition to hypogonadotropic hypogonadism, these patients have anosmia or hyposmia, color blindness, small testes and a micropenis. The olfactory function should be checked in patients with hypogonadism.

    4. The Prader-Willi syndrome consists of hypogenitalism, obesity and mental retardation.

    5. There may be an absence of the luteinizing releasing hormone or factor.

II. Gonadal

When gonadotropins are present in the urine of sexually immature patients, the secretion of pituitary gonadotropins may be considered to be adequate, especially when these values are increased above normal. The problem then becomes one of inadequate gonadal function. Urinary and plasma levels of the sex steroids may be measured.

A. Testes

Biopsy and the determination of follicle-stimulating hormone excretion are usually required for a diagnosis of testicular deficiency. As a rule, the excretion of follicle-stimulating hormone is increased. Testicular function may be impaired in the following situations.

    1. Congenital absence of testis; congenital anorchia; testicular hypoplasia

    2. Congenital deficiency of the interstitial Leydig cells

    3. Surgical castration

    4. Trauma

    5. Hemorrhage

    6. Infection, mumps

    7. Torsion of the spermatic cord

    8. Idiopathic fibrosis

    9. Klinefelter's syndrome. Except for gynecomastia in some of these patients, the secondary sexual characteristics are normal. The testes are small (less than 1.5 cm.) and firm. Spermatogenesis does not occur. The body habitus may be eunuchoid or normal male. Urinary gonadotropin excretion is increased. Plasma testosterone levels are intermediate between male and female. A chromatin-positive pattern on the buccal smear in these patients may generally be considered evidence of seminiferous tubule dysgenesis. A male chromatin pattern does not, however, exclude this diagnosis. The cytologic sex should be determined in prepuberal boys with abnormally small or hard testes, those with cryptorchidism and adolescents with gynecomastia. The most common karyotype in Klinefelter's syndrome is XXY. Other karyotypes

are XXYY or XXXY and XXXYY or XXXXY. The most frequent mosaic pattern is XY/XXY. Generally, the more X chromosomes present in a male, the greater the degree of mental retardation. It is difficult to make a clinical diagnosis of Klinefelter's syndrome before puberty.

Caldwell, P.D. and Smith, D.W.: The XXY (Klinefelter's) syndrome in childhood: detection and treatment. *J. Pediatr. 80*:250, 1972.

10. Weinstein's syndrome is characterized by hyalinization of seminiferous tubules, obesity, blindness, nerve deafness and hyperuricemia.

Weinstein, R.L., Kliman, B. and Scully, R.E.: Familial syndrome of primary testicular insufficiency with normal virilization, blindness, deafness and metabolic abnormalities. *N. Engl. J. Med. 281*:969, 1969.

B. Ovaries
  1. Turner's syndrome in phenotypic females is characterized by moderately short stature, primary amenorrhea, webbing of the neck, lymphedema of the hands and feet present at birth, coarctation of the aorta, cubitus valgus, shield-like chest and recurrent melena. Phenotypic females with stigmata of Turner's syndrome but with bilateral streak gonads and sexual infantilism are examples of "pure gonadal dysgenesis." Patients with a mosaic karyotype demonstrate fewer signs of Turner's syndrome, may menstruate and are of normal stature.

The buccal smear, useful as a screening examination, is chromatin negative in the 60 per cent of these patients who are XO. About 20 per cent of patients with Turner's syndrome are chromatin positive but they may have a smaller than normal Barr body count in terms of percentage and size. Mosaicism is frequent with a XO/XX mosaic, a frequent karyotype. Girls with deletion of the long arms of an X chromosome may have some of the clinical findings of Turner's syndrome.

McDonough, P.G.: Gonadal dysgenesis and its variants. *Pediatr. Clin. N. Amer. 19*:631, 1972.

  2. Ovarian degeneration following disease or radiation
  3. Premature menopause is extremely rare.
C. Genitalia
  1. Congenital absence of uterus and/or vagina
III. Other endocrine disorders
  A. Hypothyroidism may be characterized by hypogonadism.
  B. Delay in sexual maturation is less common in patients with hyperthyroidism.
  C. Cushing's syndrome may also be accompanied by sexual retardation.

Federman, D.D.: Disorders of sexual development. *N. Engl. J. Med. 277*:351, 1967.

## CROSS-GENDER BEHAVIOR

Cross-gender behavior is usually not a presenting complaint in girls because the "masculine" interests demonstrated by the "tomboy girl" are more admired than scorned. "Effeminate" behavior in the school-age or adolescent boy may be a reason for consultation. Some cross-gender behavior may be a normal developmental variation. In other cases, the boy openly admits his wish to be a girl, frequently dresses up in women's clothing, wears cosmetics, is interested in women's fashions, chooses girls for playmates, avoids "boy's" games, plays with dolls and demonstrates exaggerated "feminine" mannerisms, gait and gestures.

Green, R.: Childhood cross-gender identification. *J. Nerv. Ment. Dis. 147*:500, 1968.

Zuger, B.: Effeminate behavior present in boys from early childhood. I. The clinical syndrome and follow up studies. *J. Pediatr. 69*:1098, 1966.

## GENERAL REFERENCES

Gardner, L.I. (ed.): *Endocrine and Genetic Diseases of Childhood and Adolescence.* 2nd ed. Philadelphia, W. B. Saunders Co., 1975.

Root, A.W.: Endocrinology of puberty. I. Normal sexual maturation. II. Aberrations of sexual maturation. *J. Pediatr. 83*:1, 187, 1973.

Sizonenko, P.C.: Endocrinology in preadolescents and adolescents. I. Hormonal changes during normal puberty. *Am. J. Dis. Child. 132*:794, 1978.

Sizonenko, P.C.: Preadolescent and adolescent endocrinology: physiology and physiopathology. II. Hormonal changes during abnormal pubertal development. *Am. J. Dis. Child. 132*:797, 1978.

Wilkins, L.: *The Diagnosis and Treatment of Endocrine Disorders in Childhood and Adolescence.* 3rd ed., Springfield, Charles C Thomas, 1965.

## ETIOLOGIC CLASSIFICATION OF SEXUAL PRECOCITY

## ETIOLOGIC CLASSIFICATION OF INTERSEXUAL DEVELOPMENT

## ETIOLOGIC CLASSIFICATON OF DELAYED SEXUAL MATURATION; SEXUAL INFANTILISM

# CHAPTER 43

# OBESITY

Obesity, defined as excessive subcutaneous fat, is considered present if the skin-fold thickness measured by calipers in the triceps and subscapular areas exceeds two standard deviations above the mean for age.

Garn, S.M. and Clark, D.C.: Trends in fatness and the origins of obesity. *Pediatrics 57*:443, 1976

Though obesity occurs in infants and young children, it is most frequent at the end of the first decade and during adolescence. The subcutaneous tissue is normally thicker in infants and adolescents than in preschool or school children.

The term Pickwickian syndrome may be applied to patients whose obesity is accompanied by alveolar hypoventilation, arterial hypoxemia, polycythemia and somnolence.

Ward, W.A., Jr., and Kelsey, W.M.: The Pickwickian syndrome. *J. Pediatr. 61*:745, 1962.

## ETIOLOGIC CLASSIFICATION OF OBESITY

I. General causes
   A. Obesity in childhood rarely constitutes an endocrine disorder but is a
      problem of appetite and satiety. The growth and development of these

children is normal or even relatively accelerated. Obese children may experience an early adolescence.

Stunkard, A.: Satiety is a conditioned reflex. *Psychosomat. Med. 37*:383, 1975.

B. The physical explanation for obesity is usually a direct one: the child's caloric intake exceeds his energy expenditure. It is also clear that some children become or remain obese though they do not eat more than their peers. The child who gains weight excessively may be less active than other children.

C. Both the parents and the child may disclaim excessive food intake, not in a conscious attempt to make a false statement, but because they have a misconception about what constitutes an excessive amount of food.

D. There is no evidence that the specific dynamic action of food is less, that food is absorbed more easily or that fat is mobilized from the depots less readily in obese children than in others. There may, perhaps, be a constitutional or genetic tendency for some children to gain weight more rapidly than others on a similar diet.

E. The energy expenditure of children who are inactive because of illness or handicap may be decreased, especially if the metabolic rate is not elevated as a result of fever or infection. If obesity should occur in children with motor handicaps, psychologic reasons for overeating are usually operative in addition to the limitation of energy expenditure.

   The basal metabolism of obese children is either normal or increased compared with that in nonobese children of the same height and age. The obese patient must expend more energy in accomplishing work than the nonobese child. At the same time, he must eat more than a normal child to maintain his abnormal weight.

II. The endocrine glands

A. Thyroid deficiency does not lead to obesity except in rare instances. Although the decreased metabolism, activity and growth present in children with hypothyroidism cause a diminution in energy expenditure, the accompanying anorexia may lead to a decreased food intake.

B. Insulinomas may be accompanied by obesity.

C. Cushing's syndrome may present only with obesity and premature cessation of longitudinal growth. Acne and hirsutism are other common findings. The obesity is chiefly distributed in the face, the cervicodorsal area and trunk. Amenorrhea may be present. Purplish striae may occur over the abdomen and thighs. Hypertension and muscle weakness may be noted.

McArthur, R.G., Cloutier, M.D., Hayles, A.B. and Sprague, R.G.: Cushing's disease in children. *Mayo Clin. Proc. 47*:319, 1972.
Streeten, D.H.P. et al.: Hypercortisolism in childhood: shortcomings of conventional diagnostic criteria. *Pediatrics 56*:797, 1975.

D. While the presence of a suprapubic fat pad may make the genitalia appear smaller than they actually are, true hypogonadism may be present in addition to obesity in some patients with hypothlamic lesions.

E. Obesity often involves the trunk and buttocks in pituitary dwarfs.

III. The central nervous system

A. Present evidence indicates that pituitary lesions, unaccompanied by involvement of the hypothalamus, do not produce obesity.

B. The Laurence-Moon-Biedl syndrome, which consists in mental retardation, retinitis pigmentosa, hypogonadism, polydactylism and obesity, is genetic in origin.

C. Lesions in the hypothalamus that may lead to obesity by producing an intense craving for food include encephalitis, craniopharyngiomas, gliomas of the optic chiasm, histiocytosis X, pituitary tumors, congenital defects of the hypothalamus such as the Laurence-Moon-Biedl syndrome and trauma, especially basal skull fractures. Hydrocephalus, pinealomas and porencephaly may also lead to obesity.

D. Central nervous system leukemia is associated with sudden weight gain and a voracious appetite.

E. The Prader-Willi syndrome is characterized by mental retardation, neonatal hypotonia, small hands and feet, hypogenitalism, understature, compulsive hyperphagia and obesity.

Hall, B. D. and Smith, D.W.: Prader-Willi syndrome. *J. Pediatr. 81*:286, 1972.
Holm, V.A. and Pipes, P. L.: Food and children with Prader-Willi syndrome. *Am. J. Dis. Child. 130*:1063, 1976.

F. Central nervous system lesions are rare causes of obesity; however, the history should include information as to vomiting, visual disturbances, headache, ataxia, enlargement of the head and polyuria. Careful neurologic and funduscopic examinations are indicated as well as delineation of the visual fields. Roentgenograms of the skull and CAT scans may be obtained in selected patients.

IV. Socioeconomic and psychologic aspects of obesity

A. Socioeconomic factors are highly related to obesity; for example, obesity is less prevalent in adolescents in higher socioeconomic classes.

B. Obese persons are very susceptible to environmental influences on eating. Food often has a special importance in some families.

C. Overeating may occur in response to anxiety, depression and frustration.

D. Obesity leads to many secondary problems, especially in adolescents. They are often taunted and ridiculed. Reluctance or inability to engage in physical activities and sports may lead to poor muscular development and physical fitness. The poor coordination that some of these children demonstrate precludes their interest in physical activity and sports.

Heald, F.P. and Khan, M.A.: Teenage obesity. *Pediatr. Clin. N. Am. 20*:807, 1973.

E. A variety of types of parent-child relations have been described in the families of obese children. One or both parents of most overweight children are obese; however, not all the children in these families become obese.

Stunkard, A.J.: From explanation to action in psychosomatic medicine: the case of obesity. *Psychosom. Med. 37*:195, 1975.

## GENERAL REFERENCES

Bruch, H.: *Eating Disorders: Obesity, Anorexia Nervosa and the Person Within*. New York, Basic Books, 1973.
Forbes, G.B.: Obesity. *In* Green, M. and Haggerty, R.J. (eds.): Ambulatory Pediatrics II. Philadelphia, W. B. Saunders, 1977. p. 348.
Stricker, E.M.: Hyperphagia. *N. Engl. J. Med. 298*:1010, 1978.
Weil, W. B., Jr.: Current controversies in childhood obesity. *J. Pediatr. 91*:175, 1977.

## ETIOLOGIC CLASSIFICATION OF OBESITY

CHAPTER **44**

# FAILURE TO DO WELL IN SCHOOL

Failure to do well in school is a frequent presenting complaint. In this complex problem involving the child, the family and the school, diagnosis and management require an interdisciplinary medical–educational approach.

## ETIOLOGIC CLASSIFICATION OF FAILURE TO DO WELL IN SCHOOL

I. Mental retardation

Children expected to achieve beyond their cognitive abilities will experience school failure; on the other hand, appropriate educational placement permits the child to achieve within the limits of his potential. Mental retardation is discussed more fully in Chapter 45.

II. Specific learning disabilities

The Special Education for all Handicapped Children Act of 1975 (Public Law 94–142) defines a special learning disability as "a disorder in one or more of the basic psychological processes involved in understanding or in using spoken or written language. These may be manifested in disorders of listening, thinking, talking, reading, writing, spelling, or arithmetic. They include conditions which have been referred to as perceptual handicaps, brain injury, minimal brain dysfunction, dyslexia, developmental aphasia, etc. They do not include learning problems which are due primarily to visual, hearing, or motor handicaps, to mental retardation, emotional disturbance, or to environmental disadvantage."

Between 10 and 30 per cent of public school children, often with near average to above average intelligence, are estimated to have significant learning disabilities, more commonly in reading but also in writing, spelling and arithmetic. In some schools, as many as one half of the students have reading skills that are two years or more behind standard achievement levels. The most common cause of such underachievement is environmental, including poor teaching. When neurologic impairment is the etiology, the physical signs are often subtle. The history, however, may be consistent with central nervous system damage and delayed development.

Specific or developmental dyslexia occurs in 5 to 15 per cent of children, predominantly males (4:1) with normal intelligence, and often on a familial basis. Generally, there are no significant neurologic findings. On the Wechsler Intelligence Scale for Children, patients with developmental dyslexia often have a low verbal I.Q. as well as low scores on the digit-span and coding subtests.

Drew, A.L.: School underachievement: minimal cerebral dysfunction (the brain damaged child). *In* Green, M. and Haggerty, R. J. (eds.): *Ambulatory Pediatrics*. Philadelphia, W. B. Saunders Co., 1968, p. 465.

Drew, A.L. and Roach, E.G.: School underachievement: specific learning disabilities. *In* Green, M. and Haggerty, R.J. (eds.). *Ambulatory Pediatrics*. Philadelphia, W. B. Saunders Co., 1968, p. 474.

Eisenberg, L.: Reading retardation: I. Psychiatric and sociologic aspects. *Pediatrics 37*:352, 1966.

Kavanagh, J.F. and Yeni-Komshian, G.: Developmental dyslexia and related reading disorders. U.S. Dept. of HEW, No. (NIH) 78–92, Washington, D.C., U.S. Government Printing Office, 1978.

III. Emotional factors

School underachievement may be secondary to emotional disorders characterized by depression, anxiety (about himself, a sibling or a parent) or intense anger, which make it difficult for the child to attend to school work and which impair his motivation to learn. The precise etiologic factors need to be determined by interviews with the child, the mother and the father. The child may view himself as a failure. Children with specific learning disabilities, such as developmental dyslexia, often acquire secondary emotional symptoms and behavioral problems including anxiety, somatic complaints, depression, lying, stealing, delinquent behavior and feelings of frustration and low self-esteem. School phobia or resistance to attending school due to emotional factors may interfere with educational progress.

IV. Environmental factors

A. Poor teaching and the inability of some schools to be responsive in their curricula and teaching methods to the individual needs of a specific child are frequent causes of school failure, especially in economically deprived areas.

B. Frequent moves of the family may interfere with school achievement.

C. Frequent absence from school for social or emotional reasons, unless compensated for by homework, is a common cause for a child to fall behind educationally.

D. Severely disturbed home situations generally disrupt school progress.

E. Failure of the family to convey to the child a sense of the importance of education usually leads to multigenerational school underachievement.

The parental expectations for the child's school achievement may be minimal.

    F. Hyperactivity, short attention span and distractibility impede learning.

V. Neurologic factors

    A. Brain damage may be associated with a variety of learning disabilities.

    B. Undetected petit mal seizures may impede learning.

VI. Sensory factors

    A. Visual impairment

    B. Hearing impairment

VII. Speech and language delay. Delayed language and speech achievement in toddlers and preschool children may be a prelude to later reading problems.

VIII. Deterioration in previously adequate school performance is always a source of concern. Etiologic possibilities include:

    A. Emotional factors secondary to divorce, illness or other family crises

    B. Neurologic disorders

        1. Subacute sclerosing panencephalitis

        2. Wilson's disease

        3. Other degenerative disorders of the central nervous system

        4. Petit mal epilepsy

        5. Cerebral tumor

        6. Low-grade hydrocephalus (e.g., secondary to tumors of the third or fourth ventricles)

        7. Chronic cerebrospinal fluid shunt insufficiency may lead to deterioration in school performance, at times accompanied by ataxia or increased tone in the lower extremities.

    C. Hyperthyroidism; hypothyroidism

    D. Sydenham's chorea

    E. Acquired hearing loss

## THE DIAGNOSTIC PROCESS

I. The physician's role

    A. The physician reviews developmental progress, assesses the emotional status of the child and family and obtains other data that may help in understanding the causes for the school problem.

    B. In addition to screening of visual acuity, hearing and speech, a careful neurologic examination is in order. Of special interest are hard neurologic signs, e.g., hemiparesis, or asymmetrical findings, e.g., differences in fine motor movements, rapid alternating movements of the hands, and differences in the growth of the hands or thumbs.

        While, statistically, "soft" neurologic signs may be etiologically relevant, they are so much a reflection of the developmental immaturity of the neurologic system as to be of little clinical significance in an individual child. Such findings include choreiform movements of the extended hand, brief attention span, synkinesis (mirroring of fine finger and hand movements from one side to the other), clumsiness, lack of appreciation of simultaneous face-hand touch, confusion in right-left discrimination, poor performance of rapid alternating movements, immature speech and language, impaired auditory discrimination, mirror writing and strephosymbolic errors.

Barlow, C.F.: "Soft signs" in children with learning disorders. *Am. J. Dis. Child. 128*:605, 1974.

C. There are no simple screening tests that scientifically and reliably predict or detect learning disability. In the office, the physician may use a blackboard, crayons and paper, picture books, standardized reading or arithmetic problems and the Peabody Picture Vocabulary Test. The child may be asked to write, print, take dictation, draw a person and copy geometric figures. Children with a reading disability, for example, may be able to copy a sentence already printed but unable to print the same sentence if dictated. The child may read aloud slowly and with extreme effort, guess at words using the first letter or syllable of the word as a clue, make omissions and additions and be unable to convey the meaning of what he has just read.

II. School report

A school report that includes answers to questions about the child's school performance, test data, learning problems noted by the teachers and problems in adjustment is an essential element of the physician's evaluation. A variety of such report forms are available. A telephone call to the principal or teacher, and, if possible, a physician-teacher personal conference, is often helpful.

III. Psychoeducational evaluation

When intellectual retardation or a specific learning disability is a possibility, the most important diagnostic step is an adequate psychoeducational assessment. Individual intellectual assessments should be performed by the school psychologist along with other evaluations indicated, depending upon the specific learning problem. The Wechsler Intelligence Scale for Children, which can be given to children at the age of five to six years or older, is particularly helpful in children with learning disabilities, showing a scatter in the sub-test verbal or performance scores and often a 10- or 20-point discrepancy between the verbal and performance quotients. Other evaluation instruments used might include the Raven Progressive Matrices, the Peabody Picture Vocabulary Test, the Bender Visual Motor Integration, the Stanford-Binet, achievement tests in reading and mathematics and the Illinois Test of Psycholinguistic Abilities (ITPA).

IV. Sensory evaluations

A. An ophthalmologic examination for visual acuity and eye disorders is usually indicated.

B. Audiological and speech evaluation is desirable if the child has delayed language development or dysphasia.

## GENERAL REFERENCES

Grossman, H. (ed.): Symposium on learning disabilities. *Pediatr. Clin. N. Am. 20*:541, 1973.
Hammar, S.L.: School underachievement in the adolescent: a review of 73 cases. *Pediatrics 40*:373, 1967.

## ETIOLOGIC CLASSIFICATION OF FAILURE TO DO WELL IN SCHOOL

CHAPTER **45**

# MENTAL RETARDATION

## DEFINITIONS

The American Association on Mental Deficiency defines retardation as "significantly subaverage general intellectual functioning existing concurrently with deficits in adaptive behavior, and manifested during the developmental period." Significant subaverage performance is considered as more than two standard deviations from the mean of a standard intelligence test (e.g., an I.Q. of 67 or less on the Stanford-Binet and 69 or less on the Wechsler). The Cattell scale and the Kuhlmann-Binet are commonly used tests for infants or severely retarded children. Since a diagnosis of mental retardation cannot be made on the basis of the I.Q. alone, adaptive behavior must also be significantly retarded as reflected in the degree of independence and social responsibility the child has achieved. Standardized tests for adaptive behavior, such as the AAMD adaptive behavior scale and the Vineland Social Maturity Scale, have limitations and are not entirely satisfactory.

Levels of mental retardation based on measured intelligence are defined as mild, moderate, severe and profound (Table 45–1).

The term "mildly retarded" is often used interchangeably with "educable retarded" while "moderate" retardation is equated with "trainable." The term "dependent retarded" is sometimes used for the severely retarded and the "life support

TABLE 45–1  LEVELS OF MENTAL RETARDATION

|  | Stanford-Binet Cattell scales | Wechsler scale |
|---|---|---|
|  | (s.d. 16) | (s.d. 15) |
| Mild | 67–52 | 69–55 |
| Moderate | 51–36 | 54–40 |
| Severe | 35–20 | 39–25 (Extrapolated) |
| Profound | 19 and below | 24 and below (Extrapolated) |

level'' for the profoundly retarded. Table 45–2 summarizes some of the developmental characteristics, potential for training and education and social and vocational adequacy.

About 25 per cent of children with mental retardation have a syndrome that is recognizable clinically at birth or early in infancy or childhood. Most instances of mental retardation, however, are not identified until school entrance.

Developmental appraisal as a part of well-baby assessment may permit early detection of developmental retardation. When the degree of retardation is great, such determinations have prognostic significance. Their long-term predictive value is

TABLE 45–2  DEVELOPMENTAL CHARACTERISTICS, POTENTIAL FOR EDUCATION AND TRAINING AND SOCIAL AND VOCATIONAL ADEQUACY ACCORDING TO THE FOUR LEVELS OF MENTAL RETARDATION*

| Level | Preschool Age (0–5) Maturation and development | School Age (6–21) Training and education | Adult (21 and over) Social and vocational adequacy |
|---|---|---|---|
| Profound | Gross retardation; minimal capacity for functioning in sensorimotor areas; needs nursing care. | Obvious delays in all areas of development; shows basic emotional responses; may respond to skillful training in use of legs, hands and jaws; needs close supervision. | May walk, need nursing care, have primitive speech; usually benefits from regular physical activity; incapable of self-maintenance. |
| Severe | Marked delay in motor development; little or no communication skill; may respond to training in elementary self-help, e.g., self-feeding. | Usually walks barring specific disability; has some understanding of speech and some response; can profit from systematic habit training. | Can conform to daily routines and repetitive activities; needs continuing direction and supervision in protective environment. |
| Moderate | Noticeable delays in motor development, especially in speech; responds to training in various self-help activities. | Can learn simple communication, elementary health and safety habits and simple manual skills; does not progress in functional reading or arithmetic. | Can perform simple tasks under sheltered conditions; participates in simple recreation; travels alone in familiar places; usually incapable of self-maintenance. |
| Mild | Often not noticed as retarded by casual observer but is slower to walk, feed self and talk than most children. | Can acquire practical skills and useful reading and arithmetic to a 3rd to 6th grade level with special education; can be guided toward social conformity. | Can usually achieve social and vocational skills adequate to self-maintenance; may need occasional guidance and support when under unusual social or economic stress. |

*From The President's Panel on Mental Retardation: Mental Retardation, A National Plan for a National Problem: Chart Book. Washington, D.C., U.S. Department of Health, Education, and Welfare, 1963, p. 15.

much less when lesser discrepancies are found. Single-infant developmental tests do not predict later intelligence or school performance.

Oppenheimer, S. and Kessler, J.W.: Mental testing of children under three years. *Pediatrics* 31:865, 1963.

Mental retardation is a symptom of many etiologies ranging from the biomedical, usually clinically evident or diagnosable by laboratory and other procedures, to biosocial. It is often accompanied by other handicaps. Adequate diagnosis of children with mental retardation often requires multiple disciplines and reassessment over time.

Chromosome studies are obviously not indicated in most retarded children but are to be considered if a patient has multiple anomalies, especially affecting the face, ears and distal extremities or is born small for gestational age. Other indications may include a maternal history of repeated miscarriages, dermatoglyphic abnormalities, unusual facies or a clinically recognizable genetic syndrome. Lysosomal storage diseases are suggested by regression or deterioration of motor and intellectual development, hepatosplenomegaly, skeletal dysostosis, cloudy cornea, cherry red macula, retinal degeneration and similarly affected siblings. An inborn error in amino acid metabolism is suggested by positive screening tests, unusual odors, metabolic acidosis, failure to thrive, seizures, lethargy, vomiting, unusual hair, ataxia and other neurologic symptoms.

## ETIOLOGIC CLASSIFICATION OF MENTAL RETARDATION

I. Chromosomal abnormalities
   A. Down's syndrome due to trisomy 21, mosaicism or translocation (15/21; 21/22; 21/21). The diagnosis of Down's syndrome is usually readily made at birth on the basis of the following physical findings:
      Developmental retardation
      Brachycephaly
      Flat occiput
      Epicanthal folds
      Slanting palpebral fissures
      Flat nasal bridge
      Speckled iris (Brushfield's spots)
      Loose skin in the posterior neck
      Small, dysplastic ears
      Hypotonia
      Hyperextensibility of joints
      Short, broad hands
      Simian palmar creases
      Dysplastic middle phalanx of fifth finger
      Wide space between first and second toes
      Congenital heart disease in some patients
   B. Trisomy 13 (Patau's or $D_1$ syndrome) is characterized by the following findings:
      Severe developmental retardation
      Minor motor seizures

Low birth weight
Failure to thrive
Microcephaly with sloping forehead
Holoprosencephaly-type central nervous system defect
Scalp defects in parietal-occipital area
Eye defects, including microphthalmia and coloboma of iris and retina
Epicanthal folds
Loose skin on posterior neck
Cleft lip and/or palate
Prominent nose
Low-set ears
Micrognathia
Overlapping fingers
Flexion deformity of fingers with or without overlapping
Retroflexible thumb
Ulnar deviation of hands
Single palmar crease; distal palmar axial triradii
Polydactyly
Hyperconvex nails
Prominent heels
Congenital heart disease: ventricular septal defect, patent ductus, auricular septal defect
Short sternum
Hemangiomas, including capillary hemangioma on forehead
Renal anomalies

C. Trisomy 18 (Edwards' syndrome) is characterized by the following findings:

Severe developmental retardation
Low birth weight
Failure to thrive
Difficulty in feeding
High-pitched cry
Prominent occiput
Microphthalmia
Short palpebral fissures
Low-set ears
Micrognathia
Loose skin on posterior neck
Overlapping fingers
Flexion deformities of fingers with index finger overlapping third and fifth finger over fourth
Retroflexible thumbs
Rocker bottom feet
Hammer toe
Prominent heels
Congenital heart disease, especially ventricular septal defect and patent ductus arteriosus

      Hypoplastic muscles
      Hypertonia
      Single umbilical artery
      Inguinal or umbilical hernia
      Renal anomalies

D. 5p-syndrome (cri du chat syndrome) has the following characteristics:
      Severe developmental retardation
      Microcephaly
      Hypertelorism
      Oblique palpebral fissures
      Epicanthal folds
      Low-set ears
      Micrognathia
      Failure to thrive
      Hypotonia
      "Cat-like" cry

E. 4p-syndrome (Wolf-Hirschhorn syndrome)
      Developmental retardation
      Failure to thrive
      Midline scalp defect
      Microcephaly
      Low-set ears
      Nasal deformity
      Simian crease

F. 18 short arm deletion syndrome (18p-)
      Developmental retardation
      Cebocephaly
      Microcephaly
      Eye defects
      Malformed ears
      Micrognathia
      Saddle nose
      Webbed neck

G. 18 long arm deletion syndrome (18q-)
      Microcephaly
      Hypotonia
      Microcephaly
      Eye deformity
      Ear deformity

H. Other structural abnormalities of the autosomes: trisomies, deletions, duplications (partial trisomies) and translocations

I. Klinefelter's syndrome

Lewandowski, R.C., Jr., and Yunis, J.J.: New chromosomal syndromes, *Am. J. Dis. Child.* *129*:515, 1975.

Yunis, J.J. (Ed.): *New Chromosomal Syndromes.* New York, Academic Press, Inc., 1977.

II. Lysosomal storage diseases
    These disorders, caused by a deficiency of one or more lysosomal enzymes,

share a number of clinical features, including coarse facies, macrocephaly, retinal degeneration, cherry red macula, corneal clouding, hepatosplenomegaly and skeletal dysostosis. The diagnosis is based on specific laboratory examinations.

A. $G_{M1}$ gangliosidosis may appear at birth or in early infancy (infantile, type I) with a coarse facies, depressed nasal bridge, flexural contraction of fingers, kyphosis, hepatosplenomegaly and other clinical features that suggest Hurler's syndrome. A cherry red macula and cloudy cornea are often present. Type II is characterized by normal development during the first 9 to 12 months of life followed by rapid neurologic deterioration and spastic quadriparesis.

B. $G_{M2}$ gangliosidosis I (Tay-Sachs disease). The infant develops normally for the first months of life but then begins to demonstrate hyperacusis, listlessness, irritability, hypotonia, seizures and developmental regression. A cherry red macula is present.

C. $G_{M2}$ gangliosidosis II (Sandhoff's disease) is clinically indistinguishable from Tay-Sachs disease.

D. Metachromatic leukodystrophy is characterized by normal development until the age of 12 to 14 months, followed by gait disturbance, ataxia, intellectual regression, loss of reflexes, seizures and bulbar signs. Terminally, rigidity, blindness, deafness, macular degeneration and hyperpyrexia develop. A cherry red spot may be present. The cerebrospinal fluid protein is regularly elevated. Patients with the late infantile form of metachromatic leukodystrophy may have a pseudo-Hurler's appearance.

E. Krabbe's disease (globoid cell leukodystrophy) becomes clinically evident before six months of age with irritability, persistent crying, recurrent unexplained fever and myoclonic responses to light and noise. Developmental arrest is followed by regression, decerebrate posture, optic atrophy and seizures. The cerebrospinal fluid protein is regularly elevated.

F. Niemann-Pick disease in its infantile form begins in early infancy with hepatosplenomegaly, cessation of development and mental retardation. A cherry red macular spot may be present.

G. Gaucher's disease in its acute, infantile form is characterized by failure to thrive, bulbar palsy, hepatosplenomegaly, developmental regression and spastic quadriparesis.

H. Farber's syndrome

I. Wolman's syndrome is accompanied by hepatosplenomegaly and adrenal calcification.

J. Fucosidosis is characterized by normal development until one or two years of age when intellectual and physical deterioration begin. The skeletal characteristics, facial features, hepatosplenomegaly and joint contractures may suggest Hurler's syndrome. The fundi and corneae are normal.

K. Mannosidosis has many clinical features similar to Hurler's syndrome (e.g., hepatosplenomegaly, mental retardation, kyphosis, cataracts and corneal clouding).

Booth, C.W., Chen, K.K. and Nadler, H.L.: Mannosidosis: clinical and biochemical studies in a family of affected adolescents and adults. *J. Pediatr.* 88:821, 1976.

L. Aspartylglucosaminuria is a progressive disorder inherited on an autosomal recessive basis and characterized by a coarse facies with thick lips,
broad nose, anteverted nostrils and hypotonia.

M. Multiple sulfatase deficiency is manifested by slow development for the
first one or two years of life followed by neurologic deterioration with
myoclonic seizures, nystagmus, retinal degeneration and spasticity. The
facies may be suggestive of Hurler's syndrome.

N. Mucopolysaccharidoses
   1. MPS IH (Hurler's syndrome), an autosomal recessive disease, is char-
      acterized by severe mental retardation, macrocephaly, coarse facies,
      flat nasal bridge, flared nostrils, bushy eyebrows, full lips, large
      tongue, thoracolumbar gibbus, corneal clouding, skeletal deformities,
      stiff joints, hepatosplenomegaly, mucoid rhinitis and deafness.
   2. MPS II A and B (Hunter's syndrome), an X-linked recessive disorder,
      is characterized by moderate mental retardation, skeletal deformities,
      early deafness and retinal degeneration. Corneal clouding is absent.
   3. MPS III A (Sanfilippo's syndrome A), an autosomal recessive dis-
      order, is manifested by severe mental retardation and clinical features
      that simulate MPS IH but are not as marked as those of MPS IH.
   4. MPS III B (Sanfilippo's syndrome B)
   5. MPS VII β-glucuronidase deficiency
   6. MPS VIII

O. Mucolipidoses
   1. Mucolipidosis I is characterized by normal development for the first
      year of life followed by gradual intellectual deterioration. The facies
      are somewhat suggestive of Hurler's syndrome. In addition to moder-
      ate mental retardation, hepatosplenomegaly, hernias and a cherry red
      macular spot are present.
   2. Mucolipidosis II (Leroy's syndrome, I-cell disease) presents early in
      infancy with many features closely suggesting Hurler's syndrome,
      e.g., severe mental retardation, hepatosplenomegaly, a hoarse voice
      and tight skin. Corneal clouding does not occur.
   3. Mucolipidosis III becomes manifest in the second year of life with
      dwarfing, thoracic deformity, joint contractures and hearing impair-
      ment. The clinical picture resembles that of Hurler's syndrome.
   4. Mucolipidosis IV

Gordon, N.: The pseudo-Hurler syndromes. *Dev. Med. Child. Neurol. 20*:383, 1978.
Kolodny, E.H.: Current concepts in genetics. Lysosomal storage disease. *N. Engl. J. Med.
294*:1217, 1976.

III. Other cerebral degenerative disorders
   A. Ceroid lipofuscinosis (Batten's disease) has infantile, late infantile, juve-
      nile and adult variants. The late infantile form becomes clinically manifest
      between two and six years of age with intellectual deterioration, myoclon-
      ic seizures, ataxia, retinal degeneration and optic atrophy. Skin biopsy or
      tissue culture fibroblasts can be used for study of ultrastructural changes
      in fibroblasts.

Zeman, W. and Dyken, P.: Neuronal ceroid-lipofuscinosis (Batten's disease). Relationship
to amaurotic family idiocy. *Pediatrics 44*:570, 1969.

B. Spielmeyer-Vogt disease (juvenile amaurotic idiocy) begins in school-age children with progressive loss of vision, myoclonic and grand mal seizures and intellectual deterioration.

C. Pelizaeus-Merzbacher disease becomes evident in early infancy with oscillating, wheeling nystagmus, unusual eye movements and head tremor followed by regression in motor and intellectual development, ataxia, intention tremor, choreoathetosis and spasticity.

D. Subacute sclerosing panencephalitis (SSPE or Dawson's inclusion body encephalitis) has four stages. Stage 1 begins insidiously with deterioration in intellectual and school performance and personality changes that include temper outbursts, disobedience, forgetfulness, distractibility and hallucinations. In stage 2, myoclonic jerks occur along with incoordination, choreoathetosis and tremors. Personality and intellectual changes accompanied by myoclonic jerks should suggest the diagnosis. Electroencephalographic findings, spinal fluid studies and measles antibody titers are confirmatory. Stage 3 is characterized by rigidity and unresponsiveness. Intermittent periods of laughing and crying occur in stage 4 along with hypothalamic dysfunction.

Freeman, J.M.: The clinical spectrum and early diagnosis of Dawson's encephalitis. *J. Pediatr. 75*:590, 1969.
Jabbour, J.T. et al.: Subacute sclerosing panencephalitis: a multidisciplinary study of eight cases. *JAMA 207*:2248, 1969.

E. Huntington's chorea

F. Schilder's disease, which occurs in late childhood, is characterized by cortical blindness, spasticity, seizures and aphasia progressing to dementia and coma.

IV. Abnormalities of amino acid metabolism

A. Phenylketonuria. Eczema and seizures may be present. A musty body and "mousey" urine odor may be noted. All retarded children should be screened for this disorder.

*Management of Newborn Infants with Phenylketonuria.* U.S. Dept. of HEW, No. (HSA) 78–5211 Washington, D.C., U.S. Government Printing Office, 1978.

B. Hyperammonemia may cause episodic vomiting and lethargy.
   1. Carbamyl-phosphate synthetase deficiency
   2. Ornithine transcarbamylase deficiency

C. Citrullinemia may cause severe disease in the newborn with episodic vomiting, seizures, coma and mental retardation.

D. Argininosuccinicaciduria becomes manifest in the first one to two years of life with retardation of growth, trichorrhexis nodosa, hepatomegaly, seizures and ataxia.

E. Argininemia is characterized by mental retardation, seizures and spastic diplegia.

F. Maple syrup urine disease, a familial disease that is rapidly progressive if untreated, usually becomes symptomatic toward the end of the first week of life with difficulty in feeding, failure to thrive, absent Moro reflex, extreme flaccidity, irregular respirations, lethargy and myoclonic seizures. Opisthotonus and intermittent rigidity occur later. The urine has a maple syrup odor. Excessive amounts of valine, leucine and isoleucine and their alpha-keto acids are present in urine and blood.

G. Hypervalinemia causes vomiting, lethargy and feeding difficulties in new-born infants.

H. β-Alaninemia is characterized by lethargy and seizures in young infants.

I. Nonketotic hyperglycinemia is manifested by microcephaly, seizures and mental retardation.

J. Homocystinuria. In addition to mental retardation, the patient has fine, friable hair; dislocation of the lens; livedo reticularis; a malar flush; marked nervousness; and a Marfan-like habitus with genu valgum, pectus excavatum, kyphosis, scoliosis and arachnodactyly. Arterial or venous thrombotic episodes may occur. The cyanide-nitroprusside test is used for screening.

Schimke, R.N., McKusick, V.A., Huang, J. and Pollack, A.D.: Homocystinuria. *JAMA* *193*:87, 1965.

K. Saccharopinuria

L. Sarcosinemia causes a feeding problem and failure to thrive as well as mental retardation.

M. Hartnup disease is characterized by progressive mental retardation, reversible cerebellar ataxia and a pellagra-like rash on skin areas exposed to sunlight.

N. Isovaleric aciduria causes metabolic acidosis, urine with a sweaty feet odor and neurologic signs.

O. Propionic acidemia produces episodic vomiting, metabolic acidosis and ketonuria.

P. Methylmalonic aciduria is characterized by developmental retardation and infantile ketoacidosis.

Q. Lactic-pyruvic acidosis may cause metabolic acidosis in the newborn, ataxia and mental retardation.

R. β-Methylcrotonyl-glycinuria produces mental retardation, urine that has the odor of cat's urine and feeding problems.

S. α-Methyl-β-hydroxybutyric aciduria causes intermittent metabolic acidosis.

T. Carnosinemia is characterized by seizures and mental retardation.

U. Sulfite oxidase deficiency causes severe mental retardation, dislocation of the lens and blindness.

O'Brien, D. and Goodman, S.I.: The critically ill child: acute metabolic disease in infancy and early childhood. *Pediatrics 46*:620, 1970.
Scriver, C.R. and Rosenberg, L.E.: *Amino Acid Metabolism and Its Disorders*. Philadelphia, W. B. Saunders Co., 1973.

V. Other metabolic disorders associated with mental retardation

A. Hypothyroidism may cause developmental delay during early infancy.

B. Idiopathic infantile hypercalcemia

C. Hypoglycemia may cause mental retardation.

D. Galactosemia, if not diagnosed and treated early, causes mental retardation.

E. Lesch-Nyhan syndrome is characterized by developmental regression; hypotonia eventually replaced by hypertonia; athetoid posturing and choreic movements.

F. Menkes' kinky hair syndrome, or trichopoliodystrophy

G. Lowe's syndrome is characterized by severe mental retardation, glaucoma, hypotonia, cataracts, metabolic acidosis, rickets, organic aciduria and aminoaciduria.

    H. Oasthouse urine disease (methionine malabsorption) is characterized by failure to thrive, seizures, hypotonia, edema and an abnormal urinary odor (dried malt or hops).

    I. Aspartylglucosaminuria becomes manifest during the school years with coarse facial features, hypertelorism, broad nose, thick lips, large tongue, opacities of the lens, spasticity and dysarthria. Mental retardation is severe.

    J. Methemoglobin diaphorase deficiency is characterized by methemoglobinemia and mental retardation.

    K. Bartter's syndrome may cause mental and physical retardation in addition to hypokalemic alkalosis.

    L. Wilson's disease may begin with dementia and seizures.

    M. Fanconi's syndrome

    N. Adrenoleukodystrophy usually affects school-age boys, causing cortical blindness, impaired intellectual performance, ataxic or spastic gait and pigmentation of skin folds.

VI. Infections

    A. Prenatal

        1. Cytomegalovirus

        2. Rubella

        3. Toxoplasmosis

        4. Syphilis

    B. Postnatal

        1. Meningitis

        2. Viral encephalitis

        3. Postinfectious encephalopathy

VII. Toxic agents; drugs

    A. Lead poisoning

    B. Fetal alcohol syndrome

    C. Fetal anticonvulsant syndrome

    D. Maternal phenylketonuria

    E. Neonatal hyperbilirubinemia

    F. Carbon monoxide poisoning

VIII. Trauma; hypoxia

    A. Perinatal hypoxia

    B. Birth trauma

    C. Intracranial hemorrhage

    D. Head injury

IX. Other syndromes and disorders that may be associated with mental retardation

    A. Hydranencephaly. Transillumination of the head is indicated in infants seen because of mental retardation.

    B. Primary microcephaly

    C. Cerebral palsy may be accompanied by mental retardation. In the presence of severe motor and, at times, sensory handicaps, determination of the child's actual intellectual ability is often difficult.

D. Tuberous sclerosis may be accompanied by mental retardation.

E. Sturge-Weber-Dimitri syndrome

F. Neurofibromatosis

G. Laurence-Moon-Biedl syndrome consists of mental retardation, obesity, hypogenitalism, retinitis pigmentosa and polydactylism.

H. de Lange's syndrome is characterized by bradycephaly and by a pathognomonic facies with hyperconvex forehead, hypoplasia of the supraorbital ridges and zygomatic arches, small nose, depressed nasal root, flaring nostrils, micrognathia and low-set ears. The eyebrows are bushy and confluent in the midline and the eyelashes long and delicate. Scalp hair extends low on the forehead, which is covered by fine lanugo hair. There is general hypertrichosis. The fingers are short and tapering, and a simian palmar crease is often present along with proximal insertion of the thumb, clinodactyly of the little finger and poor development of the thenar muscles. Extension of the elbows is limited. Retardation is moderate to severe.

Jervis, G.A. and Stimson, C.W.: de Lange syndrome. *J. Pediatr. 63*:634, 1963.

I. The Rubinstein-Taybi syndrome is characterized by mental retardation and short, broad terminal phalanges of the thumbs and great toes. Other features include high arched palate, slight antimongoloid palpebral fissures and a prominent nose.

Rubinstein, J.H. and Taybi, H.: Broad thumbs and toes and facial abnormalities. *Am. J. Dis. Child. 105*:588, 1963.

J. Prader-Willi syndrome

K. Incontinentia pigmenti

L. Smith-Lemli-Opitz syndrome

M. Cerebral gigantism

N. Cerebrohepatorenal syndrome of Zellweger is characterized by mental retardation, severe hypotonia, hepatomegaly, jaundice, failure to thrive and a diagnostic facies consisting of a high forehead, brachycephaly, persistent metopic suture, hypertelorism, hypoplastic supraorbital ridges, micrognathia and low-set ears. Eye findings may include glaucoma, corneal clouding, epicanthal folds, Brushfield's spots and nystagmus. Epiphyseal stippling may be present.

Danks, D.M., Tippett, P., Adams, C. and Campbell, P.: Cerebro-hepato-renal syndrome of Zellweger. *J. Pediatr. 86*:382, 1975.

O. Canavan's disease is characterized by marked enlargement of the head in early infancy, splitting of the sutures, spasticity, progressive intellectual deterioration and blindness.

P. Alexander's disease is characterized by macrocephaly, muscle weakness, contractures and mental retardation.

X. Psychosis

Children who are psychotic or autistic are functionally mentally retarded. Both mental retardation and psychotic behavior may occur in the same child. The clinical manifestations of psychosis become evident during infancy or early childhood. The affected child is withdrawn, seems unaware of other persons, avoids eye contact, fails to differentiate between people and things and ignores spoken words. Even as an infant, the child may object to being picked up or cuddled. The patient may become annoyed if his activities are interrupted. Activity often consists of stereotyped, compulsive and repetitive movements such as swinging, whirling or spinning objects. The child may walk on his tip toes. There is either no speech or the child uses a secret language, gibberish or echolalia.

Aug, R.G. and Ables, B.S.: A clinician's guide to childhood psychosis. *Pediatrics 47*:327, 1971.

XI. Cultural-familial factors are the most common cause for retardation and for a disparity between a child's actual performance and his innate abilities. Insufficient physical, social and emotional stimulation from a mother or mother-substitute may lead to retarded behavior in infants and young children. Economically and socially disadvantaged children are over-represented in this group.

Haywood, H.C. (ed.): Social Retardation. New York, Appleton-Century-Crofts, 1970.

XII. Sensory deficits such as hearing and visual impairment if not detected or treated

## GENERAL REFERENCES

Beaudet, A.L.: Genetic diagnostic studies for mental retardation. *Curr. Prob. Pediatr. 7*:3 (Mar.) 1978.
Gellis, S. and Feingold, M.: *Atlas of Mental Retardation Syndromes – Visual Diagnosis of Facies and Physical Findings.* U.S. Dept. of HEW, Social and Rehabilitation Service, Rehabilitation Services Administration, Division of Mental Retardation. Washington, D.C., U.S. Government Printing Office, 1968.
Grossman, H.J. (ed.): *Manual on Terminology and Classification in Mental Retardation.* Washington, D.C., American Association on Mental Deficiency, 1973 Revision, Special Publication Series No. 2.
Grossman, H.S.: Mental retardation. *In* Green, M. and Haggery, R. J. (eds.): *Ambulatory Pediatrics II.* Philadelphia, W.B. Saunders Co., 1977, p. 271.
Holmes, L.B., Moser, H.W., Halldorsson, S., Mack, C., Pant, S.S. and Hatzilevich, B.: *Mental Retardation: An Atlas of Diseases with Associated Physical Abnormalities.* New York, The Macmillan Co., 1972.
Smith, D.W. and Simons, F.E.R.: Rational diagnostic evaluation of the child with mental deficiency. *Am. J. Dis. Child. 129*:1285, 1975.

## ETIOLOGIC CLASSIFICATION OF MENTAL RETARDATION

# CHAPTER 46

# HYPERACTIVITY

Hyperactivity is a nonspecific term that is applied to a pattern of motor behavior that the parents or teacher perceive as excessive. The complaint of hyperactivity is more common in boys than in girls. Terms such as minimal brain (cerebral) dysfunction (damage) or hyperkinetic behavior are not etiologically meaningful. Attentional deficit disorder (ADD) is the most recent diagnostic label applied to this varied clinical picture.

The child seen because of "hyperactivity" may have normal behavior that has been misinterpreted as abnormal. Other children constitutionally have a high level of motor activity. Usually, however, the "hyperactive" behavior is attributable to environmental and situational factors such as not doing well in school, having a sibling who is handicapped or has a serious illness such as leukemia, family financial problems, marital discord, divorce, parental illness, maternal depression, death of a relative, crowding, developmentally inappropriate care, with too little or too much stimulation, or anxiety. The symptom, thus, usually reflects a conduct rather than a neurologic disorder. Occasionally, the complaint may come about through a very inexperienced teacher who cannot maintain discipline in the classroom, especially in open classrooms. Some children do present with a primary attentional disorder, even if poorly defined.

Hyperactivity, distractibility, headache, vertigo, difficulty in controlling anger and sleep problems may be part of the post-traumatic syndrome following a head injury. The "little bit" syndrome refers to a clinical picture that appears to be due to a little bit of each of the following: hyperactivity, developmental retardation, brain damage and autistic-like behavior. Such children present difficult diagnostic and management problems and require longitudinal observation, preferably in a nursery school, by a multidisciplinary group.

## CLINICAL MANIFESTATIONS

I. In the history and on observation the child is unable to sit still, constantly moving around the office or classroom, picking up objects, opening drawers, climbing on chairs, touching everything in sight and bothering his classmates. He will not sit through a television program or the reading of a story. When maternal depression is present, the child's hyperactivity is often worse on those days when the mother is most depressed.

II. Short attention span and easy distractibility. The child attends better in a one-to-one situation or alone in a relatively stimulus-free room than in a group.

III. Impulsive motor and verbal behavior

IV. Overexcitability. Stimulating or exciting situations such as parties, guests, shopping centers, amusement parks, crowds, other children and Christmas activities tend to make the child much worse.

416

V. Socialization problems. The child often comes crashing in on other children as well as adults. He has poor peer relations, fights frequently and is overly aggressive.
VI. Other emotional and behavioral symptoms may include lying, stealing, fire-setting, disobedience, defiance, masturbation, destructiveness, nervousness, nail biting and fearfulness.
VII. School problems are both secondary to the child's short attention span and distractibility and to learning disabilities. Mental retardation is usually not a cause of the learning deficit. Hyperactivity does not always occur secondary to learning problems nor learning disorders secondary to hyperactivity.

## THE NEUROLOGIC EXAMINATION

On neurologic examination, a number of "soft" signs may be present (page 181). Since they usually represent a maturational lag in motor development, most soft signs in time disappear. Occasionally, there is hyper-reflexia or asymmetry of the deep tendon reflexes and extensor plantar reflexes.

## APPROACH TO DIAGNOSIS

The history should include the parents' and teacher's reports of the child's behavior in a variety of settings and a review of possible environmentally contributing factors. Interviews with the parents, child and school are critically important from a diagnostic viewpoint. In the assessment of the family, one should look for recent deaths, other acute stresses such as marital discord and divorce and long-term family vicissitudes such as alcoholism, mental illness and chaotic, crowded living arrangements. An electroencephalogram is indicated only when the history or physical examination suggests a convulsive disorder. Most of the children brought to the doctor because of hyperactivity are not unusually impulsive or distractible in the office. Rather, many are anxious or depressed.

## GENERAL REFERENCES

Bax, M.: Who is hyperactive? *Dev. Med. Child Neurol. 20*:277, 1978.
Bax, M.: The active and the over-active school child. *Dev. Med. Child. Neurol. 14*:83, 1972.
Birch, H.G., Thomas, A. and Chess, S.: Behavioral development in brain-damaged children. *Arch. Gen. Psychiatry 11*:596, 1964.
Cantwell, D. (ed.): *The Hyperactive Child—Diagnosis, Management, Current Research.* New York, Spectrum Publications Inc., 1975.
Clements, S.D.: *Minimal Brain Dysfunction in Children: Terminology and Classification.* U.S. Dept. of HEW, NINBD Monograph No. 3, PHS Publication 1415, Washington, D.C., U.S. Government Printing Office, 1966.
Eisenberg, L.: Hyperkinesis revisited. *Pediatrics 61*:319, 1978.
Fish, B.: The "one child, one drug" myth of stimulants in hyperkinesis. *Arch. Gen. Psychiatry 25*:193, 1971.
Grossman, H.J. and Grossman, P.B.: Mental retardation, school failure and hyperactivity. *In* Green, M. and Haggerty, R.J.: *Ambulatory Pediatrics II.* Philadelphia, W. B. Saunders Co., 1977, p. 271.
Miller, J.S.: Hyperactive children: a ten-year study. *Pediatrics 61*:217, 1978.
Sandberg, S.T., Rutter, M. and Taylor, E.: Hyperkinetic disorder in psychiatric clinic attendance. *Dev. Med. Child Neurol. 20*:279, 1978.
Schmitt, B.D.: The minimal brain dysfunction myth. *Am. J. Dis. Child. 129*:1313, 1975.
Walzer, S. and Wolff, P.H., (eds.): *Minimal Cerebral Dysfunction in Children.* New York, Grune and Stratton, Inc., 1973, p. 17.
Wender, P.H.: *Minimal Brain Dysfunction in Children.* New York, Wiley-Interscience, 1971.
Wender, P.H.: *The Hyperactive Child, A Guide for Parents.* New York, Crown Publishers, Inc., 1973.

# CHAPTER 47

# SLEEP DISORDERS

## PHYSIOLOGY OF SLEEP

Except in the newborn period and early infancy when the cycles are less defined, normal sleep consists of regular cycles of REM (rapid eye movement) and NREM (non-rapid eye movement) sleep. In the older child and adult, approximately five sleep cycles occur each night with about three-fourths of the night occupied in NREM sleep. The ratio of REM to NREM sleep in infants is 1:1 while in adults it is 1:4. The REM–NREM sleep cycle in infants is 50 to 60 minutes and in adults it is 90 to 100 minutes. During REM sleep, there is rapid, synchronous movement of the eyes and marked activity of the brain. Most dreaming occurs during REM sleep. NREM sleep, during which rapid eye movements do not occur and the brain assumes a resting phase, is composed of four stages: stage 1 or transitional; stage 2 during which sleep spindles are noted; and stages 3 and 4, which are characterized by high-amplitude slow waves.

## ETIOLOGIC CLASSIFICATION OF SLEEP DISORDERS

I. Hypersomnias
   A. Narcolepsy most frequently has its onset in the second decade of life. The patient experiences a sudden and irresistible urge to sleep. The attacks are brief, perhaps 30 seconds in duration if the child is standing and 1 to 2 hours if he is reclining. Occasionally, the patient can voluntarily delay the onset of an episode. Fifteen to twenty episodes may occur per day.

   Associated symptoms may also appear. Cataplexy, which is characterized by sudden weakness or loss in muscle tone that lasts from seconds to minutes, may be precipitated by affective states such as laughter, anger or surprise. The patient may experience a jaw drop, feel weak in the knees or fall to the floor, unable to move. Consciousness is maintained during these episodes.

   Sleep paralysis, which occurs either while the patient is falling asleep or awakening, is a brief attack of flaccid paralysis, perhaps accompanied by feelings of intense fear or by visual and auditory hallucinations.

   Zarcone, V.: Narcolepsy. *N. Engl. J. Med.* 288:1156, 1973.

   B. The Kleine-Levin syndrome, or periodic hypersomnia and bulimia, a disorder limited to males, is characterized by episodes of excessive sleep and overeating. The attacks occur from two to four times a year and may last several days to weeks. During the episode, the child usually sleeps continuously and awakens only to go to the bathroom or to gorge himself with food.

The cause of this syndrome is not known. Spontaneous remission is usual after two or three years.

Critchley, M.: Periodic hypersomnia and megaphagia in adolescent males. *Brain 85*:627, 1972.
Frank, Y., Braham, J. and Cohen, B.E.: The Kleine-Levin syndrome. *Am. J. Dis. Child. 127*:412, 1974.
Gilbert, G.J.: Periodic hypersomnia and bulimia. The Kleine-Levin syndrome. *Neurology 14*:844, 1964.

C. Depression is the most common cause of hypersomnia in adolescents. Other signs and symptoms associated with depression are discussed in Chapter 65.
D. Obstructive sleep apnea is an important cause of daytime hypersomnolence. The affected child reports hypersomnia and sleepiness during the daytime, headache on arising in the morning, fatigue and, secondarily, poor school performance. The child's sleep is characterized by periods of loud snoring repeatedly broken by apnea and partial awakening. The apnea spells, which appear chiefly during NREM sleep, may interrupt over one half of the sleep period.

Such apnea may be caused by a sleep-induced intermittent hypotonia of the tongue muscles causing partial or complete upper airway obstruction; obstruction associated with enlargement of the tonsils and adenoids; glossoptosis in the Pierre Robin syndrome; and extreme obesity (the obesity-hypoventilation or Pickwickian syndrome).

Prolonged apnea and sudden death may also occur during an episode of nasopharyngitis in some infants.

Guilleminault, C., Eldridge, F.L., Simmons, F.B. and Dement, W.C.: Sleep apnea in eight children. *Pediatrics 58*:23, 1976.
Guilleminault, C., Dement, W. and Alan, R. (eds.): *Sleep Apnea Syndromes*. New York, Liss Inc., 1978.
Kravath, R.E., Pollak, C.P. and Borowiecki, B.: Hypoventilation during sleep in children who have lymphoid airway obstruction treated by nasopharyngeal tube and T and A. *Pediatrics 59*:865, 1977.
Simpser, M.D. et al.: Sleep apnea in a child with the Pickwickian syndrome. *Pediatrics 60*:290, 1977.
Steinschneider, A.: Nasopharyngitis and prolonged sleep apnea. *Pediatrics 56*:967, 1975.

E. Postencephalitic
F. Post-traumatic. Sleep disorders may be part of the post-traumatic syndrome after head injury.
G. Drug induced
II. Dyssomnias
A. Somnambulism, or sleepwalking, occurs in 1 to 6 per cent of the population, most frequently in school-age boys within the first three hours of sleep in the transition from stage 3 or 4 NREM sleep to more superficial levels preceding the first REM sleep cycle period. The child suddenly awakens, sits up, climbs out of bed and walks about with his eyes open but apparently uncomprehending and poorly coordinated. Mumbled and monosyllabic responses may be given to questions. Unless protected, he may hurt himself. Episodes last from seconds to 30 minutes and are not remembered by the child. One to four episodes may occur per week. While the cause of somnambulism is not clear, the most likely etiology appears to be a develop-

mental one since sleepwalking tends to be outgrown within a few years. Psychomotor epilepsy is also a diagnostic consideration.

B. Night terrors (pavor nocturnus) occur during arousal from stage 3 or 4 NREM sleep early in the night, occasionally 90 to 100 minutes after going to sleep. Most frequent in the 3- to 8-year age group, night terrors may also occur in older infants and persist into adolescence. The child suddenly sits up, screams in terror and appears intensely anxious, with tachycardia, sweating and agitation. He cannot be consoled. Episodes last from a few seconds to 10 or 30 minutes and are not remembered by the child. Night terrors probably are a developmental phenomenon and disappear with further maturation of the central nervous system. Occasionally, a stressful environmental event can be identified as a precipitating cause.

C. Nightmares are frightening dreams that occur during REM sleep. The child is more easily aroused than with night terrors, usually becoming fully awake and vividly recalls the content of the dream. An occasional nightmare is within normal developmental limits, but persistent or frequent episodes suggest a developmental disturbance.

D. Enuresis, discussed more fully in Chapter 48, occasionally occurs as the child arouses from stage 3 or 4 NREM sleep prior to entering the first REM sleep period 1 to 3 hours after going to sleep.

Gastault, H. and Broughton, R.: A clinical and polygraphic study of episodic phenomena during sleep. *Recent Adv. Biol. Psychiatry* 7:197, 1965.

E. Somniloquy, or talking while asleep, occurs during periods of arousal from REM sleep.

III. Developmental/psychological

A. Resistance to sleep. Infants between the ages of six to nine months may object to going to sleep. This reluctance is due both to the baby's own developmental stage and to environmental events. Since sleep is a separation experience, it is understandable that the infant of this age may be uncomfortable or anxious about going to bed. If the mother is unable to set limits or if she fears that the baby's crying will disturb her husband's studying or the neighbors, the problem may persist. In the latter event, the baby develops chronic resistance to sleep.

B. Sleep awakening. After the first year of life, an occasional infant will awaken in the middle of the night and then refuse to go back to sleep. Many times, these episodes begin during an illness. If the parent is firm about her expectation that the baby go to sleep, the problem is a transient one. If, however, she is not firm or attempts to remedy the problem by taking the baby into the parental bed, sleep awakening may persist. Since one of the parents often also has a sleep problem, an appropriate question is, "Who else in your family has trouble sleeping?"

C. In the vulnerable child syndrome, sleep problems are common. The child often sleeps in the parents' bedroom, either with the mother, with both parents or in his own crib or bed, which is kept next to the mother in her direct line of vision. The parents may report that the baby does not sleep well, but a closer inquiry often reveals that it is the parent who awakens several times a night to check on the child, often managing to arouse him to be sure that he is alive. The interview in these cases may reveal that the mother is unable to sleep at night unless she feels the baby is safe and sound. It becomes apparent that many such mothers unwittingly keep the baby awake each night through a series of visual, auditory and tactile stimuli conveying her insistence that the baby not fall asleep, probably because of her fear that she would again feel the baby was dead.

D. Depressed mother. Resistance to going to sleep and sleep awakening during the night are frequent manifestations in infants of depressed mothers.

E. Mother unable to set limits. As mentioned previously, if the mother is not able to set normal developmental limits, a persistent sleep problem may develop.

F. Night-time rocking and head banging. Some babies may normally rock themselves to sleep. If this habit is exaggerated, environmental factors should be reviewed.

Sallustro, F. and Atwell, C.W.: Body rocking, head banging, and head rolling in normal children. *J. Pediatr. 93*:704, 1978.

G. Night-time wandering. Some preschool-age children, seen because of hyperactivity or destructiveness, are reported to climb out of bed during the night, wander around the house, turn on the electric or gas range and, if they can find matches, start fires. Since these children usually have major emotional disturbances, psychiatric help is generally required.

IV. Insomnia. Older children and adolescents with persistent insomnia may be tense, worried, moody or depressed. From 5 to 12 per cent of adolescents may report trouble sleeping.

Price, V.A., Coates, T.J., Thoresen, C.E. and Grinstead, O.A.: Prevalence and correlates of poor sleep among adolescents. *Am. J. Dis. Child. 132*:583, 1978.
Young people who sleep badly (Editorial). *Br. Med. J. 2*:1450, 1978.

V. Sleep reversals occur in some children with hepatic failure or postencephalitic behavior.

VI. Psychomotor seizures need to be included as a rare diagnostic possibility in children with night terrors or somnambulism episodes that appear to be more than transient developmental problems.

## GENERAL REFERENCES

Anders, T.F. and Weinstein, P.: Sleep and its disorders in infants and children: a review. *Pediatrics 50*:312, 1972.
Anders, T.F.: Night-waking in infants during the first year of life. *Pediatrics 63*:860, 1979.
Broughton, R.J.: Sleep disorders: disorders of arousal? *Science 159*:1070, 1968.
Kales, A. and Kales, J.D.: Sleep disorders. *N. Engl. J. Med. 290*:487, 1974.
Nagera, H.: Sleep and its disorders approached developmentally. *Psychoanal. Study Child 21*:393, 1966.
Parmelee, A.H., Jr., Wenner, W.H. and Schulz, H.R.: Infant sleep patterns: from birth to 16 weeks of age. *J. Pediatr. 65*:576, 1964.
Rabe, E.F.: Recurrent paroxysmal nonepileptic disorders. *Cur. Prob. Pediatr. 4*:3 (June) 1974.

CHAPTER **48**

# ENURESIS

Enuresis, defined as involuntary urination after five or six years of age, is common in children from lower socioeconomic families and in many others who appear to have a familial predisposition to bed wetting. Enuresis is more common in boys than in girls.

## ETIOLOGY

The etiology is usually a delay in neuromuscular maturation. Enuretic children often have smaller functional bladder capacities than those who are not enuretic. Enuresis may also occur in response to environmental stresses. This seems to be true especially of daytime or diurnal wetting. It is unusual, however, for primary enuresis to be the only manifestation of psychologic maladaptation. Relapse or secondary enuresis is more likely to be related to exciting events or stresses such as a separation experience. Enuresis may also be caused by obstructive uropathy, diabetes mellitus, diabetes insipidus and psychogenic water drinking. Children with myelomeningocele frequently have urinary incontinence, as do those who are mentally retarded.

## DIAGNOSIS

As with other developmental symptoms, diagnosis and treatment should proceed simultaneously, with the interview serving as the principal tool to collect data and to establish the kind of relationship between the doctor, child and family that promotes mastery of this symptom. Through the interview, the physician clarifies for himself and for the patient the multiple etiologic possibilities. He determines the familial incidence of enuresis, the family's and the child's understanding of the problem, their interest in overcoming this symptom, the methods that have already been tried and their notions about what might work. In clarifying the nature of the problem, the doctor sets the stage for the child's active participation in the mastery of his own problem. He also promotes the child's identification with the physician and the doctor's confident expectation that the child will be able to control his enuresis.

The frequency of dry nights or periods of several nights during which enuresis has not occurred has some predictive value as to the spontaneous cessation of the symptom. Frequency, urgency, dribbling, dysuria, hesitancy in beginning urination, a poor urinary stream or a history of previous urinary tract infections suggest organic etiologies. Daytime enuresis occurring more frequently than nocturnal wetting raises the possibility of an organic etiology. Observation of the boy's urinary stream by the physician may be indicated to determine whether there is difficulty in initiating urination or an interrupted urinary stream.

## LABORATORY EVALUATION

The laboratory investigation of children with enuresis should include a urinalysis for specific gravity, glycosuria, proteinuria, pyuria and culture. If symptoms suggest obstructive urologic disease, an intravenous pyelogram and voiding cystourethrogram should be strongly considered.

## GENERAL REFERENCES

Cohen, M.W.: Enuresis. *Pediatr. Clin. N. Am. 22*:547, 1975.
Imipramine for enuresis. *Med. Lett. Drugs Ther. 16*:22, 1974.
McKendry, J.B.J. and Stewart, D.A.: Enuresis. *Pediatr. Clin. N. Am. 21*:1019, 1974.
McLain, L.G.: Childhood enuresis, *Curr. Probl. Pediatr. 9*:4 (June) 1979.
Marshall, S., Marshall, H.H. and Lyon, R.P.: Enuresis: an analysis of various therapeutic approaches. *Pediatrics 52*:813, 1973.
Starfield, B.: Enuresis: its pathogenesis and management. *Clin. Pediatr. 2*:343, 1972.

# CHAPTER 49

# CONVULSIONS

Convulsive seizures affect an estimated 7 per cent of children under the age of 5 years. The underlying pathophysiologic cause of convulsive seizures is not known. Classification of convulsive seizures cannot, therefore, be based on fundamental considerations but must depend upon such factors as the age of the patient, the clinical pattern of the seizure, electroencephalographic findings, anatomic localization and the disorders that may be accompanied by this symptom. The classification given here, intended as a guide to diagnostic considerations in children with convulsive seizures, relates to a number of these etiologic factors. Some of these processes may account either for isolated acute seizures or for recurrent episodes. A patient may demonstrate more than one type of seizure. A detailed description of the seizure and possible precipitating events may be helpful diagnostically.

## ETIOLOGIC CLASSIFICATION OF CONVULSIONS IN OLDER INFANTS AND CHILDREN

I. Febrile convulsions. Convulsive seizures accompany acute febrile illnesses not infrequently in children under the age of three years, especially in the first two years and more commonly in boys. In children under the age of 5 years, these episodes have been estimated to occur with an incidence of between 3.5 and 4 per cent.

The febrile seizure, either generalized with tonic and clonic components or focal, usually follows a rapid rise in temperature to 39.4° C. (103° F.) or above. The seizure may be brief (one to ten minutes) and mild, or longer (over one-half hour) and severe.

A number of relationships exist between fever and convulsive seizures. Fever, in itself, may be the direct cause of a convulsion; on the other hand, severe convulsive seizures may cause some elevation of body temperature as a result of muscular activity. The seizure may be due primarily to an infectious or other disease and not to the fever itself. An effort should be made to determine the primary cause of the fever and of the convulsion in each child with a "febrile" convulsion. Elevation of body temperature may act as a precipitating event in a child destined to have idiopathic epilepsy. Rarely, fever may be an epileptic manifestation in itself.

Most children who have one or two febrile convulsions never experience another; however, about one third have a subsequent febrile seizure and 2 to 3 per cent will have recurrent nonfebrile seizures. Although it is impossible to prognosticate, seizures that are focal, that persist over 30 minutes or that are followed by neurologic findings such as hemiparesis are more likely to be followed by later convulsions. Children who have a history of repeated seizures with only slight elevation of temperature are also likely to have future difficulty. Other high-risk factors include a family history of seizures without fever and pre-existing neurologic impairment in the child. The electroencephalogram may provide prognostic information since there is a correlation between abnormal electroencephalographic findings and the later appearance of epilepsy.

Fishman, M.A.: Febrile seizures: the treatment controversy. *J. Pediatr. 94*:177, 1979.
Freeman, J.M.: Febrile seizures: an end to confusion. *Pediatrics 61*:806, 1978.
Nelson, K.B. and Ellenberg, J.H.: Prognosis in children with febrile seizures. *Pediatrics 61*:720, 1978.

II. Epilepsy may be defined as a recurrent symptomatic state owing to abnormal discharges from the central nervous system.
   A. Grand mal or major seizure. About half of the children who have grand mal epilepsy experience a motor, sensory or visceral aura before the convulsion. Abdominal pain is a common aura. Others include a peculiar sensation in the throat, an unusual taste or smell, chewing motions and turning of the head. The aura usually remains the same in the individual patient.

The actual seizure begins suddenly with loss of consciousness. If standing, the patient falls. The child may cry out. The first or tonic phase, which lasts about one-half to one minute and is characterized by a stiffening of the body and a fine muscular tremor, is followed by the clonic phase. The convulsive twitching and jerking movements become stronger but less rapid and gradually cease. During this time, the patient's face becomes cyanotic, and saliva may run from his mouth. Involuntary urination and defecation may occur. Vomiting commonly follows the convulsive episode.

The seizure, which may last from one to five minutes, is followed by a period of sleep from which the child is not easily aroused. On awakening, the child may appear confused and complain of a severe headache. Occasionally, transient paresis of an extremity or hemiparesis may develop (Todd's paralysis).

Young children with major convulsions may demonstrate only the tonic phase, or the clonic movements may not be as prominent as in older infants and children. This is not always the case, however.

In status epilepticus the patient has repeated or persistent convulsive seizures, usually clonic, and remains unconscious for over an hour.

B. Petit mal epilepsy. Petit mal seizures or absence attacks, which are most common between 4 and 8 years of age, are characterized by transient (5 to 20 seconds) lapses of consciousness. The patient has a blank, staring expression, or the eyes may roll up. He either becomes immobile or demonstrates rhythmic myoclonic movements such as blinking, nodding or jerking of the head, truncal swaying, twitching of the extremities or trunk and snapping of the fingers. The child may walk in circles. The patient does not fall but may drop whatever he is holding. There is no aura or postictal symptoms. Only a few seizures, or as many as a hundred, may occur per day. Petit mal episodes can often be precipitated by hyperventilation for 1 to 4 minutes. The electroencephalogram reveals a characteristic 3-per-second wave and spike pattern.

Spike-wave stupor (petit mal status) may be difficult to differentiate from psychomotor seizures. The child with this seizure pattern remains for hours in a confused, groggy state that may simulate a cerebral degenerative disease. In addition to lethargy, the child may have facial twitches and muscle jerks or he may stagger about.

Moe, P.G: Spike-wave stupor. Petit mal status. *Am. J. Dis. Child. 121*:307, 1971.

C. Myoclonic seizures
1. Myoclonic epilepsy of older children (akinetic epilepsy; petit mal variant) is characterized by sudden, spasmodic contractions, lasting only a few seconds, of the muscles of the trunk or extremities, most commonly the flexors of the arms. Extensor spasms may also occur. When they are marked, the flexor spasms may cause the child to pitch forward violently, injuring his face and head. Akinetic spells (drop fits) are characterized by a sudden loss of muscle tone with the child nodding or slumping to the floor. Grand mal seizures and staring spells may be associated kinds of convulsions. Many of these children are developmentally retarded. Myoclonic seizures are also caused by subacute sclerosing panencephalitis, other cerebral degenerative disorders and Unverricht-Lundborg progres-

sive familial myoclonic epilepsy. In myoclonic encephalopathy of infants (Kinsbourne dancing eye syndrome), the affected infant demonstrates jerking movements of the head, trunk and extremities, ataxia and dancing movements (opsoclonus) of the eyes. In sensory precipitation epilepsy, myoclonic seizures may also be precipitated by tapping or touching.

2. Massive myoclonic seizures (myoclonic epilepsy of infancy, lightning seizures and infantile spasms) are brief convulsive seizures in infants (salaam, head dropping or jackknifing) characterized by flexion and adduction or upward and outward movement of the upper extremities, flexion of the head on the chest, jackknife flexion of the thighs on the abdomen, generalized quivering and rolling of the eyes. Occasionally, extension of the head and lower extremities occurs instead. The baby may also cry out. The seizures often follow in close succession, and a hundred or so may occur in one day. Infants with this seizure pattern usually have extensive brain damage and are both microcephalic and retarded. Grand mal and focal seizures may also occur in these patients. The term "hypsarrhythmia" refers to the electroencephalographic pattern characteristically found. Disorders associated with myoclonic seizures in infants include tuberous sclerosis, Menkes' kinky hair syndrome, gangliosidosis, pyridoxine dependency or deficiency, phenylketonuria, maple syrup urine disease, cytomegalic inclusion disease, toxoplasmosis and congenital malformations of the brain.

Dyken, P. and Kolar, P.: Dancing eyes, dancing feet: infantile polymyoclonia. *Brain 91*:305, 1968.
Livingston, S.: Diagnosis and treatment of childhood myoclonic seizures. *Pediatrics 53*:542, 1974.

3. Benign myoclonus of early infancy is the term applied to a small group of infants in whom myoclonic seizures, especially involving the extensors and flexors of the neck or adversive jerking or turning of the head (cephalic myoclonus), stop spontaneously a few weeks or months after their onset.

Lombroso, C.T. and Fejerman, N.: Benign myoclonus of early infancy. *Ann. Neurol. 1*:138, 1977.

D. Diencephalic epilepsy; autonomic seizures; abdominal epilepsy; convulsive equivalent. This type of epilepsy, thought to be due to abnormal hypothalamic discharges, may be characterized by episodes of flushing, pallor, dizziness, hypertension, dilatation of the pupils, lacrimation, perspiration, tachycardia, salivation and vomiting or masticatory movements, which last from minutes to hours. Other symptoms may include paroxysmal abdominal pain, fever and headache.

Chao, D., Sexton, J. A. and Davis, S.D.: Convulsive equivalent syndrome of childhood. *J. Pediatr. 64*:499, 1964.

E. Psychomotor epilepsy, not uncommon in children, has extremely varied symptoms. They may be chiefly *motor* in the form of automatisms such as rubbing, chewing, lip smacking, drooling, spitting, hissing, muttering, swallowing, staring, blinking, muscle jerks, laughing (gelastic epilepsy); shouting, purposeless wandering and running (cursive epilepsy); *autonomic* with pallor or flushing; *psychic* in the form of confused, dream-like states, fugues, hallucinations, fearfulness, manic, aggressive or psychotic behavior and temper outbursts; or *sensory* with numbness, tingling, impaired vision or blindness, hearing loss and dizziness. Visual illusions in which objects appear small and far away, unusually large or distorted may be reported.

Irritability, hyperactivity, headache and altered appetite may be noted hours or days before episodes. Auras include epigastric discomfort or heaviness that moves up to the throat, fear, buzzing sensations, dizziness and visual and auditory illusions.

The patient may or may not have amnesia for the seizure. Consciousness may be altered if not completely lost. The electroencephalogram may show a focal seizure pattern or may be normal. Differentiation between a severe behavior disorder, schizophrenia and psychomotor epilepsy may be difficult, and they may coexist. Psychomotor epilepsy is initially sometimes confused with petit mal seizures.

Geschwind, N.: Behavioral change in temporal lobe epilepsy. *Arch. Neurol. 34*:453, 1977.
Gold, A.P.: Psychomotor epilepsy in childhood. *Pediatrics 53*:540, 1974.

F. Focal (partial) seizures, infrequent in childhood, may be either motor (clonic movements or twitching) or sensory (paresthesias). Jacksonian seizures begin with facial twitching or "march" up an extremity, perhaps continuing to involve one side of the body or progressing to a generalized seizure. Partial motor or adversive seizures may be characterized by contraversive movement of the head and eyes and lifting of the contralateral upper extremity. If accompanied by unconsciousness, the partial seizure arises from the anterior frontal lobe; without loss of consciousness, it originates from the posterior portion of the frontal lobe. Occipital seizures may cause transient blindness.

G. Sensory-precipitated seizures may be caused by a number of sensory stimuli. Photoconvulsions, the most common, are usually precipitated by watching television. They may also be self-induced by waving fingers before the eyes or blinking while looking at a bright light. Other precipitating causes are music (musicogenic epilepsy), brushing the teeth, touching, tapping and reading.

Calderon-Gonzalez, R., Hopkins, I. and McLean, W.T., Jr.: Tap seizures: a form of sensory precipitation epilepsy. *JAMA 198*:107, 1966.

H. Hyperexplexia is a hereditary disorder characterized by an excessive startle response, generalized muscle stiffness and sudden falling.

Suhren, O., Bruyn, G.W. and Tuynman, J.A.: Hyperexplexia — a hereditary startle syndrome. *J. Neurol. Sci. 3*:577, 1966.

III. Metabolic factors
   A. Hypocalcemia
      1. Newborn. Symptoms associated with hypocalcemia (serum calcium less than 7 mg./dl.) in the newborn include jitteriness, tremor, irritability, laryngospasm and seizures. The infant may also appear lethargic, fail to feed, or vomit.

    a. Birth to 72 hours
      (1) Maternal factors
         *a.* Hyperparathyroidism. The maternal serum calcium and phosphorus should be determined.
         *b.* Toxemia of pregnancy
         *c.* Diabetes mellitus
      (2) Perinatal factors
         *a.* Placenta previa, abruptio placentae
         *b.* Low birth weight; prematurity or small for gestational age
         *c.* Cesarean section
         *d.* Birth trauma with cerebral injury
         *e.* Asphyxia
         *f.* Respiratory distress syndrome
         *g.* Sepsis
         *h.* Hyperbilirubinemia
    b. After 72 hours
      (1) High phosphate intake in infants receiving cow milk or soy bean milk or other formula with high phosphate:calcium ratio
      (2) Hypomagnesemia
      (3) Hypoparathyroidism
  2. Hypoparathyroidism
    a. Transient idiopathic
    b. Familial
    c. DiGeorge's syndrome

Conley, M.E., Beckwith, J.B., Mancer, J.K.K. and Tenckhoff, L.: The spectrum of DiGeorge syndrome. *J. Pediatr. 94*:883, 1979.

    d. Acquired
    e. Pseudohypoparathyroidism
  3. Vitamin D deficiency or metabolic defect

Root, A.W. and Harrison, H.E.: Recent advances in calcium metabolism. II. Disorders of calcium homeostasis. *J. Pediatr. 88*:177, 1976.

  4. Pediatric sodium dihydrogen phosphate enemas may cause hypocalcemia secondary to hyperphosphatemia. Tetany, coma and dehydration may result.

Sotos, J.F., Cutler, E.A., Finkel, M.A. and Doody, D.: Hypocalcemia coma following two pediatric phosphate enemas. *Pediatrics 60*:305, 1977.

B. Hypomagnesemia. Serum magnesium concentrations should be obtained in infants with tetany.

Paunier, L. et al.: Primary hypomagnesemia with secondary hypocalcemia in an infant. *Pediatrics 41*:385, 1968.

C. Hypoglycemia. Symptomatic neonatal hypoglycemia is seen with a frequency of 2–3/1000 live births. Many other infants have subclinical hypoglycemia. Blood glucose determinations (Dextrostix or blood sugar) need to be repeated frequently in infants at risk as well as in those with such subtle and varied signs and symptoms as irritability, tremors, convulsions, apnea, cyanosis, listlessness, poor feeding, rolling eye movements, high-pitched cry, unstable body temperature, pallor, absent Moro reflex and limpness. A blood sugar should be obtained whenever a newborn infant seems ill. The diagnostic criteria for hypoglycemia are two or more determinations under 20 mg./dl. in infants under 2500 grams, under 30 mg. in term newborn infants and under 40 mg. in older infants and children.

1. Hypoglycemia may occur early and subclinically in infants born to diabetic mothers and in those with hemolytic disease of the newborn before and after exchange transfusion. Secondary hypoglycemia may follow such perinatal stresses as hypoxia, sepsis, respiratory distress, hypothermia, central nervous system impairment, hyperviscosity and multiple congenital anomalies. Transient neonatal hypoglycemia tends to be severe and to recur in infants, especially males, who are small for gestational age, with toxemia of pregnancy and in the smaller of twins. The metabolic, endocrine and enzymatic disorders listed may also cause neonatal hypoglycemia. In the older infant and child, the manifestations of hypoglycemia include "wilting" spells, blank stares, rolling of the eyes, episodes of pallor, periods of unexplained irritability and crying, stiffening, limpness, twitching and generalized convulsions.

2. Hyperinsulinemia
   a. Beta-cell hyperplasia: Beckwith-Wiedemann syndrome
   b. Beta-cell tumors
   c. Nesidioblastosis
   d. Functional beta-cell defects

3. Ketotic hypoglycemia, which usually becomes apparent between the ages of 18 months and 5 years and undergoes spontaneous cessation by 10 years of age, is probably the most common cause of hypoglycemia beyond the newborn period. In addition to hypoglycemia, the patient demonstrates ketonuria and ketonemia.

4. Endocrine disorders
   a. Hypopituitarism
   b. Isolated ACTH deficiency
   c. Addison's disease
   d. Hypothyroidism

5. Hepatic enzyme deficiencies
   a. Glycogenosis
      (1) Glucose-6-phosphatase (glycogenosis type I) causes marked ketosis, hypoglycemia, lactic acidosis, hepatomegaly and failure to thrive in young infants.
      (2) Amylo-1,6-glucosidase
      (3) Defects of the phosphorylase enzyme system
   b. Disorders of gluconeogenesis
      (1) Fructose-1, 6-diphosphatase. The presenting signs and symptoms are indistinguishable from those due to deficiency of glucose-6-phosphatase.
      (2) Pyruvate carboxylase
   c. Other enzymatic defects
      (1) Glycogen synthetase
      (2) Galactose-1-phosphate uridyl transferase (galactosemia)
      (3) Fructose-1-phosphate aldolase (hereditary fructose intolerance) is characterized by hypoglycemia and vomiting after fructose ingestion.

6. Other inborn errors of metabolism
   a. Maple syrup urine disease
   b. Congenital lactic acidosis
   c. Lysosomal acid phosphatase deficiency

Cornblath, M. and Schwartz, R.: *Disorders of Carbohydrate Metabolism in Infancy.* 2nd ed. Philadelphia. W. B. Saunders Co., 1976.

Guterlet, R.L. and Cornblath, M.: Neonatal hypoglycemia revisited, 1975. *Pediatrics 58*:10, 1976.

Lubchenco, L.O. and Bard, H.: Incidence of hypoglycemia in newborn infants classified by birth weight and gestational age. *Pediatrics 47*:831, 1971.

Pagliara, A.S., Karl, I.E., Haymond, M. and Kipnis, D.M.: Hypoglycemia in infancy and childhood. Parts I and II. *J. Pediatr. 82*:365,558, 1973.

Schwartz, J.F. and Zwiren, G.T.: Islet cell adenomatosis and adenoma in an infant. *J. Pediatr. 79*:332, 1971.

Stanley, C.A. and Baker, L.: Hyperinsulinism in infants and children: diagnosis and therapy. *Adv. Pediatr. 23*:315, 1976.

D. Since hyponatremia and hypo-osmolarity may occur in children with acute infections of the central nervous system, determination of the serum electrolytes is indicated in such patients who have otherwise unexplained seizures.

Varavithya, W. and Hellerstein, S.: Acute symptomatic hyponatremia. *J. Pediatr. 71*:269, 1967.

E. Uremia

F. Poisoning should be considered as an etiologic possibility with unexplained convulsive seizures. The history should include information about poisons and drugs to which the child may have had access. Seizures due to lead encephalopathy, more common in summer, may first occur during an acute infection and be mistakenly ascribed to the illness, to fever or to idiopathic epilepsy. Early symptoms of lead poisoning include vomiting, constipation, irritability and lethargy. Although parents should be specifically asked about pica, especially chewing of paint-covered surfaces, denial of such exposure does not eliminate the possibility of lead poisoning. Qualitative determination of urine coproporphyrins is a preliminary screening test. A more significant finding is increased free erythrocyte protoporphyrin. The peripheral blood may demonstrate microcytic, stippled erythrocytes. Radiopaque material may be seen in the gastrointestinal tract in a plain film of the abdomen. Glycosuria and aminoaciduria may be noted. Examination of the cerebrospinal fluid may demonstrate increased pressure and protein concentration. Early, the latter may be present without the former. Other poisons that may produce convulsive seizures include:

Strychnine
Arsenic
Sodium fluoride
Camphor
Pyrethrum
Kerosene
Gasoline
Volatile oils
Poisonous plants
Salicylate poisoning

G. Pyridoxine (vitamin $B_6$) deficiency or dependency in young infants may cause irritability, hyperacusia, colic, regurgitation and convulsive seizures.

Scriver, C.R.: Vitamin $B_6$ deficiency and dependency in man. *Am. J. Dis. Child. 113*:109, 1967.

H. Anoxia
   1. Asphyxia
   2. Carbon monoxide poisoning
   3. Near-drowning
   4. Breath-holding spells predominantly occur between the ages of six months and two years. Such episodes are precipitated by a fall or injury or an episode in which the child becomes angry or is reprimanded. He begins to cry vigorously and then holds his breath in expiration. Cyanosis, unconsciousness, rigidity, opisthotonus, and mild clonic twitching or jerking follow. Such seizures are always preceded by crying, usually vigorous, except in some children who experience large numbers of these episodes and who only gasp or cry briefly before holding their breath. While an occasional breath-holding spell is within normal limits, frequent episodes are due to maternal-infant problems.

Livingston, S.: Breathholding spells in children. A differentiation from epileptic attacks. *JAMA 212*:2231, 1970.
Lombroso, C.T. and Lerman, P.: Breathholding spells (cyanotic and pallid infantile syncope). *Pediatrics 39*:563, 1967.

   5. Respiratory failure
   6. Seizure-like states, hot flashes and episodes of weakness may be presenting complaints in children with primary pulmonary hypertension.
I. Phenothiazine tranquilizers may precipitate or increase seizures in patients with idiopathic epilepsy.
J. Newborn infants of mothers addicted to narcotics may demonstrate such withdrawal symptoms as respiratory distress, restlessness, trembling, irritability, convulsions and a shrill, high-pitched cry.
K. Phenylketonuria may be characterized by seizures.
L. Other inborn metabolic errors
IV. Cerebral factors
   A. Trauma
      1. Cerebral concussion; contusion; laceration; focal or generalized edema of the brain
      2. Extradural hematoma; subdural hematoma
   B. Infections of the central nervous system
      1. Toxoplasmosis is an important consideration in the differential diagnosis of convulsive seizures in newborn and young infants.
      2. In addition to specific types of viral encephalitis, encephalitis may precede, accompany or follow the acute exanthema of childhood.
      3. Convulsions may be an important clinical manifestation of meningitis.
      4. Subdural effusion complicating bacterial meningitis is to be considered with persistence of fever after 72 hours, positive cerebrospinal fluid culture after 48 hours, generalized convulsions during convalescence, focal convulsions, vomiting during the convalescent period, gross neuro-

logic abnormalities, hemiparesis, opisthotonus, bulging fontanel, enlargement of the head, impairment of consciousness, persistence of irritability or an otherwise unsatisfactory clinical course.

    5. Intracranial abscess

    6. Rabies

C. Intracranial hemorrhage

    1. Subdural hematoma. Generalized, unilateral or focal convulsions are a common manifestation of a subdural hematoma.

    2. Extradural hematoma

    3. Subarachnoid hemorrhage owing to rupture of a congenital aneurysm of the circle of Willis may unusually cause convulsive seizures in older children.

    4. Hemorrhagic diseases such as hemophilia or thrombocytopenic purpura may be complicated by an intracranial hemorrhage.

D. Thrombosis of cerebral vessels

    1. Congenital heart disease. Children with cyanotic heart disease and polycythemia may develop cerebral thrombosis, especially with dehydration. Syncope, coma and severe, persistent convulsions may result.

Phornphutkul, C., Rosenthal, A., Nadas, A.S. and Berenberg, W.: Cerebrovascular accidents in infants and children with cyanotic congenital heart disease. *Am. J. Cardiol.* *32*:329, 1973.

    2. Sickle cell anemia

Portnoy, B.A. and Herion, J.C.: Neurological manifestations in sickle cell disease with a review of the literature and emphasis on the prevalence of hemiplegia. *Ann. Int. Med.* *76*:643, 1972.

    3. Occlusion of the venous sinuses and cerebral veins may occur in severely dehydrated infants and young children. Clinical manifestations may include impairment of consciousness and convulsive seizures.

    4. Acute infantile hemiplegia in infants and young children is due to a sudden vascular accident such as embolism or thrombosis of the middle cerebral artery. The onset is almost always sudden with a severe convulsion, usually unilateral but occasionally generalized, followed by fever, coma and hemiparesis. Convulsions continue for one to five days, and coma may persist for seven to ten days.

Solomon, G.E., Hilal, S.K., Gold, A.P. and Carter, S.: Natural history of acute hemiplegia of childhood. *Brain 93*:107, 1970.

E. Sturge-Weber syndrome. Convulsive seizures in these children may be generalized or limited to the contralateral side.

F. Psychologic factors

    1. Breath-holding spells

    2. Children who have a low threshold to photic stimulation may induce seizures by blinking or waving their fingers in front of their eyes. Other children may produce seizures by hyperventilation. Such patients are usually mentally retarded and/or emotionally disturbed.

Green, J.B: Self-induced seizures. *Arch. Neurol. 15*:579, 1966.

    3. Emotional factors may increase the frequency of seizures.

    4. Hysteria and other psychogenic factors may cause pseudoepileptic seizures.

Finlayson, R.E. and Lucas, A.R.: Pseudoepileptic seizures in children and adolescents. *Mayo Clin. Proc. 54*:83, 1979.

G. Encephalopathy
   1. Postpertussis vaccine encephalopathy
   2. Pertussis may cause convulsions owing to cerebral hemorrhage, encephalitis or anoxia.
   3. Acute glomerulonephritis may lead to convulsive seizures caused by hypertensive encephalopathy.
   4. Toxic encephalopathy with seizures and impairment of consciousness may occur during severe systemic diseases such as bacillary dysentery.
   5. Seizures may occur with lupus erythematosus.
   6. Infectious mononucleosis may rarely cause seizures.
   7. Convulsions may be a complication of corticosteroid treatment, especially in lupus erythematosus.

H. Degenerative diseases
   1. Demyelinating encephalopathies may first become manifest with a convulsion. Often, however, seizures do not occur.
   2. $G_{M1}$ gangliosidosis (type II or late infantile) becomes manifest in the second or third year with retardation and seizures. Juvenile $G_{M1}$ gangliosidosis is characterized by ataxia, seizures and mental deterioration.
   3. Metachromatic leukodystrophy becomes symptomatic at about the end of the first year of life with ataxia followed later by intellectual deterioration and seizures.
   4. Tuberous sclerosis in infants is often accompanied by massive myoclonic seizures.
   5. Tay-Sachs disease. Convulsive seizures are a late manifestation.
   6. Other cerebromacular degenerative diseases
   7. Niemann-Pick disease
   8. Infantile Gaucher's disease
   9. Subacute sclerosing panencephalitis is initially manifested by subtle personality changes and deterioration in school performance. Behavioral changes include forgetfulness, temper outbursts, distractibility, hallucinations and insomnia. Myoclonic seizures involving the head, trunk and extremities then appear and may initially simulate ataxia. Eventually, the episodes occur every 5 to 15 seconds without loss of consciousness. The diagnosis may be made at this stage by characteristic electroencephalographic, spinal fluid and measles antibody findings. With progression of the disorder, the myoclonic jerks become exaggerated, and there is progressive intellectual deterioration.

Freeman, J.M.: The clinical spectrum and early diagnosis of Dawson's encephalitis. *J. Pediatr. 75*:590, 1969.
Noronha, M.J.: Cerebral degenerative disorders of infancy and childhood. *Dev. Med. Child Neurol. 16*:228, 1974.

I. Brain tumors. Generalized convulsive seizures may occur with supratentorial tumors as the initial symptom unaccompanied by signs of increased intracranial pressure. This is more likely to occur in late adolescence than in infancy or childhood. Convulsions are less commonly the initial symptom in patients with infratentorial tumors. Increased pressure in the posterior fossa may produce "cerebellar fits" characterized by decerebrate rigidity, opisthotonus, respiratory difficulty and cyanosis. Patients with unexplained seizures, especially focal ones, should be followed carefully with repeated neurologic examinations. In addition, changes in behavior, school performance, response to medication or type and frequency of seizures warrant consideration of a brain tumor.

Page, L.K., Lombroso, C.T. and Matson, D.D.: Childhood epilepsy with late detection of cerebral glioma. *J. Neurosurg. 31*:253, 1969.

J. Tetanus

## CONVULSIONS IN NEWBORN INFANTS

Seizures in the newborn and young infant differ from those seen in older infants and children. Since they may be subtle in their manifestations, they require special diagnostic alertness. The most frequent is the focal clonic convulsion, which may either move rapidly from one part of the body to another or remain localized. The seizure may or may not be accompanied by unconsciousness. Tonic spasms are rarely seen. Even in metabolic disorders, the seizures are focal or localized to one half of the body. In the newborn, true seizures require differentiation from the normal jitteriness precipitated by handling or startling. Such tremors are not accompanied by abnormal eye movements and are characterized by an equal rate and amplitude. Neonatal seizures, on the other hand, are usually clonic with both slow and fast components, perhaps accompanied by eye rolling, and are not stimulus responsive.

## ETIOLOGIC CLASSIFICATION OF CONVULSIONS IN NEWBORN INFANTS

I. Central nervous system disorders
   A. Asphyxia. In addition to the history and the Apgar score, infants who have experienced hypoxia are often apathetic, floppy and jittery. Seizures due to hypoxia usually begin 6 to 24 hours after birth.
   B. Intracranial hemorrhage
      1. Periventricular hemorrhage may occur 1 to 3 days after birth in premature infants, especially those who experience hypoxia.
      2. Intraventricular hemorrhage may be noted immediately after birth or become clinically manifest suddenly with a bulging fontanel in the first 24 to 48 hours. The spinal fluid is grossly bloody.
      3. Subarachnoid hemorrhage may produce focal seizures in a previously well infant. The spinal fluid demonstrates increased protein and xanthrochromic supernatant fluid.
      4. Subdural hematoma
   C. Cerebral contusion due to birth trauma
   D. Cerebral dysgenesis
   E. Infection
      1. Prenatal
         a. Toxoplasmosis
         b. Cytomegalovirus
         c. Rubella
      2. Meningitis

II. Metabolic disorders
   A. Hypoglycemia
   B. Hypocalcemia
   C. Hypomagnesemia
   D. Hyponatremia
   E. Hypernatremia
   F. Narcotic withdrawal

   Fricker, H.S. and Segal, S.: Narcotic addiction, pregnancy, and the newborn. *Am. J. Dis. Child. 132*:360, 1978.

   G. Inborn errors of metabolism (e.g., maple syrup urine disease, hyperglycinemia)
   H. Pyridoxine deficiency and dependency
   I. Administration of a local anesthetic agent in maternal anesthesia may cause seizures in the first six hours of life.

   Sinclair, J.G. et al.: Intoxication of the fetus by a local anesthetic. A newly recognized complication of maternal caudal anesthesia. *N. Engl. J. Med. 273*:1173, 1965.

   J. Hyperviscosity syndrome of the newborn
III. Sepsis

   Brown, J.K.: Convulsions in the newborn period. *Dev. Med. Child Neurol. 15*:823, 1973.
   Brown, J.K., Cockburn, F. and Forfar, J.O.: Clinical and chemical correlates in convulsions of the newborn. *Lancet 1*:135, 1972.
   Freeman, J.M.: Neonatal seizures — diagnosis and management. *J. Pediatr. 77*:701, 1970.
   Rose, A. L. and Lombroso, C.T.: Neonatal seizure states. *Pediatrics 45*:404, 1970.
   Schwartz, J.F.: Neonatal convulsions. *Clin. Pediatr. 4*:595, 1965.
   Volpe, J.: Neonatal seizures. *N. Engl. J. Med. 289*:413, 1973.

## DIAGNOSTIC APPROACH TO CONVULSIVE SEIZURES

The history, including a detailed description of the seizure, is of great diagnostic help. Special attention should be given to the perinatal period and developmental progress. Information should also be obtained about the possibility of head trauma, pica, accidental ingestion of drugs or poisons, previous seizures and other concurrent symptoms such as fever.

The physical examination should include careful developmental and neurologic evaluation. The funduscopic examination and determination of the blood pressure should be performed in every child with convulsive seizures.

The following diagnostic procedures include those that may be indicated in patients with convulsive seizures depending on the clinician's diagnostic impressions.
   I. Blood
      A. Serum calcium, phosphorus
      B. Blood urea nitrogen, serum creatinine
      C. Blood sugar
      D. Serum electrolytes
      E. Examination of erythrocytes for basophilic stippling
      F. Blood and other cultures if infection is suspected
      G. Complement fixation and neutralization tests if encephalitis is thought to be present.

H. "TORCH" screen for microbial agents if prenatal viral infection is suspected

II. Lumbar puncture is not routinely indicated but reserved for those instances in which meningitis or other intracranial lesion is suspected.

III. A subdural tap may be indicated in infants with otherwise unexplained convulsive seizures.

IV. The electroencephalogram is of great value in diagnosis of the type and location of the seizure and as a guide to therapy and prognosis.

V. Skull roentgenograms and plain film of abdomen if lead ingestion is suspected

VI. Brain and CAT scans in patients thought to have a focal lesion

VII. Urinalysis

VIII. Blood and urine studies for inborn errors of metabolism

## GENERAL REFERENCES

Dodson, W.E. et al.: Management of seizure disorders. Selected aspects. Parts I and II. *J. Pediatr.* 89:527, 695, 1976.

Golden, G.S.: Vascular diseases of the brain and tics, twitches and habit spasms. *Cur. Prob. Pediatr.* 8:3 (Apr.) 1978.

---

## ETIOLOGIC CLASSIFICATION OF CONVULSIONS IN OLDER INFANTS AND CHILDREN

I. Febrile convulsions, 424

II. Epilepsy, 424
  A. Grand mal, 424
  B. Petit mal, 425
  C. Myoclonic seizures, 425
    1. Myoclonic epilepsy of older children
    2. Massive myoclonic seizures
    3. Benign myoclonus of early infancy
  D. Diencephalic epilepsy; autonomic seizures; abdominal epilepsy; convulsive equivalent, 426
  E. Psychomotor epilepsy, 426
  F. Focal (partial) seizures, 427
  G. Sensory-precipitated seizures, 427
  H. Hyperexplexia, 427

III. Metabolic factors, 427
  A. Hypocalcemia, 427
    1. Newborn
    2. Hypoparathyroidism
    3. Vitamin D deficiency or metabolic defect
    4. Sodium dihydrogen phosphate enemas
  B. Hypomagnesemia, 428
  C. Hypoglycemia, 428
    1. Infants born to diabetic mothers; hemolytic disease before and after exchange transfusion; perinatal stresses

    2. Hyperinsulinemia
    3. Ketotic hypoglycemia
    4. Endocrine disorders
    5. Hepatic enzyme deficiencies
    6. Other inborn errors of metabolism
  D. Hyponatremia, 430
  E. Uremia, 430
  F. Poisoning, 430
  G. Pyridoxine deficiency or dependency, 431
  H. Anoxia, 431
    1. Asphyxia
    2. Carbon monoxide poisoning
    3. Near-drowning
    4. Breath-holding spells
    5. Respiratory failure
    6. Primary pulmonary hypertension
  I. Phenothiazine tranquilizers, 431
  J. Infants of mothers addicted to narcotics, 431
  K. Phenylketonuria, 431
  L. Other inborn metabolic errors, 431

IV. Cerebral factors, 431
  A. Trauma, 431
    1. Cerebral concussion; contusion; laceration; focal or generalized edema of the brain
    2. Extradural hematoma; subdural hematoma
  B. Infections of the central nervous system, 431

1. Toxoplasmosis
2. Encephalitis
3. Meningitis
4. Subdural effusion
5. Intracranial abscess
6. Rabies

C. Intracranial hemorrhage, 432
   1. Subdural hematoma
   2. Extradural hematoma
   3. Subarachnoid hemorrhage
   4. Hemorrhagic diseases

D. Thrombosis of cerebral vessels, 432
   1. Congenital heart disease
   2. Sickle cell anemia
   3. Severe dehydration
   4. Sudden vascular accident (acute infantile hemiplegia)

E. Sturge-Weber syndrome, 432

F. Psychologic factors, 432
   1. Breath-holding spells
   2. Self-induced seizures
   3. Emotional factors
   4. Hysteria and other psychogenic factors

G. Encephalopathy, 433
   1. Postpertussis vaccine encephalopathy
   2. Pertussis
   3. Acute glomerulonephritis
   4. Bacillary dysentery
   5. Lupus erythematosus
   6. Infectious mononucleosis
   7. Corticosteroid treatment

H. Degenerative diseases, 433
   1. Demyelinating encephalopathies
   2. $G_{M1}$ gangliosidosis type II
   3. Metachromatic leukodystrophy
   4. Tuberous sclerosis
   5. Tay-Sachs disease
   6. Other cerebromacular degenerative diseases ,
   7. Niemann-Pick disease
   8. Infantile Gaucher's disease
   9. Subacute sclerosing panencephalitis

I. Brain tumors, 433

J. Tetanus, 434

## ETIOLOGIC CLASSIFICATION OF CONVULSIONS IN NEWBORN INFANTS

I. Central nervous system disorders, 434
   A. Asphyxia, 434
   B. Intracranial hemorrhage, 434
      1. Periventricular
      2. Intraventricular
      3. Subarachnoid
      4. Subdural hematoma
   C. Cerebral contusion due to birth trauma, 434
   D. Cerebral dysgenesis, 434
   E. Infection, 434
      1. Prenatal
      2. Meningitis

II. Metabolic disorders, 435
   A. Hypoglycemia, 435
   B. Hypocalcemia, 435
   C. Hypomagnesemia, 435
   D. Hyponatremia, 435
   E. Hypernatremia, 435
   F. Narcotic withdrawal, 435
   G. Inborn errors of metabolism, 435
   H. Pyridoxine deficiency and dependency, 435
   I. Maternal caudal anesthesia, 435
   J. Hyperviscosity syndrome, 435

III. Sepsis, 435

CHAPTER **50**

# DELIRIUM

Delirium represents a toxic or metabolic encephalopathy characterized by a disturbance in consciousness, which ranges from extreme hyperactivity to coma. Symptoms of delirium characteristically fluctuate widely but are generally worse at night. At one moment, the child may seem to be in complete contact with his environment while, a few seconds later, he obviously does not clearly perceive or understand what is going on. At times, the impairment in consciousness is steady.

The delirious child may demonstrate great excitement and hyperactivity — running about the examining room, trying to open the door, struggling with the nurse and thrashing around on the examining table. Anxiety, fear and tremulousness may be extreme. The child may pull at his fingertips, reach for imaginary objects and pick at his clothes. Motor incoordination and ataxia may be noted. Auditory and visual hallucinations and illusions lead the child to misinterpret shadows (e.g., he may see large bugs on his bed or climbing the walls). The child's speech is often incoherent. Cognitive functions, memory and comprehension are impaired. The confused older child may be unable to answer orientation questions, to attend to a task such as sequentially subtracting 7 or 3 from 100 or to repeat backward a series of digits.

## ETIOLOGIC CLASSIFICATION OF DELIRIUM

I. Infectious disorders
   A. Any acute, febrile disease, especially the exanthemas
   B. Pneumococcal or other bacterial pneumonia. In some instances, delirium and fever may be the only presenting symptoms. A chest x-ray may be diagnostic.
   C. Inflammatory diseases of the central nervous system such as meningitis or encephalitis. Since encephalitis may be especially difficult to exclude on clinical grounds, a lumbar puncture may be necessary in most instances.
   D. Reye's syndrome is characterized by prodromal illness, protracted vomiting, lethargy and disorientation. Coma may or may not follow. Elevated levels of SGOT, SGPT and blood ammonia are found.
   E. Typhoid fever
   F. Rabies may be characterized by periods of hyperactivity, combativeness and disorientation alternating with intervals of normal mental status.
II. Drugs and poisoning
   A careful history for possible poisoning is indicated in all children with acute delirium, including a review of the contents of medicine cabinets, night tables and all medications taken currently or in the past by the parents or other adults in the household.
   A. Barbiturates

438

B. Antihistaminic preparations taken orally or contained in preparations for local application

C. Aminophylline poisoning may lead to extreme restlessness.

D. Corticosteroids taken on a continuing basis

E. Isoniazid

F. Jimson weed poisoning. Ingestion of the seeds or leaves of the Jimson weed, containing hyoscyamine and other belladonna alkaloids, may produce delirium. Convulsions are also common. Symptoms, which may begin in minutes or a few hours, initially include visual illusions, dryness of the mouth, extreme thirst, incoherent speech, confusion, disorientation, stupor, coma, incoordination and hyperactivity. The pupils are dilated and fixed, and the skin is flushed and dry. Opisthotonus may develop. A diffuse erythematous rash may be present. The temperature may be as high as 40.6° C (105° F). Recovery usually occurs in 24 to 48 hours.

Shervette, R.E., Schydlower, M., Lampe, R.M. and Fearnow, R.G.: Jimson "Loco" weed abuse in adolescents. *Pediatrics 63*:520, 1979.

G. Atropine poisoning may occur after conjunctival instillation.

H. Amphetamine intoxication due to accidental ingestion by young children.

I. LSD or other psychedelic agents. Delirium persisting for several days may be due to phencyclidine ("angel dust") intoxication. Hypertension may be present.

Cohen, S.: The "angel dust" states: phencyclidine toxicity. *Pediatr. Rev. 1*:17, 1979.

J. Gasoline sniffing

K. Alcohol

III. Hypoxia (e.g., carbon monoxide poisoning)

IV. Metabolic (e.g., uremia)

V. Burn encephalopathy, characterized by delirium, personality changes, seizures or coma, may occur with acute burns due to hypovolemia, sepsis or hyponatremia.

Antoon, A.Y., Volpe, J.J. and Crawford, J.D.: Burn encephalopathy in children. *Pediatrics 50*:609, 1972.

---

## ETIOLOGIC CLASSIFICATION OF DELIRIUM

# CHAPTER 51

# COMA

Alterations in the state of consciousness in infants and children include delirium, stupor and coma. *Delirium* is characterized by confusion, disorientation, irrationality and, perhaps, excitability. *Lethargy* is characterized by drowsiness and disinterest in the environment. *Obtundation* refers to an increase in the depth of the lethargy. *Stupor* is a state of unconsciousness, but one from which the child may be momentarily aroused. *Coma* represents prolonged and profound unconsciousness and is often preceded by stupor. Since coma presents a situation in which prompt diagnosis and management may be lifesaving, emergency management, e.g., establishment of an airway, may need to precede a specific etiologic diagnosis.

## ETIOLOGIC CLASSIFICATION OF COMA

I. Central nervous system disturbances
   A. Trauma. Since the traumatic lesions to be discussed are characterized by similar neurologic findings, clinical differentiation may not be possible. The most important sign to be observed is the patient's state of consciousness in terms of his responsiveness to questions and visual, auditory or sensory stimulation. These observations should be carefully documented.
      1. Cerebral concussion, contusion or laceration may be followed immediately by a period of unconsciousness lasting minutes or hours. Posttraumatic amnesia will encompass not only the period of unconsciousness but also the time immediately before and after. With slight head trauma, the symptoms may be limited to mild lethargy and, perhaps, one or more episodes of vomiting. Transient blindness may occur after a mild concussion.
      2. Subdural hematoma is a prominent diagnostic possibility in patients who continue to do poorly after a head injury. Headache, unilateral dilatation of the pupil and localizing neurologic signs may be present. While symptoms may appear in a few hours, coma may not occur until days or weeks later. Chronic subdural hematoma, which may be characterized in infants and children by enlargement of the head, vomiting, failure to thrive, convulsions and other neurologic signs, is not characterized by coma except terminally.
      3. Extradural hematoma. The following physical findings occur in infants and children with an extradural hematoma: swelling of the scalp, hemiparesis, drowsiness progressing to stupor, positive Babinski's sign, unequal pupils with dilatation of the pupil on the involved side, coma, decerebrate posture, convulsions, strabismus and papilledema. These signs usually appear within several minutes to a few hours after injury.

Occasionally, however, they may be delayed for a few days. Less commonly, an initial period of unconsciousness occurs immediately after the injury, followed by a lucid interval and finally by gradual reappearance of coma. Similar physical findings may be noted in patients with cerebral contusion, laceration or hemorrhage and with an acute subdural hematoma. A skull fracture may be found on roentgenographic examination. Final diagnosis may not be possible until surgical exploration. Blood loss into the extradural space may amount to as much as 100 to 150 ml. This accounts for the acute anemia and shock that may appear in some of these infants even in the absence of neurologic findings.

4. Localizing neurologic signs, convulsions and hemiparesis may occur within minutes to a few hours after head injuries in children owing to focal and generalized edema of the brain. Spontaneous recovery occurs within a few hours.

DeVivo, D.C. and Dodge, P.R.: The critically ill child: diagnosis and management of head injury. *Pediatrics 48*:129, 1971.
Singer, H.S. and Freeman, J.M.: Head trauma for the pediatrician. *Pediatrics 62*:819, 1978.

B. Disturbances in circulation
   1. Hemorrhage
      a. Subdural hematoma
      b. Cerebral hemorrhage in newborn infants
      c. Subarachnoid hemorrhage due to rupture of an intracranial arterial aneurysm. The onset is dramatic and sudden with severe suboccipital or frontal headache, perhaps pain in the neck or back, screaming, vomiting, the rapid appearance of coma and, perhaps, convulsions. The child may fall unconscious to the floor. Signs of meningeal irritation occur with nuchal rigidity and a positive Kernig's sign. The deep tendon reflexes are increased. The cerebrospinal fluid is bloody. Localizing neurologic signs are not present if the hemorrhage is entirely subarachnoid. Often, however, intracortical hemorrhage also occurs, and the patient may demonstrate focal findings.

Matson, D.D.: Intracranial arterial aneurysms in childhood. *J. Neurosurg. 23*:578, 1965.
Shucart, W.A. and Wolpert, S.M.: Intracranial arterial aneurysms in childhood. *Am. J. Dis. Child. 127*:288, 1974.

      d. Acute infantile hemiplegia is discussed on pages 432 and 442.
      e. Hemorrhagic diseases such as thrombocytopenic purpura or hemophilia may be complicated by intracranial hemorrhage.
      f. Intracranial hemorrhage may occur as an infrequent complication in patients with pertussis.
      g. Coma may be produced by sudden hemorrhage into an intracranial tumor, such as a malignant cerebral glioma. If the symptoms follow head trauma, the possibility of an intracranial neoplasm may be overlooked.
   2. Cerebral vascular occlusions
      a. Thrombosis
         (1) Cerebral thrombosis occurs not uncommonly in children who have polycythemia secondary to cyanotic congenital heart dis-

ease. Clinical manifestations include convulsive seizures, impaired consciousness and monoplegia or hemiplegia.

(2) Occlusion of the venous dural sinuses and the cerebral veins may occur in severely dehydrated infants and young children. Numerous small cerebral thrombi may also form during the course of acute infectious diseases. Thrombosis of the sagittal sinus is manifested by coma, convulsions and paraplegia. The scalp veins may be distended. Cavernous sinus thrombosis produces proptosis, papilledema, conjunctival and retinal hemorrhage and ophthalmoplegia owing to paresis of the third, fourth and sixth cranial nerves.

(3) Coma may occur in children with sickle cell anemia, presumably caused by cerebral thrombosis.

(4) Thrombotic thrombocytopenic purpura

  b. Embolism

    (1) Bacterial endocarditis

    (2) Congenital heart disease with right-to-left shunt

    (3) Pulmonary or other abscess

    (4) Fat embolism following fractures

C. Acute infantile hemiplegia, a disorder of unknown etiology, begins suddenly with a severe convulsive seizure, usually unilateral but occasionally generalized, followed by coma and hemiparesis. Fever may also occur. Convulsions recur for one or two days, and coma may persist for a week or ten days. The cerebrospinal fluid is normal. Gradual improvement in the hemiparesis may occur with flaccidity being replaced by spasticity. Cerebral arteriography may demonstrate occlusion of the middle cerebral artery.

D. Infection of the central nervous system

  1. An intracranial abscess may develop secondary to otitis media, mastoiditis or other purulent lesions elsewhwere in the body. Children with cyanotic heart disease and polycythemia are especially liable to develop this complication.

  2. Meningitis. The classic signs of purulent meningitis may not be present in young infants, and often the diagnosis must be suspected on the basis of such vague symptoms as failure to feed or vomiting. A history of unusual irritability or drowsiness may be an indication for cerebrospinal fluid examination. Alterations in the state of consciousness in patients with purulent meningitis range from hyperexcitability and delirium to stupor and coma. In patients with aseptic meningitis, there is no disturbance in level of consciousness.

  3. Encephalitis. Symptoms attributable to encephalitis include drowsiness, disorientation, stupor, coma, irritability, convulsions, headache, nuchal rigidity, hemiplegia, paralysis of cranial nerves, tremor, choreiform or athetoid movements, rigidity, aphasia and ataxia. These findings may also be caused by an intracranial neoplasm or abscess. Definitive clinical diagnosis is difficult unless these symptoms accompany measles or some other infectious disease. Examination of the cerebrospinal fluid may show an increase in the number of cells, mostly lymphocytes, and protein. Complement fixation and neutralization tests may be helpful diag-

nostically. Encephalitis may precede, accompany or follow the acute exanthematous diseases of childhood: measles, rubella, roseola, chickenpox and scarlet fever. The coma in children with measles encephalitis may persist for weeks or months. Encephalopathy may follow pertussis vaccination. Coma due to encephalitis may occasionally occur in children with mumps or pertussis. Encephalitis accompanied by unexplained lymphadenopathy may be due to cat-scratch disease.

4. Infectious mononucleosis may be characterized by disorientation, drowsiness, stupor, coma, headache, nuchal rigidity and diplopia, and by an increased number of cells in the cerebrospinal fluid.

5. Toxic encephalopathy may occur during severe systemic diseases, especially those characterized by high fever and general toxicity. The meningismus, disorientation, coma and convulsions in patients with Shigella bacillary dysentery may initially, in the absence of diarrhea, suggest encephalitis.

6. Burn encephalopathy may be characterized by delirium, seizures and coma.

7. Reye's syndrome usually has a prodromal phase characterized by symptoms of an upper respiratory tract infection followed by persistent vomiting for a day or two before the onset of encephalopathy. Chickenpox may precede these symptoms. Reye's syndrome may be classified in five stages: Stage I is characterized by vomiting, lethargy, sleepiness, hepatic dysfunction (SGOT, glucose, blood ammonia) and a type 1 EEG; stage II is manifested by delirium, combativeness, hyperventilation, hyperactive reflexes, responsivity to painful stimuli, liver dysfunction and type 2 electroencephalogram; stage III is characterized by stupor or coma, hyperventilation, decerebrate rigidity, positive pupillary light reaction, liver dysfunction and a type 2 EEG; stage IV is accompanied by deepening coma, decerebrate rigidity, loss of the doll's eye reflex, large and fixed pupils, minimal hepatic dysfunction and type 3 or 4 EEG; and stage V is characterized by seizures, loss of deep tendon reflexes, type 4 EEG and respiratory arrest.

Huttenlocher, P.R.: Reye's syndrome: relation of outcome to therapy. *J. Pediatr. 80*:845, 1972.
Kindt, G.W. et al.: Intracranial pressure in Reye's syndrome: monitoring and control. *JAMA 231*:822, 1975.
Lovejoy, F.H. et al.: Clinical staging in Reye's syndrome. *Am. J. Dis. Child. 128*:36, 1974.

E. Brain tumors. Hemorrhage into an intracranial neoplasm may cause sudden coma. Blockage of the ventricular circulation with resultant increase in the intracranial pressure may also result in unconsciousness. Tumors of the brain stem may be accompanied by coma even without an increase in the intracranial pressure. Coma occasionally occurs in children with leukemia owing to involvement of the central nervous system.

F. Hypertensive encephalopathy in patients with acute glomerulonephritis may result in impaired consciousness as well as convulsive seizures.

G. Postconvulsion coma. A period of unconsciousness, usually not prolonged, may follow convulsive seizures in children. Coma is more persistent in patients in status epilepticus.

II. Metabolic disorders
  A. Diabetic acidosis
  B. Lethargy, stupor or coma and ketoacidosis are seen in many newborn infants with hyperammonemia owing to inborn errors of metabolism, including urea-cycle deficiency syndromes. Such disorders include methylmalonic acidemia, isovaleric acidemia, carbamylphosphate synthetase deficiency, ornithine transcarbamylase deficiency, citrullinemia, argininosuccinicaciduria, propionic acidemia and maple syrup urine disease. Because of the possibility of protein intolerance, milk and other protein-containing foods should be discontinued and a balanced electrolyte glucose solution begun orally or intravenously. Urine should be examined for the presence of reducing substance, and its specific gravity, pH and ketones should be checked. A ferric chloride test should also be done. The odor of the urine (musty, maple syrup, etc.) should be checked. Electrophoresis for amino acids should be performed along with gas chromatography and mass spectrometry. Blood specimens should be analyzed for serum electrolytes, glucose, ammonia, lactate, amino acids and organic acids.

Barness, L.A.: Methylmalonic acid. *Pediatrics 51*:1012, 1973.
Campbell, A.G.M., Rosenberg, L.E., Snodgrass, P.J. and Nuzum, C.T.: Ornithine transcarbamylase deficiency. *N. Engl. J. Med. 288*:1, 1973.
Scriver, C. and Rosenberg, L.E.: *Amino Acid Metabolism and Its Disorders*. Philadelphia, W.B. Saunders Co., 1973.
Snyderman, S.E. et al.: Argininemia. *J. Pediatr. 90*:563, 1977.
Stanbury, J.B., Wyngaarden, J.B. and Fredrickson, D.S. (eds.): *Metabolic Basis of Inherited Disease*. 3rd ed. New York, McGraw-Hill Book Co., 1972.

  C. Leigh's syndrome, or subacute necrotizing encephalomyelopathy, may be characterized by lethargy and coma.

Grover, W.D., Auerbach, V.H. and Patel, M.S.: Biochemical studies and therapy in subacute necrotizing encephalomyelopathy (Leigh's syndrome). *J. Pediatr. 81*:39, 1972.

  D. Hypoglycemia. Coma caused by insulin overdosage may last for days even after the blood sugar level has been restored to normal.
  E. Renal insufficiency
  F. Hypoxia
    1. Drowning
    2. Carbon monoxide poisoning
    3. Congestive cardiac failure with circulatory inadequacy
    4. Loss of consciousness may occur during episodes of paroxysmal dyspnea in infants with cyanotic congenital heart disease. Comatose periods may last from a few minutes to two or three hours. Although loss of consciousness may be preceded by cyanosis and dyspnea, this is not always the case.
    5. Adams-Stokes attacks may be associated with atrioventricular heart block in children. Symptoms may include vertigo, syncope or coma and convulsions.

Nakamura, F.F. and Nadas, A.S.: Complete heart block in infants and children. *N. Engl. J. Med. 270*:1261, 1964.
Sissman, N.J.: Stokes-Adams syndrome in childhood. *Am. J. Dis. Child. 110*:658, 1965.

G. Tetany may lead to unconsciousness. Coma may also be due to hypercalcemia in patients with hyperparathyroidism. Tetany and coma may be a complication of pediatric sodium dihydrogen phosphate enemas.

H. Addison's disease during crises

I. Hepatic coma may occur as a complication of fulminating viral hepatitis. Initial symptomatology includes clouding of the sensorium, apathy, confusion, emotional lability and slurred speech. While coma may occur abruptly, more commonly it evolves gradually. Asterixis, a flapping tremor, may be present.

McDonald, R. and De La Harpe, P.L.: Hepatic coma in childhood. *J. Pediatr. 63*:916, 1963.

J. Acute hyponatremia; water intoxication. Hypernatremia; hyperosmolarity

K. Hyperviscosity syndrome in the newborn is characterized by lethargy.

L. Heat stroke, heat exhaustion

III. Drugs, poisons

Grade 1 coma following drug ingestion is characterized by drowsiness, with the patient reponsive to verbal command; stage 2 is characterized by coma but responsiveness to mildly painful stimuli; stage 3 denotes coma responsive only to deeply painful stimuli; and stage 4 unresponsive and areflexic.

*Poisoning is a possibility in every patient with unexplained coma.*

A. Sedatives: barbiturates

B. Phenothiazines

C. Narcotics. Miosis is classically present in noncomatose patients who have taken narcotics. Patients who have ingested barbiturates, phenothiazines or ethanol also demonstrate an increased incidence of miosis as their coma deepens. Such drug ingestion should be suspected if pupillary dilatation does not follow administration of the narcotic antagonist naloxone in a comatose patient suspected of narcotic ingestion. Hallucinogens such as LSD and mescaline may cause dilated pupils while phencyclidine ("angel dust") characteristically causes small or normal pupils.

Mitchell, A.A., Lovejoy, F.H., Jr. and Goldman, P.: Drug ingestions associated with miosis in comatose children. *J. Pediatr. 89*:303, 1976.

D. Lead poisoning. Alteration of lethargy or stupor with lucid periods is suggestive of impending lead encephalopathy, especially in a vomiting child in the summer.

E. Ethanol ingestion

Moss, M.H.: Alcohol-induced hypoglycemia and coma caused by alcohol sponging. *Pediatrics 46*:445, 1970.

F. Salicylate poisoning, especially oil of wintergreen

G. Inhalation of carbon tetrachloride, gasoline or other fluids used in cleaning

H. Mushroom poisoning

I. Kerosene poisoning

J. Organic phosphate (parathion) poisoning

IV. Narcolepsy is characterized by excessive and abnormal sleepiness. Cataplexy, which may be an associated symptom, refers to muscular weakness or paralysis precipitated by emotions such as laughter or anger. Excessive sleepiness may be due to lesions in the pituitary and hypothalamic regions.

V. Hysteria may account for the patient who is seemingly unresponsive although not physiologically comatose.

## PHYSICAL EXAMINATION OF COMATOSE PATIENTS

The depth of the coma and the status of the tendon, corneal and pupillary reflexes are usually of little diagnostic value. These reflexes, along with those of swallowing and cough, become progressively depressed as the coma deepens. Because of the absence of voluntary motor activity in comatose patients, paralysis may not be readily evident. Comatose patients should be examined for evidence of meningeal involvement, cranial trauma and for leakage of blood or cerebrospinal fluid from cranial orifices. Funduscopic examination for papilledema or retinal hemorrhage should be performed and the blood pressure taken.

## DIAGNOSTIC PROCEDURES

1. Urinalysis: microscopic. Chemical for albumin, acetone, glycosuria, salicylates. Glycosuria may be present in patients who have meningitis or other central nervous system disease.
2. Blood examinations:
   Complete blood cell count
   Evaluation of clotting mechanism
   Examination of blood smear for sickling or stippling
   Blood glucose
   Blood nonprotein nitrogen, serum creatinine
   Serum bicarbonate, chloride, sodium
   Serum calcium
   Salicylate level
   Spectrophotometry for carbon monoxide and methemoglobin
   Heterophile agglutinins
   Blood cultures
3. Examination of the cerebrospinal fluid is an important diagnostic procedure in patients with coma of unknown etiology. Shock may present a contraindication to lumbar puncture as may increased intracranial pressure.
4. Unless the patient is in shock, roentgenographic examination or computerized axial tomography of the skull should be obtained whenever there is a history or suspicion of head injury. Changes in the sella turcica, intracranial calcification or separation of the suture lines may be evident.
5. If the possibility of poisoning exists, gastric lavage may be indicated for diagnostic as well as therapeutic reasons.
6. In patients thought to have encephalitis, neutralization and complement fixation studies may be obtained.
7. An electroencephalogram may be indicated in patients with unexplained stupor or coma.

## GENERAL REFERENCE

Plum, F. and Posner, J.: *The Diagnosis of Stupor and Coma*. Philadelphia, F.A. Davis Co., 1966.

## ETIOLOGIC CLASSIFICATION OF COMA

CHAPTER 52

# FAINTING

Fainting or syncope refers to brief, usually sudden, periods of unconsciousness, loss of postural tone and falling owing to cerebral ischemia. The history is generally the most helpful diagnostic procedure. Careful attention should be given to the circumstances in which the syncope occurred, possible precipitating factors, prodromal symptoms and signs, the suddenness of onset, the duration of the episode and the occurrence of convulsive movements. A thorough history will often obviate the need for such examinations as an electroencephalogram or fasting blood sugar.

Engel, G.L.: *Fainting*. 2nd ed. Springfield, Charles C Thomas, 1962.
Friedberg, C.K.: Syncope: pathological physiology: differential diagnosis and treatment. *Mod. Concepts Cardiovasc. Dis. 40*:55, 61, 1971.

## ETIOLOGIC CLASSIFICATION OF FAINTING

I. Vasodepressor syncope (simple faint)

Vasodepressor syncope, owing to a sudden and marked fall in blood pressure, is the most common cause of fainting and is usually first noted in adolescence. It may occur when the patient becomes suddenly frightened or threatened by some real or imagined danger. Fainting may also represent a reaction to severe pain or other unpleasant stimulus such as the sight of blood or a needle puncture. Syncope is especially likely to occur in hot, humid, close quarters; after prolonged motionless standing; when the patient is fatigued; and after fasting. In patients whose syncopal attacks are emotionally induced, anxiety may be overt or evident in frightening dreams. Although psychologic factors may cause recurrent fainting spells, especially those not precipitated by apparent cause, they generally do not need to be considered in the single episode.

The simple faint almost always begins with the child standing, although in rare instances it may occur with the patient recumbent. Prodromal symptoms include a feeling of great weakness, generalized numbness, pallor, nausea, excessive salivation, warmth, sweating, lightheadedness, yawning, sighing, blurring of vision and epigastric discomfort. These antecedent complaints may suddenly terminate in the faint, or they may stop short of that either spontaneously or in response to a head-low position. The interruption of consciousness usually lasts only a few seconds but may persist for several minutes. Clonic movements may ensue if the patient remains unconscious longer than 15 to 20 seconds, or if he is held semi-erect. Symptoms may recur if the patient sits up or stands too quickly.

II. Hysteria

Syncope may also be a symbolic expression of unconscious, repressed instinctual impulses, usually of a sexual or hostile nature, and often directed toward a member of the family. Such episodes, which are most common in adolescent girls, may also be precipitated by real or fantasized heterosexual experiences. The patient may have a history of repeated episodes of syncope as well as other manifestations of hysteria. Conversion of the consciously unacceptable impulse to physical expression in the form of syncope permits a partial discharge of these feelings and helps avoid the anxiety that would be engendered by conscious expression or direct gratification of the impulse.

Whereas overt anxiety is frequently noted with vasodepressor syncope, the patient with hysterical syncope shows little concern. These episodes characteristically occur in the presence of others and are not preceded or accompanied by prodromal symptoms such as nausea, weakness, pallor and sweating. Hysterical patients may slump or fall in a dramatic fashion, but they avoid injury. They may also faint while sitting or recumbent, positions that would be unusual for vasodepressor syncope. During the episode, the patient's eyes may flutter, be held open or tightly closed. Moaning, groaning or other sounds may be noted. Unusual positions and movements may be assumed. The patient may slip in and out of unconsciousness or not be completely unconscious. Interruption of consciousness may persist for seconds or hours.

III. Epilepsy

It is occasionally difficult to differentiate in the history between vasodepressor syncope, breath-holding spells and epilepsy, since the first two disorders may be accompanied by clonic movements. Syncope caused by epilepsy usually lasts longer (generally over 30 seconds) and is more likely to occur with the patient recumbent than would be the case with simple syncope. An electroencephalogram and further studies of the causes of seizures may be necessary for differentiation.

IV. Cardiac causes

Although important to recognize, loss of consciousness from cardiac disorders is rare in comparison with the causes just listed. Occasionally, syncope occurs with exertion in patients with isolated pulmonic stenosis if the narrowing is extremely marked. Primary pulmonary hypertension may be characterized by episodes of syncope, especially on effort. Fainting may, indeed, be the presenting complaint. Congenital or acquired heart block or cardiac arrhythmias may decrease cardiac output sufficiently to produce unconsciousness.

Severe aortic stenosis may cause syncope, especially after physical exertion. Attacks of paroxysmal dyspnea in infants with congenital heart disease, e.g., tetralogy of Fallot, may terminate in syncope. Syncope may occur with paroxysmal tachycardia and with sudden obstruction of the mitral orifice by a left atrial myxoma.

Thilenius, O.G., Nadas, A.S. and Jockin, H.: Primary pulmonary vascular obstruction in children. *Pediatrics 36*:75, 1965.

V. Tussive (cough) syncope

Loss of consciousness, usually of short duration, owing to cerebral hypoxia, may occur after severe paroxysms of coughing as in children with asthma.

Katz, R.M.: Cough syncope in children with asthma. *J. Pediatr. 77*:48, 1970.

VI. Anemia

Severe anemia may be accompanied by lightheadedness, giddiness and, occasionally, syncope.

VII. Hypoglycemia

Although hypoglycemia does not lead to true syncope, the patient may complain of faintness and exhibit pallor and sweating. A meticulous history, e.g., relation to meals and careful description of symptoms, is of help in the differential diagnosis.

VIII. Hyperventilation syndrome

Hyperventilation may cause lightheadedness, generalized weakness, tingling and numbness of the hands, tetany or syncope. The physician needs to be alert to the hyperventilation syndrome as a possible cause of syncope in adolescents because patients are more likely to report "blacking-out" spells, seizures or sensations of smothering, choking or shortness of breath than overbreathing or tingling and numbness of the hands. Direct questioning or an attempt to reproduce the symptoms by having the patient hyperventilate for a couple of minutes may be necessary.

Enzer, N.B. and Walker, P.A.: Hyperventilation syndrome in childhood. *J. Pediatr. 70*:521, 1967.

IX. Breath-holding

Breath-holding spells are common in infants, especially during the latter part of the first year and the early months of the second year. They are less often seen in younger or older children, although in unusual situations they may persist until the age of four years. The breath-holding episode is triggered by some injury, often trivial, or by the child's suddenly becoming angry or frustrated. Vigorous crying is the first manifestation. After a variable period, he suddenly gasps or holds his breath until he becomes blue or pale, unconscious and limp. Convulsive movements or opisthotonus may occur if unconsciousness is prolonged.

The presenting complaint is usually convulsions or blacking out rather than breath-holding or syncope. The history and sequence of events are so characteristic that differential diagnosis generally presents no problem; however, when the precipitating event seems extremely trivial, when there appears to be no triggering circumstance, when the child is said to cry or hold his breath for only a short time or when the convulsive movements are a prominent clinical feature, differentiation from epilepsy may require an electroencephalogram and further observation.

Some babies seem especially prone to have these spells, and there may be a familial incidence. Although in some cases there appears to be no contributory disturbance in the home or in the mother-infant relation, these need to be explored carefully. Immature parents, maternal depression, inability to set limits on the child and similar difficulties in the maternal-infant interaction need to be dealt with if the spells are to be prevented. Many of these children have an iron deficiency anemia that appears to be an associated disorder rather than the causative factor.

Lombroso, C.B. and Lerman, P.: Breathholding spells (cyanotic and pallid infantile syncope). *Pediatrics 39*:563, 1967.

X. Miscellaneous
  A. Attacks of syncope lasting from a brief faint to unconsciousness for five to ten minutes are rarely associated with congenital deafness, prolonged Q–T interval and large T waves on the electrocardiogram. Sudden death has been described in the full surdocardiac syndrome or in the partial syndrome without deafness. Episodes may be precipitated by emotional stress or physical exertion.

Frank, J.P. and Friedberg, D.A.: Syncope with prolonged QT interval. *Am. J. Dis. Child. 130*:320, 1976.

  B. Attacks of unconsciousness have been reported in patients with fused cervical vertebrae. The cause is undetermined.
  C. Sudden unconsciousness may be precipitated by needle puncture of the pleural space and after drainage of fluid from the pleural or peritoneal cavities. The mechanism is probably similar to vasodepressor syncope.
  D. Postural or orthostatic hypotension is an unusual cause of syncope in children and may occur when the child has stood motionless for a long time in a military or parade formation.
  E. Takayasu's disease (primary aortitis) may cause syncope.

## ETIOLOGIC CLASSIFICATION OF FAINTING

CHAPTER 53

# VERTIGO

Vertigo, or dizziness, implies a sense of rotation or motion of the patient or his environment. Since vertigo is a subjective symptom, the clinician has to decide on the basis of the history whether the complaint accurately describes the child's symptoms. Often the patient will inaccurately use the term "dizziness" to describe lightheadedness or faintness as occurs in the hyperventilation syndrome and primary pulmonary hypertension.

The cause for vertigo is often difficult to establish even after careful study. Investigation should include a neurologic appraisal, particularly of the cranial nerves and more especially of the eighth nerve with audiometric testing and examination of vestibular functioning.

## ETIOLOGIC CLASSIFICATION OF VERTIGO

I. Labyrinthine disorders may give rise to paroxysmal, brief episodes of vertigo. The onset may be explosive, accompanied by tinnitus, decreased auditory acuity, nystagmus, nausea and vomiting. Nystagmus that persists for several days is usually central rather than labyrinthine. Toxic labyrinthitis may be caused by mumps or encephalitis. Vestibular neuronitis may occur secondary to upper respiratory and middle ear infections.

    Meniere's disease (hydrops of the labyrinth) may occur rarely in children as attacks of severe vertigo, nystagmus and a sensorineural hearing loss. There is a tendency for complete recovery between episodes.

Lindsay, J.R.: Paroxysmal postural vertigo and vestibular neuronitis. *Arch. Otolaryngol.* *85*:544, 1967.

II. Central disorders such as brain tumors may be accompanied by gradually increasing dizziness, usually less severe and more continuous than that due to labyrinthine disease. Cerebellopontine angle, supratentorial, temporal lobe and midbrain tumors may be accompanied by vertigo. Benign positional vertigo may occur a few days or weeks after cerebral concussion as part of the post-traumatic headache syndrome. Episodes of vertigo may be a sequela of meningitis. Transient dizziness may also represent a prodromal symptom of epilepsy or migraine headaches. Vertigo is a frequent symptom in basilar artery migraine. Vertiginous seizures arising from the temporal lobe cortex may cause paroxysmal episodes of vertigo, headache, nausea, vomiting and unconsciousness. Vertigo may also be a symptom of more widespread seizure activity accompanied by to-and-fro or lateral swaying of the body, falling, unconsciousness and seizures.

III. Motion sickness may be due to hyperreactivity to labyrinthine stimuli.

IV. Psychogenic factors may give rise to the complaint of dizziness.

V. Postural vertigo, imbalance and headache may be initiated by trigger areas in the sternocleidomastoid muscle.

VI. Benign paroxysmal vertigo is characterized by recurrent episodes, sudden in onset and a few seconds to minutes in duration, in which the child, usually between the ages of one to five years, appears frightened, cries out, clings for support, staggers or falls. Accompanying findings include torticollis, pallor, sweating and nystagmus. Torticollis may persist for hours or days. The electroencephalogram is normal. There is often an abnormal caloric stimulation test.

Dunn, D.W. and Snyder, C.H.: Benign paroxysmal vertigo of childhood. *Am. J. Dis. Child.* *130*:1099, 1976.

VII. Drugs. Aminoglycosides such as gentamicin may cause vertigo.

## GENERAL REFERENCE

Eviatar, L. and Eviatar, A.: Vertigo in children: differential diagnosis and treatment. *Pediatrics 59*:833, 1977.

## ETIOLOGIC CLASSIFICATION OF VERTIGO

CHAPTER $54$

# HEADACHES

Chronic, recurrent headaches, like abdominal pain, represent a pediatric problem that requires integration of both organic and psychologic etiologic possibilities. In some children, headache can be diagnosed and treated successfully without much difficulty; in others, the diagnostic and therapeutic problem remains even after thorough exploration.

## ETIOLOGIC CLASSIFICATION OF HEADACHES

I. Muscle contraction headache (tension headache)
   A. This is by far the most common chronic, recurrent headache in childhood. There are no prodromal symptoms. Although in some instances the discomfort begins in the muscles of the neck, shoulders or occiput and migrates anteriorly to the frontal region, the headache is usually generalized. At times described as a "tight band around the head," "heavy weight on the head," "pressure from the outside" or as persistent mild or severe aching, the headache may continue for days or weeks. In fact, a persistent headache is almost always psychogenic and associated with anxiety or depression. Nausea, vomiting, dizziness or feelings of anxiety are reported in some cases. Severe headaches of any cause are frequently accompanied by spasm of the neck and shoulder muscles.
   B. Occipital neuralgia, owing to instability of the first and second cervical segments, is characterized by headaches in the occipital or suboccipital area caused by muscle spasm, scalp pain, tenderness and paresthesia involving the second cervical dermatome.

Dugan, M.C., Locke, S. and Gallagher, J.R.: Occipital neuralgia in adolescents and young adults. *N. Engl. J. Med. 267*:1166, 1962.

II. Vascular headaches
   A. Migraine headaches are not uncommon in the pediatric age group. Their incidence is estimated to be in the range of 2 to 4.5 per cent. Although children above the age of seven may experience migraine headaches similar to those in adults, in very young children the gastrointestinal symptomatology may be more prominent, the headaches generalized rather than unilateral and the pain less severe. Prodromal or accompanying symptoms may include photophobia, nausea, vomiting, abdominal pain, pallor, sweating, facial flushing, transient blindness, edema of the eyelids and changes in mood. Scintillating scotomata, hemianopsia, zigzag lines, blurred vision or paresthesias are less frequent in children than in adults.

Classically, the migraine headache is periodic and unilateral, though usually but not always occurring on the same side, in the retro-orbital, frontal or temporal region. Initially throbbing or pulsing and unilateral, the headache usually becomes constant and generalized. The duration is generally 2 to 3 hours, but some attacks last as long as 48 hours, or at times, several days. Occasionally, an episode is followed by a period of sleep. Migraine headaches may awaken a child at night. Most children have only infrequent migraine headaches, but a few have several a week. A family history of migraine is almost always present.

Brown, J.K.: Migraine and migraine equivalents in children. *Dev. Med. Child Neurol.* *19*:683, 1977.
Prensky, A.L.: Migraine and migrainous variants in pediatric patients. *Pediatr. Clin. N. Am.* *23*:461, 1976.

B. Complicated migraine is accompanied by neurologic deficits. Ophthalmoplegia, usually involving the oculomotor and less frequently the abducens nerve, is a rare complication of migraine headaches in early childhood. Twelve to twenty-four hours after the onset of the headache, nausea, vomiting, sudden, usually unilateral ptosis, dilatation of the pupil and reduced mobility of the eye develop and may last for days or weeks.

Van Pelt, W. and Andermann, F.: On early onset of ophthalmoplegic migraine. *Am. J. Dis. Child.* *107*:628, 1964.

C. Hemiplegic migraine, at times familial, characterized by neurologic deficits, hemiparesis or hemiplegia, occurs rarely in children.

Verret, S. and Steele, J.C.: Alternating hemiplegia in childhood: a report of eight patients with complicated migraine beginning in infancy. *Pediatrics 47*:675, 1971.

D. Acute confusional states lasting 10 minutes to 24 hours may be the initial manifestation of or occur during a migraine episode in later childhood and adolescence. Other symptoms may include agitation, apprehension and combativeness.

Ehyai, A. and Fenichel, G.M.: The natural history of acute confusional migraine. *Arch. Neurol. 35*:368, 1978.
Emery, E.S.: Acute confusional state in children with migraine. *Pediatrics 60*:110, 1977.
Gascon, G. and Barlow, C.: Juvenile migraine, presenting as an acute confusional state. *Pediatrics 45*:628, 1970.
Golden, G.S.: The Alice in Wonderland syndrome in juvenile migraine. *Pediatrics 63*:517, 1979.

E. Basilar artery migraine, which may occur from late infancy through adolescence, begins suddenly with transient visual symptoms, vertigo, ataxia, dysarthria, tinnitus, transient bilateral blindness, blurred vision, oculomotor abnormalities and paresthesias around the mouth and the distal extremities. Severe headache and vomiting follow. While some episodes last longer, most are less than three to four hours in duration. The headache may be bifrontal, bitemporal or occipital.

Lapkin, M.L. and Golden, G.S.: Basilar artery migraine. *Am. J. Dis. Child. 132*:278, 1978.

III. Combined headache

Migraine and muscle contraction headaches may occur simultaneously.

IV. Traction headache

These headaches result from traction on intracranial contents, especially vascular structures.

A. Intracranial tumors. Headache is less commonly a symptom of intracranial tumors in children than in adults, in part because of the early separation of sutures and spontaneous decompression that occur in the young patient. More frequent with cerebellar tumors, headache is an uncommon manifestation of supratentorial neoplasms. It is, however, the most common presenting symptom in children with a meningioma. Although the headache associated with brain tumors usually appears in the morning shortly after arising and disappears after a brief time, it may occur at other times in the day or be precipitated by sudden exacerbations in intracranial pressure caused by coughing, sneezing, straining with a bowel movement or change in position. Although it is hazardous to generalize about the qualitative nature of these headaches, they are usually dull, deep, not intense and intermittent (though occasionally steady). Headache caused by an intracranial tumor may be temporarily relieved by aspirin or even by a placebo. Temporary lessening of the headache may be due to separation of the sutures. Headaches that always occur in the same area, that are both sudden in onset and severe, that no longer respond to medication and that are accompanied by changes in personality suggest a serious outlook.

B. Brain abscess may be but usually is not accompanied by a headache.

C. Intracranial aneurysm. Rupture of an intracranial aneurysm may be accompanied by excruciating headache, photophobia, meningeal signs and impaired consciousness.

D. Arteriovenous malformations may produce a sudden headache, obtundation, focal neurologic defect, signs of meningeal irritation and increased intracranial pressure.

E. Lumbar punctures may also be followed by a severe headache.

F. Pseudotumor cerebri. In addition to severe headache, patients with this syndrome may also have blurring of vision, diplopia, nausea, vomiting and papilledema. Symptoms may persist for weeks.

Weisberg, L.A. and Chutorian, A.M.: Pseudotumor cerebri of childhood. *Am. J. Dis. Child.* *131*:1243, 1977.

G. Central nervous system leukemia causes headaches, irritability, diplopia, polyphagia and weight gain.

V. Inflammatory disease of the central nervous system.

Meningitis or encephalitis may cause severe headache.

VI. Post-traumatic headache

Headaches occurring in children after a severe head injury, especially one leading to unconsciousness, may persist for months or years. The patient also complains of dizziness, nervousness, sensitivity to noise, withdrawal, inability to concentrate, hyperactivity, sleep disturbances and difficulty controlling anger. The child may have experienced an unusually severe emotional reaction to the injury; his emotional adjustment prior to the trauma may have been marginal; or he may be currently experiencing environmental problems. In these children, a diagnosis of post-traumatic neurosis may be more accurate. The litigation that is pending following involvement of the child in an accident seems to contribute to persistence of the symptoms in some cases. A chronic subdural hematoma may require consideration in the differential diagnosis.

Dillon, H. and Leopold, R.L.: Children and the postconcussion syndrome. *JAMA 175*:86, 1961.
Rune, V.: Acute head injuries in children. *Acta Paediatr. Scand. Suppl. 209*:122, 1970.

VII. Epileptic equivalent

Episodic headache may rarely be due to paroxysmal cerebral dysrhythmia without other clinical signs of a convulsive disorder; however, the concept of "epileptic equivalents" remains controversial.

VIII. Ocular disorders

Headache may be caused by eyestrain owing to uncorrected refractive errors, astigmatism, muscle imbalance or impaired convergence. Accompanying symptoms may include burning, tearing, conjunctival hyperemia, blurring and dizziness. Since photophobia and conjunctival injection may accompany severe headache of any cause, they are not necessarily indicative of eye disease.

IX. Nose and paranasal sinuses

Sinusitis or inflammation and engorgement of the nasal turbinates are not important causes of chronic headache in children.

X. Hypertension

Although an unusual cause of chronic headache in children, hypertension is a consideration in the differential diagnosis. Hypertensive encephalopathy is manifested by severe headache, nausea, vomiting, confusion, seizures and transient, focal neurologic findings.

XI. Conversion hysteria

Rarely, a headache may have some specific symbolic unconscious meaning.

XII. Headaches of unknown origin

In some cases it may be impossible to determine the exact cause of a headache even after thorough study. Continuing, careful observation is important. The possibility of a gas leak, faulty flue or other environmental factor has been suggested as a cause for some persistent headaches accompanied by anorexia and dizziness.

Sherman, B.R. and Harris, E.H.: "Gas leak syndrome." Letters to the Editor. *Pediatrics 42*:710, 1960.

## DIAGNOSIS

### HISTORY

The pediatric history that includes both organic and psychosocial considerations is the most helpful diagnostic procedure. Organic disease and emotional problems may coexist. Children with either migraine or tension headaches commonly have relatives, especially the parents, with similar symptoms. A history of headache occurs in 85 per cent of parents of children with migraine. Seventy per cent of these parents have classic migraine. Headaches of psychogenic origin are especially likely to be due to identification with a relative or other person important to the child.

The history should review exactly what precedes the headaches: what the child was thinking about and what was going on in his environment. Monday morning headaches should obviously make one think of tension causes or school phobia. Interpersonal interactions should be explored. Both migraine and tension headaches may be precipitated by stressful situations, e.g., arguments between the child and someone close to him or episodes in which the child experiences disappointment, rejection, excessive excitement, anxiety or fear of failure as in critical school examinations. Precipitating causes for migraine headaches include excessive noise, confusion, menstrual periods, emotional stress, loss of sleep, prolonged sleep and lengthy viewing of television programs or movies.

In both migraine and muscle contraction headaches, the child and, at times, the entire family may have difficulty in handling aggressive and hostile feelings, especially toward parents, siblings, teachers and close friends. Evidence of such resentment should be looked for in the interview. The patient may not be able to inform the physician of this spontaneously. Being either unaware of the relation between his complaint and such psychologic processes or even of their existence since they are often unconscious, the patient may deny such feelings. Although episodic headaches may be precipitated by events that immediately evoke hostility and anger, there may also be continuing and intense resentment that the child is unable to express directly because of strong parental disapproval.

It is always a good idea to determine from the child what kinds of things make him angry, how he handles his anger and how he would like to manage it; and from the parents how they deal with anger and what expression they permit the child. The fact that at times there may be negative feelings toward those one loves is severely repressed in some families. It is not unexpected that children in such settings may experience intense guilt as a result of such feelings and that the resultant headache may be one way of assuaging this. Depression in children may also present as a severe headache that persists for days or weeks.

Kolb, L.C.: Psychiatric aspects of the treatment of headache. *Neurology 13*:34, 1963.
Ling, W., Oftedal, G. and Weinberg, W.: Depressive illness in childhood presenting as severe headache. *Am. J. Dis. Child. 120*:122, 1970.

The physician should also look for other internalized reactions such as anxiety or shame, for continuing or recurring environmental problems and for an explanation as to why the child seems to need the secondary gain that the symptom may bring.

Although personality "profiles" have no validity as predisposing to specific symptoms or diseases, children with migraine or muscle contraction headaches often seem to be especially sensitive, overly concerned about the approval of others, shy, polite and fearful of making errors. Meticulous, serious, overconscientious and prone to worry are other adjectives commonly applied to these children.

Physical examination should include visual fields by confrontation, determination of visual acuity and ability to converge, screening for phorias and examination of the retina and optic discs.

Since it is unusual for a headache to be the only manifestation of a seizure disorder, an electroencephalogram is rarely indicated. The electroencephalogram may, however, be helpful in the evaluation of patients with the post-traumatic syndrome.

Perlo, V.P.: The use of the electroencephalogram in the evaluation of head trauma. *N. Engl. J. Med. 276*:104, 1967.

A lumbar puncture is generally not indicated in the study of persistent headache. Skull films, brain scans, computerized axial tomography or arteriography are indicated only if an intracranial lesion is suspected.

## GENERAL REFERENCES

Ad hoc Committee on Classification of Headache: Classification of headache. *JAMA 179*:717, 1962.
Friedman, A.P. and Merritt, H.H.: *Headache: Diagnosis and Treatment*. Philadelphia, F.A. Davis Co., 1959.

---

## ETIOLOGIC CLASSIFICATION OF HEADACHES

---

CHAPTER **55**

# IRRITABILITY

Irritability may accompany almost any illness in pediatric practice. Unusual irritability occurs in the following disorders either alone or along with other symptoms.

## ETIOLOGIC CLASSIFICATION OF IRRITABILITY

I. Metabolic disorders
  A. Disturbances in water and electrolyte metabolism
    1. Changes in serum sodium concentration
      a. Hypernatremia. Irritability may be heightened in these instances. Alteration in consciousness may include lethargy and coma.
      b. Hyponatremia. Restlessness, irritability and convulsions may occur with profound hyponatremia.

2. Changes in serum calcium concentration
   a. Hypercalcemia, as in idiopathic hypercalcemia of infancy
   b. Hypocalcemia, as in hypoparathyroidism
3. Hypokalemia
4. Diabetes insipidus in infancy

B. Hypoglycemia produces irritability and other symptoms in the newborn (see page 429). Older infants may develop limp spells, pallor, flushing, twitching and tremors.

C. Urea cycle disorders with hyperammonemia may initially cause irritability, poor feeding and lethargy.

D. Nutritional disturbances
   1. Underfeeding
   2. Scurvy
   3. Celiac disease
   4. Iron deficiency is an important cause of irritability. Diminution of irritability may be the first sign of response to iron therapy.

Oski, F.A.: The nonhematologic manifestations of iron deficiency. *Am. J. Dis. Child. 133*: 315, 1979.

   5. Zinc deficiency secondary to prolonged parenteral alimentation may cause such behavioral changes as irritability with excessive and unconsolable crying.

Sivasubramanian, K.N. and Henkin, R.I.: Behavioral and dermatologic changes and low serum zinc and copper concentrations in two premature infants after parenteral alimentation. *J. Pediatr. 93*:847, 1978.

II. Neurologic disorders
   A. Subdural hematoma
   B. Subdural effusion may account for persistent irritability during treatment of bacterial meningitis.
   C. Meningitis. Unusual irritability in a young infant, especially if associated with other changes in sensorium, suggests meningitis.
   D. Encephalitis
   E. Brain tumor
   F. Neurologically impaired infants may demonstrate excessive irritability and "colic."
   G. Central nervous system degenerative disorders such as Krabbe's and Batten's disease may be characterized early by unusual irritability and persistent crying.

III. Cardiac disorders
   A. Paroxysmal atrial tachycardia
   B. Congestive cardiac failure. Irritability may be an early symptom of cardiac failure in infants along with anorexia and easy tiring on feeding.
   C. Endocardial fibroelastosis. Although the onset of this disorder may be fulminant or acute, irritability, anorexia and failure to thrive may be present for some time before dyspnea and cyanosis are noted.
   D. Tetralogy of Fallot. Episodes of irritability or crying may be due to periods of hypoxia.

IV. Hematologic disorders
   A. Anemia
   B. Leukemia

V. Drugs, poisons, toxins

  A. Lead poisoning may be characterized early by extreme irritability, lethargy, drowsiness, fearfulness and unexplained crying. A high index of suspicion is indicated even without an initial history of pica.

  B. Gasoline sniffing may produce irritability, anorexia, tremor, vomiting and delirium.

    Boeckx, R.L., Postl, B. and Coodin, F.J.: Gasoline sniffing and tetraethyl lead poisoning in children. *Pediatrics 60*:140, 1977.

  C. Vitamin A poisoning owing to excessive administration may be seen in infants and young children above the age of six months. In addition to irritability, symptoms include pruritus, hepatomegaly, alopecia and painful swelling of the extremities.

  D. The fetal alcohol syndrome may be characterized by withdrawal symptoms such as irritability, tremors and seizures.

    Pierog, S., Chandavasu, O. and Wexler, I.: Withdrawal symptoms in infants with the fetal alcohol syndrome. *J. Pediatr. 90*:630, 1977.

  E. Maternal narcotic addiction may cause withdrawal symptoms in newborn infants. Manifestations include irritability, excessive and high-pitched cry, restlessness, tremors, convulsions, vomiting, drowsiness, poor feeding, nasal congestion, sneezing, dyspnea and yawning. Symptoms may begin within the first 12 hours of life or be delayed for 3 to 4 days. Withdrawal symptoms from methadone may be delayed until 2 weeks of age in some infants.

    Reddy, A.M., Harper, R.G. and Stern, G.: Observations on heroin and methadone withdrawal in the newborn. *Pediatrics 48*:353, 1971.
    Zelson, C.: Infant of the addicted mother. *N. Engl. J. Med. 288*:1393, 1973.

  F. Phenobarbital may cause irritability in some children. Infants born to mothers who have taken barbiturates throughout pregnancy may manifest withdrawal symptoms.

    Desmond, M.M. et al.: Maternal barbiturate utilization and neonatal withdrawal symptomatology. *J. Pediatr. 80*:190, 1972.

VI. Mothering disabilities. Excessive irritability in an infant may be attributable to psychologic factors (e.g., situations in which the baby's need for nurture is not adequately met, underfeeding, overfeeding and restriction of movement). Maternal depression or excessive tension in the home may cause irritability in an infant.

VII. Miscellaneous

  A. Atopic eczema

  B. Cow milk allergy

  C. Unrecognized skeletal trauma; traumatic periostitis; child abuse

  D. Inguinal hernia

  E. Unrecognized ingestion of a foreign body such as an open safety pin

  F. Unrecognized deafness

  G. Infantile cortical hyperostosis

    Staheli, L.T., Church, C.C. and Ward, B.H.: Infantile cortical hyperostosis (Caffey's disease). *JAMA 203*:96, 1968.

H. Pheochromocytoma. Some of these patients may be markedly irritable.

I. Persistent irritability occurs with the Smith-Lemli-Opitz syndrome.

J. Anal fissures are an important cause of crying and irritability in young infants.

K. Teething

L. Colic, a syndrome of many etiologies, is characterized by the episodic occurrence of vigorous and persistent crying. The infant appears to be in pain with his hands clenched, arms and thighs flexed, face beet red and abdomen distended. Some infants have colic almost every evening or night for two to three months. Usually, no specific cause can be established. Poor feeding technique may be etiologic in some instances. Emotional tension in the home may be related in a few cases. Cow milk allergy may be a factor in a few other babies. In general, however, the cause is obscure.

Paradise, J.L.: Maternal and other factors in the etiology of infantile colic. *JAMA 197*:123, 1966.

## ETIOLOGIC CLASSIFICATION OF IRRITABILITY

I. Metabolic disorders, 458
  A. Disturbances in water and electrolyte metabolism, 458
    1. Changes in serum sodium concentration
    2. Changes in serum calcium concentration
  B. Hypoglycemia, 459
  C. Urea cycle disorders with hyperammonemia, 459
  D. Nutritional disturbances, 459
    1. Underfeeding
    2. Scurvy
    3. Celiac disease
    4. Iron deficiency
    5. Zinc deficiency

II. Neurologic disorders, 459
  A. Subdural hematoma, 459
  B. Subdural effusion, 459
  C. Meningitis, 459
  D. Encephalitis, 459
  E. Brain tumor, 459
  F. Neurologic impairment, 459
  G. Central nervous system degenerative disorders, 459

III. Cardiac disorders, 459
  A. Paroxysmal atrial tachycardia, 459
  B. Congestive cardiac failure, 459
  C. Endocardial fibroelastosis, 459
  D. Tetralogy of Fallot, 459

IV. Hematologic disorders, 459
  A. Anemia, 459
  B. Leukemia, 459

V. Drugs, poisons, toxins, 460
  A. Lead poisoning, 460
  B. Gasoline sniffing, 460
  C. Vitamin A poisoning, 460
  D. Fetal alcohol syndrome, 460
  E. Maternal narcotic addiction, 460
  F. Phenobarbital, 460

VI. Mothering disabilities, 460

VII. Miscellaneous, 460
  A. Atopic eczema, 460
  B. Cow milk allergy, 460
  C. Unrecognized skeletal trauma; traumatic periostitis; child abuse, 460
  D. Inguinal hernia, 460
  E. Unrecognized ingestion of a foreign body, 460
  F. Unrecognized deafness, 460
  G. Infantile cortical hyperostosis, 460
  H. Pheochromocytoma, 460
  I. Smith-Lemli-Opitz syndrome, 460
  J. Anal fissures, 460
  K. Teething, 460
  L. Colic, 460

# CHAPTER 56

# CYANOSIS

## CLINICAL CONSIDERATIONS

Cyanosis refers to a bluish color of the skin, attributable in most cases to an abnormally large amount of reduced (ferrous) hemoglobin (5 gm./dl.) in the capillaries. Methemoglobin, an oxidized derivative of hemoglobin, also produces cyanosis when its concentration exceeds 15 per cent of the total hemoglobin. Carboxyhemoglobin, formed as a result of carbon monoxide intoxication, is bright red, so it produces a reddish rather than a bluish discoloration of the skin.

The presence of cyanosis may, at times, be difficult to be certain about clinically. Because cyanosis is more easily seen in bright light, newborn infants should be kept in a well-lighted room during the initial observation period.

Cyanosis may be *central* (tongue, mucous membranes and peripheral skin) owing to arterial desaturation or an abnormal hemoglobin. *Peripheral* cyanosis, confined to the extremities, is due to an increased arteriovenous oxygen difference in the presence of normal arterial saturation. Precise differentiation between central and peripheral cyanosis may depend upon the determination of arterial oxygen saturation, or $Pao_2$. The cyanosis may be considered central if the $Pao_2$ is under 75 mm. Hg at one day of age or if the oxygen saturation is under 94 per cent.

Cyanosis is first apparent and most evident where the epidermis is thin, pigmentation minimal and capillaries numerous, that is, in the tips of the fingers and toes (nail beds), the ear lobes, the tip of the nose, the lips, the tongue and the buccal mucous membrane. In deeply pigmented persons, cyanosis may be apparent only in the tongue and mucous membranes. In patients in whom arterial unsaturation is not severe, redness rather than blueness may be noted in the lips, cheeks, nose and fingers. In polycythemia or hyperviscosity syndrome of the newborn, the cyanosis may appear bluish-red and have a blotchy rather than uniform distribution. The color of true cyanosis disappears if blood is expressed from the capillaries by diascopic pressure.

## PHYSIOLOGY OF CYANOSIS

In the newborn infant, central cyanosis may be noted in the tongue and mucous membranes with only 3 gm. of reduced hemoglobin and an arterial saturation of 75 to 88 per cent. An anemic patient with less than 5 gm. of hemoglobin/dl. of blood cannot become cyanotic since 5 gm. of reduced hemoglobin in 100 ml. of capillary blood is necessary.

Owing to the high affinity of fetal hemoglobin for oxygen and the large amount of such hemoglobin in the newborn, serious degrees of anoxia may be present in the absence of cyanosis. It is improper, therefore, to wait for cyanosis before considering hypoxia. Measurement of the oxygen tension may be more helpful than oxygen saturation in such instances.

Duc, G.: Assessment of hypoxia in the newborn. Suggestions for a practical approach. *Pediatrics 48*:469, 1971.

## ETIOLOGIC CLASSIFICATION OF CYANOSIS

Please see also chapters on respiratory distress and respiratory disease. Some of the disorders discussed there could also have been included here.

I. Cyanosis owing to abnormal forms of hemoglobin. The diagnosis in these cases depends upon a careful history and on spectrophotometry.

   A. Congenital methemoglobinemia. Familial methemoglobinemia may be due either to an abnormality of erythrocyte energy-dependent mechanisms for reducing methemoglobin or inherited defects in hemoglobin structure, as in the hemoglobin M group. Methemoglobin diaphorase deficiency and deficiency of cytochrome $b_5$ reductase is characterized by both methemoglobinemia and mental retardation. With methemoglobinemia, the blood is chocolate-brown when drawn and does not become red when mixed.

Gerald, P.S.: The clinical implications of hemoglobin structure. *Pediatrics 31*:780, 1963.
Jaffé, E.R.: Hereditary methemoglobinemias associated with abnormalities in the metabolism of erythrocytes. *Am. J. Med. 41*:786, 1966.

   B. Methemoglobinemia may be caused by well-water (nitrate) ingestion in young infants, especially those with diarrhea and with coliform organisms in the upper intestine. Vegetables with a known high nitrate content (beets, cabbage and spinach) may lead to methemoglobinemia under special circumstances. The nitrates are converted to nitrites by bacteria. With absorption of nitrite, methemoglobin is produced.

Keating, J.P. et al.: Infantile methemoglobinemia caused by carrot juice. *N. Engl. J. Med. 288*:824, 1973.
Report of the Committee on Nutrition of the American Academy of Pediatrics: Infant methemoglobinemia: the role of dietary nitrate. *Pediatrics 46*:475, 1970.

   C. Methemoglobinemia in young infants has been caused by aniline dyes used in marking shirts and diapers. Ingestion of wax crayons has caused methemoglobinemia in older children. Methemoglobinemia has also been attributed to benzocaine ointment or rectal suppositories.

   D. Hemoglobin Kansas and Hemoglobin Beth Israel, hemoglobin mutants with an abnormal affinity for oxygen, are associated with cyanosis.

Nagel, R.L. et al.: Hemoglobin Beth Israel. *N. Engl. J. Med. 295*:125, 1976.

   E. Cyanosis from carbon monoxide poisoning is more red than blue.

II. Cyanosis due to abnormal amounts of reduced hemoglobin.

   A. Cyanosis in which the primary factor is an increased amount of hemoglobin passing in reduced form through aerated portions of the lung. The essential change is an increase in the value for arterial oxygen unsaturation in the blood returning from the lungs. If inhalation of 100 per cent oxygen increases the partial pressure of oxygen in the alveoli and aids diffusion, arterial oxygen unsaturation is diminished and cyanosis improved. Cyanosis does not appear until alveolar ventilation has been reduced.

1. Decreased alveolar ventilation caused by failure of the respiratory center secondary to prematurity, intrauterine hypoxia, intracranial hemorrhage, drug administration or Ondine's curse.

Fishman, L.S., Samson, J.H. and Sperling, D.R.: Primary alveolar hypoventilation syndrome (Ondine's curse). *Am. J. Dis. Child. 110*:155, 1965.

2. Decreased alveolar ventilation from obstruction of the respiratory tract
   a. Congenital obstructive lesions
      (1) Atresia of the posterior nasal choanae
      (2) Macroglossia
      (3) Hypoplasia of the mandible with glossoptosis (Pierre Robin syndrome). Posterior displacement of the tongue in these babies causes obstruction of the airway and may precipitate episodes of cyanosis.
      (4) Thyroglossal duct cyst
      (5) Laryngeal web or cyst
      (6) Congenital absence of the cartilaginous rings of the trachea; tracheal stenosis
      (7) Congenital vascular ring
   b. Acquired intrinsic obstruction
      (1) Nasal mucus in the newborn. The young infant may lack the ability to open his mouth reflexly during sleep.
      (2) Meconium aspiration syndrome
      (3) Bilateral paresis of the vocal cords due to intracranial hemorrhage at birth
      (4) Obstetrical damage to the cricothyroid or cricoarytenoid cartilages
      (5) Retropharyngeal abscess; infections of the deep spaces of the neck
      (6) Acute laryngotracheobronchitis; spasmodic croup
      (7) Laryngeal edema; angioneurotic edema; serum sickness; nephrotic syndrome
      (8) Laryngospasm
      (9) Foreign body in the larynx or trachea
      (10) Laryngeal neoplasm: papilloma, hemangioma, fibrolipoma
      (11) Cystic fibrosis
      (12) Acute bronchiolitis
   c. Acquired extrinsic obstruction
      (1) Pneumomediastinum
      (2) Congenital goiter
      (3) Cystic hygroma
      (4) Enterogenous cyst in the chest
      (5) Lymphadenopathy: lymphoma, tuberculosis, sarcoidosis
3. Decreased alveolar ventilation due to structural changes in the lungs, impairment of diffusion, ventilation/perfusion unevenness and shunting.
   a. Cystic fibrosis
   b. Asthma
   c. Pulmonary fibrosis
   d. Congenital pulmonary cysts

    e. Interstitial pulmonary emphysema

    f. Diaphragmatic hernia

    g. Hyaline membrane disease; respiratory distress syndrome

    h. Transient tachypnea of the newborn

    i. Bronchopulmonary dysplasia

    j. Atelectasis in the newborn

    k. Aspiration pneumonitis. An isolated tracheoesophageal fistula is a diagnostic consideration when cyanotic episodes accompany feedings in infancy. A history of choking and repeated episodes of aspiration pneumonia may also be obtained.

    l. Pneumonia. Since the blood is shunted to aerated portions of the lung in patients with pneumonia, only a small portion of the total hemoglobin is exposed to unaerated, consolidated lung. Group A beta-hemolytic streptococcal pneumonia is a special consideration in the newborn.

    m. Pulmonary edema. In cardiac failure, pulmonary edema may interfere with the diffusion of gases.

    n. Idiopathic pulmonary hemosiderosis may be characterized by repeated attacks of cyanosis, pallor, dyspnea, cough and fatigue.

    o. Congestive heart failure

    p. Pneumothorax. Since blood is shunted to the remaining aerated lung, cyanosis may not appear if the lung collapse is unilateral.

    q. Empyema; pyopneumothorax; hemothorax; chylothorax; pleural effusion

    r. Lobar emphysema

    s. Abdominal distention with pressure on the diaphragm may cause attacks of cyanosis.

    t. Pulmonary alveolar proteinosis

    u. Congenital cystic adenomatoid malformation of the lung may cause cyanosis and tachypnea in infants. The mediastinum is displaced to the opposite side. Roentgenographic examination demonstrates a mass of soft-tissue density containing scattered radiolucent areas.

    v. Desquamative interstitial pneumonitis

    w. Congenital lobar emphysema

    x. Pulmonary lymphangiomatosis

    y. Wilson-Mikity syndrome

    z. Pneumocystis carini pneumonia

  4. Decreased alveolar ventilation due to neuromuscular dysfunction

  5. Breath-holding spells

  6. Decreased alveolar exchange caused by lowered barometric pressure. Rapid ascent to high altitudes may cause pulmonary edema in susceptible children.

B. Cyanosis in which the primary factor is the amount of hemoglobin passing in reduced form through unaerated, venoarterial shunts from the right side of the heart to the arterial blood in the lungs or through the foramen ovale or the ductus arteriosus. The essential change is an increased arterial oxygen unsaturation in the systemic arteries. The value for arterial oxygen unsaturation in blood returning from the lungs is normal.

The inhalation of 100 per cent oxygen will cause only a slight diminution in the cyanosis in these patients because the hemoglobin passing through the lungs is normally oxygenated. Inhalation of 100 per cent oxygen increases the oxygenation of pulmonary blood only ½ to 1 volume/dl. in normal persons. An additional 2 volumes/dl. may be dissolved in the plasma, but this oxygen is slowly released and has little effect on the amount of reduced hemoglobin. The minimal decrease in arterial oxygen unsaturation gained by oxygen therapy is usually not sufficient to counteract the effect of a large amount of venous blood shunted into the arterial circulation. In most of these patients, the extent of oxygen unsaturation is further increased with exercise. In infants with increased pulmonary vascular resistance, however, there may be a direct effect of oxygen to dilate the pulmonary vessels and reduce venoarterial shunting.

1. Cyanotic congenital heart disease
    a. Transposition of the great vessels is the most frequent cause of cyanotic congenital heart disease in infants. Severe cyanosis is usually present within two to three days after birth. Pulmonary vascular markings are increased. If oxygenated blood is shunted to the systemic circulation through a persistent ductus, the hands are more cyanotic than the feet since the ductus arteriosus enters the aorta distal to the origin of the arteries to the arms.
    b. Tricuspid atresia with a nonfunctioning, rudimentary right ventricle is associated with severe cyanosis from birth and decreased pulmonary vascular markings.
    c. Pseudotruncus arteriosus, a severe form of tetralogy with pulmonary atresia, is a cause of neonatal cyanosis. Pulmonary vascular markings are decreased.
    d. Pulmonary atresia causes severe cyanosis during the first week of life. Pulmonary vascular markings are decreased.
    e. Hypoplastic left heart syndrome causes cyanosis and congestive failure in the first 24 to 48 hours of life. Pulmonary vascular markings are increased.
    f. Persistent pulmonary hypertension of the newborn infant (fetal circulation syndrome) owing to continuing postnatal pulmonary hypertension is characterized by abnormal right-to-left shunting through a patent foramen ovale or patent ductus arteriosus. This hemodynamic pattern may occur in full-term infants with pulmonary disease, hypoglycemia, polycythemia, asphyxia or for unknown reasons. The infant, usually term or near term, may appear normal at birth but then develops cyanosis accompanied by tachypnea and acidemia in the first 24 hours of life. The second sound is often loud. The chest x-ray shows normal pulmonary parenchymal markings.

Gersony, W.M.: Persistence of the fetal circulation: a commentary. *J. Pediatr. 82*:1103, 1973.
Levin, P.L. et al.: Persistent pulmonary hypertension of the newborn. *J. Pediatr. 89*:626, 1976.

    g. Single ventricle may not be accompanied by early cyanosis. Pulmonary vascular markings are increased.

h. Truncus arteriosus is characterized by a delayed appearance of cyanosis. Pulmonary vascular markings are increased.

i. Tetralogy of Fallot consists of pulmonary stenosis or atresia, a ventricular septal defect, a dextroposed aorta that overrides the septal defect, and right ventricular hypertrophy. Pulmonary vascular markings are decreased. Although cyanosis is present at birth in about one third of these patients, in most instances it does not appear or become persistent until the child begins to walk or run. Cyanosis is accentuated by exercise or exertion.

j. Pulmonary stenosis, if sufficiently severe, may be accompanied by cyanosis. Pulmonary vascular markings are decreased.

k. Ebstein's anomaly of the tricuspid valve is accompanied by decreased pulmonary vascular markings.

l. Total anomalous pulmonary venous return is characterized by an increase in pulmonary vascular markings. The infant frequently is asymptomatic during the first month of life.

m. Pulmonary hypertension and patent ductus arteriosus. When the pressure in the pulmonary circulation exceeds that in the systemic circulation, the descending aorta receives blood from the pulmonary artery. As a result, cyanosis is greater in the feet than in the hands. Because of its proximity to the ductus arteriosus, the subclavian artery may also receive venous blood from the pulmonary artery. As a result, cyanosis may be greater in the left than in the right hand.

n. Primary pulmonary hypertension caused by an abnormality in the pulmonary vascular bed may be characterized by cyanosis, dyspnea and fatigue. Cyanosis may result from a right-to-left shunt through a patent foramen ovale secondary to elevation of the pressure in the right ventricle and atrium. In other children, cyanosis has occurred in the absence of a septal defect. Some of these instances may be attributable to an arteriovenous aneurysm or pulmonary shunt. Primary pulmonary hypertension may occur in children who live at high altitudes.

o. Eisenmenger complex. Cyanosis frequently does not appear until adolescence.

p. A preductile coarctation of the aorta with a patent ductus arteriosus may be associated with differential cyanosis between the upper and lower extremities, blood from the right ventricle being shunted through the ductus.

Nadas, A.S. and Fyler, D.C.: *Pediatric Cardiology*. 3rd ed. Philadelphia, W.B. Saunders Co., 1972.

Rudolph, A.: *Congenital Disease of the Heart*. Chicago, Year Book Medical Publishers, 1974.

2. Cyanosis from a pulmonary arteriovenous fistula. With this lesion, unoxygenated blood is shunted from the pulmonary arteries to the pulmonary veins. The degree of cyanosis and dyspnea depends upon the extent of the shunt. Symptoms usually begin in childhood. A murmur may be audible over the shunt. Polycythemia and clubbing of the fingers gradually develop.

3. Hyaline membrane disease produces hypoxia because of alveolar hypoventilation and right-to-left shunts.
4. Cyanosis possibly caused by portopulmonary anastomoses or pulmonary arteriovenous fistulas in patients with chronic hepatic disease and portal hypertension

Silverman, A., Cooper, M.D., Moller, J.H. and Good, R.A.: Syndrome of cyanosis, digital clubbing, and hepatic disease in siblings. *J. Pediatr. 72*:70, 1968.

5. Intermittent cyanosis may occur in the cardiorespiratory syndrome of obesity. In addition to extreme obesity, symptoms and findings include dyspnea, polycythemia, somnolence, right ventricular hypertrophy and right-sided heart failure. The exact cause of the cyanosis is unknown.

C. Cyanosis in which the primary factor is the amount of hemoglobin converted to the reduced form while passing from the arteries to veins, i.e., the extent of deoxygenation in the capillaries. This is usually due to capillary stasis, and the essential change is an increased venous oxygen unsaturation. The oxygen saturation of the arterial blood is normal. Oxygen therapy cannot reduce cyanosis unless capillary stasis results from arterial hypoxia.
   1. Peripheral, or localized cyanosis
      a. Acrocyanosis of the circumoral region and distal extremities in the first few hours after birth
      b. Local cyanosis due to constriction of an extremity with a tourniquet
      c. Obstruction of the superior vena cava
      d. Livedo reticularis
      e. Raynaud's disease is characterized by paroxysmal cyanosis or pallor of the fingers and toes. In many instances, only the fingers are involved. Characteristically, involvement is bilateral and symmetrical. Symptoms occur more frequently in girls then in boys and may be precipitated by cold or emotional stress. Raynaud's syndrome may be an early manifestation of lupus erythematosus.
   2. Generalized cyanosis due in part to increased venous pressure
      a. Cardiac failure
         (1) Paroxysmal atrial tachycardia
         (2) Coarctation of the aorta of the infantile type. Failure may develop when the ductus arteriosus closes.
         (3) Hypoplastic left heart syndrome
         (4) Endocardial fibroelastosis
         (5) Anomalous origin of the left coronary artery may be characterized by episodes of cyanosis (especially in relation to feedings), colicky pain, tachycardia, dyspnea and drenching perspiration.
         (6) Myocarditis
         (7) Rheumatic valvular disease
         (8) Patients with left-to-right shunts may demonstrate cyanosis with the onset of congestive heart failure.
      b. Constrictive pericarditis
      c. The cyanosis that occurs during major convulsive seizures may, in part, be due to the increased venous pressure that develops at that time.
      d. Cyanosis due to crying

3. Generalized cyanosis due to poor peripheral perfusion
   a. Capillary stasis owing to polycythemia or hyperviscosity may be an important secondary cause of cyanosis, (e.g., in patients with congenital heart disease with hematocrit over 70 per cent).

Wirth, F.H., Goldberg, K.E. and Lubchenco, L.O.: Neonatal hyperviscosity: I. Incidence. *Pediatrics 63*:833, 1979.

   b. Localized cyanosis in the newborn (e.g., cord around the neck)
   c. Shock or hypotension may be characterized by cyanosis or an ashen gray color as well as by pallor. Dehydration is a major cause of shock and capillary stasis in infants and young children with severe diarrhea, adrenal hemorrhage and hypoadrenalism. Shock may also be due to acute blood loss. Mottled cyanosis may occur in infants and children with severe, acute infectious diseases such as sepsis (Group B beta-hemolytic streptococcus in the newborn infant), as a result of low cardiac output, hypotension, peripheral vascular collapse and pooling of blood in the skin. Cyanosis associated with profound circulatory collapse may be seen in the Waterhouse-Friderichsen syndrome. The "gray syndrome," characterized by peripheral vascular collapse and a gray pallor, occurs in newborn infants who receive inappropriately large doses of chloramphenicol.

Sommerville, R.J., Nora, J.J., Clayton, G.W. and McNamara, D.G.: Adrenal insufficiency mimicking heart disease in infancy. *Pediatrics 42*:691, 1968.

   d. Hypoglycemia in the newborn
   e. Poor perfusion occurs in the hypoplastic left heart syndrome and with primary myocardial disease. Profound congestive heart failure with dyspnea and mild or moderate cyanosis (ashen gray color) occurs in the first hours or days of life in infants with the hypoplastic left heart syndrome.
   f. Congestive heart failure. Cyanosis in the infant with heart failure may be due, in part, to a low cardiac output. In addition to congenital heart defects, congestive heart failure and cyanosis may be caused by pulmonary disease, sepsis, anemia, myopathy, hypoxia and hypoglycemia.
   g. Peripheral cyanosis caused by chilling of the skin and venostasis. This is often a familial characteristic.
D. Peripheral cyanosis in which the primary factor is an increase in the total hematocrit
   1. Polycythemia and hyperviscosity syndromes in the newborn infant. Polycythemia in the newborn infant is present when the venous hematocrit is above 60 to 65 per cent. Viscosity increases markedly above a hematocrit of 65. Presenting signs and symptoms include peripheral cyanosis, respiratory distress, cardiomegaly, lethargy or seizures. Several disorders may be associated with neonatal polycythemia, including infants small for gestational age, infants of diabetic mothers, chromosomal abnormalities such as Down's syndrome, and placental-cord, maternal-fetal and twin-twin transfusion. Since the hyperviscosity syndrome may also occur when the hematocrit is within the upper limits of normal, the blood viscosity

should be measured with a microviscometer in infants with suggestive symptoms. Hyperviscosity may also be associated with acidosis and hypothermia.

Gross, G.P., Hathaway, W.E. and McGaughey, H.R.: Hyperviscosity in the neonate. *J. Pediatr. 82*:1004, 1973.
Kontras, S.B.: Polycythemia and hyperviscosity syndromes in infants and children. *Pediatr. Clin. N. Am. 19*:919, 1972.

2. Polycythemia secondary to chronic hypoxia. Chronic hypoxia invariably produces polycythemia if the bone marrow is normal. Hypoxia and polycythemia accompany most forms of cyanotic heart disease and are present in patients with a pulmonary arteriovenous fistula. Polycythemia usually accentuates the cyanosis in these cases.
3. Polycythemia vera

## DIAGNOSIS OF CYANOSIS IN THE NEWBORN

The differentiation of pulmonary and cardiac causes of cyanosis in the newborn, a frequent problem in the newborn intensive care unit, may be difficult or impossible. Indeed, both etiologies may be simultaneously involved. A few generalizations may be made. The response of cyanosis to crying in the newborn period does not permit differentiation between a pulmonary or a cardiac etiology. Severe cyanosis usually implies a congenital heart disorder such as transposition of the great vessels. Similarly, tachypnea accompanied by intense cyanosis without apparent respiratory distress is more characteristic of cyanotic congenital heart disease. Arterial blood gases and pH should be promptly obtained in the infant with cyanosis. The chest x-ray is probably the next most helpful examination since it may demonstrate the radiologic features of respiratory distress syndrome, the cardiomegaly due to cardiac disease and the increased or decreased pulmonary vascular markings associated with specific congenital cardiac disorders. The increase in $Pco_2$ and the decrease in $Pao_2$ and pH secondary to severe pulmonary disease may also lead to moderate cardiomegaly.

While both alveolar hypoventilation and a right-to-left shunt may be accompanied by a low $Pao_2$, the $Pco_2$ is generally increased in the former but not the latter. In the case of hyaline membrane disease with right-to-left shunting, the low $Pao_2$ may be accompanied by a normal or decreased $Pco_2$. The response of the $Pao_2$ to breathing of 100 per cent oxygen for 10 to 30 minutes is also of differential interest: in alveolar hypoventilation the $Pao_2$ will rise, whereas there will be no effect with a right-to-left shunt. A $Pao_2$ over 50 or 60 while breathing 100 per cent oxygen almost always rules out a cyanotic congenital cardiac defect. Response to oxygen with clinical improvement in color does not always permit differentiation between pulmonary and congenital heart disease. Some babies with right-to-left shunts improve with oxygen; some infants with marked pulmonary disease do not. Infants who remain cyanotic beyond three hours after birth should be evaluated by a pediatric cardiologist.

The diagnostic work-up of a cyanotic infant should generally include the following: arterial blood gases ($Po_2$, $Pco_2$), pH, chest x-ray, hematocrit, blood sugar, cultures, possibly an electrocardiogram and response to 100 per cent oxygen ($Pao_2$ in 100 per cent $Fi0_2$). Cardiac catheterization with angiocardiography and/or echocardiography may also be indicated.

# GENERAL REFERENCES

Emmanouilides, G.C. and Baylen, B.G.: Neonatal cardiopulmonary distress without congenital heart disease. *Curr. Probl. in Pediatr. 9*:4 (May) 1979.

Hipona, F.A. and Sanyal, S.K.: Differential cyanosis in congenital heart disease. *J. Pediatr. 72*:194, 1968.

Lees, M.H.: Cyanosis of the newborn infant. *J. Pediatr. 77*:484, 1970.

Sahn, D.J. and Friedman, W.F.: Difficulties in distinguishing cardiac from pulmonary disease in the neonate. *Pediatr. Clin. N. Am. 20*:293, 1973.

---

# ETIOLOGIC CLASSIFICATION OF CYANOSIS

I. Abnormal forms of hemoglobin, 463
   A. Congenital methemoglobinemia, 463
   B. Methemoglobinemia from well-water (nitrate) ingestion, 463
   C. Methemoglobinemia from aniline dyes, wax crayons, benzocaine ointment or suppositories, 463
   D. Hemoglobin mutants (Hemoglobin Kansas, Hemoglobin Beth Israel), 463
   E. Carbon monoxide poisoning, 463

II. Abnormal amounts of reduced hemoglobin, 463
   A. Increased amount of hemoglobin passing in reduced form through aerated portions of the lung, 463
      1. Decreased alveolar ventilation from prematurity, intrauterine hypoxia, intracranial hemorrhage, drug administration or Ondine's curse
      2. Decreased alveolar ventilation from respiratory tract obstruction
      3. Decreased alveolar ventilation from lung structural changes, diffusion impairment, ventilation/perfusion unevenness, shunting
      4. Decreased alveolar ventilation from neuromuscular dysfunction
      5. Breath-holding spells
      6. Decreased alveolar exchange from lowered barometric pressure
   B. Amount of hemoglobin passing in reduced form through unaerated, venoarterial shunts from the heart's right side to the arterial blood in the lungs or through the foramen ovale or ductus arteriosus, 465
      1. Cyanotic congenital heart disease
      2. Pulmonary arteriovenous fistula
      3. Hyaline membrane disease
      4. Portopulmonary anastomoses or pulmonary arteriovenous fistula in patients with chronic hepatic disease and portal hypertension
      5. Cardiorespiratory syndrome of obesity
   C. Extent of deoxygenation in the capillaries, 468
      1. Peripheral cyanosis
      2. Generalized cyanosis from increased venous pressure
      3. Generalized cyanosis from poor peripheral perfusion
   D. Peripheral cyanosis from an increase in the total hematocrit, 469
      1. Polycythemia and hyperviscosity syndrome in newborn
      2. Polycythemia secondary to chronic hypoxia
      3. Polycythemia vera

# CHAPTER 57

# RESPIRATORY° DISTRESS; DYSPNEA; APNEA

## CLINICAL CONSIDERATIONS

Dyspnea is a subjective feeling of respiratory discomfort. In the infant and young child, the term *dyspnea* is probably not semantically correct and *respiratory distress* may be preferable. Orthopnea is a form of dyspnea present in the recumbent position but absent when the patient is sitting up. In infants, respiratory distress is usually accompanied by tachypnea with a respiratory rate greater than 60 per minute. Normally, the respiratory rate in a newborn infant averages 40 with a range of 35 to 50. The respiratory rate should be determined at regular intervals in all newborn infants and every 15 minutes during the first hour if a problem is suspected. A fall in the respiratory rate may mean that the tachypnea is improving or that the infant is beginning to experience respiratory failure.

Downes, J.J., Fulgencio, T. and Raphaely, R.C.: Acute respiratory failure in infants and children. *Pediatr. Clin. N. Am. 19*:423, 1972.
Haddad, G.G., and Mellins, R.B.: The role of airway receptors in the control of respiration in infants. A review. *J. Pediatr. 91*:281, 1977.
Polgar, G.: Practical pulmonary physiology. *Pediatr. Clin. N. Am. 20*:303, 1973.

The three chief factors that have an effect on the respiratory centers and on the control of respiration are *chemical*, including hypoxemia, hypercapnia and acidosis; *reflex,* owing to the Hering-Breuer reflex; and *cerebral,* or central. Although pressoreceptors in the wall of the carotid sinus and the aortic arch are probably not concerned with the regulation of respiration, a fall in blood pressure may act to increase pulmonary ventilation. Thermoreceptors in the hypothalamus and in the skin may provide a minimal stimulus to respiration in the presence of fever.

Though one of these factors may initiate an alteration in respiration, others usually come in to contribute to respiratory control. It is unusual for one factor to act alone.

Asphyxiation of the newborn should be evaluated immediately at birth by the Apgar score (Table 57–1). A score of 0 to 3 implies severe distress and is an

TABLE 57–1  SIGNS USED IN DETERMINING APGAR SCORE (0−2)

| Sign | 0 | 1 | 2 |
|------|---|---|---|
| Heart rate | Absent | Slow (below 100) | Over 100 |
| Respiratory effort | Absent | Slow, irregular | Good, crying |
| Muscle tone | Flaccid | Some flexion of extremities | Active motion |
| Reflex irritability | No response | Grimace | Vigorous cry |
| Color | Blue, pale | Body pink, extremities blue | Completely pink |

indication for immediate resuscitation. Apgar scores of 4 to 7 indicate moderate respiratory distress. With a score of 7 to 10, continued observation is all that is required. When the respiratory problem is urgent and intervention cannot be delayed to wait for 1- and 5-minute Apgar scores, evaluation of the respiratory effort and heart rate will suffice. If respiratory effort is good and the heart rate above 100, continued observation is proper. If respiration is inadequate or labored and the heart rate is over 100 per minute, oxygen by mask or positive pressure by resuscitator (Ambu) bag may be used. If the heart rate is under 100, intubation and positive pressure ventilation is indicated.

## ETIOLOGIC CLASSIFICATION OF RESPIRATORY DISTRESS

I. Chemical factors
  A. Hypoxia
    1. Respiratory disorders. The chest x-ray is the most important examination in an infant in respiratory distress.
      a. Atelectasis. Some degree of atelectasis exists normally at birth and may persist for days. The atelectasis may be asymptomatic or extensive enough to cause retractions and intermittent cyanosis. Atelectasis or pneumonitis of the right upper lobe may occur with esophageal atresia.

        Cohesiveness of the alveolar walls is an important factor in neonatal atelectasis. The elastic resistance of the lung itself must also be overcome if adequate initial expansion of the lungs is to occur. The newborn infant transiently exerts pressures of 40 to 60 cm. water and occasionally higher in order to expand his lungs. Factors that may limit pulmonary expansion in newborn infants include the poorly developed, weak and yielding thoracic skeleton and musculature and incoordination of the respiratory movements secondary to damage or immaturity of the respiratory centers.

Purves, M.J.: Onset of respiration at birth. *Arch. Dis. Child. 49*:333, 1974.

      b. Respiratory distress syndrome (hyaline membrane disease) is due to surfactant deficiency associated either with (1) immaturity and an inadequate number of type II pneumocytes or surfactant-producing cells or (2) stress, e.g., asphyxia, hypovolemia, acidosis, hypothermia, hypoglycemia, sedation and maternal hemorrhage that impairs the surfactant-producing pneumocytes. A history of fetal distress is common. The Apgar score may be low; however, it may be moderately good.

        Hyaline membrane disease is more common in premature than in full-term infants. The second of a set of twins is more likely than the first to have hyaline membrane disease. The greatest incidence occurs in infants who weigh between 1000 and 2000 gm.

        Clinical features are suggestive but not diagnostic. Expiratory grunting, rapid respiratory rate, flaring of the alae nasi, inspiratory retractions and cyanosis may be noted at delivery or shortly thereafter. The full-blown picture is apparent within 6 to 12 hours after birth. The respiratory rate may be greater than 100 per minute. Edema, especially of the hands and feet, may develop.

Respiratory failure in an infant with hyaline membrane disease is present when more than a 50 to 60 per cent inspired oxygen concentration is required to maintain arterial oxygen tension at 50 mm. Hg. Respiratory acidosis, reflected by an increasing $Pa_{CO_2}$ or apnea, are other indications for mechanical ventilation. If supplemental oxygen is not required for a period exceeding 24 hours, hyaline membrane disease is not present.

A characteristic diffuse reticulogranular appearance with air bronchograms and hypoaeration is noted on the chest roentgenogram. A patent ductus arteriosus may complicate the course of respiratory distress syndrome, producing a need for augmented oxygen therapy and ventilation. Group B beta-hemolytic streptococcus or other bacterial pneumonia may simulate or complicate the respiratory distress syndrome. Differences frequently noted between the two include (1) the diminished lung volume in hyaline membrane disease in contrast to the normal volume with pneumonia and (2) the patchy infiltrates, pleural effusion and fluid in the fissure in pneumonia.

Ablow, R.C. et al.: A comparison of early onset group B streptococcal neonatal infection and the respiratory distress syndrome of the newborn. *N. Engl. J. Med. 294*:65, 1976.

   c. Respiratory distress syndrome type II, or transient tachypnea of the newborn, occurs in both premature and full-term infants. Symptoms begin shortly after birth with respiratory distress manifested chiefly by tachypnea but, at times, also by grunting, flaring of the alae nasi and retractions. The respiratory rate, often 80 to 140 per minute, may remain elevated for 2 to 5 days. The chest film shows slight cardiomegaly, an increased lung volume, hyperinflated peripheral lung fields with accentuated central vascular markings or patchy infiltrates, edematous interlobar septa, an increased anterior-posterior chest diameter and, possibly, a pleural effusion. $P_{CO_2}$ and blood pH are compatible with normal alveolar ventilation. There may be a history of heavy maternal medication, anesthesia or cesarean section.

Avery, M.E., Gatewood, O.B. and Grumley, G.: Transient tachypnea of newborn. *Am. J. Dis. Child. 111*:380, 1966.

   d. The meconium aspiration syndrome, a largely preventable complication, is seen in term or post-term infants who have experienced hypoxia owing to intrauterine distress or placental insufficiency. There is a history of meconium-stained amniotic fluid. Findings are due to plugging of the distal airways by meconium-containing amniotic fluid. Roentgenographic examination of the chest demonstrates an uneven pattern of atelectasis, consolidation and emphysema. The lung fields may appear hyperinflated and the anterior-posterior diameter increased. Interstitial emphysema or pneumomediastinum may also be noted. There is right-to-left shunting and ventilation perfusion is abnormal. The infant is at special risk of developing pneumonia.

Bacsik, R.D.: Meconium aspiration syndrome. *Pediatr. Clin. N. Am. 24*:463, 1977.

e. Pulmonary hemorrhage may lead to dyspnea and hemoptysis. This complication may be associated with erythroblastosis, central nervous system damage, pneumonia, septicemia, hemorrhagic disease of the newborn and other neonatal disorders.

McAdams, A.J.: Pulmonary hemorrhage in the newborn. *Am. J. Dis. Child. 113*:255, 1967.

f. Bronchopulmonary dysplasia, the most common chronic respiratory disease of infants who have been treated with mechanical ventilation and supplemental oxygen for over 150 hours because of respiratory distress, is characterized by cyanosis when the infant cries outside of supplemental oxygen and by fine, diffuse rales.

Edwards, D.K., Dyer, W.M. and Northway, W.H., Jr.: Twelve years' experience with bronchopulmonary dysplasia. *Pediatrics 59*:839, 1977.
Northway, W.H., Jr. and Rosan, R.C.: Radiographic features of oxygen toxicity in the newborn: bronchopulmonary dysplasia. *Radiology 91*:49, 1968.

g. Mikity-Wilson syndrome may develop insidiously in premature infants after the first week of life without a history of severe respiratory distress syndrome of the newborn. Symptoms, which include recurrent episodes of respiratory distress and cyanosis, reach their maximal severity in four to eight weeks and then clear slowly over a period of months. Apnea occurs frequently late in the course of the disease. The chest x-ray is distinctive with diffuse, streaky infiltrates and small cystic areas present initially, followed by basilar hyperaeration with residual stranding in the upper lobes.

Hodgman, J.E., Mikity, V.G., Tatter, D. and Cleland, R.S.: Chronic respiratory distress in the premature infant. Wilson-Mikity syndrome. *Pediatrics 44*:179, 1969.
Mikity, V.G., and Taber, P.: Complications in treatment of respiratory distress syndrome: bronchopulmonary dysplasia, oxygen toxicity, and the Wilson-Mikity syndrome. *Pediatr. Clin. N. Am. 20*:419, 1973.

h. Congenital anomalies
   (1) Hypoplasia of the mandible with glossoptosis (Pierre Robin syndrome). Respiratory distress dates from birth with stridor, cyanosis, retractions and, at times, opisthotonus. Feeding is difficult, and the infant fails to thrive. Cardiorespiratory complications may include cardiomegaly, cor pulmonale and pulmonary edema. The Pierre Robin syndrome is present in some patients with the Stickler syndrome of myopia, cleft palate and spondyloepiphyseal dysplasia. Characteristic x-ray changes may be present in the distal tibial epiphyses.

Schreiner, R.L. et al.: Stickler syndrome in a pedigree of Pierre Robin syndrome. *Am. J. Dis. Child. 126*:86, 1973.

   (2) Macroglossia

(3) Atresia of the posterior nasal choanae. Since infants usually sleep with their mouths closed and breathe through their noses, patent airways are important for normal respiration. Obstruction caused by congenital occlusion of the posterior nares may lead to irritability, intermittent cyanosis and dyspnea, especially during feeding.

(4) Tracheoesophageal fistula with esophageal atresia is characterized by excessive mucus, choking and intermittent cyanosis.

(5) Atresia of bronchus; pulmonary agenesis or hypoplasia; congenital anomalies of larynx

(6) Primary mediastinal cysts and neoplasms; superior mediastinal syndrome

Hope, J.W., Borns, P.F. and Koop, C.E.: Radiologic diagnosis of mediastinal masses in infants and children. *Radiol. Clin. N. Am. 1*:17, 1963.

(7) Congenital pulmonary cyst; cystic adenomatoid hyperplasia

(8) Asphyxiating thoracic dystrophy

(9) Lobar emphysema caused by massive overinflation of a single lobe of the lung. Involvement is limited to the upper or middle lobes. Lobar emphysema is a diagnostic consideration in newborn and young infants who present with tachypnea and dyspnea, often intermittent, without preceding respiratory infection or disease. About one half of the patients have symptoms on the first day or two of life. The dyspnea, which often becomes rapidly worse, may be accompanied by wheezing, coughing and cyanosis. Physical examination may demonstrate hyperresonance and decreased breath sounds over the affected side. Lobar emphysema is confirmed on roentgenographic examination. Bronchoscopy, which may be indicated in older infants to exclude a foreign body or other obstruction within the bronchus, is unnecessary in the newborn infant.

Eigen, H., Lemen, R.J. and Waring, W.W.: Congenital lobar emphysema: long-term evaluation of surgery and conservatively treated children. *Am. Rev. Res. Dis. 113*:823, 1976.
Leape, L.L. and Longino, L.A.: Infantile lobar emphysema. *Pediatrics 34*:246, 1964.

(10) Congenital vascular ring. Episodes of dyspnea and cyanosis may occur. Respiratory symptoms may also be due to compression of bronchi by pulmonary arteries or the left atrium.

Stanger, P., Lucas, R.V., Jr. and Edwards, J.E.: Anatomic factors causing respiratory distress in acyanotic congenital cardiac disease: special reference to bronchial obstruction. *Pediatrics 43*:760, 1969.

(11) Pulmonary sequestration may cause respiratory distress in the newborn infant as well as in the adolescent. The extralobar form of sequestration usually occurs on the left side in association with a diaphragmatic hernia. The intralobar sequestration occurs in the posterior basal segment of a lower lobe, usually the left.

deParedes, C.G. et al.: Pulmonary sequestration in infants and children: a 20-year experience and review of the literature. *J. Pediatr. Surg.* 5:136, 1970.
Pearl, M.: Sequestration of the lung. *Am. J. Dis. Child. 124*:706, 1972.

(12) Diaphragmatic hernia or diaphragmatic eventration caused by hypoplasia, atrophy or paralysis secondary to unilateral phrenic nerve injury must be considered in newborn and young infants with respiratory distress. Most instances of phrenic nerve paralysis are associated with Erb's palsy. A scaphoid abdomen in an infant with respiratory distress should suggest a diaphragmatic hernia. In infants with a hernia on the right, the ipsilateral lung may be hypoplastic. In the presence of a defect in the cervicodorsal spine, a jejunal enteric canal extending into the chest, a neuroenteric cyst or a thoracic kidney is to be considered. Fluoroscopy with barium swallow and an intravenous pyelogram are indicated.

Neuhauser, E.B.D.: Right diaphragmatic hernia with thoracic kidney. *Postgrad. Med.* 48:57, 1970.

(13) Congenital bronchobiliary fistula causes recurrent aspiration pneumonia, atelectasis and bile-stained sputum.

Weitzman, J.J., Cohen, S.R., Woods, L.O., Jr. and Chadwick, D.L.: Congenital bronchobiliary fistula. *J. Pediatr. 73*:329, 1968.

i. Pneumonia. (See also Chapter 59.)
  (1) Group B beta-hemolytic streptococcus pneumonia may be confused with hyaline membrane disease. The presence of pleural effusion in the former and its absence in the latter may be of diagnostic help. There may be a history of premature rupture of the membranes or maternal fever. Symptoms usually begin suddenly a few hours after birth with such signs of respiratory distress as apnea, grunting respiration, retraction, cyanosis and shock. The white blood count is often less than 5000/mm³.

Baker, C.J.: Group B streptococcal infections in neonates. *Pediatrics in Review 1*:5, 1979.

  (2) Pneumonia due to *Chlamydia trachomatis* may begin in the second and third weeks of life with a distinctive pertussis-like cough and respiratory rates above 50 to 60.
  (3) Pneumocystis carinii pneumonia most commonly presents with dyspnea followed by fever and nonproductive cough.
  (4) Rheumatic pneumonia is characterized by extreme tachypnea and marked pulmonary consolidation.

Serlin, S.P., Rimsza, M.E. and Gay, J.H.: Rheumatic pneumonia: the need for a new approach. *Pediatrics 56*:1075, 1975.

j. Acute bronchiolitis in infants may be characterized by severe dyspnea.
k. Pulmonary edema in infants, associated with left ventricular fail-

ure or an obstruction to pulmonary venous flow, is characterized by tachypnea with respiratory rates over 60. Rales may not be evident until considerable fluid is present in the alveoli. Retraction of the head and grunting respirations occur when the edema is marked. Differentiation from dyspnea caused by primary pulmonary disease may be difficult. Rales and rhonchi may be heard in both situations. The chest film may not be differentially helpful.

Pulmonary edema may also occur as a complication of croup and epiglottitis, heroin overdose and head trauma.

Milley, J.R., Nugent, S.K. and Roger, M.C.: Neurogenic pulmonary edema in childhood. *J. Pediatr. 94*:706, 1979.

Travis, K. W., Todres, I.D., and Shannon, D.C.: Pulmonary edema associated with croup and epiglottitis. *Pediatrics 59*:695, 1977.

Pulmonary edema may occur in susceptible children within a day or two after a rapid ascent to a high altitude. Symptoms include pallor, fatigue, cyanosis, dyspnea, cough, hemoptysis, wheezing and chest pain. Physical and roentgenographic findings are characteristic of pulmonary edema.

Frates, R.C., Jr., Harrison, G.M. and Edwards, G.A.: High-altitude pulmonary edema in children. *Am. J. Dis. Child. 131*:687, 1977.

l. Pulmonary fibrosis and chronic obstructive pulmonary disease due to alpha$_1$-antitrypsin deficiency.

m. Acquired atelectasis

n. Pulmonary emphysema

o. Pleural effusion, empyema, hemothorax, chylothorax

p. Pneumomediastinum may complicate pneumonia, measles, pertussis, asthma, acute laryngotracheobronchitis or foreign body aspiration. In the newborn, it may occur spontaneously with the respiratory distress syndrome, especially in infants on mechanical ventilation. Symptoms include dyspnea and, perhaps, cyanosis. Pneumomediastinum is a diagnostic consideration in every newborn infant with otherwise unexplained dyspnea. Pneumomediastinum and pneumothorax may occur with bilateral renal agenesis or other major renal malformations.

q. Pneumothorax. A small pneumothorax in the newborn may be asymptomatic or associated with mild apnea, irritability or restlessness. With larger amounts of pleural air, dyspnea may be extreme and accompanied by marked tachypnea, cyanosis, grunting, restlessness and collapse. Pneumothorax is a diagnostic consideration whenever dyspnea suddenly occurs in a newborn infant with the respiratory distress syndrome (especially when treated with mechanical ventilation), severe renal malformation (including total renal agenesis) and the meconium aspiration syndrome. It should also be considered in an infant with staphylococcal pneumonia or an adolescent with cystic fibrosis. Frequent determination of the vital signs and blood gases help identify the onset of a pneumothorax. The blood pressure, heart rate, respiratory rate and $Po_2$ are usually decreased.

Boat, T.F., Di Sant'Agnese, P.A., Warwick, W.J., and Handwerger, S.A.: Pneumothorax in cystic fibrosis. *JAMA 209:*1498, 1969.
Chernick, V. and Reed, M.H.: Pneumothorax and chylothorax in the neonatal period. *J. Pediatr. 76:*624, 1970.
Ogata, E.S. et al.: Pneumothorax in the respiratory distress syndrome: incidence and effect on vital signs, blood gases, and pH. *Pediatrics 58:*177, 1976.
Stern, L., Fletcher, B.D. and Dunbar, J.S.: Pneumothorax and pneumomediastinum associated with renal malformations in newborn infants. *Am. J. Roentgenol. Rad. Ther. Nucl. Med. 66:*785, 1972.

r. Acquired pneumatoceles, usually asymptomatic, may occur during the course of pneumonia, especially that caused by the staphylococcus, streptococcus and Klebsiella organisms. Sudden enlargement of a pneumatocele may cause acute respiratory distress. Most lesions regress spontaneously over a period of weeks. Interstitial pulmonary emphysema occurs in some infants with respiratory distress syndrome, especially those treated with mechanical respirators. Chest roentgenograms demonstrate large cysts surrounded either by normal pulmonary parenchyma or by diffuse multicystic involvement of all lobes.

Stocker, J.T. and Madewell, J.E.: Persistent interstitial pulmonary emphysema: another complication of the respiratory distress syndrome. *Pediatrics 59:*847, 1977.

s. Pulmonary lymphangiectasia is a congenital abnormality often symptomatic at birth with respiratory distress and cyanosis. In one form, complex cardiac disease and obstructed pulmonary venous return are associated anomalies. Some children with noncardiac-associated pulmonary lymphangiectasia may appear normal and have an unremarkable chest roentgenogram before the delayed onset of the disorder. The x-ray may resemble stage III bronchopulmonary dysplasia.

Felman, A.H., Rhatigan, R.M. and Pierson, K.K.: Pulmonary lymphangiectasia. *Am. J. Roentgenol Rad.·Ther. Nucl. Med. 66:*548, 1972.

t. Asthma
   (1) Infectious asthma occurs in infants and children up to the age of five to eight years. An asthma attack follows respiratory infections, but the child is asymptomatic between infections.
   (2) Atopic asthma may also be triggered by infection.
u. Obstruction to airways. (See Chapter 58.)
v. Smoke inhalation. Respiratory complications may be delayed up to 24 hours in patients subjected to smoke inhalation. Serious respiratory damage may occur in the absence of facial burns. Symptoms include tachypnea, stridor, hoarseness, retractions and cough. Auscultation reveals decreased breath sounds, wheezes and rales.

Mellins, R.B. and Park, S.: Respiratory complications of smoke inhalation in victims of fires. *J. Pediatr. 87:*1, 1975.

w. Idiopathic pulmonary hemosiderosis. Patients with this disorder may have episodes of coughing, occasionally with blood-tinged sputum, slight exertional dyspnea, pallor, failure to gain weight

and easy fatigability. Acute episodes are characterized by dyspnea, tachycardia, cough, hemoptysis, hematemesis, pallor and
fever. Bilateral perihilar, patchy infiltration is noted on the chest
roentgenogram. Sputum or gastric washings may contain
hemosiderin-laden macrophages, a diagnostic finding in the absence of other causes of pulmonary passive congestion.

   x. The "chest syndrome," a common complication of sickle cell
anemia, may be caused either by multiple microinfarcts or pulmonary infection from Diplococcus pneumoniae. These two etiologies cannot be differentiated clinically. Symptoms include acute
fever, pain on respiration and dyspnea. Leukocytosis is present.

Barrett-Connor, E.: Pneumonia and pulmonary infarction in sickle cell anemia. *JAMA*
*224*:997, 1973.
Powars, D.R.: Natural history of sickle cell disease — the first ten years. *Semin. Hematol.*
*12*:267, 1975.

   y. Desquamative interstitial pneumonia in which there is a proliferation and desquamation of alveolar pneumocytes is manifested by
gradually progressive dyspnea, nonproductive cough, anorexia,
weight loss and easy fatigability. The physical examination is not
striking except for an increased respiratory rate. Chest roentgenographic changes are not specific. Lung biopsy may be necessary.

Howatt, W.F. et al.: Desquamative interstitial pneumonia. *Am. J. Dis. Child. 126*:346,
1973.

   z. Pulmonary alveolar proteinosis occurs generally in infants under
one year of age. Initially, the symptoms may be gastrointestinal
with diarrhea and vomiting; however, respiratory symptoms soon
develop with dyspnea, cyanosis, cough and clubbing.

Colon, A.R. et al.: Childhood pulmonary alveolar proteinosis (PAP). *Am. J. Dis. Child.
121*:481, 1971.

2. Circulatory disturbances
   a. Congenital heart disease. Depending upon the degree of hypoxemia associated with the cardiac lesion, dyspnea on exertion may
range from mild to severe. Infants with congenital heart disease
of the cyanotic type, especially those in whom pulmonary stenosis is extreme, may experience attacks of paroxysmal dyspnea
owing to an increase in right-to-left shunting or an increased peripheral demand for oxygen. During these episodes, the cyanosis
becomes much more intense. The infant gasps for breath and may
become unconscious for a time. Though the attacks may occur
spontaneously, they are often precipitated by feeding, bathing,
crying or defecation. When dyspnea occurs with the minimal exertion of nursing, adequate nutrition may be difficult to maintain.
Anomalous origin of the left coronary artery, among other cardiac
lesions of the noncyanotic type in infants, may be characterized
by dyspnea, at times paroxysmal. Children who have an isolated
pulmonary stenosis with an intact interventricular septum may
have dyspnea on exertion.

b. Congestive cardiac failure. Dyspnea, especially during nursing, and tachypnea, with respiratory rates of 50 to 100 during sleep, are usually the first clinical manifestations of cardiac failure in infants. These episodes of respiratory distress may last several hours, often occur with only mild cyanosis and may be misdiagnosed as pneumonia, asthma or bronchiolitis.

Goldring, D., Hernandez, A. and Hartmann, A.F., Jr.: The critically ill child: care of the infant in cardiac failure. *Pediatrics* 47:1056, 1971.
Rudolph, A.M.: Diagnosis and treatment: respiratory distress and cardiac disease in infancy. *Pediatrics* 35:999, 1965.

c. Chronic constrictive pericarditis
d Paroxysmal tachycardia
e. Myocarditis. Dyspnea may be a prominent clinical feature in infants and children with acute interstitial myocarditis. Tachycardia, a change in the quality of the heart sounds, and enlargement of the liver may point to this disease. Because of the severe dyspnea, the diagnosis of myocarditis is sometimes overlooked and the child is thought to have pneumonia.
f. Endocardial fibroelastosis. Onset of symptoms is usually in the first six months of life with dyspnea, irritability, cough, anorexia and failure to thrive. Respiratory distress, cyanosis, tachycardia and vomiting may appear abruptly, followed by a fulminant course. On the other hand, the symptoms may occur intermittently. Abdominal pain may appear to be present during these episodes.
g. Anemia. Dyspnea on exertion may occur in patients who are severely anemic. Shortness of breath may appear during a hemolytic crisis.
h. Polycythemia and hyperviscosity syndromes in the newborn may cause respiratory distress.
i. Pulmonary embolism
j. Fat embolism may cause acute dyspnea, tachypnea and cyanosis.

Shulman, S.T. and Grossman, B.J.: Fat embolism in childhood. *Am. J. Dis. Child.* 120:480, 1970.

k. Dyspnea may also occur in patients in shock and in those with acute adrenal insufficiency.
1. Primary pulmonary hypertension may be characterized by dyspnea, especially on exertion, easy fatigability and, at times, cyanosis and episodes of syncope. Diagnosis is made by cardiac catheterization. Primary pulmonary hypertension may occur in children who live at high altitude.

Khoury, G.H. and Hawes, C.R.: Primary pulmonary hypertension in children living at high altitude. *J. Pediatr.* 62:177, 1963.

m. Congenital pulmonary arteriovenous aneurysm may be characterized by dyspnea, usually on exertion, as well as by cyanosis, polycythemia and clubbing of the fingers. Symptoms may begin in childhood.

n. The cardiorespiratory syndrome of obesity is characterized by extreme obesity, polycythemia, periodic respiration, intermittent cyanosis, somnolence, right ventricular hypertrophy and cardiac decompensation.

Finklestein, J.W. and Avery, M.E.: The Pickwickian syndrome. *Am. J. Dis. Child.* *106*:251, 1963.

### 3. Hypersensitivity lung disease

McCombs, R.P.: Diseases due to immunologic reactions in the lungs. *N. Engl. J. Med.* *286*:1186, 1245, 1972.

a. Asthma
   (1) Infectious asthma
   (2) Atopic (extrinsic) asthma
   (3) Loeffler's syndrome is characterized by recurrent respiratory illness with wheezing, pulmonary infiltrates and marked eosinophilia. Allergens include Aspergillus, Candida albicans and ascariasis.
b. Extrinsic allergic alveolitis
   (1) Lycoperdonosis due to inhalation of large quantities of spores from the puffball mushroom.

Strand, R.D., Neuhauser, E.B.D. and Sornberger, C.F.: Lycoperdonosis. *N. Engl. J. Med.* *277*:88, 1976.

   (2) Pigeon breeder's lung caused by hypersensitivity to pigeon dust is characterized by severe interstitial pneumonia with progressive dyspnea, fever, chest pain, chronic cough, cyanosis and weight loss.

Chandra, S. and Jones, H.E.: Pigeon fancier's lung in children. *Arch. Dis. Child.* *47*:716, 1972.

c. Pulmonary vasculitis may occur with periarteritis nodosa, lupus erythematosus and Goodpasture's syndrome.

O'Connell, E.J. et al.: Pulmonary hemorrhage-glomerulonephritis syndrome. *Am. J. Dis. Child.* *108*:302, 1964.

d. Sensitivity to ingestants
   (1) Nitrofurantoin sensitivity may cause a diffuse chronic interstitial pneumonia.

David, R.B., Andersen, H.A. and Stickler, G.B.: Nitrofurantoin sensitivity. *Am. J. Dis. Child.* *116*:418, 1968.

   (2) Hypersensitivity to cow milk (Heiner's syndrome) may cause recurrent pulmonary infiltrates, chronic cough, wheezing, pulmonary hemosiderosis, eosinophilia and iron-deficiency anemia.

Boat, T.F.: Hyperreactivity to cow milk in young children with pulmonary hemosiderosis and cor pulmonale secondary to nasopharyngeal obstruction. *J. Pediatr.* *87*:23, 1975.
Lee, S.K., Kniker, W.T., Cook, C.D. and Heiner, D.C.: Cow's milk-induced pulmonary disease in children. *Adv. Pediatr.* *25*:39, 1978.

4. Impairment of respiratory musculature
   a. Neurologic
   (1) Unilateral congenital diaphragmatic paralysis following injury to the phrenic nerve
   (2) Respiratory irregularity due to depression, immaturity or injury of respiratory centers
   (3) Poliomyelitis or the Guillain-Barré syndrome. Early diagnosis of intercostal and/or diaphragmatic paralysis is important if mechanical ventilation is to be used promptly and fatigue and hypoxia prevented. Early findings in patients with respiratory paralysis include irregular, shallow respiration; perhaps an increase in the respiratory rate; use of the accessory muscles of respiration; dilatation of the alae nasi; slight grunting; unwillingness to talk, interrupted or monosyllabic speech; restlessness; anxiety; fear of falling asleep; mental confusion and disorientation. Decreased vital capacity may be demonstrated by asking the patient to count rapidly to ten. Patients with respiratory difficulty cannot do this. A vital capacity of less than 12 ml./kg. and a $PaO_2$ of less than 70 mm. Hg in air are physiologic criteria for respiratory failure. Cyanosis is a late symptom, as is the forced use of the accessory muscles of respiration with gasping for each breath. With involvement of the deltoid muscles, the diaphragm may also be paralyzed, either unilaterally or bilaterally. Fluoroscopy may be helpful in determining the extent of this paralysis. The diaphragm on the involved side is elevated and demonstrates paradoxical movement, moving upward during inspiration. A shift of the mediastinum may occur toward the opposite side. In patients with intercostal muscle weakness, splinting of the abdomen by the examiner will accentuate the use of accessory respiratory musculature; conversely, splinting of the chest wall in patients with diaphragmatic involvement leads to overt dyspnea.
   (4) Myasthenia gravis
   (5) Diphtheritic neuritis
   (6) Werdnig-Hoffmann disease
   (7) Acute parathion poisoning is manifested by the rapid onset of respiratory distress owing to muscle paralysis or impairment of the central respiratory center. Clinical features include excessive salivation, constricted pupils, muscle tremors and weakness, cough, wheezing, dyspnea and pulmonary edema.

Eitzman, D.V. and Wolfson, S.L.: Acute parathion poisoning in children. *Am. J. Dis. Child. 114*:397, 1967.
Sim, V.M.: Diagnosis and therapy for anticholinesterase poisoning. *JAMA 192*:143, 1965.

   (8) Bulbar paralysis. The pooling of saliva in the pharynx leads to respiratory difficulty.

    b. Mechanical
       (1) Because of poorly developed and yielding thoracic skeleton and musculature in premature and some term infants, contraction of the diaphragm may be accompanied by retraction of the thoracic wall instead of a simultaneous elevation of the ribs and expansion of the chest.
       (2) In patients with emphysema and in certain other dyspneic states, expiration becomes an active instead of a primarily passive process. Contraction of the abdominal muscles helps push up the diaphragm, and contraction of the internal intercostal muscles facilitates depression of the ribs. Instead of remaining negative throughout the entire respiratory cycle, the intrapleural pressure at the end of forced expiration may become positive. This may impair venous return. On the other hand, in patients whose dyspnea is associated with asthma or other disease in which the air passages are constricted, the negative intrapleural pressure may actually be increased, owing, perhaps, to failure of the lungs to expand during inspiration as rapidly as the thoracic cage.
       (3) Chylothorax is the most common form of pleural effusion in the newborn. Thoracentesis reveals serous pleural fluid if milk feedings have not been begun and chylous fluid after initiation of feedings.
       (4) Pleural effusion
       (5) Diaphragmatic hernia or eventration of the diaphragm in infants may lead to tachypnea, dyspnea and cyanosis.
       (6) Ascites
       (7) Abdominal distention in infants may cause dyspnea, rapid respiration and cyanosis. The respiratory distress becomes especially noticeable in the presence of pneumonia or patchy atelectasis.
       (8) Large abdominal tumor masses
       (9) Peritonitis. Respiratory movements in these patients are chiefly thoracic. Grunting may occur because of the pain associated with abdominal respiration.
       (10) Dermatomyositis
    c. Chemical. Paralysis of the respiratory musculature may occur in patients with hypopotassemia.
B. Hypercapnia causes an increase in depth and, to a less extent, in the rate of respiration. Carbon dioxide in itself is excitatory to the chemoreceptors. The concomitant acidosis that it effects is an additive stimulus. Carbon dioxide is not a respiratory stimulus at all concentrations since in excessive amounts it causes depression of the respiratory center, especially when hypoxia, anesthesia or narcosis is also present.
    1. Poliomyelitis. In the presence of medullary involvement from poliomyelitis, the respiratory centers may demonstrate decreased sensitivity to carbon dioxide. Since pulmonary ventilation may also be diminished, elevation of carbon dioxide tension may occur. Symptoms of

carbon dioxide intoxication include confusion, stupor, hypertension and, perhaps, shock. This has been termed the hypoventilation syndrome. The abrupt administration of oxygen to such patients may cause cessation of respiration.

2. Asphyxia
3. Emphysema. These patients may have chronic carbon dioxide retention.
4. Asthma
5. Any airway obstruction
6. Pneumonia. Some retention of carbon dioxide may occur in patients with extensive pneumonia.
7. Cystic fibrosis in which there is extensive pulmonary involvement may be accompanied by carbon dioxide retention.

Wood, R.E., Boat, T.F. and Doershuk, C.F.: Cystic fibrosis. *Am. Rev. Res. Dis.* *113*:833, 1976.

C. Acidosis and other metabolic factors. Chemoreceptors in the medullary respiratory center respond to acidosis or lowering of the blood pH with an increase in the depth and, to a lesser extent, in the rate of respiration. Alkalosis has the opposite effect. Severe acidosis, however, has a depressing rather than an excitatory effect on respiration and may cause respiratory failure.

1. Carbon dioxide inhalation or retention may also cause respiratory acidosis.
2. Silo filler's disease owing to inhalation of nitrogen dioxide in fumes from freshly filled silos may cause only an episode of bronchitis or moderately severe dyspnea, cough and chest pain. A relapse may occur in about ten days and may lead to death from pulmonary edema and bronchiolitis obliterans.

Olson, E.T.: Occurrence of silo fillers' disease in children. *J. Pediatr. 64*:724, 1964.

3. Anoxia or severe hypoxia is associated with metabolic acidosis.
4. Nephritis. Dyspnea in patients with nephritis and renal insufficiency is more likely due to myocarditis and cardiac failure than to acidosis.
5. Diabetic acidosis
6. Acute acetylsalicylic acid intoxication. Hyperpnea, or deep and rapid respirations, occurs three to eight hours after ingestion of salicylates in toxic amounts. Salicylate poisoning should be suspected in a child who presents with hyperventilation, even in the absence of a history of salicylate ingestion. The ferric chloride urine test may be useful. A burgundy-red color persists after boiling in the presence of salicylate, but not in the case of acetoacetic acid.
7. Acidosis associated with inborn errors of metabolism. (e.g., glycogenosis, congenital lactic acidosis, fructose-1,6 diphosphatase deficiency, organic acidemias and disorders in the urea cycle).
8. Hypothermia or hyperthermia increases oxygen needs tremendously, the former especially so in the newborn infant.
9. Exercise
10. Hypoglycemia may cause apnea.

11. Anemia

12. Hypovolemia and shock

13. Hyperviscosity syndrome in newborns may cause tachypnea.

II. Reflex factors due to increased sensitivity of the Hering-Breuer reflex. At the end of a normal inspiratory excursion, the Hering-Breuer reflex serves to inhibit further distention of the lungs. Receptors in the alveolar ducts are activated by stretching and inflation. Impulses are sent through the vagus to the expiratory center, which in turn interrupts efferent discharges from the inspiratory center. The sensitivity of this reflex mechanism, important in regulating the depth of inspiration, is exaggerated by any factor that decreases pulmonary distensibility or places part of the lung on a stretch. These factors include pulmonary engorgement, inflammation, fibrosis and edema.

   A. Emphysema. Chronic obstructive pulmonary disease due to a deficiency of alpha$_1$-antitrypsin may cause progressive dyspnea. Emphysema may occur in Marfan's syndrome.

Bolande, R.P. and Tucker, A.S.: Pulmonary emphysema and other cardiorespiratory lesions as part of the Marfan abiotrophy. *Pediatrics 33*:356, 1964.

Talamo, R.C. et al.: Symptomatic pulmonary emphysema in childhood associated with hereditary alpha-1-antitrypsin and elastase inhibitor deficiency. *J. Pediatr. 79*:20, 1971.

   B. Cardiac dyspnea. Pulmonary engorgement is a primary cause of the respiratory distress in these patients.

   C. Atelectasis

   D. Asthma. Vagal stimulation may occur as a result of the alveolar pressure changes associated with the exchange of air through narrowed orifices. The decrease in pulmonary elasticity may increase the sensitivity of the Hering-Breuer reflex.

   E. Tracheal obstruction. Vagal stimulation may result from the exchange of air through a narrowed orifice.

   F. Pneumonia

   G. Pneumothorax

III. Cerebral and other central factors. The lesions listed here may involve the respiratory centers directly or indirectly through their proximity. The centers may also be affected indirectly as a result of an increase in the intracranial pressure or by interference with medullary circulation.

   A. Immaturity of the respiratory center.

   B. Depression of respiratory centers due to intrauterine hypoxia, anesthesia, barbiturates, morphine, carbon dioxide intoxication and anoxia

   C. Seizures may interfere with respiration in newborn infants.

   D. Cerebral neoplasm

   E. Cerebral hemorrhage

   F. Cerebral edema

   G. Encephalitis, meningitis

   H. Poliomyelitis

   I. Hyperventilation syndrome is to be considered in children, especially girls, who complain of shortness of breath, "smothering" spells, inability to breathe, dizziness, blackout episodes or fainting. The complaint of rapid breathing is virtually never volunteered. The hyperventilation episode may be accompanied by tetany or syncope. Some children experience numerous episodes of hyperventilation syndrome owing to anxiety.

Enzer, N.B. and Walker, P.A.: Hyperventilation syndrome in childhood. A review of 44 cases. *J. Pediatr. 70*:521, 1967.

Missri, J.C. and Alexander, S.: Hyperventilation syndrome. *JAMA 240*:2093, 1978.

# APNEA

I. Newborn
   A. Prolonged apnea is defined as cessation of respiration for 20 or more seconds or for briefer time periods if accompanied by bradycardia, cyanosis or pallor. The differential diagnosis includes immaturity, seizure disorder, hypothermia, hyperthermia, intracranial hemorrhage and hypoxic brain damage. Severe infections including pneumonia, meningitis and sepsis are important considerations when apnea occurs within the first 24 hours of life. Group B streptococcus sepsis frequently causes severe apnea on the first day of life. Apnea is also associated with severe respiratory distress syndrome and with pulmonary hemorrhage. Significant anemia, patent ductus arteriosus, hypotension, gastroesophageal reflux, acidosis, hypoglycemia, hypocalcemia, hypomagnesemia, hypernatremia and hyponatremia, upper airway obstruction, hyperviscosity, pneumothorax, necrotizing enterocolitis, impaired regulating of breathing, posterior pharyngeal reflexes with suction catheters or nipple may also produce apnea. Apnea occurs in about 80 per cent of infants with a birth weight of less than 1000 gm. and in about 25 per cent of those who weigh less than 2500 gm.

Kattwinkel, J.: Neonatal apnea: pathogenesis and therapy. *J. Pediatr. 90*:342, 1977.

   B. Periodic breathing, characterized by apneic spells of five to ten seconds, occurs frequently in premature and some term infants. The cause is unknown.

Rigatto, H. and Brady, J.P.: Periodic breathing and apnea in preterm infants. I and II. *Pediatrics 50*:202, 219, 1972.

   C. Ondine's curse or apnea due to failure of automatic control of ventilation during sleep.

Haddad, G.G. et al.: Congenital failure of automatic control of ventilation, gastrointestinal motility and heart rate. *Medicine 57*:517, 1978.

II. Older infants
   A. "Sudden infant death syndrome" is the leading cause of death in infants after the first week of life. Death occurs most frequently between the second and fourth months of life with 90 per cent of instances by 6 months of age. Death usually occurs while the infant is asleep. Fewer instances are reported in the summer. There is an increased incidence in males, low-birth-weight infants and lower socioeconomic groups.
   B. "Near-miss" sudden infant death. Apneic spells lasting over 20 seconds may occur in otherwise normal older infants, probably due to decreased chemoresponsiveness to carbon dioxide. The frequency of such apneic spells is greatest during episodes of nasopharyngitis.

Steinschneider, A.: Nasopharyngitis and prolonged sleep apnea. *Pediatrics 56*:967, 1975.

III. Children
  A. Sleep apnea
    1. Extreme obesity may be associated with airway obstruction during sleep. The sleep deprivation caused by repeated apnea and recurrent awakening leads to excessive somnolence.

Simpser, M.D. et al.: Sleep apnea in a child with the Pickwickian syndrome. *Pediatrics* *60*:290, 1977.

    2. Sleep apnea may result from functional upper airway obstruction induced by sleep. Symptoms include loud nocturnal snoring and periodic apnea. Because of the interruptions of sleep, the child is excessively sleepy during the day.

Guilleminault, C., Eldridge, F.L., Simmons, F.B. and Dement, W.C.: Sleep apnea in eight children. *Pediatrics 58*:23, 1976.

    3. Chronic upper airway obstruction owing to enlarged tonsils and adenoids or to the glossoptosis in the Pierre Robin syndrome is characterized by stertorous respiration while sleeping, marked periodic breathing, lethargy and, eventually, pulmonary hypertension and congestive heart failure.

Bland, J.W., Jr., Edwards, F.K. and Brinsfield, D.: Pulmonary hypertension and congestive heart failure in children with chronic upper airway obstruction. *Am. J. Cardiol.* *23*:830, 1969.
Shannon, D.C., Kelly, D.H. and O'Connell, K.: Abnormal regulation of ventilation in sudden-infant-death syndrome. *N. Engl. J. Med. 297*:747, 1977.

## GENERAL REFERENCES

Avery, M.E. and Fletcher, B.D.: *The Lung and Its Disorders in the Newborn Infant.* Philadelphia, 3rd ed. W. B. Saunders Co., 1974.
Kendig, E. L., Jr. and Chernick, V. (eds.): *Disorders of the Respiratory Tract in Children.* 3rd ed. Philadelphia, W.B. Saunders Co., 1977.

---

# ETIOLOGIC CLASSIFICATION OF RESPIRATORY DISTRESS

I. Chemical factors, 473
  A. Hypoxia, 473
    1. Respiratory disorders
    2. Circulatory disturbances
    3. Hypersensitivity lung disease
    4. Impairment of respiratory musculature
  B. Hypercapnia, 484
    1. Poliomyelitis
    2. Asphyxia
    3. Emphysema
    4. Asthma
    5. Airway obstruction
    6. Pneumonia
    7. Cystic fibrosis
  C. Acidosis and other metabolic factors, 485

    1. Carbon dioxide inhalation or retention
    2. Silo filler's disease
    3. Metabolic acidosis
    4. Nephritis
    5. Diabetic acidosis
    6. Acute acetylsalicylic acid intoxication
    7. Inborn errors of metabolism
    8. Hypothermia or hyperthermia
    9. Exercise
    10. Hypoglycemia
    11. Anemia
    12. Hypovolemia and shock
    13. Hyperviscosity syndrome
II. Reflex factors, 486
  A. Emphysema, 486

CHAPTER 58

# STRIDOR, NOISY BREATHING, SNORING, WHEEZING

## CLINICAL CONSIDERATIONS

Stridor is a harsh, vibratory, high-pitched, sometimes shrill, crowing noise, usually most distinct during inspiration. Children reported to have stridor or other evidence of respiratory obstruction and distress should be seen promptly.

Clinical manifestations of respiratory obstruction include hoarseness, dyspnea, inspiratory retractions, brassy cough, tachycardia, apprehensiveness, increased respiratory rate and use of the accessory muscles of respiration. Restlessness is an early indication of hypoxia and occurs before overt cyanosis. Increasing restlessness in an infant or child with respiratory obstruction may indicate the need for a tracheostomy or intubation. Since it may mask the manifestations of hypoxia and inhibit needed accessory respiratory efforts, sedative medication should not be given to children in respiratory distress. Once an adequate airway has been established, restlessness is followed almost dramatically by sleep.

That the incidence of respiratory obstruction is relatively greater in infants than in older children may, in part, be ascribed to three anatomic features: the small size of the infant larynx, the presence of loose submucous connective tissue in the supraglottic and subglottic regions and the rigid encirclement of the subglottic area by the cricoid cartilage.

The triangular glottic opening of the infant larynx is approximately 7 mm. in length and 4 mm. in width at the base. Though in infants edema produces a reduction in the size of this opening and signs of respiratory obstruction, a similar degree of edema in the adult would result only in hoarseness. The laryngeal mucosa is loosely fixed to the epiglottis anteriorly and along the aryepiglottic folds laterally. Edema in the supraglottic spaces secondary to inflammation causes downward pressure on the epiglottis and laryngeal obstruction. A similar process may occur in the narrow subglottic area with swelling of the submucosal tissue and acute respiratory obstruction. Since this space is completely encircled by the cricoid cartilage, swelling due to edema impinges upon the airway.

## ETIOLOGIC CLASSIFICATION OF STRIDOR

I. Intrinsic obstruction of airways
   A. Congenital anomalies
      1. Inspiratory laryngeal collapse (congenital laryngeal stridor, laryngomalacia) generally becomes apparent in the first weeks of life and is again asymptomatic by the end of the first year. Caused by flaccidity of the epiglottis, aryepiglottic folds and arytenoids, this disorder is characterized by retractions and stridor that are usually inspiratory but occasionally also expiratory. Stridor may appear only with excitement or crying and often diminishes or disappears in the prone position. Without laryngoscopy, this process cannot be differentiated from other, more serious causes of stridor.
      2. Congenital laryngeal web. A mucous membrane web across the anterior half to two-thirds of the vocal cords or around the glottis may produce signs of respiratory obstruction and absence of a cry.
      3. Laryngeal cyst. Enlargement of a laryngeal cyst may produce progressive respiratory obstruction.
         a. Cysts of laryngeal ventricle
         b. Cysts of aryepiglottic fold
      4. Subglottic stenosis
      5. Tracheal stenosis
      6. Absence of or defect in tracheal cartilaginous rings
      7. Calcification of laryngeal and tracheal cartilage may cause congenital stridor.

Ferguson, C.F: Congenital abnormalities of the infant larynx. *Otolaryngol. Clin. N. Am.* *3*:185, 1970.

   B. Laryngeal paralysis
      1. Bilateral laryngeal paralysis in the newborn may go unsuspected because of a normal, though weak, cry. With unilateral paralysis, the cry is usually weak or absent. Inspiratory stridor, dyspnea and intercostal retractions are common.
      2. Congenital cardiovascular anomalies may produce unilateral recurrent nerve paralysis, usually on the left, with minimal laryngeal obstruction. Hoarseness and slight stridor may occur.
      3. Birth trauma
      4. Bilateral abductor vocal cord paralysis with severe stridor may occur suddenly in infants with increased intracranial pressure associated with Arnold-Chiari malformation and hydrocephalus. Since the paralyzed cords are flaccid, the cry is normal.

Holinger, P.C., Holinger, L.D., Reichert, T.J. and Holinger, P.H.: Respiratory obstruction and apnea in infants with bilateral abductor vocal cord paralysis, meningomyelocele, hydrocephalus, and Arnold-Chiari malformation. *J. Pediatr. 92*:368, 1978.

C. Tumors
1. Laryngeal papilloma, the most common benign laryngeal neoplasm, may cause croupy cough, hoarseness or aphonia. The occurrence of stridor and retractions depends upon the degree of laryngeal obstruction. Although symptoms may appear in young infants, they are most common between the ages of two and four years.
2. Fibrolipoma
3. Hemangioma of the trachea is a common cause of subglottic obstruction. Since the lesion may be covered by mucosa, it may be difficult to see by direct visualization.

Hudson, H.L. and McAlister, W.H.: Obstructing tracheal hemangioma in infancy. *Am. J. Roentgenol. Rad. Ther. Nucl. Med. 93*:428, 1965.

D. Trauma
1. Repeated and inexpert tracheal aspiration may cause laryngeal edema.
2. Dislocation of the cricothyroid or cricoarytenoid articulations as a result of obstetric injury may cause partial inspiratory obstruction.
3. Intubation
E. Infections
1. Laryngitis, laryngotracheobronchitis, infectious croup. Most cases of laryngotracheobronchitis are of viral etiology with parainfluenza virus type 1 the most common cause. Other etiologic viral agents include parainfluenza 2 and 3, influenza A and B, respiratory syncytial virus and adenoviruses. Hemophilus influenzae type B is a common etiologic agent, especially likely to produce epiglottitis.

Glezen, W.P. et al.: Epidemiologic patterns of acute lower respiratory disease of children in a pediatric group practice. *J. Pediatr. 78*:397, 1971.

Infectious croup is an important problem in infants and, to some extent, in young children. This respiratory infection constitutes, in many cases, a threat to life. The process may extend abruptly from mild to severe involvement. Management of these patients requires continued, close observation.
2. Epiglottitis. Epiglottitis is a medical emergency. The disease may progress extremely rapidly. The onset is abrupt with severe sore throat, dysphagia, drooling, hoarseness, stridor, dyspnea and muffled voice. Appearing very ill and anxious, the patient sits up with his mouth open, tongue protruded, head forward and neck slightly flexed. The inflamed and edematous epiglottis may appear like a bright red cherry sitting at the base of the tongue. Vigorous attempts to see the epiglottis are, however, absolutely contraindicated, since forceful depression of the tongue may cause sudden respiratory arrest. A simple lateral roentgenogram of the neck is diagnostic, but the child's posture of comfort should not be compromised by laying him down or other manipulations during this examination.
F. Acute spasmodic laryngitis usually begins suddenly during the night, awakening the child. The symptoms, which are often alarming to the child and his parents, include hoarseness; a tight, barking, brassy, sepulchral cough;

stridor; and suprasternal and infrasternal retractions. Acute spasmodic laryngitis occurs almost exclusively in the preschool age period and some children tend to have many episodes.

G. Laryngeal edema
   1. Angioneurotic edema
   2. Trauma due to foreign body or laryngeal intubation
   3. Corrosives, such as lye
   4. Nephrosis
   5. Infectious mononucleosis

H. Laryngospasm
   1. Tetany
   2. Acute infantile Gaucher's disease

 I. Foreign bodies. A foreign body in the respiratory tract should always be considered in the differential diagnosis of respiratory obstruction and unexplained chest lesions in infants and children. Symptoms include hoarseness or aphonia; persistent, perhaps barking cough; wheezing; hemoptysis; and, at times, cyanosis. A laryngeal foreign body may cause manifestations that simulate those of laryngitis. There may be a history of choking or gagging at the time of aspiration, but this is often absent or indirect; for example, the mother may find the infant placing safety pins in his mouth or may suddenly miss a small object.

   Usually, a foreign body does not remain lodged in the larynx, but progresses to the trachea or is coughed back into the pharynx. Eggshell is the most common laryngeal foreign body. The signs of tracheal foreign body include stridor, wheezing and retractions. Bronchial foreign bodies may be largely asymptomatic unless obstruction occurs.

J. Rarely, an esophageal foreign body may cause only stridor.

Tauscher, J.W.: Esophageal foreign body: an uncommon cause of stridor. *Pediatrics 61*:657, 1978.

K. Cri du chat syndrome is characterized by an inspiratory stridor and a cat-like cry. Other symptoms and signs include microcephaly, hypertelorism, hypotonia, epicanthal folds and severe mental retardation.

L. Cricoarytenoid arthritis may cause stridor in patients with juvenile rheumatoid arthritis.

Jacobs, J.C. and Hui, R.M.: Cricoarytenoid arthritis and airway obstruction in juvenile rheumatoid arthritis. *Pediatrics 59*:292, 1977.

II. Extrinsic obstruction of airway
  A. Congenital anomalies
    1. Thyroglossal duct cyst. In infants with stridor, the base of the tongue should always be palpated for this lesion, which produces dysphagia and respiratory obstruction by forcing the epiglottis into the laryngeal aperture.
    2. Micrognathia with glossoptosis
    3. Macroglossia
    4. Diaphragmatic hernia
    5. Compression of the trachea by vascular anomalies
      a. Double aortic arch usually produces symptoms in the first six months of life.

    b. Right aortic arch with left ligamentum arteriosum. Symptoms may not appear until the end of the first year or a few months later.

    c. Anomalous innominate artery

    d. Anomalous left common carotid artery

    e. Aberrant subclavian artery

A vascular anomaly is to be considered in infants who present with wheezing; stridor, usually both inspiratory and expiratory; apnea; rattling and gurgling respiratory noises; hyperextension of the head; inspiratory retractions; a history of recurrent pneumonia; and hesitancy in swallowing, especially when offered solid foods. Respiratory symptoms may become worse during feeding, with the appearance of cyanosis.

  B. Infections

    1. Retropharyngeal abscess

    2. Infections of the closed spaces of the neck

  C. Tumors

    1. Thyroid tumors

    2. Cystic hygroma

    3. Mediastinal masses

    4. Lymphomas: lymphosarcoma, leukemia, Hodgkin's disease

  D. Organ enlargement

    1. Mediastinal lymphadenopathy — tuberculosis, sarcoidosis or chronic inflammatory disease

    2. Congenital goiter

III. Slight stridor is not uncommon during periods of crying in many normal babies.

## DIAGNOSTIC STUDIES

**Roentgenographic Studies.** Anteroposterior and lateral soft tissue roentgenograms of the neck and chest may be helpful in patients with respiratory obstruction.

Dunbar, J.S.: Upper respiratory tract obstruction in infants and children. *Am. J. Roentgenol. Rad. Ther. Nucl. Med.* 59:227, 1970.

**Foreign Bodies.** Opaque foreign bodies may easily be visualized. Non-opaque objects may also be detected in left anterior oblique chest films if they create a defect in the column of radiolucent air or if there is evidence of obstructive atelectasis or emphysema. Fluoroscopy and films in both full inspiration and expiration may be helpful.

**Vascular Anomalies.** Plain lateral films of the chest may demonstrate narrowing and forward displacement of the trachea. Fluoroscopy with barium swallow reveals posterior esophageal compression at the level of the third or fourth thoracic vertebra. Arteriography may be diagnostically helpful.

**Laryngoscopy.** Direct visualization of the larynx is indicated if respiratory obstruction cannot otherwise be explained.

## NOISY BREATHING AND SNORING

Snoring or snorting noises occasionally arise from the nasopharynx in young infants, perhaps owing to imperfect functioning of the soft palate. Noisy breathing may also occur in infants with stenosis of the posterior choanae. Children with sleep apnea also snore loudly at night.

Guilleminault, C., Eldridge, F.L., Simmons, F.B. and Dement, W.C.: Sleep apnea in eight children. *Pediatrics 58*:23, 1976.

The stertorous breathing that occurs in some children with cerebral palsy is due to narrowing of the airway secondary to tonic contractions of the muscles at the base of the tongue and in the posterior pharynx.

Stertorous breathing while asleep may be associated with upper airway obstruction caused by enlarged tonsils and adenoids. Over a period of time, such obstruction may lead to alveolar hypoventilation, pulmonary hypertension and congestive heart failure.

Bland, J.W., Edwards, F.K. and Brinsfield, D.: Pulmonary hypertension and congestive heart failure in children with chronic upper airway obstruction. *Am. J. Cardiol. 23*:830, 1969.

## WHEEZING

Wheezing may occur in the following disease states:
1. Asthma
2. Infants with viral pneumonia or acute bronchiolitis may demonstrate wheezing with considerable dyspnea, chiefly expiratory, and perhaps cyanosis. These symptoms are associated with generalized obstructive emphysema.
3. Aspiration pneumonitis
4. Cystic fibrosis
5. Lobar emphysema
6. Extrabronchial pressure caused by enlarged hilar and mediastinal nodes or tumor. Endobronchial tuberculosis may be suggested by persistent coughing or wheezing.
7. Foreign bodies
8. Compression of the trachea by vascular anomalies. An anomalous course of the left pulmonary artery may cause compression of the right main stem bronchus, resulting in respiratory distress in newborn infants. Symptoms include prolongation of expiration, wheezing and suprasternal and subcostal retractions. The right lung is emphysematous. Barium swallow reveals indentation or constriction of the anterior esophagus and right main stem bronchus.
9. Isolated tracheoesophageal fistula may cause wheezing.
10. Wheezing may occur secondary to pulmonary congestion in patients with large left-to-right shunts.
11. Audible wheezing may occur in patients with left heart failure caused by transudate in the bronchioles. The clinical picture may resemble bronchiolitis with obstructive airway disease.
12. Visceral larva migrans may be characterized by recurrent wheezing, dyspnea, pulmonary infiltration, eosinophilia and hepatomegaly.
13. The middle lobe syndrome, characterized clinically by wheezing and cough, occurs most commonly in children with allergic airway disease. Chest x-rays show atelectasis of the right middle lobe. Patients with this

syndrome may experience recurrent episodes of asthma and pneumonia.

Dees, S.C. and Spock, A.: Right middle lobe syndrome in children. *JAMA 197*:8, 1966.

14. Wheezing may be associated with recurrent aspiration secondary to gastroesophageal reflux.

---

## ETIOLOGIC CLASSIFICATION OF STRIDOR

I. Intrinsic obstruction of airways, 490
  A. Congenital anomalies. 490
    1. Inspiratory laryngeal collapse
    2. Congenital laryngeal web
    3. Laryngeal cyst
    4. Subglottic stenosis
    5. Tracheal stenosis
    6. Absence of or defect in tracheal cartilaginous rings
    7. Calcification of laryngeal and tracheal cartilage
  B. Laryngeal paralysis, 490
    1. Bilateral laryngeal paralysis
    2. Congenital cardiovascular anomalies
    3. Birth trauma
    4. Bilateral abductor vocal cord paralysis
  C. Tumors, 491
    1. Laryngeal papilloma
    2. Fibrolipoma
    3. Hemangioma
  D. Trauma, 491
    1. Repeated and inexpert tracheal aspiration
    2. Dislocation of the cricothyroid or cricoarytenoid articulations as a result of obstetric injury
    3. Intubation
  E. Infections, 491
    1. Laryngitis, laryngotracheobronchitis, infectious croup
    2. Epiglottitis
  F. Acute spasmodic laryngitis, 491
  G. Laryngeal edema, 492
    1. Angioneurotic edema
    2. Foreign body or laryngeal intubation
    3. Corrosives
    4. Nephrosis
    5. Infectious mononucleosis
  H. Laryngospasm, 492
    1. Tetany
    2. Acute infantile Gaucher's disease
  I. Foreign bodies, 492
  J. Esophageal foreign body, 492
  K. Cri du chat syndrome, 492
  L. Cricoarytenoid arthritis, 492
II. Extrinsic obstruction of airway, 492
  A. Congenital anomalies, 492
    1. Thyroglossal duct cyst
    2. Micrognathia with glossoptosis
    3. Macroglossia
    4. Diaphragmatic hernia
    5. Compression of trachea by vascular anomalies
  B. Infections, 493
    1. Retropharyngeal abscess
    2. Infections of closed spaces of neck
  C. Tumors, 493
    1. Thyroid tumors
    2. Cystic hygroma
    3. Mediastinal masses
    4. Lymphomas: lymphosarcoma, leukemia, Hodgkin's disease
  D. Organ enlargement, 493
    1. Mediastinal lymphadenopathy
    2. Congenital goiter
III. Periods of crying in normal babies, 493

# CHAPTER 59

# RESPIRATORY INFECTIONS

## CLINICAL CONSIDERATIONS

Respiratory infection is the most frequent kind of childhood illness for which the physician is consulted, accounting for 50 per cent of sick-child visits. Diseases of the respiratory tract produce a number of signs and symptoms, including fever, stridor, tachypnea, dyspnea, cough, failure to thrive and cyanosis. These are discussed individually in other chapters.

Accurate diagnosis and rational therapy of respiratory diseases is based on knowledge of their specific etiology, pathology and symptomatology. In recent years, much progress has been made in the understanding of these factors. At the same time, it is evident that an individual etiologic agent may cause several clinical respiratory illnesses.

Growth and developmental considerations influence the clinical manifestations and complications noted in infants and children. The incidence and severity of certain respiratory diseases are greater in some age periods than in others; such complications of respiratory disease as otitis media and pneumonia are more common in infants and young children than in older age groups; and vomiting and diarrhea are more likely to accompany respiratory infections in infants. In addition, the relatively narrow caliber of the laryngotracheobronchial tree and the absence of an effective cough reflex in infants predispose to airway obstruction.

## ETIOLOGIC CLASSIFICATION OF UPPER RESPIRATORY TRACT INFECTIONS

I. The common cold, or nasopharyngitis, causes symptoms that are well known. With the exception of the first two or three months, infants and young children may have a significant elevation of temperature with the common cold. In infants, the first evidence of a cold may be sudden anorexia; otherwise, clinical manifestations are usually mild in infants but may persist somewhat longer than in older children and adults. Nasal obstruction caused by rhinitis is, of course, annoying, especially since this obstruction may make it difficult for the infant to nurse.

Children experience, on the average, eight colds during the second year of life. The frequency decreases to three or four a year by adolescence. Some children, however, appear to have a cold almost constantly during the winter. Complications of the common cold, especially during infancy and early childhood, include otitis media, cervical adenitis, sinusitis, laryngitis, acute spasmodic laryngitis and pneumonia.

The etiologic agents include rhinoviruses, respiratory syncytial virus, Mycoplasma pneumoniae, coronaviruses, influenza, parainfluenza and some adenoviruses and enteroviruses.

Symptoms simulating those of the common cold may occur in the prodromal phases of measles and pertussis. Epidemic nausea, vomiting and diarrhea may be accompanied by respiratory symptoms and abdominal pain. Frequent or chronic colds may be due to seasonal or perennial allergic rhinitis, repeated exposure to infectious contacts, sinusitis and cystic fibrosis.

II. Chronic sinusitis may be characterized by "frequent colds," cough, nasal obstruction, fatigue and anorexia. Acute sinusitis may be accompanied by high or spiking fever. A nasal discharge is not always observed. In addition to bacterial pathogens (e.g., Group A beta-hemolytic streptococcus, Hemophilus influenzae, staphylococcus and pneumococcus), respiratory viral agents may be etiologic. Ethmoid sinusitis may develop as a serious complication in patients with the common cold or one of the acute exanthematous diseases. The maxillary and the ethmoid sinuses are the ones that become infected during infancy and early childhood. Although the sphenoid sinus is developed at birth, infection usually does not occur during infancy. The frontal sinuses, which arise from an anterior ethmoid cell during the preschool period, may not develop in children who have had repeated episodes of ethmoid sinusitis. Frontal sinusitis, however, usually does not occur until later childhood.

III. Pharyngitis and tonsillitis are prevalent childhood diseases and probably the most common cause of fever in children. Clinical differentiation between bacterial and viral pharyngitis cannot be made on physical examination alone. Tonsillar exudates, which occur in both viral and bacterial pharyngitis, range from pinpoint to pinhead in size and from a thin, translucent membrane, easily missed on superficial examination, to thick, crumpled, opaque patches. A specific diagnosis can be made only by throat culture. Only 5 to 15 per cent of instances of pharyngitis with fever are due to the Group A beta-hemolytic streptococcus, in which event the throat culture will show most of the colonies to be streptococcal. About 50 per cent of patients with pharyngitis and a positive streptococcus culture are likely to be chronic carriers with the symptoms caused by another etiologic agent. With carriers, fewer streptococcal colonies grow out. A streptococcal etiology can be proved by culture within 24 hours using commercially available disposable sheep blood agar plates.

Mortimer, E.A., Jr.: The role of the pediatrician in rheumatic fever control. *Pediatrics* *47*:1, 1971.
Wannamaker, L.W.: Perplexity and precision in the diagnosis of streptococcal pharyngitis. *Am. J. Dis. Child. 124*:352, 1972.

Pharyngitis is not always accompanied by the complaint of a sore throat, especially in preschool children. Instead, the child may refuse to eat. Complications of pharyngitis include otitis media, cervical adenitis, retropharyngeal abscess, peritonsillar abscess, acute glomerulonephritis and rheumatic fever. An undocumented history of frequent sore throats does not permit prognostication as to future experience. Accepted indications for tonsillectomy and/or adenoidectomy include cor pulmonale secondary to chronic, severe upper airway obstruction (tonsillectomy or adenoidectomy); enlargement of the tonsils sufficient to cause difficulty (tonsillectomy); nasal obstruction causing speech distortion and difficulty breathing (adenoidectomy); and chronic or recurrent otitis media.

Paradise, J.L. et al.: History of recurrent sore throat as an indication for tonsillectomy. *N. Engl. J. Med. 298*:409, 1978.
Paradise, J.L: Clinical trials of tonsillectomy and adenoidectomy: limitations of existing studies and a current effort to evaluate efficiency. *South. Med. J. 69*:1049, 1976.
Paradise, J.L. and Bluestone, C.D.: Toward rational indications for tonsil and adenoid surgery. *Hosp. Pract. 11*:79 (Feb.) 1976.

A. Viral
  1. Pharyngitis may be caused by the adenovirus, parainfluenza, influenza, Coxsackie, echovirus and respiratory syncytial viruses. The tonsillitis may be characterized, perhaps not until several hours after the onset of fever, by grayish or yellow-white, pinhead-sized or larger, discrete areas of exudate on the tonsils. Enlargement of the cervical lymph nodes may occur in some cases. Viral pharyngitis usually lasts three or four days.
  2. Herpangina due to Coxsackie and echoviruses is the term applied to papulovesicular pharyngeal lesions that occur in the summer and cause dysphagia and a mildly sore throat. The lesions are few in number and appear chiefly on the anterior tonsillar pillars, occasionally on the tonsils and the soft palate and, more unusually, on the tongue. The individual lesion, which ranges in size from 1 to 4 mm., is surrounded by a zone of intense erythema. Rupture of the vesicles may leave a grayish-yellow ulcer. The pharynx may be diffusely injected. The buccal mucosa and gingivae are not involved.

Cherry, J.D. and Jahn, C.L.: Herpangina: the etiologic spectrum. *Pediatrics 36*:632, 1965.

  3. Infectious mononucleosis caused by the Epstein-Barr virus may be characterized by a diffusely red pharynx, follicular tonsillitis, a pharyngeal membrane or ulcerative pharyngitis. Streptococcal pharyngitis not uncommonly accompanies infectious mononucleosis.

Andiman, W.A.: The Epstein-Barr virus and EB virus infections in childhood. *J. Pediatr. 95*:171, 1979.

  4. Pharyngoconjunctival fever, an epidemic disease caused by type 3 adenovirus, is characterized by low-grade fever, follicular conjunctivitis, sore throat and cervical lymphadenopathy.
B. Bacterial pharyngitis
  1. Group A beta-hemolytic streptococcus pharyngitis may be characterized by exudate on the tonsils and enlarged, tender cervical nodes.

Peter, G. and Smith, A.L.: Group A streptococcal infections of the skin and pharynx. *N. Engl. J. Med. 297*:311, 365, 1977.

  2. Pneumococcus
  3. Staphylococcus
  4. Hemophilus influenzae
  5. Pharyngeal diphtheria may be characterized by one or more dirty gray or yellowish-white, moderately thick, adherent, membranous, tonsillar

patches. The patches may become confluent and spread to the contiguous mucous membrane of the soft palate and pharynx. Removal of the membrane leads to oozing from the underlying mucous membrane.

C. Mycoplasma pneumoniae is an infrequent cause of pharyngitis in early adolescence.

Glezen, W.P. et al.: Group A streptococci, mycoplasmas, and viruses associated with acute pharyngitis. *JAMA 202*:119, 1967.

IV. Nasopharyngeal obstruction and/or hypertrophy of adenoid tissue cause mouth breathing and may, over a period of time, produce bony distortion of the face, maxilla, palate and chest. The child often has a poor appetite, some difficulty in feeding, sleeps poorly and is easily fatigued and irritable. Otitis media may recur.

V. Otitis media in infants and young children occurs frequently as a complication of the common cold. Bacterial otitis media is a frequent finding in the newborn intensive care unit. Etiologic agents in the premature and term newborn infant include Staphylococcus aureus, Escherichia coli, group B streptococcus and Klebsiella pneumonia. In infants and young children, bacterial etiologic organisms include the Group A beta-hemolytic streptococcus, pneumococcus, staphylococcus and Hemophilus influenzae. Other etiologic agents include Mycoplasma pneumoniae, Coxsackie B and respiratory syncytial viruses. The relatively high incidence of otitis media in infants may be explained, in part, by their short, almost horizontal, relatively wide eustachian tubes. This anatomic feature may facilitate progression of infection from the nasopharynx to the middle ear, a process augmented by the proximity of abundant lymphoid tissue to the eustachian orifices in the nasopharynx. Complications of otitis media may include mastoiditis, petrositis, meningitis, arachnoiditis, lateral sinus thrombosis, brain abscess, facial nerve paralysis and impairment of hearing.

Berman, S.A., Balkany, T.J. and Simmons, M.A.: Otitis media in the neonatal intensive care unit. *Pediatrics 62*:198, 1978.

## ETIOLOGIC CLASSIFICATION OF UPPER RESPIRATORY DISEASE

## ETIOLOGIC CLASSIFICATION OF LOWER RESPIRATORY DISEASE

I. Acute laryngotracheobronchitis, or infectious croup, which occurs chiefly in infants and young children, usually has a viral etiology, especially parainfluenza type 1. Other viral agents include parainfluenza type 2 and 3, influenza A and B, respiratory syncytial virus, adenovirus and the same agents that cause nasopharyngitis. (See Chapter 58.)

II. Tracheobronchitis may occur in patients with measles or pertussis and as an extension of upper respiratory tract infections, especially during the first years of life. Rhinoviruses, influenza, parainfluenza virus type 3, Coxsackie viruses, respiratory syncytial virus and adenovirus may be etiologic agents. Persistent bronchitis may be present with chronic sinusitis, respiratory allergy, bronchiectasis, cystic fibrosis and typhoid fever. Asthmatic bronchitis is a form of respiratory disease seen in toddlers and preschool children. Symptoms include cough, wheezing and respiratory distress.

III. Bronchiolitis, a common illness in infants, is characterized by cough and severe expiratory dyspnea owing to bronchiolar obstruction caused by edema and mucus. The respiratory syncytial virus is the most common etiologic agent. Other agents include parainfluenza virus type 3, influenza B and adenovirus. Typable H. influenzae strains may also have an etiologic role.

Glezen, W.P. and Denny, F.W.: Epidemiology of acute lower respiratory disease in children. *N. Engl. J. Med. 288*:498, 1973.

Henderson, F.W. et al.: The etiologic and epidemiologic spectrum of bronchiolitis in pediatric practice. *J. Pediatr. 95*:183, 1979.

Wohl, M.E.B. and Chernick, V.: Bronchiolitis. *Am. Rev. Resp. Dis. 118*:759, 1978.

IV. Pneumonia

Clinical differentiation between viral and bacterial pneumonia is difficult or impossible. In the newborn infant, pneumonia may be part of a transplacental systemic infection caused by rubella, cytomegalovirus, type II herpesvirus, Treponema pallidum, toxoplasmosis, influenza virus and listerosis. Group B beta-hemolytic streptococcus is a major cause of pneumonia in newborn infants. A little later, Staphylococcus aureus, Chlamydia trachomatis and Klebsiella pneumoniae are etiologic. In older children, about 95 per cent of pneumonias have a viral etiology. The alveolar spaces may be principally involved, as in bacterial pneumonia, or the interstitial tissues, as in viral pneumonia.

The onset of bacterial pneumonia is usually more sudden and the child likely to be more toxic and in greater respiratory distress than with viral infections. Bacterial pneumonia may also be accompanied by pleural effusion or empyema. Although slight pleural effusion may be seen with Mycoplasma pneumonia, this finding is not associated with viral pneumonia. Lobar or segmental consolidations are predominantly due to the pneumococcus and less likely to Klebsiella or Group A streptococci. Blood cultures or tracheal aspirates may permit identification of the etiologic bacterial agent. Bone marrow cultures may be performed in patients thought to have histoplasmosis. Lung puncture has been used as a diagnostic measure in children who are seriously ill, not responding to antibiotics or immunodeficient.

Klein, J.O.: Diagnostic lung puncture in the pneumonias of infants and children. *Pediatrics 44*:486, 1969.

Bronchoscopy and culture of aspirated secretions for bacteria and fungi are usually reserved for patients who have chronic pneumonitis or who are not responding to therapy. Bronchial secretions may also be inoculated into guinea pigs if tuberculosis is suspected. Tuberculin, histoplasmin, blastomycin or coccidioidin skin tests may be indicated.

The physical findings on percussion and auscultation may not be abnormal in some infants with pneumonia. In the presence of rapid, shallow breathing, flaring of the alae nasi, decreased pulmonary excursions, a short inspiratory phase and expiratory grunting, pneumonia is a likely diagnosis. The child with pneumonia may attempt to splint his chest, perhaps by lying on the involved side. He is disinclined to talk and may use monosyllabic speech.

Eichenwald, H.F.: Pneumonia syndromes in children. *Hosp. Pract. 11*:89 (Apr.) 1976.

A. Bacterial pneumonia
   1. Pneumococcal is the most frequent type of bacterial pneumonia in infants and children. Children with sickle cell anemia have an increased risk of pneumococcal pneumonia. Pneumococcal pneumonia in children under two years of age may not be evident on the basis of the history and physical examination; therefore, a chest roentgenogram is recommended in a child under two years of age who presents with high fever and who is found to have an elevated white blood count and/or sedimentation rate.

McCarthy, P.L.: Controversies in pediatrics: what tests are indicated for the child under 2 with fever. *Pediatr. Rev. 1*:51, 1979.
Smith, A.L.: The febrile infant. *Pediatr. Rev. 1*:35, 1979.

   2. Staphylococcal pneumonia, which has its greatest incidence in early infancy, may be characterized by a paroxysmal, pertussiform cough and severe dyspnea. Pyopneumothorax may develop suddenly. Multiple pulmonary abscesses and bacteremia may also occur.
   3. Tuberculosis is always a diagnostic consideration in infants and children with pulmonary disease. With periodic tests, a conversion of the tuberculin test indicates a recent exposure to tuberculosis since the tuberculin test becomes positive some three to five weeks after exposure. The reactivity of the tuberculin test may be diminished in the presence of hyperpyrexia and, at times, during measles. It may also be negative in patients with active tuberculosis if tuberculin allergy has not had time to develop or if the child is anergic.
   4. Group A beta-hemolytic streptococcal pneumonia occurs in children above the age of five or six. The onset is abrupt and the symptoms severe. In addition to fever, chills, lethargy, myalgia, dyspnea, cough, chest pain and hemoptysis, cyanosis occurs in more than 50 per cent and empyema in 100 per cent of patients. Streptococcal pharyngitis may occur concomitantly. Fever and chest pain persist for eight to ten days. Group B beta-hemolytic pneumonia is a major etiologic agent in the newborn.

Molten, R.A.: Group A beta-hemolytic streptococcal pneumonia. *Am. J. Dis. Child. 131*: 1366, 1977.

5. Hemophilus influenzae. Meningitis may occur as a complication in infants with this type of pneumonia.
6. Pseudomonas
7. Friedlander's bacillus
8. Klebsiella pneumonia usually occurs in infants, but it may also develop in an older immunodeficient child. Characteristic radiologic findings include bulging of the lung fissures, absence of pleural effusion and presence of lung abscesses or pneumatoceles.
9. Children with cystic fibrosis have frequent episodes of pneumonitis. In the early episodes, the etiologic agent is usually the hemolytic Staphylococcus aureus.
10. Tularemia

B. Viral pneumonia has a varied symptomatology. Cough may be a prominent feature. Dyspnea, cyanosis, inspiratory retractions and expiratory wheezing may be present in infants. The chest x-ray often demonstrates involvement more extensive than that suspected on physical examination, and the involvement tends to be more interstitial than alveolar, as in bacterial and fungal pneumonias. Hyperinflation, not seen with bacterial pneumonias, may be present. Clinical differentiation of viral and Mycoplasma pneumonia may not be possible.

1. Adenovirus, especially types 3, 7 and 21, may cause a severe necrotizing bronchopneumonia with chronic sequelae such as bronchiectasis, bronchiolitis obliterans and lobar emphysema.
2. Parainfluenza virus, types 1, 2 and 3. Type 3 causes viral pneumonia in infants.
3. Respiratory syncytial virus is an etiologic agent in infants under one year of age.
4. Rhinoviruses
5. Influenza A and B usually occur with epidemic incidence.
6. Infectious mononucleosis
7. Measles, chickenpox

Olson, R.W. and Hodges, G.R.: Measles pneumonia. *JAMA 232*:363, 1975.
Young, L.W., Smith, D.I. and Glasgow, L.A.: Pneumonia of atypical measles. *Am. J. Roentgenol. Rad. Ther. Nucl. Med. 60*:439, 1970.

8. Psittacosis, ornithosis
9. Lymphocytic choriomeningitis
10. Giant cell pneumonia (Hecht's disease), a chronic, interstitial pneumonia, may develop in patients with measles or as an isolated disease.
11. Cytomegalovirus infection may be characterized by a chronic interstitial pneumonia. Gastrointestinal symptoms or hepatosplenomegaly may also be present.

C. Mycoplasma pneumoniae is the chief cause of pneumonia in school-age children. Headache is usually severe. Other symptoms include sore throat, anorexia, malaise, fever, chills and a paroxysmal, dry cough. Physical findings are generally minimal. The chest roentgenogram shows bronchopneumonia.

Denny, F.W., Clyde, W.A., Jr. and Glezen, W.P.: Mycoplasma pneumoniae disease: clinical spectrum, pathophysiology, epidemiology and control. *J. Infect. Dis. 123*:74, 1971.

D. Chlamydia trachomatis is a frequent etiologic agent in young infants with pneumonia. Symptoms generally begin in the second or third week, with the principal manifestations being tachypnea and a characteristic pertussis-like staccato cough. Nasal obstruction and discharge may also be present. While paroxysms may end in cyanosis and vomiting, the series of coughs do not occur during a single inspiration. Rather, each is separated by a brief inspiration. Inspiratory crepitant rales are usually present. The patient is afebrile. Hyperexpansion with diffuse interstitial and patchy alveolar infiltrates is noted on the chest x-ray. Serum immunoglobulins G and M are elevated.

Tipple, M.A., Beem, M.O. and Saxon, E.M.: Clinical characteristics of the afebrile pneumonia associated with Chlamydia trachomatis infection in infants less than 6 months of age. *Pediatrics 63*:192, 1979.

E. Spirochetal. Congenital syphilis may be accompanied by pneumonitis.
F. Rickettsial
    1. Q fever
    2. Rocky Mountain spotted fever
    3. Typhus
G. Fungal infection
    1. Histoplasmosis
    2. Moniliasis
    3. Blastomycosis

Powell, D.A. and Schuit, K.E.: Acute pulmonary blastomycosis in children. *Pediatrics 63*: 736, 1979.

    4. Coccidioidomycosis

Richardson, H.B., Jr., Anderson, J.A. and McKay, B.M.: Acute pulmonary coccidioidomycosis in children. *J. Pediatr. 70*:376, 1967.

    5. Aspergillus
    6. Sporotrichosis
    7. Actinomycosis
H. Protozoan
    1. Toxoplasmosis
    2. Pneumocystis carinii
I. Aspiration
    1. Lipoid
    2. Kerosene or hydrocarbon poisoning. Respiratory distress following the ingestion of furniture polish containing mineral seal oil is usually more severe than that produced by ingestion of other hydrocarbon products.
    3. Foreign bodies
    4. Recurrent aspiration pneumonia may occur after repair of an esophageal atresia or may be associated with gastroesophageal reflux.

Whitington, P.F. et al.: Role of lower esophageal sphincter incompetence in recurrent pneumonia after repair of esophageal atresia. *J. Pediatr. 91*:550, 1977.

    5. Milk and other food substances. Persistent pneumonitis may occur in infants with a tracheoesophageal fistula, in infants who are severely retarded and in children with cerebral palsy who are unable to swallow normally.
J. Eosinophilic infiltration

1. Löffler's syndrome, or eosinophilic pneumonia, may be asymptomatic; on the other hand, it may cause severe episodes of coughing and respiratory distress.
2. Visceral larva migrans in infants and young children is characterized by eosinophilia, leukocytosis, elevation of serum globulins, pulmonary infiltration and hepatomegaly.
3. Pneumocystis carinii pneumonia occurs in immunosuppressed or immunodeficient children. Dyspnea is the most common presenting symptom, followed by fever, cough, tachycardia, cyanosis and chest pain. Physical findings are minimal or absent. Rales are not heard. The chest x-ray shows bilateral, diffuse haziness or patchy interstitial infiltrates. The disease may be fulminant. Diagnosis is best made by open-lung biopsy.

Hughes, W.T.: Pneumocystis carinii pneumonia. *N. Engl. J. Med. 297*:1381, 1977.
Walzer, P.D. et al.: Pneumocystis carinii pneumonia in the United States. Epidemiologic, diagnostic, and clinical features. *Ann. Intern. Med. 80*:83, 1974.

K. Familial dysautonomia is characterized by frequent episodes of pulmonary disease. Chest roentgenograms show widespread changes suggestive of cystic fibrosis.
L. Lupus erythematosus may cause an interstitial pneumonitis.

V. Pleurisy
   A. Acute or fibrinous pleurisy
      1. Pleurisy may accompany upper respiratory tract infections.
      2. The pneumococcus may cause fibrinous pleurisy.
      3. Rheumatic fever
      4. Rheumatoid arthritis
      5. Tuberculosis
   B. Pleurisy with effusion
      1. Serofibrinous
         a. Tuberculosis is the most common cause of serofibrinous pleurisy.
         b. Rheumatic fever
         c. Lupus erythematosus. The pleurisy in these patients may also be dry.
      2. Purulent empyema
         a. Pneumococcus
         b. Staphylococcus
         c. Group A beta-hemolytic streptococcus. The effusion is initially serous, then serosanguineous and finally fibrinopurulent.
         d. Hemophilus influenzae type B
         e. E. coli
   C. Pleural effusions caused by malignancies
      Diagnostic measures include a pleural tap with culture, smear (Gram and methylene blue), cell count, protein determinations and cell block.

## GENERAL REFERENCE

Cherry, J.D.: Newer respiratory viruses: their role in respiratory illnesses of children. *Adv. Pediatr. 20*:225, 1973.

## ETIOLOGIC CLASSIFICATION OF LOWER RESPIRATORY DISEASE

CHAPTER **60**

# COUGH AND HEMOPTYSIS

## CLINICAL CONSIDERATIONS

Coughing begins with a short inspiratory phase followed by closure of the glottis and a forceful expiration. With opening of the glottis, there is a sudden release of air under pressure, and the child coughs. This process is controlled by a medullary cough center. Excitatory stimuli arise from respiratory, central or other extrapulmonary sources. Afferent impulses from the pharynx, larynx, trachea (especially at the bifurcation), bronchi of the first and second order, and from the pleura are transmitted through the vagi. Stimuli from the ear traverse the same pathway (auricular branch of the vagus, Arnold's nerve). The glossopharyngeal nerve may transmit some of the impulses that arise in the pharynx. The efferent arc of the cough reflex is through the motor innervation of the respiratory and laryngeal musculature.

Afferent stimuli occur secondary to alteration in the respiratory secretions or changes in the mucosa. Not all portions of the respiratory tree have the same stimulus threshold. Cough may be absent, at times, even with a foreign body in the tracheobronchial tree. Tolerance or decreased reflex excitability may also develop. Coughing in patients with bronchiectasis and in some instances of atelectasis is not continuous.

In general, cough is an important defense mechanism that excludes infected secretions from the tracheobronchial tree and dislodges and removes secretions, exudates and foreign bodies from the lower respiratory tract. The relatively narrow caliber of the laryngotracheobronchial tree and the absence of an effective cough reflex in young infants predispose to aspiration of nasopharyngeal secretions and to obstruction of the airways. The elongation and widening of the tracheobronchial tree during inspiration, alternating with shortening and narrowing during expiration, serve to propel secretions from the periphery to the larger bronchi. This expiratory compression is even more forceful during cough.

Although cough is usually an important physiologic mechanism, and therapy is best designed to enhance its effectiveness, persistent coughing causes fatigue, interrupts sleep, interferes with feeding and may precipitate vomiting.

The cough reflex is absent in very young infants. Effective coughing may also be impossible in emaciated children, in those with weakness or paralysis of the respiratory musculature and in those with massive ascites.

## ETIOLOGIC CLASSIFICATION OF COUGH

I. Respiratory
   A. Infections
      1. Common cold. A profuse nasal discharge may cause pharyngeal irritation and cough that is worse at night.
      2. Chronic sinusitis is a common cause for persistent cough due to a postnasal mucus drip. Cough may be especially bothersome on arising and after going to bed.
      3. Hypertrophy of adenoid tissue and nasopharyngeal obstruction may prevent normal warming and moistening of inspired air. As a result, laryngeal irritation and cough may occur. Pharyngeal cough receptors may also be stimulated by a postnasal drip.
      4. Pharyngitis may cause an irritative cough.
      5. Laryngitis. The cough in these patients is tight, barking and brassy.
      6. Tracheobronchitis, bronchitis. The cough in these patients is deep and is often paroxysmal.
         a. Bronchitis may accompany upper respiratory tract infections, especially sinusitis.

   b. Measles. A hoarse, barking or hacking, nonproductive cough may be present in patients with measles.

   c. Pertussis is classically characterized by paroxysms of hacking, expiratory cough followed by a sudden, deep, tight, crowing inspiration or whoop. The child's face may become suffused or cyanotic during these episodes, especially in young infants. Vomiting of stringy mucoid material may occur after the paroxysms of coughing. In young infants, the episodes may consist more of choking then coughing. The severity and frequency of cough vary widely in individual patients. Some older infants and children do not vomit or whoop, and the atypical illness may be misdiagnosed as persistent bronchitis. Since atypical forms of the disease are difficult to diagnose clinically, the physician has to rely on a history of exposure, the white blood cell count (lymphocytosis) and fluorescent antibody staining of nasopharyngeal smears. False-positive smears may occur if the technician is not experienced. The cough usually begins to diminish after three or four weeks, but paroxysmal episodes may continue for weeks or months.

   d. Parapertussis

   e. Adenoviruses may cause a pertussis-like syndrome with recurrent episodes of paroxysmal coughing followed by mucus production, vomiting, whooping and cyanosis. These manifestations may reflect reactivation of a latent adenoviral infection by Bordetella pertussis.

Baraff, L.J., Wilkins, J. and Wehrle, P.F.: The role of antibiotics, immunizations, and adenoviruses in pertussis. *Pediatrics 61*:224, 1978.
Nelson, K.E. et al.: The role of adenoviruses in the pertussis syndrome. *J. Pediatr. 86*:335, 1975.

   f. Typhoid fever

   g. Scarlet fever

   h. Respiratory allergy accompanying respiratory infections

  7. Cystic fibrosis is a diagnostic consideration in infants who have a persistent cough or frequent respiratory infections. The cough, at times, is paroxysmal and resembles that of pertussis.

Shwachman, H.: Cystic fibrosis. *Cur. Prob. Pediatr. 8*:5 (Aug.) 1978.
Waring, W.W.: Current management of cystic fibrosis. *Adv. Pediatr. 23*:401, 1976.

  8. Pneumonia. Because of the accompanying pain, cough may be a distressing symptom in older children with pneumonia. Cough does not always occur, however, especially in young infants. The cough in babies with staphylococcal or viral pneumonia may be paroxysmal and resemble that of pertussis. Pneumocystis carinii may cause cough due to an interstitial pneumonia.

  9. Tuberculosis

 10. Fungal infections

   a. Histoplasmosis

   b. Moniliasis

   c. Coccidioidomycosis

11. Lung abscess

Marks, P.H. and Turner, J.A.P.: Lung abscess in childhood. *Thorax 23*:216, 1968.

12. Pleurisy. Because of pain, the child with pleurisy may attempt to suppress coughing.
B. Parasitic infections
1. Ascariasis
2. Strongyloidiasis
3. Hookworm infection
4. Visceral larva migrans. In young children with a history of pica, this disorder may present with a chronic cough, often paroxysmal and worse at night, wheezing and irritability. Such symptoms may suggest acute bronchiolitis, asthma or pneumonitis. Fever, leukocytosis, eosinophilia and hepatomegaly may also be present.

Schantz, P.M. and Glickman, L.T.: Toxocaral visceral larva migrans. *N. Engl. J. Med. 298*:436, 1978.

C. Congenital or acquired anomalies or alteration in pulmonary tissue
1. Bronchiectasis secondary to cystic fibrosis, agammaglobulinemia or endobronchial tuberculosis. The cough in these children is often paroxysmal and may be initiated or accentuated by changes in posture.
2. Kartagener's syndrome, which consists of bronchiectasis, chronic sinusitis and situs inversus, is frequently accompanied by cough.
3. Middle lobe syndrome
4. Intralobar bronchopulmonary sequestration is associated with chronic cough, recurrent pneumonia, hemoptysis and roentgenographic evidence of a mass in the basilar segments of the lower lobe.

Durnin, R.E. et al.: Bronchopulmonary sequestration. *Chest 57*:454, 1970.

5. Diaphragmatic hernia
6. Esophageal atresia with tracheoesophageal fistula. A brassy cough may be present for several months after surgical correction of this anomaly.
D. Allergy; allergic airway disease
1. Allergic rhinitis with a postnasal drip
2. Asthma. A short, deep, annoying cough may occur during asthmatic episodes. Initially, a persistent nonproductive cough after lying down at bedtime or during the night may be the only symptom of allergic airway disease. Although wheezing is not reported or noted on auscultation, pulmonary function tests and bronchodilator treatment may demonstrate reversible airway obstruction. Coughing and shortness of breath in these children may be precipitated by running and other vigorous exercise.
3. Respiratory "allergy" accompanying respiratory infections may be a cause of cough.
E. Pulmonary edema; congestive heart failure

F. Idiopathic pulmonary hemosiderosis is characterized by iron deficiency anemia and recurrent mild hemoptysis. A chest film may suggest the diagnosis.

Repetto, G. et al.: Idiopathic pulmonary hemosiderosis. *Pediatrics 40*:24, 1967.

G. Pulmonary alveolar proteinosis may be suspected in infants with failure to thrive, cough and increasing dyspnea. A fine perihilar increase in pulmonary density is noted on the chest roentgenogram. The diagnosis is established by cytologic examination of the sputum.

Wilkinson, R.H., Blanc, W.A. and Hagstrom, J.W.C.: Pulmonary alveolar proteinosis. *Pediatrics 41*:510, 1968.

H. Mechanical obstruction
1. Intrinsic
    a. Foreign body. The initial symptoms produced by foreign bodies in the air and food passages, which include paroxysms of coughing, choking and gagging, may be followed by a symptom-free period.
    b. Copious secretions associated with bronchiectasis and cystic fibrosis
    c. Atelectasis
    d. Children with an isolated tracheoesophageal fistula may cough, choke and, perhaps, become cyanotic during feedings, especially of liquids.
    e. Middle lobe syndrome, which occurs most commonly in young children with allergic airway disease, is characterized by recurrent or persistent coughing and wheezing.

Caplin, I., Haynes, J.T. and Green, M.: Middle lobe syndrome and intractable asthma. *J. Asthma Res. 8*:57, 1970.

    f. Congenital bronchopulmonary-foregut malformation with accessory lung tissue communicating with the gastrointestinal tract can cause cough during feedings.

Gerle, R.D., Jaretzki, A., III, Ashley, C.A. and Berne, A.S.: Congenital bronchopulmonary-foregut malformation. *N. Engl. J. Med. 278*:1413, 1968.

    g. Recurrent bronchitis with cough, especially on lying down at night, and wheezing may be caused by recurrent bronchitis and aspiration pneumonitis secondary to gastroesophageal reflux.

Danus, O., Casar, C., Larrain, A. and Pope, C.E., II: Esophageal reflux — an unrecognized cause of recurrent obstructive bronchitis in children. *J. Pediatr. 89*:220, 1976.

2. Extrinsic
    a. Retropharyngeal abscess
    b. Mediastinal tumor
    c. Enlargement of mediastinal lymph nodes owing to infection or neoplasm may cause a brassy cough.
    d. Pleurisy with effusion; empyema

II. Extrarespiratory
  A. Ear. The auricular branch of the vagus nerve (Arnold's nerve) may be stimulated by impacted cerumen, foreign body or external otitis.
  B. Esophageal duplication
  C. Psychogenic
      1. Psychogenic cough tic accounts for recurrent, severe episodes of coughing in older children and adolescents. Paroxysms do not occur during sleep. The nonproductive cough is loud, deep and barking.
      2. Cough tics also occur in the Gilles de la Tourette's syndrome.

Kravitz, H. et al.: Psychogenic cough tic in children and adolescents. *Clin. Pediatr.* *8*:580, 1969.

## DIAGNOSIS

1. In patients with cough, the history should contain information about exposure to contagious diseases, especially pertussis and tuberculosis, the presence and nature of cough in close contacts and the possibility of aspiration of a foreign body. In the physical examination, special attention should be given to the ears, nose, pharynx and chest. Inspection of the pharynx may demonstrate a postnasal discharge owing to sinusitis or chronic nasopharyngeal infection.
2. Tuberculin skin test. If the tuberculin test is positive, the child and all contacts should have chest roentgenograms. The second-strength Mantoux test should be performed if the first-strength test is negative.
3. Histoplasmin skin test and perhaps tests for other fungus infections.
4. If cough persists and cannot be explained by the history and physical examination, anteroposterior and lateral roentgenograms of the chest should be obtained.
5. Bacteriologic studies
    a. Throat culture if there is clinical evidence of pharyngitis
    b. Nasopharyngeal swab with fluorescent antibody stain for pertussis
    c. Examination of gastric washings and inoculation of guinea pig if tuberculosis is suspected. Infants and young children swallow the sputum that they have coughed up.
    d. Examination of bronchoscopic secretions
6. Leukocyte count and differential. A leukocyte count of 15,000 to 20,000 with a relative and absolute lymphocytosis is characteristically present before and during the early paroxysmal stage of pertussis.
7. A high, cold agglutinin titer may be present in patients with Mycoplasma pneumonia.
8. Bronchoscopy is indicated
    a. In patients with unexplained hemoptysis
    b. When aspiration of a foreign body is suspected. This possibility always exists with unexplained chest lesions in children.
    c. To obtain bronchial secretions for culture and guinea pig inoculation: bacterial, tuberculous and fungal infections
9. Bronchography may be indicated if bronchiectasis is suspected.
10. In infants with chronic respiratory infections and cough, the sweat chloride should be checked.

11. The stools should be examined for ova and parasites in children with persistent or chronic cough.
12. Pulmonary function tests may be helpful in children with cough caused by allergic airway disease.
13. In selected instances, studies for gastroesophageal reflux should be obtained.

## GENERAL REFERENCES

Irwin, R.S., Rosen, M.J. and Braman, S.S.: Cough. A comprehensive review. *Arch. Intern. Med. 137*: 1186, 1977.

## ETIOLOGIC CLASSIFICATION OF COUGH

I. Respiratory, 506
  A. Infections, 506
    1. Common cold
    2. Chronic sinusitis
    3. Hypertrophy of adenoid tissue and nasopharyngeal obstruction
    4. Pharyngitis
    5. Laryngitis
    6. Tracheobronchitis, bronchitis
    7. Cystic fibrosis
    8. Pneumonia
    9. Tuberculosis
    10. Fungal infections
    11. Lung abscess
    12. Pleurisy
  B. Parasitic infections, 508
    1. Ascariasis
    2. Strongyloidiasis
    3. Hookworm infection
    4. Visceral larva migrans
  C. Congenital or acquired anomalies or alteration in pulmonary tissue, 508
    1. Bronchiectasis secondary to cystic fibrosis, agammaglobulinemia or endobronchial tuberculosis
    2. Kartagener's syndrome
    3. Middle lobe syndrome
    4. Intralobar bronchopulmonary sequestration
    5. Diaphragmatic hernia
    6. Esophageal atresia with tracheoesophageal fistula
  D. Allergy; allergic airway disease, 508
    1. Allergic rhinitis with postnasal drip
    2. Asthma
    3. Respiratory "allergy" accompanying respiratory infections
  E. Pulmonary edema; congestive heart failure, 508
  F. Idiopathic pulmonary hemosiderosis, 509
  G. Pulmonary alveolar proteinosis, 509
  H. Mechanical obstruction, 509
    1. Intrinsic
    2. Extrinsic
II. Extrarespiratory, 510
  A. Ear, 510
  B. Esophageal duplication, 510
  C. Psychogenic, 510
    1. Psychogenic cough tic
    2. Gilles de la Tourette's syndrome

## HEMOPTYSIS

Massive pulmonary hemorrhage may occur in low-birth-weight newborn infants who have been hypoxemic.

Massive pulmonary hemorrhage may also occur in newborn infants with hyperammonemia.

Sheffield, L.J., Danks, D.M., Hammond, J.W. and Hoogenraad, N.J.: Massive pulmonary hemorrhage as a presenting feature in congenital hyperammonemia. *J. Pediatr. 88*:450, 1976.

Group A beta-hemolytic streptococcus pneumonia
Pertussis, after severe paroxysms of coughing
Bronchiectasis

Cystic fibrosis in young adults. Bronchial arteriography may be helpful in localizing the site of bleeding.

Holsclaw, D.S., Grand, R.J. and Shwachman, H.: Massive hemoptysis in cystic fibrosis. *J. Pediatr. 76*:829, 1970.
Levitsky, S., Lapey, A. and Di Sant'Agnese, P.A.: Pulmonary resection for life-threatening hemoptysis in cystic fibrosis. *JAMA 213*:125, 1970.

Bronchial adenoma, papilloma, hemangioma. Although rare in children, the possibility of a bronchogenic tumor should be included in the differential diagnosis of cough and hemoptysis. Chest x-rays and bronchoscopy are helpful diagnostically.

De Paredes, C.G., Pierce, W.S., Gruff, D.B. and Waldhausen, J.A.: Bronchogenic tumors in children. *Arch. Surg. 10*:574, 1970.

Lung abscess
Tuberculosis
Foreign body in the laryngotracheobronchial tree
Esophageal duplication
Idiopathic pulmonary hemosiderosis. Hemoptysis in these cases is usually not massive but consists of blood-stained sputum.
Hemorrhagic disorders
Extreme pulmonary stenosis (chiefly tetralogy with outflow atresia); enlarged bronchial arteries
Pulmonary vascular obstructive diseases: primary pulmonary hypertension; Eisenmenger reaction in right-to-left shunt or single ventricle; following systemic-pulmonary anastomosis.

Haroutunian, L.M. and Neill, C.A.: Pulmonary complications of congenital heart disease: hemoptysis. *Am. Heart J. 84*:540, 1972.

Mitral stenosis
Fungus infection involving bronchus
Wegener's granulomatosis
Goodpasture's syndrome, rare in children, is characterized by hemoptysis, pulmonary infiltration, anemia and renal failure.
Lupus erythematosus


## PERSISTENT HICCOUGHS

Acute renal failure

# CHAPTER 61

# CHEST PAIN

## ETIOLOGIC CLASSIFICATION OF CHEST PAIN

I. Cardiopulmonary
   A. Pericarditis of various etiologies may be characterized by chest pain, usually sudden in onset and localized substernally over the precordium, in the epigastrium, in the interscapular region or over the entire thorax. Accentuation of the pain may occur with deep breathing, coughing, swallowing or twisting of the thorax. The child may have grunting respirations.
   B. Pulmonary vascular obstructive syndrome or primary pulmonary hypertension may be characterized, in part, by pain on exertion.
   C. Rheumatic fever may be accompanied by precordial pain.
   D. Ruptured congenital aneurysm of the sinuses of Valsalva.
   E. Anginal pain may occur in children with sickle cell anemia, severe aortic stenosis, pulmonic stenosis and hypertrophic subaortic stenosis.

   Hamilton, W., Rosenthal, A., Berwick, D. and Nadas, A.S.: Angina pectoris in a child with sickle cell anemia. *Pediatrics 61*:911, 1978.

   F. Mitral valve prolapse is an unusual cause for sharp or dull, intermittent pain or angina on the left side of the chest.
II. Pleura and diaphragm
   Since the posterior third and the lateral parts of the diaphragm are innervated by the lower six intercostal nerves, pain arising from these areas is referred to the lower part of the thorax or upper part of the abdomen. The central and anterior portions of the diaphragm are innervated by the phrenic nerve, with pain referred to the shoulder and trapezial ridge.
   A. Pleurisy may occur alone or as a complication of pneumonia. Well-localized over the involved area and perceived as superficial, the pain is sharp in intensity and accentuated by deep breathing, coughing and movements of the arms. The patient attempts to splint the involved side. Some localized tenderness may be noted.
   B. Epidemic pleurodynia is characterized by sharp or stabbing pain similar to that of pleurisy. Involvement may be unilateral or bilateral. Tenderness and some swelling may be noted over the involved area. The pain may last two or three days and recur.
   C. Familial paroxysmal polyserositis (Mediterranean fever) may be characterized by paroxysmal pleuritis with severe, sharp, stabbing pain. These episodes may occur independently or with paroxysmal peritonitis.
   D. Spontaneous pneumothorax may cause acute chest pain.
   E. Trichinosis involving the diaphragm is characterized by chest pain as well as systemic manifestations.

III. Musculoskeletal
   A. Muscle strain and fatigue are probably the most common causes of chest pain in children. The involved muscles may be tender. Weight-lifting and other vigorous sports may be etiologic.
   B. Trauma to the chest wall
   C. Tumors or other infiltrative processes involving the bony skeleton may give rise to pain.
   D. Fracture of ribs
   E. Tietze's syndrome or costochondritis. See page 103
   F. Severe paroxysms of coughing or asthma may cause chest pain.
IV. Esophageal
   A. Cardiospasm with diffuse spasm of esophagus
   B. Hiatal hernia and gastroesophageal reflux

   Darling, D.B., Fisher, J.H. and Gellis, S.S.: Hiatal hernia and gastroesophageal reflux in infants and children: analysis of the incidence in North American children. *Pediatrics 54*:450, 1974.

V. Psychogenic
   A. Occasionaliy, children seen because of pain over the precordium will be found to have a psychologic basis for the symptom. The interview will frequently disclose that a parent or other relative has angina or some other cardiac disorder.

   Friedman, S.: Conversion symptoms in adolescents. *Pediatr. Clin. N. Am. 20*:873, 1973.

   B. Hyperventilation syndrome may present with the complaint of chest pain.
VI. Neurologic
   A. Radicular pain due to compression of the spinal cord by tumor, epidural abscess or vertebral collapse
   B. Prodromal phase of herpes zoster

## GENERAL REFERENCE

Driscoll, D.J., Glicklich, L.B. and Gallen, W.J.: Chest pain in children: a prospective study. *Pediatrics 57*:648, 1976.

# CHAPTER 62

# FREQUENT INFECTIONS

## CLINICAL CONSIDERATIONS

In considering the presenting complaint of "frequent infections," the physician must differentiate among parental overestimation of the number and severity of the illnesses, an above-average but normal number of infections, allergic airway disease, and a true immunodeficiency illness. Whereas the first three can be readily managed in an office setting, the child with true immunodeficiency generally requires referral to a regional center.

Dingle's classic study demonstrated that during the second year of life children experience, on the average, eight respiratory infections a year. The frequency of such infections gradually decreases until an average of three to four a year is reached in the adolescent years. More than 10 per cent of children have over 12 respiratory infections per year. These are generally the patients seen for "frequent colds." Other studies suggest that children, on the average, experience 100 infections, most asymptomatic, by the age of 10 years. Environmental factors predisposing to frequent infections include crowding, especially in sleeping areas, contact with siblings of school age, or attendance in nursery school, kindergarten or the primary grades. Respiratory airway disease is a common cause of frequent colds. A history of frequent sore throats is often misleading, as prospective experience will usually document fewer episodes than a retrospective history.

Paradise, J.L. et al.: History of recurrent sore throat as an indication for tonsillectomy. Predictive limitations of histories that are undocumented. *N. Engl. J. Med. 298*:409, 1978.

The possibility of an immunodeficiency syndrome exists in cases that have any one of the following four characteristics: (1) infections are especially frequent, severe, or persistent; (2) there are multiple sites of infection with many etiologic agents, especially organisms not commonly pathogenic; (3) there is recurrence of infections to which the child should have acquired immunity; or (4) a common disease has an unusually severe and progressive course.


## ETIOLOGIC CLASSIFICATION OF IMMUNODEFICIENCY DISORDERS

I. Neutrophil disorders
   A. Neutropenia (absolute granulocyte count under 1500/mm³)
      1. Cyclic neutropenia is manifested by periodic (approximately every three weeks) episodes characterized by fever, mouth ulcers, arthralgia and recurrent mild infections such as furunculosis or pneumonia. Each episode lasts about one week. Unless the neutropenia is detected sooner, the diagnosis may be established by obtaining white blood cell and differential counts three times a week for two months.
      2. Chronic infantile agranulocytosis, an autosomal recessive and usually fatal disease occurring in the first year of life, is characterized by chronic, recurrent pyogenic infections of the skin and respiratory tract or by other serious, recurrent infectious diseases. Although the total white blood count may be normal, the neutrophil count is usually under 300 neutrophils per mm³.
      3. Chronic benign granulocytopenia of childhood, which usually becomes symptomatic by the end of the first year and continues for months to years, is characterized by mild infections, mouth ulcers and stomatitis.
      4. Exocrine pancreatic insufficiency and neutropenia, dwarfism, severe infections and, at times, metaphyseal dysostosis constitute a fatal disorder in infancy or childhood.
      5. Ineffective myelopoiesis causes chronic neutropenia in children. Appropriate leukocytosis develops in response to infections.

6. Drug-induced neutropenia results from a profound bone marrow suppression involving the myeloid cells.
7. Aplastic anemia
8. Acute leukemia
9. Neutropenia may occur secondary to vitamin $B_{12}$ or folic acid deficiency.
10. Neonatal isoimmune neutropenia
11. Congestive splenomegaly
12. Chronic granulocytopenia in childhood, usually a self-limited disorder, is characterized by susceptibility to localized infections such as paronychia, subcutaneous abscesses, impetigo, gingivitis and genital ulcers. With infection, the bone marrow responds with the release of immature but functionally adequate white blood cells.
13. Cartilage-hair hypoplasia is characterized by chronic neutropenia and depression of cell-mediated immunity.

Kauder, E. and Mauer, A.M.: Neutropenias of childhood. *J. Pediatr. 69*:147, 1966.
Lang, J.E. and Cutting, H.O.: Infantile genetic agranulocytosis. *Pediatrics 35*:596, 1965.
Lux, S.E. et al.: Chronic neutropenia and abnormal cellular immunity in cartilage-hair hypoplasia. *N. Engl. J. Med. 282*:231, 1970.
Shwachman, H. et al.: The syndrome of pancreatic insufficiency and bone marrow dysfunction. *J. Pediatr. 65*:645, 1964.
Zuelzer, W.W. and Bajoghli, M.: Chronic granulocytopenia in childhood. *Blood 23*:359, 1964.

B. Phagocytic dysfunction syndromes
   1. Defective chemotaxis; the "lazy leukocyte" syndrome
   2. Defective opsonization
      a. Complement deficiencies. Dysfunction of the fifth component of complement causes Leiner's disease, with generalized seborrheic dermatitis, persistent diarrhea, gram-negative infections and failure to thrive.
      b. Sickle cell anemia may be accompanied by deficient heat-labile opsonic function against pneumococci.
   3. Defective intracellular bacterial killing
      a. Chronic granulomatous disease is characterized by a qualitative defect in polymorphonuclear leukocytes so that intracellular killing of phagocytosed or ingested bacteria does not occur. The disorder, which occurs in a male-to-female ratio of 7:1, is genetically transmitted in an X-linked recessive and, more uncommonly, an autosomal recessive form. Marked suppurative lymphadenopathy and draining cutaneous fistulas usually occur by the end of the first year of life. Other findings include pneumonia, hepatosplenomegaly, eczematous lesions around the mouth and ears, chronic pyoderma, hepatic abscesses, persistent diarrhea, perianal abscesses and osteomyelitis, usually of the small bones of the hands and feet. The peripheral blood leukocytes fail to reduce nitroblue tetrazolium dye during phagocytosis.

Johnson, R.B., Jr. and Baehner, R.L.: Chronic granulomatous disease: correlation between pathogenesis and clinical findings. *Pediatrics 48*:730, 1971.
Johnson, R.B., Jr.: Unusual forms of an uncommon disease (chronic granulomatous disease). *J. Pediatr. 88*:172, 1976.
Quie, P.G.: Chronic granulomatous disease of childhood. *Adv. Pediatr. 16*:287, 1969.

b. Job's syndrome, which occurs in light-skinned, red-haired girls, is characterized by recurrent cold staphylococcal abscesses and relatively mild infections without a granulomatous reaction. The phagocytic functional defect is similar to that in chronic granulomatous disease.

Bannatyne, R.M. et al.: Job's syndrome — a variant of chronic granulomatous disease. *J. Pediatr. 75*:236, 1969.
Hill, H.R. et al.: Defect in neutrophic granulocyte chemotaxis in Job's syndrome of recurrent "cold" staphylococcal abscesses. *Lancet 2*:617, 1974.

c. Familial lipochrome histocytosis is also characterized by defective phagocytic function similar to that of chronic granulomatous disease.

4. Myeloperoxidase deficiency
5. Chédiak-Higashi syndrome, probably transmitted as a simple autosomal recessive trait, is manifested by partial ocular and cutaneous albinism with pale gray or blond hair, photophobia, nystagmus and frequent pyogenic infections, especially with gram-positive organisms. Many patients develop massive hepatosplenomegaly and generalized lymphadenopathy. Abnormally large granules are present in the neutrophils, eosinophils and basophils.

Blume, R.S. and Wolff, S.M.: The Chédiak-Higashi syndrome: studies in four patients and a review of the literature. *Medicine 51*:247, 1972.
Hayward, A.R. et al.: Delayed separation of the umbilical cord, widespread infections and defective neutrophil mobility. *Lancet 1*:1099, 1979.
Quie, P.G.: Infections due to neutrophil malfunction. *Medicine 52*:411, 1973.
Winkelstein, J.A. and Drachman R.H.: Phagocytosis. *Pediatr. Clin. N. Am. 21*:551, 1974.

II. T-cell deficiency syndromes may be suspected in infants and children who have persistent or recurrent thrush in spite of appropriate treatment, a negative skin test response to monilial antigen and failure of lymphocyte response to phytohemagglutinin.
A. DiGeorge's syndrome (congenital aplasia of thymus, pharyngeal pouch syndrome) is manifested by a characteristic facies and recurrent infections. Neonatal tetany is usually the first clinical manifestation. Facial features include micrognathia; low-set, poorly formed ears; a short philtrum of the upper lip; a "fish" mouth; hypertelorism; and clefts in the midline of the nose. Congenital heart disease may also be present. Symptoms include extreme susceptibility to infection with Pneumocystis carinii, pneumonia, diarrhea, moniliasis and failure to thrive. The humoral immunity and serum immunoglobulins are normal. Impairment of cellular immunity is reflected in failure to demonstrate delayed hypersensitivity to such agents as monilia, trichophyton or streptokinase and streptodornase. Delayed hypersensitivity cannot be produced with dinitrofluorobenzene, and the lymphocyte response to phytohemagglutinin is deficient.

Kretschmer, R., Say, B., Brown, D. and Rosen, F.S.: Congenital aplasia of the thymus gland (DiGeorge's syndrome). *N Engl. J. Med. 279*:1295, 1968.
Rosen, F.S.: The lymphocyte and the thymus gland—congenital and hereditary abnormalities. *N. Engl. J. Med. 279*:643, 1968.

B. Wiskott-Aldrich syndrome, a sex-linked recessive disorder with abnormal cellular immunity, is characterized by marked thrombocytopenia, abnormal platelet function, eczema, skin infections, otitis media and pneumonia. Other findings in these boys are low numbers of circulating lymphocytes, low IgM and absent isohemagglutinins.

Cooper, M.D. et al.: Wiskott-Aldrich syndrome. *Am. J. Med. 44*:499, 1968.

C. Ataxia telangiectasia, which affects both boys and girls, begins with ataxia, dysarthric speech, tremors and choreoathetosis. Infections, usually of the respiratory tract, begin between three and eight years of age. Conjunctival and facial telangiectasia often appears between two and eight years of age. IgA is absent in 80 per cent of these patients. Delayed hypersensitivity may be impaired.

McFarlin, D.E., Strober, W. and Waldmann, T.A.: Ataxia-telangiectasia. *Medicine 51*:281, 1972.

D. Children with intrauterine growth retardation have impaired cellular immunity at birth and for at least five years. These patients have an increased susceptibility to infection and an inadequate response to immunization.

Ferguson, A.C.: Prolonged impairment of cellular immunity in children with intrauterine growth retardation. *J. Pediatr. 93*:52, 1978.

E. Type 2 short-limbed dwarfism may occur with cell-mediated immunodeficiency. Some of these patients have cartilage-hair hypoplasia.

Ammann, A.J., Sutliff, W. and Millinchick, E.: Antibody-mediated immunodeficiency in short-limbed dwarfism. *J. Pediatr. 84*:200, 1974.
Virolainen, M. et al.: Cellular and humoral immunity in cartilage-hair hypoplasia. *Pediatr. Res. 12*:961, 1978.

F. Purine nucleoside phosphorylase deficiency may be associated with defective T-cell function.

Biggar, W.D., Giblett, E.R., Ozere, R.L. and Grover, B.D.: A new form of nucleoside phosphorylase deficiency in two brothers with defective T-cell function. *J. Pediatr. 92*:354, 1978.

III. B-cell or antibody deficiency syndromes are characterized by recurrent, severe pyogenic infections of the skin, bones, joints, lungs, meninges, sinuses and middle ear. Etiologic agents include pneumococci, Hemophilus influenzae, Staphylococcus aureus, meningococci and, occasionally, beta-hemolytic streptococci. While these infections respond to antibiotics, there is a high recurrence rate.

A. Transient hypogammaglobulinemia, attributable to delayed maturation of B-cell function, begins in both sexes between two and six months of age. Diagnosis may be made by screening the serum of relatives of patients who have a primary immunodeficiency or in the course of study in patients with recurrent fever, repeated or severe pyogenic infections, chronic mucocutaneous candidiasis and bronchitis. Low levels of IgG, IgA and IgM are found. Patients identified on the basis of screening are asymptomatic whereas those with a history of recurrent infections usually have no further major problems after six months of age. In the former group, the immunoglobulin levels in time become completely normal while the values in the latter gradually improve but may remain below normal.

Tiller, T.L., Jr. and Buckley, R.H.: Transient hypogammaglobulinemia of infancy: review of the literature, clinical and immunologic features of 11 new cases, and long-term follow-up. *J. Pediatr. 92*:347, 1978.

B. X-linked agammaglobulinemia, which occurs only in boys in the first three years of life, is characterized by recurrent pyogenic infections. Since the tonsils and adenoids are absent or underdeveloped, lateral pharyngeal x-rays do not have an adenoid shadow. The levels of IgG are very low, less than 100 mg. per cent, while the IgA levels are either very low or very high. Delayed hypersensitivity tests are normal, and the patients demonstrate a positive Shick test after diphtheria immunization. About one third of these patients develop a nonbacterial arthritis that closely simulates rheumatoid arthritis.

C. Common variable or acquired forms of antibody deficiency syndrome are characterized by a low level of IgG and variable amounts of IgA and IgM. Clinical manifestations include pyoderma, pneumonia, meningitis, tonsillitis, otitis media, sinusitis and a sprue-like syndrome. Both sexes are affected, and manifestations may appear at any age. Children with the nephrotic syndrome may develop secondary hypogammaglobulinemia owing to urinary protein loss and increased catabolism. Such hypogammaglobulinemia may contribute to the increase in susceptibility to bacterial infection that characterizes these children. Hereditary lymphopenic agammaglobulinemia may be associated with short-limbed dwarfism and ectodermal dysplasia.

Gatti, R.A. et al.: Hereditary lymphopenic agammaglobulinemia associated with a distinctive form of short-limbed dwarfism and ectodermal dysplasia. *J. Pediatr.* 75:675, 1969.

D. Partial or selective deficiency of one of the major immunoglobulin classes or of one of the subclasses of IgG
   1. The clinical significance of IgA deficiency is uncertain. Children with this finding may be clinically normal or they may have recurrent upper respiratory infections or intermittent diarrhea.

Ammann, A.J. and Hong, R.: Selective IgA deficiency: presentation of 30 cases and a review of the literature. *Medicine 50*:223, 1971.

   2. In partial gamma globulin deficiency, one or more of the four IgG subclasses may be absent. This disorder occurs in both boys and girls and is characterized by recurrent pyogenic infections that are less severe than those secondary to agammaglobulinemia.

E. Type 3 short-limbed dwarfism may be associated with antibody-mediated immunodeficiency.

F. Complement disorders
   1. C3 or beta$_1$ C globulin deficiency
   2. Dysfunction of the fifth component of complement (C5)

Alper, C.A. et al.: Increased susceptibility to infection associated with abnormalities of complement-mediated functions and of the third component of complement (C3). *N. Engl. J. Med.* 282:349, 1970.

Jacobs, J.D. and Miller, M.E.: Fatal familial "Leiner's disease": a deficiency of the opsonic activity of serum complement. *Pediatrics 49*:225, 1972.

Miller, M.E. and Nilsson, U.R.: A familial deficiency of the phagocytosis-enhancing activity of serum related to a dysfunction of the fifth component of complement (C5). *N. Engl. J. Med. 282*:354, 1970.

IV. Severe, combined immune deficiency, a rare disorder in infants, may be inherited in either a sex-linked or an autosomal fashion. T and B lymphocytes are markedly defective in both number and function. Affected infants are markedly susceptible to all types of infections. Clinical characteristics include marked failure of growth or runting, chronic pneumonitis, persistent diarrhea and extensive moniliasis. Laboratory findings include lymphopenia, hypo-gammaglobulinemia, lack of ABO group antibodies and absence of lympho-cyte response to phytohemagglutinin. A fatal graft-versus-host reaction may be precipitated by transfusions.

Bortin, M.M. and Rimm, A.A.: Severe combined immunodeficiency disease. *JAMA 238*:591, 1977.

Gatti, R.A. et al.: Hereditary lymphopenic agammaglobulinemia associated with a distinctive form of short-limbed dwarfism and ectodermal dysplasia. *J. Pediatr. 75*:675, 1969.

Type 1 short-limbed dwarfism may be associated with combined antibody-and cell-mediated immunodeficiency.

V. Secondary immunodeficiency disorders
  A. Splenectomy may make a child susceptible to overwhelming sepsis, re-current meningitis and other serious infections. Howell-Jolly bodies may be present in the peripheral blood.

Diamond, L.K.: Splenectomy in childhood and the hazard of overwhelming infection. *Pediatrics 43*:886, 1969.

---

## ETIOLOGIC CLASSIFICATION OF IMMUNODEFICIENCY DISORDERS

B. Severe protein-caloric malnutrition

Katz, M. and Stiehm, E.R.: Host defense in malnutrition. *Pediatrics* 59:490, 1977.

C. Measles and Epstein-Barr virus infections
D. Long-term, high-dose corticosteroid treatment
E. Lymphomatous disease
F. Use of immunosuppressive drugs for treatment of neoplasia
G. Immunologic diseases such as lupus erythematosus
H. Transplantation rejection reactions
I. Sickle cell anemia patients have an increased susceptibility to pneumo-coccal meningitis, bacteremia and/or pneumonia. Their functional asplen-ia may increase susceptibility to pyogenic infections.

## GENERAL REFERENCES

Janeway, C.A.: Recurrent infections. *In* Green, M. and Haggerty, R.J. (eds.): *Ambulatory Pediatrics II*. Philadelphia, W.B. Saunders Co., 1977.
Miller, M.E.: *Host Defenses in the Human Neonate*. New York, Grune and Stratton, 1978.
Mortimer, E.A., Jr.: Frequent colds. *In* Green, M. and Haggerty, R.J. (eds.): *Ambulatory Pediatrics*. 1st ed. Philadelphia, W.B. Saunders Co., 1968.
Stiehm, E.R. and Fulginiti, V.A. (eds.): *Immunologic Disorders in Infants and Children*. Philadelphia, W.B. Saunders Co., 1973.

CHAPTER 63

# LYMPHADENOPATHY

Lymph nodes, often small and firm or shotty, are palpable to a variable degree in normal infants and children in the cervical, axillary, inguinal and occipital areas. They are not palpable in the newborn infant.

Apart from enlargement, lymphadenopathy may be accompanied by local pain and tenderness. If suppuration occurs, the overlying skin becomes reddened. Other symptoms depend upon the location of the adenopathy. Stiffness of the neck and torticollis may accompany cervical adenopathy. Suppuration of retropharyngeal nodes (retropharyngeal abscess) leads to dysphagia and obstructive breathing. Mediastinal adenopathy may cause stridor, cyanosis, dyspnea, dysphagia, cough, pleural effusion, edema of the face and venous congestion. Mesenteric and retroperitoneal adenopathy may be characterized by abdominal pain. Iliac adenitis may cause abdominal pain; tenderness, especially above Poupart's ligament; and a limp.

## ETIOLOGIC CLASSIFICATION OF LYMPHADENOPATHY

I. Infections. Bacterial, mycotic and especially viral infections are common causes of adenopathy in infants and children. Lymph nodes mechanically remove cellular debris, bacteria and other foreign matter from the lymph stream but are not efficient barriers for viruses. Chronic, localized adenopathy is usually attributable to a persistent regional infection. Cervical adenitis commonly accompanies tonsillitis and pharyngitis. Submaxillary adenopathy may develop secondary to stomatitis or periapical dental abscess. Occipital and postauricular adenopathy may accompany infections, seborrheic dermatitis or pediculosis of the scalp. Epitrochlear and axillary lymphadenopathy may result from infections on the arms while inguinal and femoral adenopathy may be due to those on the lower extremities. The upper eyelid drains into the preauricular node. Uniocular granulomatous conjunctivitis with preauricular adenopathy (Parinaud's syndrome) may be caused by cat-scratch disease, tularemia or tuberculosis. Adenovirus type 3 causes pharyngeal-conjunctival fever characterized by follicular conjunctivitis and enlarged preauricular and/or posterior cervical nodes. Epidemic keratoconjunctivitis, caused by adenovirus type 8, is also accompanied by preauricular adenopathy.

Mediastinal or hilar adenopathy may occur in patients with tuberculosis, chronic sinusitis, histoplasmosis, tularemia, infectious mononucleosis, sarcoidosis, moniliasis, coccidioidomycosis and bronchiectasis. Lymphosarcoma and Hodgkin's disease are noninfectious causes of mediastinal adenopathy.

Zeanah, C.H. and Zusman, J.: Mediastinal and cervical histoplasmosis simulating malignancy. *Am. J. Dis. Child. 133*:47, 1979.

Acute unilateral pyogenic adenitis is the most common type of lymphadenopathy. The involved node may be walnut-sized, firm and tender, with erythema of the overlying skin. Etiologic agents are predominantly Group A betahemolytic streptococcus, staphylococci and viruses. Bilateral acute cervical adenitis is usually due to viral pharyngitis or infectious mononucleosis.

Dajani, A.S., Garcia, R.E. and Wolinsky, E.: Etiology of cervical lymphadenitis in children. *N. Engl. J. Med. 268*:1329, 1963.
Hieber, J.P. and Davis, A.T.: Staphylococcal cervical lymphadenitis in young infants. *Pediatrics 57*:424, 1976.

A. Cat-scratch disease is a common cause of localized adenopathy. Depending upon the site of the scratch, axillary, epitrochlear, supraclavicular, femoral, inguinal or submaxillary nodes may be affected. Nodes may appear in unusual sites — under pectoral, trapezius or sternomastoid muscles. The involved node is characteristically nontender, discrete, movable and moderately or greatly enlarged. On occasion, tenderness, redness, warmth and even suppuration may occur. Lymphadenopathy may persist for weeks or months. Other symptoms include malaise, fever and skin lesions that resemble erythema multiforme or erythema nodosum. A red papule, 2 to 5 mm. in diameter, may appear at the site of the scratch a few days or weeks before the adenopathy and later may become pustular or crusted. This primary lesion persists for one to four weeks.

Carithers, H.A., Carithers, C.M. and Edwards, R.O., Jr.: Cat-scratch disease. Its natural history. *JAMA 207*:312, 1969.
Warwick, W.J.: The cat-scratch syndrome: many diseases or one disease? *Prog. Med. Virol.* 9:256, 1967.

B. Rubella is characterized by enlargement and tenderness of the posterior auricular, posterior cervical and occipital lymph nodes. Scarlet fever may also be accompanied by cervical adenitis. Generalized superficial lymphadenopathy may occur in patients with measles, chickenpox, mumps and other infectious diseases.

C. Generalized adenopathy may be noted after immunization with typhoid vaccine. Regional adenitis may follow immunization with pertussis vaccine, diphtheria toxoid and tetanus toxoid.

D. Tularemia. The primary lesion in patients with tularemia may be accompanied by regional adenopathy with local tenderness, pain, perhaps suppuration and fever. Generalized lymphadenopathy may also develop.

Hughes, W.T.: Tularemia in children. *J. Pediatr.* 62:495, 1963.

E. Toxoplasmosis may cause an acquired infection simulating infectious mononucleosis and characterized by cervical, suboccipital, supraclavicular or generalized adenopathy and fever.

Jones, T.C., Kean, B.H. and Kimball, A.C.: Toxoplasmic lymphadenitis. *JAMA 192*:87, 1965.
Rafaty, M.F.: Cervical adenopathy secondary to toxoplasmosis. *Arch. Otolaryngol. 103*: 547, 1977.

F. The Gianotti-Crosti syndrome consists of generalized lymphadenopathy, hepatomegaly, nonicteric hepatitis and crops of papular lesions that form plaques.

G. Infectious mononucleosis. The lymph nodes in patients with infectious mononucleosis are discrete, firm, resilient, usually nontender and ½ to 3 inches in size. Enlarged anterior and cervical nodes are present. Postauricular and suboccipital lymphadenopathy are also frequent. Generalized lymphadenopathy may also occur. Hepatosplenomegaly is common.

Fernbach, D.J. and Starling, K.A.: Infectious mononucleosis. *Pediatr. Clin. N. Am. 19*:957, 1972.
Ginsburg, C.M., Henle, W., Henle, G. and Horwitz, C.A.: Infectious mononucleosis in children. Evaluation of Epstein-Barr virus-specific serological data. *JAMA 237*:781, 1977.

H. Cytomegalovirus infection may be characterized by lymphadenopathy, fever and atypical lymphocytes in the peripheral blood.

I. Coxsackie virus may cause a syndrome of cervical or axillary lymphadenopathy, conjunctivitis, painful hepatomegaly and/or splenomegaly, fever, nausea and vomiting.

Siegel, W. et al.: Two new variants of infection with Coxsackie virus group B, type 5, in young children. *N. Engl. J. Med. 268*:1210, 1963.

J. Echovirus may cause mild to moderate lymphadenitis.

K. Tuberculosis. Generalized lymphadenopathy in a child with tuberculosis may indicate that a hematogenous spread of tubercle bacilli has occurred. Localized involvement is most common in the mediastinal, mesenteric or anterior cervical nodes. Early, tuberculosis of the cervical nodes may be confused with lymphadenitis secondary to pharyngitis or with Hodgkin's disease. Tuberculous nodes are initially discrete, firm, mobile and tender. Later, they become soft, fluctuant, matted and adherent to the overlying skin. The skin may become erythematous. Draining sinuses may develop. Bilateral involvement is the rule, and pulmonary disease is commonly present. A tuberculous etiology is unlikely if the tuberculin test is negative.

L. Atypical mycobacteria also leads to cervical adenitis clinically similar to that caused by tuberculosis, except that involvement is usually unilateral.

M. Rat-bite fever may be characterized by regional lymphadenopathy secondary to the primary lesion. Generalized lymphadenopathy may also occur.

N. Bacteremia frequently leads to generalized lymphadenopathy.

O. Histoplasmosis. With the exception of mediastinal lymphadenopathy, lymph node enlargement is not a prominent feature of this disease.

P. Brucellosis. Lymphadenopathy may be chronic or intermittent.

Q. Sarcoidosis. Almost all patients with sarcoidosis demonstrate lymphadenopathy, either generalized or hilar. The bilaterally enlarged cervical nodes are firm, rubbery and discrete, with little tendency to coalesce. Other symptoms include fatigue, cough, fever, dyspnea and weight loss. Hyperglobulinemia and eosinophilia are common laboratory findings.

Kendig, E.L.: The clinical picture of sarcoidosis in children. *Pediatrics 54*:289, 1974.

R. Salmonella infection. Generalized lymphadenopathy may be a prominent symptom in salmonellosis.

S. Eczema. Infants with atopic eczema may demonstrate generalized lymphadenopathy, with axillary nodes possibly 2 to 3 cm. in diameter.

T. Bubonic plague due to Yersinia pestis may cause tender lymphadenitis and fever.

II. Diseases of hypersensitization

A. Juvenile rheumatoid arthritis should be considered in children with unexplained fever and chronic lymphadenopathy.

B. Serum sickness is often accompanied by generalized, tender lymphadenopathy. The serum-sickness type of reaction to penicillin may be characterized by lymphadenopathy, splenomegaly, myalgia and arthritis.

C. Mesantoin medication may cause enlargement of lymph nodes, most commonly those in the cervical region; fever; eosinophilia; rash; and hepatosplenomegaly. Hydantoin may also lead to lymphadenopathy.

Snead, C., Siegel, N. and Hayslett, J.: Generalized lymphadenopathy and nephrotic syndrome as a manifestation of mephenytoin (mesantoin) toxicity. *Pediatrics 57*:98, 1976.

III. Primary disease of lymphoid or reticuloendothelial tissue; metastatic lymphadenopathy

A. Leukemia. Although it may be an early manifestation of leukemia, lymphadenopathy often does not become prominent until the disease is advanced. In many children, it never becomes remarkable.

B. Lymphosarcoma. The cervical and the mediastinal lymph nodes are commonly involved by lymphosarcoma. Initially firm, rubbery, painless and discrete, the nodes soon become matted, owing to invasion of the capsule and infiltration of the surrounding tissue by lymphosarcoma cells. Involvement may be unilateral or bilateral.

C. Reticulum cell sarcoma arises from the sinus endothelium of the lymph nodes.

Murphy, S.B.: Current concepts in cancer: childhood non-Hodgkin's lymphoma. *N. Engl. J. Med. 299*:1446, 1978.

D. Hodgkin's disease is usually characterized by an insidious, painless enlargement of regional lymph nodes, most frequently the cervical and less commonly the supraclavicular, mediastinal, axillary, epitrochlear or inguinal nodes. Adenopathy is usually unilateral. Rarely, preauricular nodes may be involved. The right supraclavicular node may be enlarged secondary to mediastinal involvement while enlargement of the left node may occur secondary to abdominal disease. At first, the nodes are soft, but later they become firm and rubbery. Although discrete, their large size and close proximity may cause them to seem adherent and fixed. Pain may occur if axillary or inguinal nodes become enlarged. Superimposed infections, such as pharyngitis, may cause further enlargement and pain. Early diagnosis may be difficult. The central nodes in an involved area should be selected for biopsy since peripheral nodes may show only follicular hyperplasia.

E. Malignant histiocytosis or histiocytic lymphoma may present as an inflammatory disorder with fever, lymphadenopathy, hepatosplenomegaly and weight loss.

F. Rhabdomyosarcoma of the nasopharynx may first present as cervical adenopathy in the upper one third of the neck.

G. Neuroblastoma may cause a mass in the neck that may simulate enlarged cervical nodes. In metastatic neuroblastoma, the left supraclavicular (Virchow's) node may be involved secondary to extension up the thoracic duct. Such adenopathy may be the first sign of disease.

H. Carcinoma of the thyroid. Careful palpation of the thyroid is indicated in patients with cervical adenopathy. Enlarged, firm, discrete cervical lymph nodes may be the initial complaint with carcinoma of the thyroid. At times, the thyroid malignancy is recognized only after biopsy of enlarged cervical nodes.

I. Benign sinus histiocytosis is characterized by massive enlargement of the cervical lymph nodes, which develops insidiously and persists for months or years.

Becroft, D.M.D. et al.: Benign sinus histiocytosis with massive lymphadenopathy: transient immunological defects in a child with mediastinal involvement. *J. Clin. Pathol.* 26:463, 1973.

IV. Metabolic and storage diseases may be accompanied by generalized lymphadenopathy. That the reticuloendothelial cells present on the reticulum and lining the lymph sinuses have phagocytic and storage functions perhaps accounts for the lymphadenopathy associated with the storage diseases.

A. Gaucher's disease
B. Niemann-Pick disease
C. Histiocytosis X
D. Cystinosis

V. Primary hematopoietic disease may be accompanied by generalized lymphadenopathy.

A. Sickle cell anemia
B. Thalassemia
C. Congenital hemolytic anemia
D. Autoimmune hemolytic anemia may be accompanied by massively enlarged, nontender nodes. Cytomegalovirus may be present in the enlarged nodes.

VI. Miscellaneous
   A. Cystic fibrosis is a frequent cause of submandibular node enlargement.
   B. Chronic granulomatous disease of childhood is characterized by chronic suppurative lymphadenitis, especially involving the cervical nodes; hepato-splenomegaly; pulmonary infiltration; and recurrent infections.
   C. Kawasaki disease, or mucocutaneous lymph node syndrome, is a febrile illness of one to two weeks' duration, occurring usually in children under the age of five years. Clinical characteristics include congestion of the ocular conjunctivae, redness of the lips and oral mucosa, a "strawberry" tongue and, frequently, tender, nonpurulent, cervical lymphadenopathy. The lips become dry and fissured. Cutaneous manifestations include marked reddening of the palms and soles, swelling of the hands and feet and desquamation that begins during the second week at the junction of the nails and skin on the finger tips and toe tips. Myocarditis is frequent and myocardial infarction occurs in 1 to 2 per cent of patients.

   Kawasaki, T., Kosaki, F., Okawa, M.D., Shigematsu, I. and Yanagawa, H.: A new infantile acute febrile mucocutaneous lymph node syndrome (MLNS) prevailing in Japan. *Pediatrics 54*:271, 1974.

## DIAGNOSTIC APPROACH

In the presence of regional or localized adenopathy, the areas drained by the involved nodes should be screened for evidence of infection. In the absence of obvious infection, another explanation should be sought. Investigation of significant generalized adenopathy may require the performance of selected procedures, including blood cell counts; examination of the peripheral blood smear; bone marrow study; throat culture; needle aspiration and culture (aerobic and anaerobic) of enlarged cervical nodes; blood cultures; serologic test for syphilis; agglutination titers for tularemia, brucellosis and salmonella; toxoplasma titers; heterophile antibody; tuberculin, histoplasmin, coccidioidin and cat-scratch skin tests; stool cultures; and roentgenograms of the chest and long bones. In the physical examination, attention should be given to the detection of other adenopathy, tumor masses, hepatomegaly or splenomegaly. If a diagnosis cannot be made within a relatively short time, biopsy of involved nodes may be necessary, especially with generalized or supraclavicular adenopathy. In addition to microscopic examination of biopsy material, the tissue should be cultured for bacteria, tubercle bacilli and fungi. A portion of the material should also be injected into a guinea pig. If diagnostic studies do not lead to a specific diagnosis, careful follow-up is indicated.

## GENERAL REFERENCES

Barton, L.L. and Feigin, R.D.: Childhood cervical lymphadenitis: a reappraisal. *J. Pediatr. 84*:846, 1974.
Kissane, J.M. and Gephardt, G.N.: Lymphadenopathy in childhood: long-term follow-up in patients with nondiagnostic lymph node biopsies. *Hum. Pathol. 5*:431, 1974.
Lake, A.M. and Oski, F.A.: Peripheral lymphadenopathy in childhood. Ten-year experience with excisional biopsy. *Am. J. Dis. Child. 132*:375, 1978.
Saltzstein, S.L.: The fate of patients with nondiagnostic lymph node biopsies. *Surgery 58*:659, 1965.
Schmitt, B.D.: Cervical adenopathy in children. *Postgrad. Med. 60*:251, 1976.
Sinclair, S., Beckman, E. and Ellman, L.: Biopsy of enlarged superficial lymph nodes. *JAMA 228*:602, 1974.
Zuelzer, W.W. and Kaplan, J.: The child with lymphadenopathy. *Semin. Hematol. 12*:323, 1975.

## ETIOLOGIC CLASSIFICATION OF LYMPHADENOPATHY

I. Infections: bacterial, mycotic and viral, 521
  A. Cat-scratch disease, 522
  B. Rubella, 522
  C. Generalized adenopathy, post-immunization, 523
  D. Tularemia, 523
  E. Toxoplasmosis, 523
  F. Gianotti-Crosti syndrome, 523
  G. Infectious mononucleosis, 523
  H. Cytomegalovirus, 523
  I. Coxsackie virus, 523
  J. Echovirus, 523
  K. Tuberculosis, 523
  L. Atypical mycobacteria, 524
  M. Rat-bite fever, 524
  N. Bacteremia, 524
  O. Histoplasmosis, 524
  P. Brucellosis, 524
  Q. Sarcoidosis, 524
  R. Salmonella infection, 524
  S. Eczema, 524
  T. Bubonic plague, 524

II. Diseases of hypersensitization, 524
  A. Juvenile rheumatoid arthritis, 524
  B. Serum sickness, 524
  C. Mesantoin medication, 524

III. Primary disease of lymphoid or reticuloendothelial tissue; metastatic lymphadenopathy, 524
  A. Leukemia, 524
  B. Lymphosarcoma, 524
  C. Reticulum cell sarcoma, 524
  D. Hodgkin's disease, 524
  E. Malignant histiocytosis or histiocytic lymphoma, 525
  F. Rhabdomyosarcoma, 525
  G. Neuroblastoma, 525
  H. Carcinoma of the thyroid, 525
  I. Benign sinus histiocytosis, 525

IV. Metabolic and storage diseases, 525
  A. Gaucher's disease, 525
  B. Niemann-Pick disease, 525
  C. Histiocytosis X, 525
  D. Cystinosis, 525

V. Primary hematopoietic disease, 525
  A. Sickle cell anemia, 525
  B. Thalassemia, 525
  C. Congenital hemolytic anemia, 525
  D. Autoimmune hemolytic anemia, 525

VI. Miscellaneous, 526
  A. Cystic fibrosis, 526
  B. Chronic granulomatous disease of childhood, 526
  C. Kawasaki disease, 526

CHAPTER **64**

# BIOSOCIAL AND PSYCHOLOGIC SYMPTOMS

Psychologic or biosocial symptoms may be approached by understanding the significance of the developmental and psychologic challenges that a child is attempting to solve at a given age. Certain psychosocial symptoms are more commonly seen in one age period than another. Table 64–1 illustrates this developmental spectrum of problems from infancy to adolescence.

Biosocial symptoms are largely ambulatory or office problems; they require a family orientation; their management utilizes the physician himself and his usual tools of history-taking, physical examination, performance of procedures, and the giving of advice; and they presume knowledge and experience in relation to both psychosocial and organic etiologies.

## TABLE 64–1  DEVELOPMENTAL SPECTRUM OF BIOSOCIAL PROBLEMS FROM INFANCY TO ADOLESCENCE

Developmental delay
Failure to thrive
Feeding problem
Anorexia
Rumination
Breath-holding spells
Excessive rocking and head banging
Resistance to going to sleep; sleep awakening
Unmanageable behavior
Biting, scratching or hitting the mother
Temper tantrums
Pica
Autistic behavior
Resistance to separation from mother
Problems in toilet training
Constipation with withholding of stools
Delayed speech
Phobias
Destructiveness
Hyperactivity
Night terrors and fears
Shyness
Withdrawn behavior
Cruelty to animals
Fire setting
Nervousness
Childhood schizophrenia
Resistance to attending school; school phobia
Failure to do well in school
Encopresis
Enuresis
Excessive or public masturbation
Effeminate behavior in boys
Anxiety attacks
Lying
Stealing
Excessive fighting
Prolonged grief reaction
Poor peer relations
Hyperventilation syndrome
Somatic complaints such as abdominal pain and headaches
Conversion symptoms
Difficulty in expressing anger
Depression
Treatment noncompliance of children with long-term disorders such as diabetes, asthma, epilepsy and cystic fibrosis
Excessive daydreaming
Low self-esteem
School underachievement
Truancy
Delinquency
Vandalism
Running away
Alcohol and drug abuse
Anorexia nervosa
Suicide attempts
Homicide

To exemplify this diagnostic approach, this chapter is concerned with infants in the first year of life and with their parents, who are usually in their late adolescence or early adulthood, though often younger. Some of the signs and symptoms and observations listed are associated in infants with "mothering disabilities" or in impairment of mother-infant interaction.

Other chapters in this volume discuss other symptoms prominent in certain age periods, e.g., hyperactivity (page 416) in preschool children; failure to do well in school (page 399) in school-aged children; recurrent abdominal pain (page 335) and headache (page 453) in school-aged children and adolescents; and depression (page 533) and chronic fatigue (page 537) in adolescents. Other symptoms such as stealing or fire setting are not specifically discussed.

## BIOSOCIAL SIGNS AND SYMPTOMS AS REFLECTED IN THE INFANT

1. Failure to thrive or slow weight gain. Whether failure to thrive is attributable to inadequate caloric intake or to anorexia, mothering disability is the most frequent cause for this condition. Indeed, periodic determination of an infant's weight and length offers a simple screening method that can alert the physician to difficulties in mother-infant interaction.
2. Feeding problems such as anorexia and refusal of solid or unfamiliar foods. (See Chapter 36.)
3. Developmental delay, especially in vocalization and smiling and use of large muscles. The baby may show other evidences of environmental deprivation, such as "hot cube" behavior, a reluctance to accept from the examiner one of the one-inch cubes used in infant testing.

> Provence, S. and Lipton, R.C.: *Infants in Institutions*. New York, International Universities Press, Inc., 1962.

4. Recurrent vomiting or rumination
5. Recurrent diarrhea
6. Irritability or excessive crying
7. Listlessness or lethargy
8. Sleep disturbances
9. Increased visual alertness with "radar-like" behavior
10. Decreased cuddling behavior
11. Infant not well cared for physically
12. Evidence of physical abuse
13. Stereotypic behavior in the infant
14. Breath-holding episodes
15. Nutritional anemia
16. The mother is a poor historian who seems unable to report what has been going on.
17. Infant held stiffly away from the mother

Mothering disabilities often represent the current sequelae of many historically predisposing factors. These past life experiences do not always lead to problems, but they increase the odds against successful mothering. They represent, in a sense, high-risk factors analogous to maternal diabetes or hypertension. The list below includes those commonly reported by women who experience difficulties in their mothering roles.

## HISTORICALLY PREDISPOSING FACTORS IN THE INFANT'S ENVIRONMENT

1. A history of a poor relationship between the mother and her own mother is a frequent antecedent to a mothering disability. The experiencing of emotional deprivation, rejection, derogation, lack of affection and constant criticism appears to be a major handicap to successful mothering. The parents of physically abused children almost always seem to have had highly unsatisfactory rearing experiences when they were young.

> Steele, B.F. and Pollock, C.B.: A psychiatric study of parents who abuse infants and small children. *In* Kempe, C.H. and Helfer, R.E. (eds.): *The Battered Child.* Chicago, University of Chicago Press, 1974, pp. 103–147.

2. Lack of social supports for the mother from spouse or boyfriend, other relatives, friends and neighbors and an inability to turn to others for help
3. Long-term emotional disturbance or maladaptation such as alcoholism, drug abuse, intellectual limitation, immaturity, psychosis or character disorder
4. Unresolved maternal grief, perhaps over the previous loss of an infant to the "sudden infant death syndrome" or over the recent death of her husband or one of her parents. More unusually, the mother may be handicapped in her mothering ability because the new baby comes to represent for her an important person from her past (e.g., her own mother, who had died prematurely). The mother is secretly convinced that the new baby will also die prematurely.
5. Marital discord or separation
6. Maternal physical illness, especially illness thought possibly injurious to the baby or to the mother
7. Many pregancies and children at short intervals
8. A very much unwanted pregnancy
9. Family illness, especially when the expectant mother has had to provide care for the sick relative
10. A disruptive geographic move late in pregnancy

The current life situation of a pregnant woman or new mother affects greatly her child-rearing behavior. Such women may be vulnerable to a breakdown in their mothering capacities when overwhelmed by unexpected perinatal contingencies. The pediatrician should be especially diagnostically alert in the following contemporary situations in which mothering may be vulnerable.

## PERINATAL CONTINGENCIES

1. Prematurity. The potentially deleterious effects that the birth of a premature baby may have on mothering arise from such considerations as the receiving of a guarded prognosis, the anticipatory mourning that may occur, the sense of failure that the woman may endure and the separation and infrequent contact with the baby that may be experienced. Such babies also appear to be at higher risk of being physically abused than those who are full-term.
2. The birth of an infant with a congenital anomaly or birth injury. The birth of a handicapped infant may lead to parental feelings of inadequacy, distortion of child-rearing practices, lack of communication within the family, increased physical demands on the mother and social isolation of the parents. If a baby is

severely retarded, the feedback and positive reinforcement that mothering requires are seriously hampered. With the birth of a malformed baby, the parents' previously formed notion of what their baby would be like — the infant's anticipated identity — is either modified strikingly or lost almost completely, depending upon the character of the malformation.

3. The occurrence of an early critical illness or of a long-term life-threatening illness. Serious illnesses are dangerous psychologically as well as physically. Unexpected recovery from an illness during which the mother thought the baby would die may be followed by the "vulnerable child syndrome." This constellation of symptoms includes difficulty in separation of the infant or child from the mother, sleep problems, delay in the child's acquisition of self-help skills, inability of the mother to discipline the child and maternal overconcern about the child's health. Because such mothers are unable to tell whether the baby is well or ill, they may call the physician frequently about symptoms that appear to the doctor to be trivial or about signs such as rapid respiration, which the physician does not regard as abnormal.

Green, M., and Solnit, A.J.: Reactions to the threatened loss of a child: a vulnerable child syndrome. *Pediatrics 34*:58, 1964.

4. Maternal depression in the first year of the infant's life. Depression in mothers during the first year is frequently associated with characteristic symptoms in the child. There is a marked lack of discipline, and the child demonstrates severe temper tantrums, negativism and abusive behavior toward the mother. Hyperactivity, crying and harrassing irritability — worse on days when the mother is most depressed — difficulty in separation, overprotection and delay in acquisition of self-help skills are other prominent symptoms. These are the problems that bring the mother to the pediatrician; her depression is usually not disclosed unless the physician makes appropriate inquiry. Because of their depression, these women appear to lose their *mothering presence,* that nonverbal projection of an effective mother somewhat analogous to *command presence* in the military. As a result, the mother becomes unable to provide the leadership and sense of security that children require. While these women may not appear to be depressed enough to require psychiatric hospitalization, they are too ill to function effectively as mothers.

Coleman, R.W. and Provence, S.: Environmental retardation (hospitalism) in infants living in families. *Pediatrics 19*:285, 1957.

5. A difficult delivery in which complications threatened the life of the mother or baby
6. Multiple births
7. Psychologic or physical absence of the father
8. Marital discord
9. Social isolation. Many young mothers and fathers are isolated from the support that comes from friends, neighbors or older relatives experienced in mothercraft. Families who abuse their children have great difficulty in turning to others for help in crisis situations. Some women are alienated from their own parents or from community agencies.
10. Failure of the infant to meet parental expectations. The infant or young child's temperment, sex, activity, and style of responsiveness obviously have major

influences on mothering. Some mothers who abuse their children seem to expect the child, in a kind of role reversal, to reassure and comfort the parent.

11. Financial insecurity, sudden loss of a job, unexpected expenses and other financial crises obviously have an important impact on parenting.
12. If she finds motherhood unrewarding, a mother may have little interest in infant and child care.
13. Illness of the mother or of a relative for whom the mother must provide care

Prevention of developmental problems manifested in the first year necessitates that the clinician identify those high-risk mothers vulnerable to the development of a parenting disability. This requires that mothers be screened for these possibilities just as they are evaluated for other biologic vulnerabilities or problems. This kind of comprehensive evaluation, encompassing both psychosocial and organic considerations, needs to be integrated into the routine care given by the obstetrician, the family physician, the pediatrician or appropriately prepared physician associates seeing expectant mothers prenatally. Such prenatal evaluations would include attention to those predisposing factors just listed. Such screening data could also lead to specific diagnostic alertness on the part of the physician.

Detection and secondary prevention require that the physician and other health professionals be alert for early evidence of disturbance in the infant. Such signs and symptoms in relation to the baby may provide the only clue, since a mother will not usually spontaneously volunteer that she is depressed or that there are other stresses that limit her functioning. It is not difficult to recognize mothering disturbances when one knows that the child has lived in an institution, but it may be a diagnostic challenge to be aware of the same problems when the infant lives with his own family.

Whenever possible, the father should be seen along with the mother to promote communication within the family. Mothers who are having difficulties need to sense the physician's empathy for how they are feeling and what they are experiencing. Expressions of interest by the physician such as, "How are *you* feeling?" or "You sound kind of tired. . . ." or "You seem a little blue. . . ." may open a channel for communication and support. Clarification and identification of the problem linked to the offering of an accepting relationship impressively facilitate successful mothering. The right word or phrase at the appropriate time may be extremely effective in early intervention.

Once full-blown symptoms such as failure to thrive or severe sleep or discipline problems are present in the baby, one may anticipate secondary reactions in the mother such as feelings of inadequacy, extreme frustration, guilt, anxiety and anger. These nonverbalized feelings may masquerade as overt hostility or apparent disinterest such as failure to visit the baby in the hospital. Such defenses need to be understood. Such mothers are extremely sensitive to any implication of blame. They need acceptance and support, not criticism.

# CHAPTER 65

# DEPRESSION

Depression, a common problem in pediatric patients, causes a variety of symptoms and signs in infants, children and adolescents. The implications of such presenting complaints need to be recognized by the pediatrician and family physician because of the significant morbidity and occasional mortality associated with depression. Accordingly, in this chapter the effects of maternal depression on infants and children and the manifestations of acute and chronic depression in children are reviewed.

## MATERNAL DEPRESSION

Depression in the mother may be suspected by the physician from symptoms and signs in the infant or child. Almost never does a mother initially report that she herself is depressed. Neither does she relate the symptoms in her child to her own affective state. ("You mean a baby knows how *I* feel?") That the mother's emotional state is only rarely perceived by others is perhaps due to the pioneer heritage in the United States that expects a mother to keep going as a matter of course without complaints, regardless of her condition. Unable themselves to understand the reason for their incapacitating symptoms, historically they could expect little understanding or help from others.

Maternal depression may begin in the postpartum period, follow the death of a significant person, accompany a chronic or life-threatening illness in the mother or be due to marital difficulties. Since the mother tends to conceal her depression outside of the house and may appear to do well with adults, there is no substitute for the physician's astute observation of the baby as well as the mother. The infant's or young child's behavior may provide the only clue to maternal depression. Once suspected, depression is usually confirmed by a question such as, "How have *you* been feeling?" or "Have you been feeling run down and tired?" or "Have you been kind of blue?"

Symptoms and signs in the infant and child that may alert the physician to the possibility of maternal depression include the following:
I. In the infant and toddler
  A. Marked lack of discipline. The child, who has come to dominate the household, resents and ignores the mother's disciplinary efforts. Although victimized by the child, she appears powerless and afraid to deal firmly with the child's behavior.
  B. Severe temper tantrums occur with great frequency and often end with both the mother and child in tears.
  C. Negativism is marked.
  D. Abusive behavior toward the mother, e.g., scratching, slapping, pinching and kicking, is often reported or observed.

E. Hyperactivity is a frequent presenting complaint.

F. Crying and harassing irritability, most marked in the presence of the mother and worse on days when the mother is most depressed, is a common symptom.

G. Difficulty in separation is often such that the mother is rarely, if ever, away from the child.

H. Sleep problems, especially resistance to going to sleep, is often the precipitating cause for the visit to the doctor.

I. Delay in achievement of self-help skills such as feeding

J. Rumination may occur secondary to unsatisfying maternal-infant interactions.

K. Developmental delay may be manifested by slow gross motor development.

L. Maternal anxiety about the child's health is manifested by frequent calls to the doctor or visits to the office or emergency room because of complaints that cannot be verified or that seem inconsequential to the physician.

II. School-aged child.

A. School phobia or resistance to going to school always raises the possibility of maternal depression.

B. Chronic depression in a child is usually accompanied by chronic or recurrent depression in one of the parents.

C. Hyperactivity in the child may be secondary to depression in the mother in some instances.


## ACUTE DEPRESSION IN CHILDREN

Experiences and contingencies that may make children vulnerable to an acute depressive reaction include the following:

I. Separation experiences, especially clusters of losses

A. Death of a loved relative, friend or pet

B. Serious illness in a relative

C. Recent move of the family or of an especially close friend

D. Onset in the child of a chronic illness or handicap with loss of health and change in the child's self-image

E. Unilateral termination of a close boyfriend-girlfriend relationship

F. Separation or divorce of parents

II. Stresses, especially clusters of stresses

A. Entrance to a new school (e.g., a large, consolidated junior high school)

B. The first year in college, especially when the adolescent is a long distance from home and without close friends

C. Learning problems in school

D. "Phantom" parents: mothers and fathers with whom the child has relatively little physical contact or close relationship

E. Lack of friends

F. A generally unhappy life with few or no experiences of joy or success

G. Inability of a child to maintain a high level of achievement or accomplishment

H. Severe acne

I. Remarriage of a parent to a spouse whom the child does not like or with whom the child is not comfortable

J. Birth of a sibling with a handicap or the onset of a chronic or life-threatening illness in a sibling

K. Out-of-wedlock pregnancy in an adolescent

III. Depression in a parent

## THE INTERVIEW AND PHYSICAL EXAMINATION

Since a child generally does not initially volunteer that he or she is depressed, the doctor must sense this on the basis of the patient's appearance and affect and the pediatric interview. Usually, the parents have not recognized that the child is depressed, and they sometimes find it difficult to believe or accept that depression causes symptoms such as fatigue, hyperactivity and headache. ("How can you tell since you haven't done any tests?")

Symptoms of acute depression in children include withdrawal and isolation from friends, family and social or extracurricular school activities. The history may also reveal weeping "for no reason," fear of dying, hyperactivity, boredom, irritability, insomnia, hypersomnia, anorexia or overeating, moodiness, tiredness, fatigue, "loss of energy," "weakness," decline in the quality of school work and resistance to attending school. Depressed children feel inadequate, worthless, helpless, stupid, no good and unloved by their parents.

The patient's facial expression, especially if he is unaware of being observed, may be almost diagnostic. Other clues include somber and dark dress, flat affect, slow speech and a mendicant posture. While the child may sit erect at the onset of the interview, as time goes on he slowly leans forward with his head downcast. The patient may cry whenever the physician touches upon a significant subject, situation or person.

## CHRONIC AND MASKED DEPRESSION

Whereas children who are acutely depressed usually have been previously emotionally healthy, some children have a long history of poor adjustment. Symptoms in the patient include school failure, resistance to attending school, repeated truancy and weight loss due to anorexia. Usually, one of the parents is chronically or recurrently depressed and the family is disorganized. Generally, there is no history of a recent loss or separation.

Since children try to avoid conscious expression of the feelings associated with chronic depression, these feelings are often *masked*. In this event, the child is brought to the doctor because of frequent temper tantrums, disobedience, truancy, running away, hyperactivity, aggressive behavior, delinquency, intense anger, promiscuity and substance abuse. It is estimated that one-fourth to one-third of delinquent children are depressed. Persistent school phobia and underachievement may be reported. Somatic complaints such as chronic or recurrent headache, abdominal pain, chest pain or anorexia are frequent. Indeed, chronic depression is probably the most frequent cause of persistent headaches in adolescent children.

Since the child will not usually initially volunteer that he or she is depressed or consciously recognize this to be the problem, the physician should avoid phrasing his question in an intrusive manner, e.g., "What are *you* depressed about?" Rather a physician's statement such as, "I would guess that things aren't going so well for you," will be answered by a glance or other nonverbal affirmation on the part of the child. The physician can then invite the child to "Tell me about it. . . ."

If the child denies depression, the doctor, with a nod to convey his awareness of the child's hesitancy to talk about such upsetting feelings, may simply say, "Well, OK. . . . I just thought that maybe you were kind of down. We can talk about it some other time. . . ." This statement conveys the doctor's understanding and his availability to be of help when the child is ready to discuss more openly his or her unhappiness.

## SUICIDE RISKS, GESTURES AND ATTEMPTS

In the presence of depression, the physician needs to determine whether the child is at risk of suicide. High-risk situations are those in which the child feels helpless, hopeless and trapped in an intolerable situation from which there seems no way of extrication; has thought out in detail how he or she would commit suicide; seems extremely guilty; or has not given thought to the devastating impact of the suicide on the family. The management of children at risk of suicide or those who make actual suicide attempts is optimally a joint pediatric-child psychiatric enterprise. One skilled physician should do the primary interview, with ad lib interviewing or probing by other staff members discouraged.

Early recognition and intervention in the case of a child at risk of suicide is enhanced if the physician has seen the child or adolescent regularly during the school and teenage years and has a prior relationship that permits him to be psychologically accessible to the child. The physician needs also to be alert to the child who is especially vulnerable to depression (e.g., the adolescent who has lost a parent).

## GENERAL REFERENCES

Cytryn, L. and McKnew, D.H.: Proposed classification of childhood depression. *Am. J. Orthopsychiatry 129*:149, 1972.

Malmquist, C.P.: Depression in childhood and adolescence. *N. Engl. J. Med. 284*:887, 155, 1971.

Marks, A.: Management of the suicidal adolescent on a nonpsychiatric adolescent unit. *J. Pediatr. 95*:305, 1979.

Mattson, A., Seese, L.R. and Hawkins, J.W.: Suicidal behavior as a child psychiatric emergency. *Arch. Gen. Psychiatr. 20*:100, 1969.

Schulterbrandt, J.G. and Raskin, A. (eds.): *Depression in Children: Diagnosis, Treatment and Conceptual Models.* New York, Raven Press, 1977.

Simmons, J.E.: School phobia and depression. *In* Green, M. and Haggerty, R.J. (eds.): *Ambulatory Pediatrics II.* Philadelphia, W.B. Saunders Co., 1977, p. 208.

CHAPTER 66

# CHRONIC FATIGUE

Chronic fatigue, lassitude or "lack of energy," not a common primary complaint in pediatric practice, tends to be seen more in older children and adolescents.

## ETIOLOGIC CLASSIFICATION OF CHRONIC FATIGUE

I. Emotional factors
   A. Depression is probably the most common cause of chronic fatigue in children and adolescents. The patient reports being tired on awakening and the need to rest frequently during the day. (See Chapter 65.)
   B. Masked school phobia should be considered in older children and adolescents seen because of chronic fatigue.
   C. Grief is characterized by feelings of overwhelming fatigue and lassitude.
   D. Hyperventilation syndrome is characterized by fatigue, precordial pain and light-headedness.
II. Infections
   A. Infectious mononucleosis is commonly accompanied by easy fatigability.
   B. Infectious hepatitis. Subclinical hepatitis may account for fatigue. Determination of SGOT may be indicated.
   C. Chronic aggressive hepatitis
   D. Tuberculosis
   E. Histoplasmosis
   F. Chronic infections in general
III. Hematology/oncology
   A. Anemia
   B. Leukemia
   C. Lymphoma
IV. Endocrine disorders
   A. Cushing's disease
   B. Addison's disease
   C. Hypothyroidism
   D. Hyperthyroidism
   E. Primary hyperaldosteronism
V. Collagen-vascular disorders
   A. Lupus erythematosus
   B. Dermatomyositis
   C. Rheumatoid arthritis
VI. Allergic conditions
   A. Allergic rhinitis, if severe, causes the child to complain of being tired.

B. "Tension-fatigue" syndrome, a term applied to a somewhat vague group of symptoms and ascribed to food allergy, is not an established disorder.

VII. Sleep disorders. (See Chapter 47.)

A. Insufficient sleep is a common cause of fatigue in school-aged children permitted to stay up late.

B. Obstructive sleep apnea is an unusual but important cause of fatigue. The history is one of loud snoring and repeated episodes of apnea during sleep.

C. Insomnia may occur in the older adolescent patient.

VIII. Cardiac disorders

A. Congenital heart disease: cyanotic, left-to-right shunt

B. Primary pulmonary hypertension

IX. Miscellaneous

A. Sarcoidosis

B. Myasthenia gravis

C. Chronic renal disease

D. Chronic pulmonary disease (e.g., cystic fibrosis)

# CHAPTER 67

# EDEMA

Edema represents an abnormal increase in the amount of extravascular, extracellular fluid. Recording of the daily weight permits an appraisal of the accumulation or loss of edema. A number of factors are usually concurrently or sequentially involved in edema production. The following presentation reviews some of these complex and ill-defined mechanisms.

## FACTORS CONTRIBUTING TO EDEMA FORMATION

I. Increased hydrostatic pressure. Increased hydrostatic pressure usually contributes to edema in patients with constrictive pericarditis, portal hypertension, congestive heart failure, Chiari's syndrome, thrombophlebitis and other lesions that impede venous return. Increase in the hydrostatic pressure promotes the filtration of fluid from the intravascular to the interstitial spaces. The increased hydrostatic pressure in localized inflammatory states results from capillary dilatation with transmission of a greater than normal head of pressure.

Increased hydrostatic pressure is not always accompanied by edema formation. Congenital absence of a portion of the inferior vena cava may not lead to edema of the lower extremities. Patients with constrictive pericarditis and chronic elevation of the venous pressure may not demonstrate edema. The role of an elevated venous pressure in patients with congestive cardiac failure is not always clear.

II. Decreased oncotic pressure. A fall in the concentration of serum albumin permits escape of fluid from the vascular system. The resultant decrease in the circulatory volume leads to an increase in the reabsorption of sodium, perhaps to an increase in the secretion of antidiuretic hormone, and to an activation of other compensatory mechanisms. A decrease in the oncotic pressure may be found in patients with protein-caloric malnutrition (kwashiorkor), hepatic disease, the nephrotic syndrome, or ascites caused by inflammatory states and malignancy. The oncotic pressure, however, may not be the major contributing factor in edema formation in these diseases. Nutritional edema may occur without much change in serum protein concentration. The administration of salt-poor albumin may not produce diuresis in patients with cirrhosis or nephrosis, and spontaneous diuresis may occur in the presence of reduced oncotic pressure. The production of serum proteins may be impaired in patients with chronic constrictive pericarditis. Edema caused by hypoproteinemia may rarely be an early manifestation of celiac disease and of cystic fibrosis.

Fleisher, D.S., DiGeorge, A.M., Barness, L.A. and Cornfeld, D.: Hypoproteinemia and edema in infants with cystic fibrosis of the pancreas. *J. Pediatr. 64*:349, 1964.

Lee, P.A., Roloff, D.W. and Howatt, W.F.: Hypoproteinemia and anemia in infants with cystic fibrosis. A presenting symptom complex often misdiagnosed. *JAMA 228*:585, 1974.

Protein loss into the gastrointestinal tract occurs in protein-losing gastroenteropathy. This nonspecific disorder occurs in patients with intestinal lymphangiectasia; regional enteritis; ulcerative colitis; constrictive pericarditis; gastrointestinal allergy, including intolerance to cow milk; celiac disease; lymphoma; and congenital ileal stenosis. Findings include hypoproteinemia, hypogammaglobulinemia, edema, ascites and pleural effusion. Infants with intolerance to cow milk may show iron deficiency anemia, occult blood in the stools and eosinophilia. Most patients with intestinal lymphangiectasia have mild diarrhea or steatorrhea at some time.

Gorske, K., Winchester, P. and Grossman, H.: Unusual protein-losing enteropathies in children. *Radiology 92*:739, 1969.

Lahey, M.E.: Protein-losing enteropathy. *Pediatr. Clin. N. Am. 9*:689, 1962.

Plauth, W.H., Jr. et al. Protein-losing enteropathy secondary to constrictive pericarditis in childhood. *Pediatrics 34*:6536, 1964.

Pomerantz, M. and Waldmann, T.A.: Systemic lymphatic abnormalities associated with gastrointestinal protein loss secondary to intestinal lymphangiectasia. *Gastroenterology 45*:703, 1963.

Waldmann, T.A., Wochner, R.D., Laster, L. and Gordon, R.S., Jr.: Allergic gastroenteropathy. A cause of excessive gastrointestinal protein loss. *N. Engl. J. Med. 276*:761, 1967.

III. Increased capillary permeability. The control of capillary permeability is incompletely understood. Increased permeability may be one of the causes for edema in allergic and chemical, thermal, bacterial or rickettsial inflammatory states. Edema in infants with severe hemolytic disease of the newborn is not entirely explained but may be due to severe hypoxia or cardiac failure.

The explanation for the relatively high protein content of ascitic or pleural fluid may be that the capillaries in these serous cavities are relatively more permeable or that lymphatic drainage from these areas is less efficient than elsewhere in the body.

IV. Tissue tension. Before edema can become evident, tissue tension must be relatively lowered. Low tissue tension may account for the localization of slight edema in the periorbital region, scrotum or vulva and the dorsum of the hands and feet in young infants.

V. Sodium reabsorption and excretion. Sodium plays an etiologic role in most instances of edema. Accounting for nearly half of the electrolyte osmotic activity in the extracellular fluid, it exerts an important effect on the distribution of body water and cellular hydration. Retention of sodium is generally accompanied by that of water. Sodium retention is of special clinical importance in congestive heart failure; in the ascites accompanying hepatic cirrhosis; in chronic, severe anemia; in nephritis; and in the nephrotic syndrome.

VI. The excretion of water. Renal reabsorption of water occurs by obligatory and facultative processes. Eighty to 90 per cent of the glomerular filtrate undergoes obligatory reabsorption in the proximal tubules, along with such electrolytes as sodium and chloride. The remainder of the water is subject to facultative reabsorption in the distal tubule in response to the action of the antidiuretic hormone. An increased excretion of antidiuretic hormone occurs in some patients with hepatic cirrhosis and ascites, congestive cardiac failure and nephrosis. Peripheral edema and variable hepatomegaly have been reported in a few children with newly discovered diabetes mellitus during the first three weeks of treatment. The cause is unknown but may be related to increased deposition of glycogen accompanied by retention of water.

Klein, R. et al.: The occurrence of peripheral edema and subcutaneous glycogen deposition following the initial treatment of diabetes mellitus in children. *J. Pediatr. 60*:807, 1962.

## ETIOLOGIC CLASSIFICATION OF EDEMA

The factors contributing to edema formation and the disease states in which they are operative may be summarized as follows:

I. Increased hydrostatic pressure
   A. Constrictive pericarditis
   B. Portal hypertension
   C. Congestive heart failure
   D. Chiari's syndrome
   E. Thrombophlebitis
   F. Extrinsic pressure upon veins owing to tumor masses

II. Decreased oncotic pressure
   A. Inadequate intake, impaired alimentation, failure of utilization or loss of protein from the gastrointestinal tract as in protein-losing enteropathy. Hypercatabolic hypoproteinemia is due to an increase in rate of plasma protein degradation, as in the nephrotic syndrome.
   B. Impaired production of protein caused by liver disease or in association with chronic constrictive pericarditis
   C. Loss of protein in patients with nephrosis or those with ascites, especially from inflammatory or malignant disorders. Loss of protein also occurs through the skin, as in Leiner's disease.

III. Increased capillary permeability
  A. Allergic reactions
  B. Inflammatory reactions: chemical, thermal, bacterial, rickettsial
IV. Impairment of lymphatic drainage
 V. Retention of sodium chloride and water
  A. Congestive cardiac failure
  B. Hepatic cirrhosis
  C. Chronic anemia
  D. Acute glomerulonephritis
  E. Nephrotic syndrome
  F. Excessive administration of saline
  G. Administration of corticosteroids
VI. Tissue tension
VII. Colloid osmotic pressure of tissue fluid associated with inflammatory reactions.

## ASCITES

Ascites, the accumulation of serous fluid in the peritoneal cavity, may occur in the following disease states:
  A. Congestive cardiac failure
  B. Chronic constrictive pericarditis

Idriss, F.S., Nikaidoh, H. and Muster, A.J.: Constrictive pericarditis simulating liver disease in children. *Arch. Surg. 109*:223, 1974.
Simcha, A. and Taylor, J.F.N.: Constrictive pericarditis in childhood. *Arch. Dis. Child. 46*:515, 1971.

The nephrotic syndrome
Hepatic cirrhosis; chronic active hepatitis
Portal hypertension with congestive splenomegaly
Chiari's syndrome, obliterative endophlebitis of the hepatic veins
Malnutrition
Malignancy
Bile ascites or bile peritonitis owing to the perforation of the common bile duct may simulate a surgical abdomen with distention, pain and toxicity. Chronic bile ascites is characterized by abdominal distention; acholic stools; fluctuating, mild jaundice; ascites; and inguinal hernias. Rose bengal excretion is absent or very low but the direct bilirubin is under 4 mg./dl. The ascitic fluid may not be bile-stained early.

Hansen, R.C., Washnich, R.D., DeVries, P.A. and Sunshine, P.: Bile ascites in infancy: diagnosis with [133]I-rose bengal. *J. Pediatr. 84*:719, 1974.

Protein-losing enteropathy
Ascites may occur secondary to pancreatitis. In children with otherwise unexplained ascites, serum and ascitic fluid amylase and lipase determinations should be obtained.

Kalwinsky, D., Frittelli, G. and Oski, F.A.: Pancreatitis presenting as unexplained ascites. *Am. J. Dis. Child. 128*:734, 1974.

Pressure on lymphatic or venous channels

Inflammatory peritoneal reaction

Leukemia, Hodgkin's disease

Chylous ascites is diagnosed by the finding on paracentesis of milky fluid that clears with ether and that contains sudan red-staining fat particles.

Vollman, R.W., Keenan, W.J. and Eraklis, A.J.: Post-traumatic chylous ascites in infancy. N. Engl. J. Med. 275:875, 1966.

Peritonitis, especially the ascitic form of tuberculous peritonitis

Ascites may rarely develop in patients with peritonitis due to tularemia.

Congenital ascites may be associated with bilateral hydronephrosis and hydroureters in newborn infants. The cause is not known.

## CARDIAC FAILURE

Edema as a manifestation of congestive cardiac failure is much less common in infants and children than in adults. With right-sided failure, there is sodium retention and fluid retention, but edema is usually confined to the sacrum and around the eyes.

## ACUTE GLOMERULONEPHRITIS

Glomerular function is relatively more impaired than tubular activity in most patients with acute glomerulonephritis. Normal tubular function in the presence of a decreased glomerular filtration rate provides an opportunity for increased tubular reabsorption of sodium and water. If the tubular ability to reabsorb sodium is also impaired, abnormal sodium retention may not occur. The congestive cardiac failure present in some of these patients may contribute to edema formation.

## THE NEPHROTIC SYNDROME

The explanation for the occurrence of edema in the nephrotic syndrome is complex and involves a number of contributory factors. Increased permeability of the glomerulus permits loss of protein into the urine. The resulting hypoproteinemia and decreased plasma colloid osmotic pressure contributes to the formation of edema by permitting the transudation of fluid into the interstitial spaces. Another is the increase in tubular reabsorption of sodium, possibly secondary to increased renin secretion and aldosterone excretion. Water retention may be due to secretion of antidiuretic hormone.

## EDEMA OF PREMATURITY: EDEMA OF THE NEWBORN

Transitory edema involving the hands, feet, face and genitalia occurs occasionally in premature infants on the second or third day of life. Development of generalized edema is less frequent. The cause is not known.

Hydrops fetalis is usually due to hemolytic disease of the newborn with high output failure secondary to anemia. Other disorders that may be associated with generalized edema of the newborn include thalassemia, Bart's hemoglobin, intrauterine infection, feto-maternal hemorrhage, major congenital anomalies and chorioangioma of the placenta.

Infants born to diabetic or toxemic mothers may be edematous at birth.

Edema of the hands and feet may occur in infants with hyaline membrane disease.

Widespread edema, most evident on the lower extremities, labia and eyelids, along with hemolytic anemia, may be due to vitamin E deficiency.

Driscoll, S.G.: Hydrops fetalis. *N. Engl. J. Med. 275*:1432, 1966.

Ritchie, J.H., Fish, M.B., McMasters, V. and Grossman, M.: Edema and hemolytic anemia in premature infants. A vitamin E deficiency syndrome. *N. Engl. J. Med. 279*:1185, 1968.

Sweet, L., Reid, W.D. and Roberton, N.R.C.: Hydrops fetalis in association with chorioangioma of the placenta. *J. Pediatr. 82*:91, 1973.

Thumasathit, B. et al.: Hydrops fetalis associated with Bart's hemoglobin in Northern Thailand. *J. Pediatr. 73*:132, 1968.

## GENERAL REFERENCE

Fisher, D.A.: Obscure and unusual edema. *Pediatrics 37*:506, 1966.

## ETIOLOGIC CLASSIFICATION OF EDEMA

I. Increased hydrostatic pressure, 540
   A. Constrictive pericarditis, 540
   B. Portal hypertension, 540
   C. Congestive heart failure, 540
   D. Chiari's syndrome, 540
   E. Thrombophlebitis, 540
   F. Extrinsic pressure upon veins from tumor masses, 540

II. Decreased oncotic pressure, 540
   A. Inadequate uptake, impaired alimentation, failure of utilization or loss of protein from the gastrointestinal tract, 540
   B. Impaired production of protein owing to liver disease or in association with chronic constrictive pericarditis, 540
   C. Loss of protein in nephrosis or ascites owing to inflammatory or malignant disorders, 540

III. Increased capillary permeability, 541
   A. Allergic reactions, 541
   B. Inflammatory reactions: chemical, thermal, bacterial, rickettsial, 541

IV. Impairment of lymphatic drainage, 541

V. Retention of sodium chloride and water, 541
   A. Congestive heart failure, 541
   B. Hepatic cirrhosis, 541
   C. Chronic anemia, 541
   D. Acute glomerulonephritis, 541
   E. Nephrotic syndrome, 541
   F. Excessive administration of saline, 541

VI. Tissue tension, 541

VII. Colloid osmotic pressure of tissue fluid associated with inflammatory reactions, 541

CHAPTER 68

# LIMB AND SKELETAL PAINS

Nonarticular limb pains that occur at night, usually in the thighs or the calves and at times in the arms, are common in preschool children, but they may also occur in school-aged children and adolescents. The pain, which varies considerably in frequency and intensity, may be accompanied by restlessness. While some children awaken crying with pain, others complain much less. Usually, massage of the extremities or the application of heat relieves the symptom. Nocturnal limb pains may be due to muscle fatigue or minor orthopedic defects and almost never to rheumatic fever; however, the exact cause usually cannot be determined. Muscle cramps, especially in the gastrocnemius and soleus muscles and in the feet, occasionally occur at night in older children and adolescents.

Øster, J.: Recurrent abdominal pain, headache and limb pains in children and adolescents. *Pediatrics 50*:429, 1972.
Øster, J. and Nielsen, A.: Growing pains. *Acta Paediatr. Scand. 61*:329, 1972.
Peterson, H.A: Leg aches. *Pediatr. Clin. N. Am. 24*:731, 1977.

## ETIOLOGIC CLASSIFICATION OF LIMB PAINS

I. Orthopedic or postural defects
   A. Pes planus
   B. Pronated feet
   C. Genu valgum
   D. Bowlegs
   E. Tight Achilles tendon
   F. Contracted or shortened hamstring muscles
   G. Children with generalized ligamentous relaxation may complain of leg pains following exercise.
II. Diseases of the joints
   A. Arthritis. (See page 212.)
   B. Osteochondritis dissecans. (See page 218.)
III. Diseases that involve the hip joint. *A roentgenogram of the hip is indicated in all patients who have unexplained pain in the knee.*
   A. Osteochondrosis of the femoral capital epiphysis (Legg-Calvé-Perthes disease) is characterized by the insidious appearance of an almost imperceptible limp. Pain, which may be referred along the distribution of the obturator nerve to the medial aspect of the thigh and knee, is usually relatively slight and may simulate that of myalgia or muscle stiffness.
   B. Slipped femoral epiphysis. Pain in the knee or in the medial aspect of the thigh above the knee, referred along the course of the obturator nerve from the hip, is the earliest sign of a slipped epiphysis.

IV. Bone tumors. Persistent bone pain is suggestive of a bone tumor.
    A. Ewing's tumor
    B. Osteogenic sarcoma
    C. Osteochondroma
    D. Osteoid osteoma. Pain is often present at night and is relieved by aspirin.
    E. Children with leukemia may complain of severe bone pain.

O'Regan, S., Melhorn, D.K. and Newman, A.J.: Methotrexate-induced bone pain in childhood leukemia. *Am. J. Dis. Child. 126*:489, 1973.

    F. Neuroblastoma metastases may cause bone pain, limp and painful joints.
    G. Primary lymphosarcoma of the bone may present with bone pain.

V. Trauma
    A. Sprains
    B. Fractures, especially bone chipping and greenstick fractures
    C. Traumatic periostitis

Singer, J. and Towbin, R.: Occult fractures in the production of gait disturbance in childhood. *Pediatrics 64*:192, 1979.

VI. Other diseases affecting bone
    A. Scurvy
    B. Infantile cortical hyperostosis
    C. Vitamin A poisoning
    D. Hyperparathyroidism
    E. Osteomyelitis
    F. Gaucher's disease may be associated with generalized skeletal pain, or the pain may be localized in the large joints and spine.
    G. Osseous lesions accompanied by bone pain and soft tissue swelling, polyarthritis, fever, and tender erythematous subcutaneous nodules may be seen with disseminated fat necrosis associated with pancreatitis.

Shackelford, P.G.: Osseous lesions and pancreatitis. *Am. J. Dis. Child. 131*:731, 1977.

VII. Muscle involvement. Pain caused by involvement of muscle is often referred to the adjacent joint.
    A. Myositis, infectious or traumatic
    B. Children with Rocky Mountain spotted fever may cry with pain if their thigh or calf muscles are squeezed.
    C. Endemic myalgia (Bornholm disease)
    D. Trichinosis
    E. Dermatomyositis
    F. Poliomyelitis
    G. Guillain-Barré syndrome
    H. Leptospirosis

VIII. Diseases of the blood
    A. Severe anemia from any cause, e.g., thalassemia, may be accompanied by limb pain, especially during periods of active hemolysis. The possibility of sickle cell anemia should be considered when limb pains occur in a black child.

B. Leukemia may cause limb pain as an early manifestation. This possibility should be especially considered if anemia and purpura are also present.

IX. Rheumatic fever. Although patients with rheumatic fever may have red, hot, painful and swollen joints, these physical signs, with the exception of pain, may be minimal or absent, especially in young children. The diagnosis of rheumatic fever cannot be established on the basis of arthralgia or limb pain alone. Limb pains that occur during the night are almost never due to rheumatic fever. Those that occur during the day and cause the child to come in from play may be more important in this regard.

X. Collagen-vascular diseases

A. Periarteritis nodosa, serum sickness and dermatomyositis may also be characterized by limb pain.

B. Takayasu's disease may cause claudication in the lower extremities.

XI. Infectious diseases are commonly accompanied by myalgia and limb pains.

XII. Reflex neurovascular dystrophy in childhood is a syndrome characterized by pain and tenderness, at times exquisite, in an extremity or joint accompanied by swelling or vasomotor changes. The pain is constant and increased by weight bearing or movement.

Bernstein, B.H. et al.: Reflex neurovascular dystrophy in childhood. *J. Pediatr. 93*:211, 1978.

## ETIOLOGIC CLASSIFICATION OF LIMB PAINS

# CHAPTER 69

# TUMORS, SWELLINGS, MASSES

The initial symptom in a child with a malignancy may be an unexplained swelling or mass. Superficial swellings on the forehead, over the eye or elsewhere may at first be thought to be a hematoma owing to trauma. If the swelling does not regress within a few days, the possibility of malignancy must be seriously considered and roentgenographic studies, excision or biopsy performed. The child with an abdominal or other tumor mass represents an emergency problem. Diagnostic procedures should be completed within 48 hours, followed by surgical removal of the mass or institution of other therapy. Palpation of the tumor should be limited to those immediately involved in diagnosis and therapy.

CHAPTER **70**

# SYMPTOMS REFERABLE
# TO THE URINARY TRACT

Disease of the urinary tract may account for a number of symptoms, including abdominal pain, abdominal tumor, growth retardation, failure to thrive, fever, edema, convulsions and hypertension. An urinalysis is indicated as a routine procedure in each child who is ill. It is important that urine specimens be examined shortly after voiding. Casts and red blood cells may disintegrate in dilute, alkaline urine. A random urinalysis does not eliminate the possibility of renal disease.

## CHARACTERISTICS OF URINATION

**Frequency.** Although over 90 per cent of term and premature infants void during the first day of life, occasionally a newborn infant will not urinate for 36 to 48 hours.

> Moore, E.S. and Galvez, M.B.: Delayed micturition in the newborn period. *J. Pediatr.* *80*:867, 1972.

The frequency of urination during infancy shows considerable variation. Infants may void between 6 and 30 times a day. During an illness, the number of diapers an infant wets may be a good index of his hydration. Dehydrated infants usually do not urinate often. During the second year, many infants are able to remain dry for two or more hours. Children between the ages of 3 to 5 years urinate 8 to 14 times a day. The frequency decreases to 6 to 12 times per day in the 5- to 8-year age group and to 6 to 8 in children 8 to 14 years of age. The frequency of urination increases during cold weather and with excitement. Children under considerable acute or chronic emotional stress may have frequency (pollakiuria) and urgency in the absence of urinary tract infection. Such symptoms respond to therapy directed to lessen the stress. The "sham" syndrome has been suggested as a term to indicate the situation in which such symptoms as frequency, urgency, daytime wetting, cross-leg squeezing to stop wetting, nighttime enuresis and dysuria occur in the absence of infection. The wetting, which may be almost continuous, is exaggerated by excitement or other emotional factors.

> Stephens, F.D., Whitaker, J. and Hewstone, A.: True, false and sham urinary tract infection in children. *Med. J. Aust. 2*:840, 1966.

Frequency and dribbling may be reported by the parents in even a very young child with a urinary tract infection.

> Randolph, M.F., Morris, K.E. and Gould, E.B.: The first urinary tract infection in the female infant. *J. Pediatr. 86*:342, 1975.

Polyuria owing to any cause is, of course, accompanied by frequency. Disease states that may be characterized by frequency include urinary tract infections, obstruction, megaloureter, foreign bodies and calculi. An inflamed appendix in contact with the right ureter or the bladder may also cause urinary frequency.

Asnes, R.S. and Mones, R.L.: Pollakiuria. *Pediatrics* 52:615, 1973.

## Oliguria, Anuria.

Renal failure
Acute glomerulonephritis
Hyperuricemia secondary to treatment of leukemia
Hemolytic-uremic syndrome
Severe dehydration
Shock
Acute tubular necrosis
Bilateral renal cortical necrosis
Unilateral or bilateral renal vein thrombosis
Bladder neck obstruction
Transfusion reaction

Dobrin, R.S., Larsen, C.D. and Holliday, M.A.: The critically ill child: acute renal failure. *Pediatrics* 48:286, 1971.

*Retention of urine* may occur in patients with meningitis, poliomyelitis, the Guillain-Barré syndrome, transverse myelitis, in patients who are comatose, stuporous or postoperative. Phimosis, superficial ulceration of the urethral meatus in infant boys, balanitis, posthitis, hematocolpos or vulvovaginitis may also lead to urinary retention. Rarely, urinary retention may be a manifestation of emotional disturbance.

## Polyuria.

Diabetes mellitus
Diabetes insipidus
Ingestion of large quantities of water
Diuresis in patients with edema
Renal tubular acidosis
Fanconi syndrome
Chronic renal failure
Hypokalemic nephropathy
Primary aldosteronism
Urinary tract infection
Sickle cell disease or trait. The defect in concentration may be evident by six months of age.
Low specific gravity of the urine may be noted in infants with cystic fibrosis who have metabolic alkalosis and hypokalemia as a major presenting manifestation.

Beckerman, R.C. and Taussig, L.M.: Hypoelectrolytemia and metabolic alkalosis in infants with cystic fibrosis. *Pediatrics* 63:580, 1979.

Hypercalcemia
Acute tubular necrosis
Nephrogenic diabetes insipidus
Psychogenic water drinking occurs in young children as a result of a disturbed

maternal-child relationship. The child asks for liquids almost constantly. Usually, there is no history of dehydration, fever or growth failure. Laboratory examination reveals a normal serum sodium, serum osmolality and urine concentration. Rarely, psychogenic water drinking may accompany diabetes insipidus.

Linshaw, M.A., Hipp, T. and Gruskin, A.: Infantile psychogenic water drinking. *J. Pediatr.* *85*:520, 1974.

**Urinary Stream.**   Inability of a male infant or child to urinate or to produce a forceful, sustained urinary stream warrants urgent urologic investigation. With partial obstruction in the posterior urethra, the urinary stream may be interrupted and without force. It is a good practice during well-baby visits of boys in early infancy to ask mothers routinely about the nature of the infant's urinary stream. If a urethral obstruction is suspected, it is well to observe the urinary stream for spraying or dribbling. Distention of the urinary bladder may be evident as a lower abdominal mass in infants who have a posterior urethral obstruction.

Leadbetter, G.W., Jr.: The etiology, symptoms, and treatment of urethral strictures in male children. *Pediatrics 31*:80, 1963.

**Incontinence.**   Children with chronic bladder distention may dribble constantly or intermittently. Urologic investigation for posterior urethral valves or other partial obstruction is urgently indicated.

Exstrophy of the bladder is, of course, characterized by incontinence.

Feinberg, T. et al.: Questions that worry children with exstrophy. *Pediatrics 53*:242, 1974.

Incontinence may occur during convulsive seizures. With nocturnal seizures, the urinary incontinence may be mistaken for enuresis.

Severely retarded children may dribble almost constantly.

Involuntary wetting in girls may be due to an ectopic ureter opening near the urethral meatus. This is a diagnostic consideration in instances of combined day and night enuresis.

Myelodysplasia or agenesis of the sacrum may be characterized by paralysis, impaired functioning of the bladder with urinary incontinence or orthopedic abnormalities. A tight filum terminale associated with spina bifida occulta may lead to urinary frequency, urgency and enuresis.

Thompson, I.M., Kirk, R.M. and Dale, M.: Sacral agenesis. *Pediatrics 54*:236, 1974.

*Enuresis* is discussed in Chapter 48, p. 422.

## URINE pH

Determination of the pH of *freshly* passed urine with nitrazine paper may be diagnostically helpful. The finding of an alkaline urine in a patient with systemic acidosis is significant. Patients with such disorders as renal tubular acidosis, idiopathic hypercalcemia or primary aldosteronism may have a neutral or alkaline urine.

## BACTERIURIA, PYURIA

Urine to be examined for bacteriuria or polymorphonuclear leukocytes should be collected with careful avoidance of contamination. In most instances, a cleanly voided specimen will suffice so that catheterization may be avoided. Patients should be as carefully prepared as for catheterization before the voided specimen is collected in a sterile container. In uncircumcised boys, the foreskin should be retracted, and the area around the meatus cleansed. After the initial few cubic centimeters of urine have been voided, the specimen may be collected. A midstream specimen may be an unrealistic expectation in young girls, but school-aged girls can usually obtain a clean midstream specimen when given careful instructions. Suprapubic bladder puncture is the only reliable method to obtain urine for culture in infants. Catheterization should be avoided if at all possible, although it may be necessary when the patient is acutely ill and immediate therapy is indicated and when the patient's cooperation cannot be obtained.

In an uncentrifuged specimen, the presence of more than five to ten polymorphonuclear leukocytes per high power field is usually considered an abnormal finding in a cleanly voided specimen.

Urinary tract infection may be defined as the growth of bacteria in the urinary tract. Such infections are commonly asymptomatic but they may also cause fever, irritability, vomiting, diarrhea, neonatal jaundice, failure to thrive, frequency, burning, urgency and a foul urine odor. Except for the newborn period when the prevalence of urinary tract infection is higher in boys than in girls, the incidence in girls is 30 times that in boys. The prevalence rate in newborn infants is about 1 per cent. In girls between the ages of 2 and 5 years, it is also about 1 per cent. The rate increases about 0.5 per cent over each of the next 5 years. It is estimated that 5 to 10 per cent of girls have a urinary tract infection before 18 years of age.

E. coli is the most common etiologic agent, accounting for 75 to 80 per cent of initial and recurrent infections. Klebsiella and enterobacter account for 10 to 15 per cent, staphylococcus and enterococci for 5 to 10 per cent and proteus and pseudomonas for a small percentage.

A number of simple and relatively inexpensive office tests are available for detection of urinary tract infection. Dip-slides (Uricult, Oxoid, Clinicult) have differential bacteriologic media on each side of the slide. While both gram-negative and gram-positive bacteria will grow on one side of the slide, only gram-negative organisms will grow on the other. Although the dip-slide is as accurate as standard bacteriologic culture techniques, these standard methods are needed for identification and antimicrobial sensitivity of the etiologic organism, a desirable procedure once the diagnosis of a urinary tract infection is established. Microstix is a dipstick that turns pink within a few seconds if nitrite is present in the urine. Almost all bacteria associated with urinary tract infections reduce nitrate. Optimal results are obtained with the first morning specimen. Since only 80 to 90 per cent of infected patients will have a positive test, it may be more helpful diagnostically if three morning samples are checked unless the first or second is positive. The Microstix strip can also be incubated and used for a colony count. These methods permit the mother to obtain the specimen at home and bring it to the office for processing.

All children with an initial urinary tract infection should have an intravenous pyelogram. A voiding cystourethrogram is indicated in all preschool and older children in whom there is evidence of upper tract disease. These studies should not usually be repeated if they are normal, if no surgical problem is identified and if reflux is only minimal or moderate. Cystoscopy is indicated only if there are positive x-ray findings of obstructive disease.

Not sufficient, in itself, for diagnosis of a urinary tract infection, pyuria may be found only intermittently and is frequently absent in the presence of bacteriuria. The diagnosis of a urinary tract infection requires the presence of a significant number of bacteria in the urine. The presence of any bacteria in a specimen obtained by suprapubic aspiration is significant. Usually, 10,000 or more colonies per milliliter are found in urine collected by this method if an infection is present.

Differentiation between contamination and a true urinary tract infection can usually be made on the basis of bacterial counts of uncentrifuged "clean catch" urine. Less than 10,000 colonies/ml. suggests contamination, while more than 100,000 colonies per milliliter indicates infection. In the asymptomatic child, the diagnosis of significant bacteriuria should be based on two consecutive colony counts of 100,000/ml. or more with the same organism. Intermediate counts raise the suspicion of infection and are an indication for repeat examination. Early morning specimens are optimal for culturing. Specimens should be cultured within one hour of voiding or refrigerated for a maximum of 48 hours until culture.

A drop of clean, uncentrifuged urine that has been dried and Gram-stained may also be examined. Organisms are noted on such a preparation in 80 to 95 per cent of cases when colony counts are 100,000 or more per milliliter. No bacteria are seen when the colony count is less than 1000/ml.

Urinary tract infection in infants and children is often due to a congenital anomaly with secondary partial obstruction and stasis. Hydronephrosis, megaloureters or a ureterocele may also be responsible for persistent or recurrent pyuria. Figure 70–1 is a flow diagram (Kunin) for the management of children seen with a symptomatic urinary tract infection.

Berger, M., Warren, M.M. and Hayden, C.K.: Urinary tract infection in the infant: the unsuspected diagnosis. *Pediatrics 62*:610, 1978.
Kunin, C.M.: Urinary tract infections. *In* Green, M. and Haggerty, R.J. (eds.): *Ambulatory Pediatrics II*. Philadelphia, W. B. Saunders Co., 1977, p. 165.
Kunin, C.M.: *Detection, Prevention and Management of Urinary Tract Infections*. 2nd ed. Philadelphia, Lea and Febiger, 1974.
Kunin, C.M.: Urinary tract infections; flow charts (algorithms) for detection and treatment. *JAMA 233*:458, 1975.
Kunin, C.M. and DeGroot, J.: Self-screening for significant bacteriuria: evaluation of a dip-strip combination nitrite/culture. *JAMA 231*:1349, 1975.
Microstix and other office tests for detection of urinary tract infection. *Med. Lett. 1*:13, 1974.
Randolph, M.F., Woods, S.E., Hudson, C.J. and Klauber, G.T.: Home screening for the detection of urinary tract infection in infancy. *Am. J. Dis. Child. 133*:713, 1979.
Screening school children for urologic disease. Statement by the Section on Urology, American Academy of Pediatrics. *Pediatrics 60*:239, 1977.

## HEMATURIA

In the presence of massive hematuria, the urine may be bright red or smoky in color. When the urine is grossly red, the bleeding is usually extraglomerular. Clots may be present, but red cell casts should be absent. Brown or reddish-brown (tea- or cola-colored) urine usually denotes glomerular bleeding. Red blood cell casts may be found. No color change occurs with microscopic hematuria. The presence of hematuria may be established by the microscopic examination of a freshly voided centrifuged urine sediment or the use of a hemoglobin dipstick. Since hematuria may be transient, the urinalysis should be repeated. A family history of renal disease or recent respiratory infection should be checked.

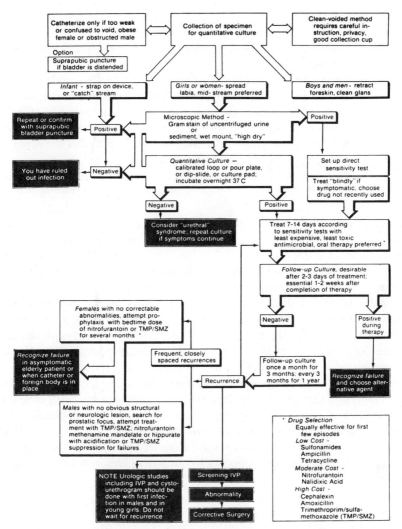

**Figure 70–1** Algorithm of sequence of events for a patient first seen in an office practice and signs and symptoms suggestive of urinary infection. IVP indicates intravenous pyelogram. (From *JAMA 233*:460, 1975. Kunin, C.M.)

If hematuria persists in the absence of proteinuria and casts, serum C3 or total complement, urine culture, tuberculin test, intravenous pyelogram and cystourethrogram are indicated. Tests for sickle cell trait should be obtained in black children who have gross hematuria. If these examinations are normal, the patient should be followed at intervals, with renal biopsy and/or cystoscopy reserved for hematuria that persists beyond six months. Family members should also be checked for hematuria. This can be done by providing the family with dipsticks. The finding of significant proteinuria in addition to hematuria indicates the presence of a glomerular lesion. Gross extraglomerular bleeding should be checked by cystoscopy to localize its source. If persistent microhematuria is accompanied by proteinuria in a number of specimens, renal biopsy may be indicated.

**Causes of Hematuria.**

Acute postinfectious (poststreptococcal) glomerulonephritis

Membranous glomerulonephritis may present with the nephrotic syndrome accompanied by microhematuria.

IgA–IgG mesangial nephropathy (Berger disease) begins with sudden gross hematuria associated with a respiratory infection. With subsidence of the infection, the gross hematuria clears, but intermittent or constant microscopic hematuria and 1+ level of proteinuria may persist. Gross hematuria may recur with further infections. Proteinuria accompanying these findings is an indication for renal biopsy.

Berger, J.: IgA glomerular deposits in renal disease. *Transplant Proc. 1*:939, 1969.

Roy, L.P., Fish, A.J., Vernier, R.L. and Michael, A.F.: Recurrent macroscopic hematuria, focal nephritis, and mesangial deposition of immunoglobulin and complement. *J. Pediatr. 82*:767, 1973.

Nephritis of chronic bacteremia (shunt nephritis) owing to chronic bacteremia associated with subacute bacterial endocarditis and infected catheters. The serum complement level is depressed.

Membranoproliferative glomerulonephritis (hypocomplementeric persistent glomerulonephritis) is characterized by proteinuria, micoscopic and gross hematuria and, occasionally, by the nephrotic syndrome. In its silent phase, this disorder may be clinically evident only by transient hematuria. The serum C3 concentration is often but not invariably depressed. This disorder may present with the nephrotic syndrome, hematuria or proteinuria. In some cases, especially type II, the onset may simulate acute glomerulonephritis with azotemia and a rapidly progressive course. On the basis of the pathologic findings, this disorder has been subdivided into MPGN type I (membranoproliferative glomerulonephritis with subendothelial deposits). MPGN type II (membranoproliferative glomerulonephritis with dense intramembranous deposits; dense deposit disease) and MPGN type III (MPGN with mixed deposits). The three types are clinically indistinguishable. Membranoproliferative glomerulonephritis occurs frequently in children with partial lipodystrophy.

Sissons, J.G.P. et al.: The complement abnormalities of lipodystrophy. *N. Engl. J. Med. 294*:461, 1976.

Rapidly progressive glomerulonephritis may be of the poststreptococcal or idiopathic type. Findings include gross hematuria, oliguria, anuria and hypertension. With a low C3, the disorder is likely to be poststreptococcal.

Lupus nephritis. Proteinuria and microscopic hematuria may be present at onset of this disorder. The hematuria may be indistinguishable from that in acute glomerulonephritis. The serum complement level is characteristically low. Since renal changes may occur in the absence of hematuria, a renal biopsy is indicated.

Glomerulonephritis of Henoch-Schönlein purpura occurs in about one half of these patients. Hematuria and proteinuria may be mild or the kidney involvement may progress to the nephrotic syndrome or renal insufficiency.

Meadow, S.R. et al.: Schönlein-Henoch nephritis. *Am. J. Med. 41*:241, 1972.

West, C.D. and McAdams, A.J.: The chronic glomerulonephritides of childhood. *J. Pediatr. 93*:1, 167, 1978.

Goodpasture's syndrome is characterized by hemoptysis, glomerulonephritis, anemia, cough, dyspnea and fever.

Polycystic disease of the kidney is frequently accompanied by hematuria.

Acute urinary tract infection may be accompanied by signs of bladder irritation. Although asymptomatic hematuria is rarely caused by such infection, a culture should be obtained.

Neoplasm. While relatively rare, gross hematuria may be the initial symptom in patients with a Wilms' tumor. An intravenous pyelogram is indicated. A bladder tumor is usually accompanied by signs of bladder irritation.

Renal hemangioma may cause severe bleeding, passage of clots and renal colic.

Trauma. Because of the possibility of pre-existing renal anomaly or disease, the urinary tract should be carefully investigated whenever hematuria follows trauma. A previously silent hydronephrosis may be identified in this fashion.

Football hematuria. Both gross and microscopic bleeding may occur transiently after playing football.

Renal calculi

Unilateral or bilateral thrombosis of the renal veins

Periarteritis nodosa

Bacterial endocarditis; other types of bacteremia

Renal tuberculosis is an unusual cause.

Foreign bodies in urethra or bladder

Hemorrhagic disorders: thrombocytopenia, hemophilia

Interstitial nephritis caused by methicillin and cephalosporins. Eosinophiluria may be present early.

Sulfonamide medication

Congestive heart failure

Leptospirosis

Infectious mononucleosis

Transient hematuria may develop during acute febrile episodes.

Prolapse of the urethra in young girls

Megaloureter

Superficial ulceration of the external urethral meatus in circumcised infant boys

Gross hematuria may occur in children with sickle cell trait, sickle cell hemoglobin C disease and, occasionally, sickle cell disease. Infarction of the renal papillae with papillary necrosis may occur.

Hemolytic-uremic syndrome

Acute hemorrhagic cystitis is characterized by a sudden onset of bright red hematuria accompanied by symptoms of bladder irritation such as marked dysuria and lower abdominal discomfort. Adenovirus (types 11 and 21) is the usual cause in children, especially boys between 6 and 15 years of age.

> Numazaki, Y. et al.: Further study on acute hemorrhagic cystitis due to adenovirus type 11. *N. Engl. J. Med. 284*:344, 1973.

Cyclophosphamide may cause hemorrhagic cystitis.

> Johnson, W.W. and Meadows, D.C.: Urinary-bladder fibrosis and telangiectasia associated with long-term cyclophosphamide therapy. *N. Engl. J. Med. 284*:290, 1971.

Benign recurrent hematuria is characterized by repeated episodes of microscopic or gross hematuria without proteinuria often precipitated by respiratory infections or exercise. Usually, no cause can be found. Red cell casts may be present. Since the diagnosis is always a tentative one, the child should be re-evaluated at intervals, with repeated urinalyses performed for proteinuria.

Ayoub, E.M. and Vernier, R.L.: Benign recurrent hematuria. *Am. J. Dis. Child. 109*:217, 1967.
McConville, J.M., West, C.D. and McAdams, A.J.: Familial and nonfamilial benign hematuria. *J. Pediatr. 69*:207, 1966.

Familial hematuria, inherited as an autosomal dominant, is characterized by constant microscopic hematuria with gross hematuria. Episodes may be associated with infections. Family members should be screened for hematuria. Proteinuria is not present either in the patient or family members. Renal biopsy is not necessary.

Glomerulonephritis of Alport's syndrome (hereditary nephritis) is an uncommon cause of hematuria. Neurosensory hearing loss may be an associated finding. Hearing impairment may be overlooked unless audiometric studies are done. Proteinuria is usually present. There may be a history of nephritis or microscopic hematuria in other family members.

Emanual, B. and Aronson, N.: Neonatal hematuria. *Am. J. Dis. Child. 128*:204, 1974.
Ingelfinger, J.R., Davis, A.E., and Grupe, W.B.: Frequency and etiology of gross hematuria in a general pediatric setting. *Pediatrics 59*:557, 1977.
Sherman, R.L., Churg, J. and Yudis, M.: Hereditary nephritis with a characteristic renal lesion. *Am. J. Med. 56*:44, 1974.

## PROTEINURIA

Multiple test reagent strips are generally employed to test for proteinuria. A false-positive reaction may be obtained if the urine is strongly alkaline. The finding of trace amounts of proteinuria by dipsticks may be checked by the sulfosalicylic acid precipitation method.

The normal upper limit of proteinuria is between 100 and 200 mg./m²/24 hours. Proteinuria that exceeds 1 gm./24 hours usually implies glomerular disease. Persistent proteinuria is clinically significant and requires investigation. Transient proteinuria in the absence of other urine abnormalities is a common finding, usually of no clinical significance, in adolescents and, less frequently, in preschool and school-aged children. In benign persistent asymptomatic proteinuria, a diagnosis made by exclusion, laboratory findings, intravenous pyelogram and biopsy are normal except for the proteinuria, which ranges from 0.5 to 1.8 gm./24 hours.

Orthostatic proteinuria occasionally occurs in older children and adolescents. Proteinuria is absent or nearly so when the child is recumbent but is regularly or intermittently present up to 1 gm./24 hours when the child is upright. Other causes of proteinuria should be ruled out by history and urinalyses. The child is asked to empty his bladder at bedtime. The first morning specimen obtained either in bed or immediately upon arising and the second sample obtained two hours later after the child has been normally active are checked for proteinuria. Specimens should be obtained on three separate mornings at home, marked for identification and frozen until brought to the office. If only the second specimens demonstrate proteinuria, the diagnosis of orthostatic proteinuria is established. If both specimens are positive, persistent proteinuria is present.

Investigation of persistent proteinuria includes determination of the 24-hour excretion of protein, urine culture, intravenous pyelogram and determination of serum proteins, creatinine, complement and cholesterol. If total protein excretion over 1 gm./day, hypocomplementemia or persistent microscopic hematuria is present, renal biopsy may be indicated.

Proteinuria may accompany infectious and other febrile diseases, exercise, emotional stress and exposure to cold.

*Other disease processes* in which proteinuria may occur include:

Acute and chronic glomerulonephritis. Microscopic hematuria is also often present.

Membranous and membranoproliferative glomerulonephritis may cause asymptomatic proteinuria. Hematuria is also usually present. The diagnosis is established by renal biopsy.

Nephrotic syndrome is the most likely cause of asymptomatic proteinuria in children from one to six years of age. Proteinuria may be present for weeks before manifest edema appears. Serum proteins, albumin and IgG levels may be depressed and serum cholesterol elevated. Renal biopsy is unnecessary except in congenital nephrosis.

Chronic pyelonephritis

Renal hypoplasia

Hydronephrosis

Polycystic disease of the kidney

Dehydration

Congestive cardiac failure

Galactosemia

Fanconi's syndrome

Dodge, W.F., West, E.F., Smith, E.H. and Bunce, H., III: Proteinuria and hematuria in school children: epidemiologic and early natural history. *J. Pediatr. 88*:327, 1976.

James, J.A.: Proteinuria and hematuria in children: diagnosis and assessment. *Pediatr. Clin. N. Am. 23*:807, 1976.

McLaine, P.N. and Drummond, K.N.: Benign persistent asymptomatic proteinuria in childhood. *Pediatrics 46*:548, 1970.

Wagner, M.G., Smith, F.G., Tinglof, B.O. and Cornberg, E.: Epidemiology of proteinuria. A study of 4,807 school children. *J. Pediatr. 73*:825, 1968.

## REDUCING SUBSTANCES

Glycosuria
  Diabetes mellitus
  Cushing's disease
  Excessive glucose ingestion
  Fanconi's syndrome
  Lead poisoning
  Following convulsive seizures
  Central nervous system infections, trauma, tumors, hemorrhage
  Glycosuria may occasionally occur during acute febrile illnesses.
  Advanced tubular damage

Pentosuria may be noted after ingestion of fruit or may be a manifestation of an inborn error of metabolism. The Benedict's reaction is positive (Clinitest), but the glucose oxidase dipstick (Clinistix) is negative.

Fructosuria may appear after ingestion of large amounts of fruit or may represent an inborn error of metabolism. The Benedict's test is positive, but the glucose oxidase dipstick (Clinistix) is negative.

Galactosuria is found in infants with galactosemia. The Benedict's test (Clinitest) is positive, but the glucose oxidase dipstick is negative.

## POSITIVE FERRIC CHLORIDE TEST

Phenylketonuria
Histidinemia
Maple syrup urine disease
Oasthouse urine disease

## ABNORMAL URINARY PIGMENTS

Bile produces a golden yellow color.

The red diaper syndrome, characterized by the appearance of a red color in soiled diapers after 24 to 36 hours, is due to Serratia marcescens.

The blue diaper syndrome may be associated with hypercalcemia and nephrocalcinosis with production of the dye indigotin or with Pseudomonas aeruginosa as the predominant organism in the stool.

> Drummond, K.N., Michael, A.F, Ulstrom, R.A. and Good, R.A.: The blue diaper syndrome: familial hypercalcemia with nephrocalcinosis and indicanuria. *Am. J. Med.* 37:928, 1964.
>
> Libit, S.A, Ulstrom, R.A. and Doeden, D.: Fecal Pseudomonas aeruginosa as a cause of the blue diaper syndrome. *J. Pediatr. 81:547*, 1972.

Hemoglobinuria, usually caused by massive intravascular hemolysis, produces pink, reddish-brown, smoky or black urine. Tests for hemoglobin are positive, but red blood cells are not seen on microscopic examination. Spectroscopic examination of the urine confirms the presence of hemoglobin.

Hematuria causes the urine to have a bright red or smoky appearance.

Urates may cause slight pink or reddish staining of the diaper in newborn and young infants. Orange sand in the diapers may be an early finding in the Lesch-Nyhan syndrome.

Beets (beeturia or anthocyaninuria) may cause red pigmentation of the urine. Iron deficiency may be present.

Porphyria, either congenital or intermittent and acute, causes a burgundy red or dark reddish-brown color that may develop in the urine on standing.

Homogentisic acid, excreted in the urine of patients with alcaptonuria, causes the urine to turn dark on standing or after alkalinization. If it is alkaline, freshly passed urine may be black or dark brown.

Paroxysmal myoglobinuria is characterized by muscle pain, weakness or paralysis and red or burgundy-colored urine. Myoglobinuria usually is noted 12 to 24 hours after the onset of muscle pain but may appear sooner or later. Both myoglobin and hemoglobin produce a positive test for hemoglobin in the absence of red cells in the urine. Acute porphyria may be excluded by a negative Watson test. The serum is pink or red in patients with hemoglobinuria. Myoglobin may be identified spectroscopically.

> Cone, T.E., Jr.: Diagnosis and treatment: some syndromes, diseases, and conditions associated with abnormal coloration of the urine or diaper. *Pediatrics 41*:654, 1968.

Meconium or gas may be present in the urine of the infant with a rectovesical fistula.

## KETONURIA

(Positive Acetest or Ketostix.)
Diabetic acidosis
Persistent vomiting
Starvation
Ketotic hypoglycemia
Fructose 1,6–diphosphatase deficiency
Lead poisoning
Acetonuria may occur during acute febrile illnesses in children.
Glycogenosis types I and III
Isovaleric acidemia
Propionic acidemia
Pyruvate carboxylase deficiency
Pyruvate dehydrogenase disorders
Methylmalonic aciduria
*Unusual odors* may suggest an inborn error of metabolism. (See p. 559)

### GENERAL REFERENCE

Edelmann, C.M., Jr. (ed.): *Pediatric Kidney Disease*. Boston, Little, Brown and Co., 1978.

CHAPTER 71

# UNUSUAL BODY OR URINE ODOR

| *Odor* | *Disease* |
| --- | --- |
| Maple syrup or burnt sugar | Maple syrup urine disease |
| Musty, mousy | Phenylketonuria<br>Tyrosinemia |
| Dried malt, celery or yeast-like | Oasthouse urine disease (methionine malabsorption) |
| Boiled cabbage, rancid butter or decaying fish | Hypermethioninemia<br>Tyrosinemia |
| Cheesy or sweaty feet | Isovaleric acidemia<br>Absence of the enzyme green acyl dehydrogenase |
| Cat urine | Beta-methylcrotonyl-CoA carboxylase deficiency |
| Acetone | Diabetic ketoacidosis<br>Other disorders characterized by ketosis |

# CHAPTER 72

# PALLOR: ANEMIA

## CLINICAL CONSIDERATIONS

Among other factors, the symptom of pallor is conditioned by the concentration of hemoglobin in the blood, the distribution and state of contraction or dilatation of cutaneous blood vessels and the presence or absence of edema. Although pallor is often attributable to an abnormally low concentration of hemoglobin, it may be due to other causes. Many infants and children appear pale even though they have a normal red blood cell count and hemoglobin concentration. A sallow complexion is often a familial characteristic. Some light-complexioned or fair-skinned children are thought by their parents to be anemic.

Pallor may be noted, even in the absence of anemia, in patients with rheumatic fever, acute glomerulonephritis, urinary tract infection, hypothyroidism, malabsorption syndromes, infantile cortical hyperostosis, chronic ulcerative colitis and other long-term diseases. It is also present in bacterial endocarditis, Henoch-Schönlein purpura, nephrosis and other diseases characterized by edema. Pallor is also a manifestation of shock. It may occur episodically in patients with pheochromocytoma, hypoglycemia, paroxysmal atrial tachycardia and anomalous origin of the left coronary artery. Newborn infants who are deeply sedated or severely hypoxic are also pale.

Anemia is characterized by a diminution in the hemoglobin concentration or oxygen-carrying capacity of the blood. For general purposes, a hemoglobin level below 10 gm./dl. of blood or a red blood cell count below 4 million indicates the presence of anemia.

In addition to pallor, a number of other symptoms may occur in anemic patients. The nature of these symptoms depends upon the primary cause of the anemia, its severity, the rapidity with which it developed and the length of time it has been present. Symptoms may include headache, vertigo, faintness, weakness, easy fatigability, irritability, palpitation, tachycardia, dyspnea, anorexia and edema. Children with hemolytic types of anemia may demonstrate nausea, vomiting, diarrhea, abdominal pain, arthralgia, leg pains, fever, jaundice, restlessness and, in some instances, hemoglobinuria. Splenomegaly may occur in patients with hemolytic anemia and, occasionally, in those with an iron deficiency anemia. Enlargement of the spleen becomes less prominent in patients with sickle cell anemia as that organ becomes fibrotic. The liver may be enlarged and tender in patients with hemolytic anemia. Hemolytic anemia may be present in the absence of jaundice. Anemia of long duration may cause retardation of physical development. Physiologic adjustments may be surprisingly compensatory, however, as far as physical activity is concerned.

Since normally the destruction or loss of erythrocytes is balanced by production, anemia may be caused by one of three basic mechanisms: (1) decreased production of erythrocytes, (2) increased destruction of erythrocytes or (3) blood loss.

The diagnosis of anemias in infants and children is not difficult in the great majority of instances and usually requires but few laboratory procedures. The presence of anemia may first be established by a determination of the hemoglobin concentration, the hematocrit or by a red blood cell count. Normal hematologic findings are given in Table 72–1. Directed history and physical examination may assist in classification of the anemia. A history of anemia in other members of the family, of blood loss or of poor diet is diagnostically helpful. Physical examination may reveal evidence of purpura, jaundice, lymphadenopathy or splenomegaly. Other procedures that may be helpful include examination of a stained blood smear, white blood cell count and a reticulocyte count. Determination of the mean corpuscular volume (MCV) may also be helpful. This figure is low with iron deficiency anemia, chronic disease, thalassemia minor and lead poisoning; normal in the anemia of chronic disease and malignancy as well as in the acute aplastic and hypoplastic anemias; and high with folate or vitamin $B_{12}$ deficiency, chronic hypoplastic anemia and active hemolysis. The urine and stool may be checked for the presence of blood, and the urine for bile and urobilinogen. These readily available procedures permit categorization of the anemia according to one of the three basic mechanisms.

## ETIOLOGIC CLASSIFICATION OF ANEMIA

I. Decreased production of erythrocytes
   A. Physiologic anemia of infancy; anemia of prematurity. With the increase in oxygen saturation at birth, less red cell mass is needed. An augmented oxygen unloading capability also develops owing to the change from fetal to adult hemoglobin. Because of physiologic marrow limitations, the rapid increase in blood volume that occurs in early infancy is unaccompanied by a proportionate increase in erythrocyte production. At 2 months of age, a hemoglobin value of 10.5 gm./dl. is normal. At 3 months of age, the red blood cell count may be about 4 million per cubic millimeter, the hemoglobin concentration about 11 gm./dl., and the hematocrit about 35. Other than the occurrence of pallor in some infants, symptoms attributable to anemia are not present. The erythrocyte count has usually risen again by the seventh month and the hemoglobin by the eighth or ninth month. Until this time, the red cells may demonstrate slight hypochromia.

   Anemia of prematurity begins shortly after birth and in its first phase extends to about the seventh week. During this time, there is a proportionate fall in both the hemoglobin concentration and red blood cell count. The resultant anemia is normochromic. The hemoglobin concentration ranges from 8.0 gm./dl. for infants with birth weights between 1000 and 1500 gm. to 9.5 gm./dl. 100 ml. for those with birth weights of 2000 to 2500 gm. The fall in hemoglobin concentration is due to a decrease in erythropoietic activity along with a slight decrease in the red cell life span.

   The intermediate phase, which lasts about two months, is characterized by a steady increase in total circulating hemoglobin mass. The peripheral hemoglobin concentration does not rise because of the rapid expansion of blood volume that accompanies the rapid growth at this time.

## TABLE 72–1 NORMAL BLOOD VALUES IN INFANTS AND CHILDREN*

| | Cord blood | Day 1 | 2 weeks | 6 weeks | 12 weeks | 1 year | 4 years | 8 to 12 years |
|---|---|---|---|---|---|---|---|---|
| Hemoglobin (gm.%) | 16–18 | 19.0±2.8 | 17.3±2.0 | 12.0±1.5 | 11.3±0.9 | 11.6±0.8 | 12.6±0.8 | 13.1±1.2 |
| Hematocrit (%) | 53–58 | 61±7 | 54±8 | 36±5 | 33±3 | 35±3 | 37±3 | 41±3 |
| Red Cells ($\times 10^6$/mm$^3$) | 5.25 | 5.14±0.7 | 4.80±0.8 | 3.40±0.4 | 3.70±0.3 | 4.60±0.4 | 4.70±0.4 | 4.90±0.5 |
| MCV (u$^3$) | 115 | 119±9 | 112±19 | 105±12 | 88±8 | 77±6 | 80±6 | 81±7 |
| MCHC (%) | 32 | 32±2 | 32±3 | 34±2 | 35±2 | 33±2 | 34±2 | 34±2 |
| Reticulocyte (%) | 3.7 | 3.2±1.4 | 0.8±0.6 | 1.2±0.7 | 0.7±0.3 | 0.9±0.5 | 0.9±0.5 | 1.1±0.6 |

*Modified from Albritton, E. C.: Standard Values in Blood. Philadelphia, W. B. Saunders Co., 1952. p. 38. and Matoth et al.: Acta Paediatr. Scand. *60*:317, 1971.

In the late phase, an iron deficient, hypochromic and microcytic type of anemia develops unless the diet has been supplemented with iron.

B. Iron deficiency anemia in infants and children is almost always due to a long-standing dietary inadequacy, infection or blood loss in the stools. Anemia is a late manifestation of iron deficiency. Irritability is a much earlier complaint. The ingestion of large amounts of milk without other iron-containing foods is usually a reflection of a parenting problem. (See Chapter 64, p. 529.) With infection, iron is poorly utilized in hemoglobin synthesis, and much of it is stored in the tissues. The anemia accompanying infection may at first be normochromic and normocytic. With the development of iron deficiency, however, the erythrocytes become predominantly hypochromic and microcytic. Maternal iron deficiency, multiple births or rapid growth in early infancy may predispose to iron deficiency anemia. The adolescent growth spurt and loss of blood during menstruation may contribute to iron deficiency and anemia.

The term "relative anemia" describes the hematologic findings in some children with cyanotic congenital heart disease who demonstrate polycythemia in the presence of an average or below-average hemoglobin concentration. The red blood cells in these patients are microcytic and hypochromic. After the administration of iron, the hemoglobin concentration rises to a level commensurate with the red blood cell count.

In patients with iron deficiency anemia, the erythrocytes have a central pallor. Poikilocytosis and anisocytosis may also be noted. The hematocrit level and the hemoglobin concentration may reflect the extent of iron deficiency anemia more closely than does the red blood cell count. The plasma supernatant in the hematocrit tube is colorless in iron deficiency. In some infants, the red cell count may be normal or even elevated in the presence of moderately low hemoglobin and hematocrit levels. The mean corpuscular volume will be less than 70 cubic microns in patients under age 2. There will also be a low serum transferrin saturation (16 per cent or less), a decreased serum iron level and a reduced transferrin level. The effectiveness of iron therapy may be gauged by the reticulocyte response, which occurs in 72 hours. Failure of a patient with a hypochromic, microcytic anemia to demonstrate a reticulocyte response after receiving adequate doses of iron in the absence of a large milk intake suggests that the patient has an infectious, chronic inflammatory or neoplastic disease. The hypochromic anemia of thalassemia, which early may be difficult to differentiate from iron deficiency anemia, does not respond to iron therapy. Also, the serum transferrin saturation in thalassemia is normal. Patients with juvenile rheumatoid arthritis may have an anemia caused by either iron deficiency or inflammation.

Koerper, M.A., Stempel, D.A. and Dallman, P.R.: Anemia in patients with juvenile rheumatoid arthritis. *J. Pediatr. 92*:930, 1978.

Although breast milk has a low content of iron, it is readily absorbed and iron supplementation is not essential. Cow milk, however, leads to iron deficiency anemia for two reasons: (1) it has low iron content and (2) the gastrointestinal system is sensitive to cow milk with resultant occult blood loss. Both these factors affect infants who ingest a quart or more of homogenized pasteurized cow milk a day. Pallor, edema, hypoproteinemia and irritability, in addition to anemia, may occur along with hypoferremia, hypocupremia and a reduced iron-binding capacity. A rise in the hemoglobin concentration follows the administration of iron or the substitution of a soy bean or proprietary milk formula.

Shumway, C.N.: Iron deficiency in children. *Pediatr. Clin. N. Am. 19*:855, 1972.
Wilson, J.F., Lahey, M.E. and Heiner, D.C.: Studies on iron metabolism. V. Further observations on cow's milk — induced gastrointestinal bleeding in infants with iron deficiency anemia. *J. Pediatr. 84*:335, 1974.

C. Copper deficiency may occur in premature infants, in infants on prolonged intravenous alimentation and in those wtih chronic diarrhea and malnutrition. Presenting signs and symptoms include failure to thrive, apathy, hypotonia, developmental retardation, underpigmented skin and hair and seborrheic dermatitis. Laboratory examinations reveal hypochromic anemia unresponsive to iron, leukopenia, low serum copper and low ceruloplasmin. X-rays show osteoporosis with metaphyseal flaring, cupping, spurs and pathologic fractures.

Ashkenazi, A. et al.: The syndrome of neonatal copper deficiency. *Pediatrics 52*:525, 1973.
Cordano, A., Baertl, J.M. and Graham, G.G.: Copper deficiency in infancy. *Pediatrics 34*:324, 1964.

D. Megaloblastic anemia of infants and children is usually due to $B_{12}$ or folic acid deficiency, occurring in some patients who have a history of intestinal resection, repeated infections, chronic diarrhea or chronic hemolytic anemia. Folic acid is absorbed in the small intestine, principally in the jejunum. The red blood cells may be macrocytic, normocytic or, at times, microcytic. Hypersegmentation of polymorphonuclear neutrophils may also occur. Bone marrow examination is diagnostic.

Hereditary orotic aciduria is a rare hereditary disorder of pyrimidine metabolism associated with megaloblastic anemia, leukopenia, retarded growth and the urinary excretion of excessive amounts of orotic acid. Sideroblastic anemias, malignancies of the Di Guglielmo variety and thiamine dependency are other causes. Megaloblastic anemia may occur during chemotherapy and in patients receiving anticonvulsants. Liver disease may cause a decrease in folic acid stores. $B_{12}$ absorption may be impaired in malabsorption disorders, regional enteritis and intestinal resection.

Rogers, L.E., Porter, F.S. and Sidbury, J.B., Jr.: Thiamine-responsive megaloblastic anemia. *J. Pediatr. 74*:494, 1969.
Smith, L.H., Jr.: Hereditary orotic aciduria — pyrimidine auxotrophism in man. *Am. J. Med. 38*:1, 1965.

Juvenile pernicious anemia, an extremely unusual disease in children, may be due to (1) a congenital lack of intrinsic factor accompanied by gastric achlorhydria, (2) failure of secretion of intrinsic factor with normal gastric acidity or (3) familial malabsorption of $B_{12}$.

Fakatselli, N.M., Delta, B.C., Hudauerdi, E.Y. and Liakoff, D.: Pernicious anemia in children. *Am. J. Med. Sci. 276*:144, 1978.
Miller, D.R. et al.: Juvenile "congenital" pernicous anemia. *N. Engl. J. Med. 275*:978, 1966.

E. Pyridoxine deficiency is a rare cause of a hypochromic microcytic or sideroblastic anemia.

F. Hypoplastic and aplastic anemias
1. Congenital hypoplastic anemia (Blackfan-Diamond) may have its onset
within the first months of life. The anemia is normochromic and normocytic. Production of leukocytes and platelets is not diminished.
2. Fanconi's syndrome consists of pancytopenia, mental retardation, understature, cafe-au-lait spots, microcephaly, strabismus and absence of
the thumbs and radii. The pancytopenia usually does not appear until
age 4.

Alter, B.P. and Nathan, D.G.: Red cell aplasia in children. *Arch. Dis. Child. 54*:263, 1979.
Bloom, G.E., Warner, S., Gerald, P.S. and Diamond, L.K.: Chromosome abnormalities in
constitutional aplastic anemia. *N. Engl. J. Med. 274*:8, 1966.

3. Osteopetrosis is characterized by a hypoplastic anemia.
4. Erythropoiesis may be transiently depressed (aplastic crisis) during the
course of sickle cell anemia, thalassemia major, congenital hemolytic
anemia and in patients who receive repeated blood transfusions.
5. Lead poisoning causes a hypochromic, microcytic anemia. The transferrin saturation is normal, and the free erythrocyte porphyrin level is
increased.
6. Chronic renal disease leads to impaired bone marrow response and
decreased production of erythropoietin. Determination of the blood
urea nitrogen or nonprotein nitrogen level is essential in the study of
unexplained anemia. Other chronic infections or inflammatory diseases
that may lead to anemia because of sequestration of iron in the reticuloendothelial system include juvenile rheumatoid arthritis, chronic
pulmonary disease, Crohn's disease and chronic granulomatous disease
of childhood. The anemia in these children may be either hypochromic-
microcytic or normochromic-normocytic. The serum iron level is decreased as is transferrin and the iron-binding protein. The saturation of
transferrin is over 30 per cent.
7. Aplastic anemias are normochromic and normocytic. Leukopenia and
thrombocytopenia also occur. Megakaryocytes, myeloid and erythroid
precursors are absent from the marrow. Though the diagnosis of aplastic anemia can often be postulated from the appearance of the peripheral blood, biopsy of the bone marrow is essential for verification.
a. Drugs and chemicals: chloramphenicol, insecticides and benzene
compounds
b. Radiation
c. Infection
d. Malignancy
(1) Neuroblastoma
(2) Leukemia is most frequent between two and five years of age.
The presenting complaint may be pallor, often accompanied by
fever, tiredness, easy bruising, lymphadenopathy and limb pain.
Gingival inflammation may occur in myelomonocytic leukemia
and in cases in which the absolute granulocyte count is less than
1000/mm$^3$. Early in the disease, acute leukemia may be a difficult

diagnostic problem. The anemia is usually normocytic-normochromic. Thrombocytopenia is a frequent finding. The peripheral blood in some cases may reveal few or no abnormal cells. Normal or low white blood cell counts are common but the WBC may be greater than 50,000/mm³. Abnormal cells may be found only after diligent search. Occasionally, on study of the marrow, agranulocytosis, thrombocytopenic purpura or aplastic anemia is found to be due to acute leukemia. The diagnostic appraisal of children with anemia, leukopenia and thrombocytopenia requires a bone marrow examination.

    e. Hepatitis may be followed by an aplastic anemia.

Schwarz, E. Baehner, R.L. and Diamond, L.K.: Aplastic anemia following hepatitis. *Pediatrics 37*:681, 1966.

    f. Idiopathic

  8. Marrow displacement by leukemia, neuroblastoma or granuloma may cause a normocytic, normochromic anemia with teardrop red cells, nucleated red cells, increased platelets and left shift of the white blood cells.

  9. Congestive splenomegaly, Gaucher's disease and, at times, other causes of splenomegaly may be accompanied by an anemia.

 10. Thyroid deficiency may be accompanied by anemia.

 11. Sideroblastic anemias, caused by defective iron or heme metabolism, are characterized by hypochromic and microcytic erythrocytes in the peripheral blood and sideroblasts in the bone marrow. The serum ferritin level is elevated.

II. Increased destruction/shortened life span of erythrocytes

    The normal life span of the erythrocyte is between 100 and 120 days. In the presence of hemolytic disease, survival time is shortened, at times markedly. This abnormal shortening may be due to an inborn error in the red cell membrane, a hemoglobinopathy, an abnormality of the intracellular enzymes or an acquired extracorpuscular mechanism. Increased red cell destruction is accompanied by a fall in free plasma haptoglobin.

Miller, D.R.: The hereditary hemolytic anemias. Membrane and enzyme defects. *Pediatr. Clin. N. Am. 19*:865, 1972.

A. Erythrocyte membrane defects. Because of physical characteristics, red blood cells with membrane defects do not survive as long as normal red cells. Such erythrocytes may be retained by the spleen for a relatively prolonged time, thus accelerating their destruction.

  1. Congenital hemolytic anemia may be symptomatic in newborns and during the first year of life but often not until the latter part of the first decade or later. If the hemolytic process is mild and the marrow activity normal, anemia may not occur. Peripheral blood examination usually reveals spherocytes. The mean corpuscular hemoglobin concentration (MCHC) is over 35 per cent. Reticulocytosis may be very active. The osmotic fragility of the red cells, commonly increased, may begin at concentrations of about 0.50 instead of at the normal level of 0.45.

When the osmotic fragility as determined by the standard procedure is normal, fragility of incubated red blood cells may provide additional information. It may be difficult, at times, to determine whether a patient has an acquired or a congenital hemolytic anemia. The demonstration of spherocytosis in one of the patient's parents makes congenital hemolytic anemia a likely diagnosis. In 10 to 20 per cent of patients, no familial incidence can be ascertained.

Aplastic crises in patients with congenital hemolytic anemia, usually caused by a viral infection, are characterized by depression of erythropoiesis, disappearance of reticulocytosis and increased hemolysis of cells.

2. Hereditary elliptocytosis, a disorder in which the erythrocytes are elliptical or cigar-shaped with possible crenated or spiculated surfaces, is accompanied by a hemolytic anemia in about 10 per cent of patients.

3. Infantile pycnocytosis is a hemolytic anemia occurring during the first three months of life and characterized by numerous distorted and contracted erythrocytes or burr cells. In the newborn, this disorder may cause hyperbilirubinemia.

4. Hereditary stomatocytosis, an autosomal dominant trait, is characterized by erythrocytes with an area of central pallor that resembles a basket, mushroom cap or pinch bottle.

5. Paroxysmal nocturnal hemoglobinuria, caused by an intrinsic erythrocyte defect, is a chronic hemolytic anemia. Hemolysis is increased at night and hemoglobinuria is noted in the morning.

6. Erythropoietic porphyria

Gross, S.: Hematologic studies on erythropoietic porphyria: a new case with severe hemolysis, chronic thrombocytopenia, and folic acid deficiency. *Blood* 23:762, 1964.

7. Abetalipoproteinemia is characterized, in part, by acanthocytosis, reticulocytosis and hemolytic anemia.

B. Hemoglobinopathies. The most frequently encountered hemoglobinopathies in the United States are sickle cell disease, thalassemia and the variants of hemoglobin C disease.

1. Sickle cell hemoglobin disorders. Sickle cell disease may occur as sickle cell trait or anemia or as a variant in association with hemoglobins C, D Punjab, E, G, J, N and O Arab, with beta-thalassemia, hereditary spherocytosis and hereditary persistence of F hemoglobin. Patients with the sickle cell trait are asymptomatic. The "trait" cells have a normal life span while the sickle cell anemia cells have an abbreviated life span of 15 to 60 days. Both parents of a child with sickle cell anemia demonstrate sickling, but it is present in only one parent of a child with the trait. The patient with sickle cell anemia is homozygous with respect to the abnormal sickle cell gene. The "trait" cells contain a mixture of both "A" and "S" types of hemoglobin while the sickle cell anemia cells are composed of "S" and "F" hemoglobin.

Hemoglobin C in combination with sickle cell hemoglobin is responsible for a hemolytic syndrome ("sickle cell-hemoglobin C disease") characterized by mild anemia, sickling and slowly developing hepato-splenomegaly that usually disappears after the age of five years. The hemoglobin concentration in these children ranges between 9 and 10 gm. and the red blood cell count between 3.5 and 4.5 million. The erythrocytes are small and rarely sickle on the routine smear. A striking number (40 to 85 per cent) of target cells are present. One parent demonstrates the sickling trait while the other is an asymptomatic carrier of hemoglobin C. Crises may occur, but they are infrequent and not severe. Patients may demonstrate arthralgia, abdominal pain and jaundice. Large numbers of target cells on the peripheral smear of a patient thought to have mild sickle cell anemia raises the possibility of sickle cell-hemoglobin C disease. Patients with the hemoglobin C trait (hemoglobin C plus normal hemoglobin) have many target cells on the peripheral smear. Rarely, homozyous hemoglobin C disease occurs as a compensated hemolytic anemia with a large number of target cells on the peripheral smear.

Transient "aplastic" crises, which may persist for about 10 days, follow acute infectious diseases in children with sickle cell anemia. During these periods, almost no red blood cells are released from the marrow. The child becomes weak, pale and demonstrates high output failure. Acute sequestration may cause sudden enlargement of the spleen.

Sickle cell anemia is normochromic and normocytic. In addition to sickling, the peripheral blood may show polychromasia, nucleated red blood cells, spherocytes, siderocytes, Howell-Jolly bodies and target cells. The reticulocyte count is increased. The hemoglobin ranges from 5.5–9.5 gm./dl. Because of failure of rouleau formation, the sedimentation rate is not increased. Although sickling usually cannot be regularly demonstrated in infants under three or four months of age, occasionally a few sickled cells may be seen. The quickest method for the demonstrtion of sickling consists of mixing 1 or 2 drops of a fresh solution of sodium metabisulfite (2 per cent) with a drop of blood on a glass slide, applying a cover slip, and examining the slide at 15-minute intervals. The Sickledex test, based on the precipitation of hemoglobins in alkali, may also be used. Hemoglobin electrophoresis permits early diagnosis of a hemoglobinopathy.

In infants, painful swelling of the hands and feet (hand-foot syndrome) or dactylitis may occur. Hemolytic crises may be manifested by fever, pain, jaundice, increased anemia and dark urine. Arthralgia, muscle pain, cardiac dilatation and murmurs may simulate acute rheumatic fever. Severe abdominal pain and abdominal rigidity (abdominal crises) may be difficult or impossible to differentiate from an acute surgical abdomen. Severe pain in an extremity may be due to a vaso-occlusive complication or to osteomyelitis or, at times, to salmonella. Neurologic manifestations include hemiparesis and seizures. Children with sickle cell anemia are very susceptible to pneumococcal bacteremia. Because the child may not initially appear ill, the clinician must be alert to this possibility. Dyspnea, high fever, leukocytosis and pain on breathing are usually due to Diplococcus pneumoniae. Pulmonary infarction may also occur.

Powars, D.R.: Natural history of sickle cell disease — the first ten years. *Semin. Hematol.* *12*:267, 1975.
Scott, R.B. and Ferguson, A.D.: Studies in sickle cell anemia. XXVII. Complications in infants and children in the United States. *Clin. Pediatr. 5*:403, 1966.

2. The thalassemia syndromes are a heterogenous group of hereditary anemias, caused by impaired synthesis of adult hemoglobin, and occurring chiefly in persons of Mediterranean extraction. Classification is based on the specific globin chain that is diminished or absent. Accordingly, beta globin is decreased or absent in beta-thalassemia and alpha globin in alpha-thalassemia. Hereditary persistence of fetal hemoglobin is another variant.

Beta-thalassemia, the most frequent type, occurs in either a heterozygous or homozygous form. The heterozygous form, termed thalassemia trait or minor, is asymptomatic except for slight splenomegaly. The red blood cells are microcytic and hypochromic. Poikilocytosis, target cells, basophilic stippling and ovalocytosis are present. HbA$_2$ is increased, and HbF is normal or slightly increased. The mean corpuscular volume and mean corpuscular hemoglobin are very low, 60 and 22, respectively. Serum ferritin and transferrin saturation are normal.

Homozygous beta-thalassemia (thalassemia major or Cooley's anemia) becomes evident in infancy with a hemoglobin concentration frequently under 5 gm., marked poikilocytosis, anisocytosis, hypochromasia, polychromatophilia, basophilic stippling, target cells, oval cells, macrocytes and microcytes. Hepatosplenomegaly appears early. Osseous changes are apparent on roentgenographic examination. Usually, HbF is increased to 30 to 60 per cent with a range from 3 to 100 per cent. The iron-binding capacity is fully saturated.

Thalassemia intermedia, a milder form of homozygous beta-thalassemia characterized by slight splenomegaly and hemoglobin over 6.5 gm., does not require blood transfusions.

Alpha-thalassemia, more frequently occurring in the Chinese, is seen, in order of increasing severity, in an asymptomatic carrier state with normal erythrocyte morphology; alpha-thalassemia trait characterized by either hypochromic microcytosis or normal morphology without anemia; and HbH disease or fatal hydrops fetalis, in which only HbBarts and HbH are present. Sickle cell-thalassemia disease (microdrepanocytic anemia) results when the gene for thalassemia is inherited from one parent and that for sickle cell from the other. The peripheral blood smear simulates that of Cooley's anemia. Only a few sickle cells may be noted on the fixed smear, but up to 100 per cent sickling is noted on special preparations.

Bank, A.: The thalassemia syndromes. *Blood 51*:369, 1978.
Orkin, S.H. and Nathan, D.G.: The thalassemias. *N. Engl. J. Med. 295*:710, 1976.

3. Hemoglobin variants (hemoglobin Zurich, Koln), some 40 in number

and known as "unstable" hemoglobins, may be associated with a chronic severe or a compensated hemolytic state.

Zinkham, W.H.: Unstable hemoglobins and the selective hemolytic action of sulfonamides. *Arch Int. Med. 137*:1365, 1977.

4. Hereditary persistence of fetal hemoglobin through life causes no problems in the heterozygote and mild polycythemia in the homozygote.

C. Hereditary enzymatic defects of the erythrocytes produce nondeformable cells; this characteristic causes them to be entrapped in the reticuloendothelial system. Although the term "congenital nonspherocytic" anemia has been applied to these disorders in the past, that designation should be discarded owing to increased understanding of etiologic mechanisms and to the occasional presence of spherocytes. The hereditary enzymatic defects may be classified into three groups.

1. Defects of the Embden-Meyerhof or anaerobic pathway.
   a. Pyruvate kinase deficiency, transmitted in an autosomal recessive fashion, is the most common enzymatic defect of this group. The severity of the hemolytic process is variable. Hemolytic anemia and jaundice in newborn infants is common. Splenomegaly may be present.
   b. Diphosphoglyceromutase deficiency
   c. Glucosephosphage isomerase deficiency
   d. Hexokinase deficiency
   e. Phosphofructokinase deficiency
   f. Phosphoglycerate kinase deficiency
   g. Triosephosphate isomerase deficiency

2. Defects of the hexose monophosphate shunt
   a. Glucose-6-phosphate dehydrogenase (G6PDH) deficiency, likely the most common inborn error of metabolism and linked in its transmission to the X chromosome, has been described in over 70 variants. This deficiency occurs most frequently in blacks (10 to 15 per cent of black Americans), Chinese, Italians, Greeks and Sephardic Jews. When present, the hemolysis may be acute or chronic, spontaneous or precipitated by exposure to oxidant drugs such as phenacetin, acetylsalicylic acid, sulfonamides, nitrofurans and naphthalene; and to fava beans, vitamin K and antimalarials. Acute hemolysis appears two to four days after drug exposure with a drop in hemoglobin concentration, hemoglobinuria, jaundice, reticulocytosis, decreased or absent haptoglobin and a peripheral smear characterized by fragmented erythrocytes, crenated forms, Heinz bodies and occasional spherocytes. Hemolytic reactions may also be precipitated by infections. G6PDH deficiency is a cause of neonatal hyperbilirubinemia.
   b. 6-phosphogluconic dehydrogenase deficiency

3. Defects in GSH synthesis, peroxidation and reduction
   a. GSH synthetase deficiency
   b. GSH reductase deficiency
   c. GSH perioxidase deficiency

Gilman, P.A.: Hemolysis in the newborn infant resulting from deficiencies of red blood cell enzymes: diagnosis and management. *J. Pediatr. 84*:625, 1974.

D. Extracorpuscular mechanisms. In this group of hemolytic anemias, extrinsic factors cause intrinsically normal erythrocytes to be destroyed or increase their susceptibility to destruction. Transfused red blood cells are also rapidly destroyed. Occasionally, acquired extracorpuscular mechanisms complicate the cause of anemia owing to an intrinsic erythrocyte abnormality, perhaps as a result of repeated blood transfusions. While the exact nature of these extracorpuscular mechanisms is not fully known, some are immunologic.

  1. Immune hemolytic anemias
    a. Isoimmune
      (1) Mismatched blood transfusion
      (2) Rh or ABO sensitization (hemolytic disease of the newborn)
    b. Autoimmune. Hemolytic anemias of this etiology may be transient or chronic. The onset is usually so acute or hyperacute that the degree of anemia is severe enough to require transfusions, at least initially. Thrombopenia, thrombopenic purpura or hemoglobinuria may also occur. The direct Coombs test is positive.

Habibi, B., Homberg, J-C., Schaison, G. and Salmon, C.: Autoimmune hemolytic anemia in children. A review of 80 cases. *Am. J. Med.* 56:61, 1974.
Zuelzer, W.W. et al.: Autoimmune hemolytic anemia. Natural history and viral-immunologic interactions in childhood. *Am. J. Med.* 49:80, 1970.

      (1) Idiopathic
      (2) Secondary
          *a.* Viral infection: (infectious mononucleosis, influenzae, Coxsackie B, measles, varicella, cytomegalovirus)
          *b.* Bacterial infection (E. coli, streptococcal sepsis, typhoid fever); Mycoplasma pneumonia infection
          *c.* Malaria
          *d.* Drugs (phenacetin, Keflin, penicillin)
          *e.* Collagen vascular disorders (lupus erythematosus, periarteritis nodosa, scleroderma, dermatomyositis, rheumatoid arthritis)
          *f.* Hematologic and oncologic disorders (leukemia, lymphoma, idiopathic thrombocytopenic purpura, paroxysmal cold hemoglobinuria)
          *g.* Miscellaneous (ulcerative colitis)
  2. Nonimmune hemolytic anemias
    a. Idiopathic
    b. Secondary
      (1) Infections (as listed in (2) above plus histoplasmosis)
      (2) Drugs (vitamin K, benzene, phenacetin). The hemolytic action of drugs may be due to an enzymatic deficiency of the red cell, a hemoglobinopathy or the formation of antibodies against the drug.

Zinkham, W.H.: The selective hemolytic action of drugs: clinical and mechanistic considerations. *J. Pediatr.* 70:200, 1967.

(3) Hematologic disorders (leukemia, megaloblastic anemia, congestive splenomegaly, histiocytosis)

(4) Thermal burns

(5) The venom of certain reptiles and arachnids may act as hemolysins. The bite of the brown recluse spider (Loxosceles reclusus) causes both a local necrotic lesion and a severe systemic reaction with fever, nausea, hemolytic anemia, hemoglobinuria and thrombocytopenia.

Minton, S.A., Jr. and Olson, C.: A case of spider bite with severe hemolytic reaction. *Pediatrics* *33*:283, 1964.

(6) Porphyria

(7) Microangiopathic hemolytic anemia

    *a.* The hemolytic uremic syndrome in infants and young children commonly begins with vomiting, diarrhea, mild fever and an upper respiratory infection followed by a severe hemolytic anemia, thrombocytopenia, hemoglobinuria, bleeding, acute renal failure, hypertension, irritability, seizures and stupor. The red blood cells may be distorted, fragmented, contracted and deeply stained. Burr and helmet cells may be noted.

Hammond, D. and Lieberman, E.: The hemolytic uremic syndrome. Renal cortical thrombotic microangiopathy. *Arch. Int. Med. 126*:816, 1970.

    *b.* Disseminated intravascular coagulation

    *c.* Cardiac hemolytic anemia may rarely occur after surgical repair of an endocardial cushion defect or of tetrology of Fallot.

Maurer, H.M.: Hematologic effects of cardiac disease. *Pediatr. Clin. N. Am. 1 9*:1083, 1972.

    *d.* Marked neonatal microangiopathic hemolytic anemia, thrombocytopenia and persistent hemolysis may occur in association with a large placental chorioangioma.

Bauer, C.R., Fojaco, R.M., Bancalari, E. and Fernandez-Rocha, L.: Microangiopathic hemolytic anemia and thrombocytopenia in a neonate associated with a large placental chorioangioma. *Pediatrics 62*:574, 1978.

(8) Vitamin E deficiency may cause a hemolytic anemia by four to six weeks of age. There is a predilection for premature infants who weigh less than 1500 gm. The hemoglobin in these patients is 6 to 9 gm./dl. and the reticulocyte count ranges between 4 and 20 per cent. The blood smear shows spherocytes, red cell fragments and spiculated red blood cells. The platelet count is markedly elevated. Because of formula supplementation, vitamin E-dependent anemia is now rare.

Oski, F.A. and Barness, L.A.: Vitamin E deficiency: a previously unrecognized cause of hemolytic anemia in the premature infant. *J. Pediatr. 70*:211, 1967.

III. Blood loss. Acute hemorrhage causes a normochromic, normocytic anemia, leukocytosis and an increase in the percentage of polymorphonuclear leukocytes. Reticulocytosis develops within a day or two. Chronic hemorrhage causes a hypochromic, microcytic anemia with moderate reticulocytosis. Further discussion of blood loss is included in Chapter 73 on Hemorrhage (p. 575). Performance of a stool guaiac test should be routine in patients with an unexplained anemia.

Idiopathic pulmonary hemosiderosis may be characterized by iron deficiency anemia and episodes of fatigue, dyspnea, cyanosis, fever and cough, progressive pulmonary changes and reticulocytosis.

The possibility of intrauterine fetal-fetal or fetal-maternal hemorrhage is an important consideration in infants with pallor or shock at birth or in the first few hours of life. Blood loss may also occur secondary to placenta previa, placenta abruptio or tears in the placental vessels during delivery. Maternal blood may be examined for fetal erythrocytes.

Gill, F.M. and Schwartz, E.: Anemia in early infancy. *Pediatr. Clin. N. Am. 19*:841, 1972.

## LABORATORY EXAMINATIONS

Special examinations that may be indicated in patients thought to have increased blood destruction include the following:

1. Blood smear. Examination of the peripheral blood smear may demonstrate polychromasia, nucleated red cells, immature myeloid cells and an increase in the percentage of polymorphonuclear leukocytes. The morphologic characteristics of the red cells may be diagnostic or very suggestive in patients with red cell membrane defects or hemoglobinopathies. Spherocytes may occur in hereditary spherocytosis, autoimmune hemolytic anemias, ABO incompatibility, congestive splenomegaly and microangiopathic hemolytic anemias. In the presence of an active hemolytic process, spherocytes are usually readily evident on the stained smear. Target cells are frequently present in patients with abnormal types of hemoglobin (e.g., sickle cell anemia and thalassemia), in liver disease and after splenectomy. Twenty to 95 per cent of the erythrocytes may appear as target cells in patients with hemoglobin C or sickle cell hemoglobin C disease. Basophilic stippling of red cells may be noted in patients with lead poisoning. Stippling, which becomes even more evident when the smear is stained with brilliant cresyl blue, is not specific for lead poisoning but may be seen in other hematologic disorders. Heinz bodies, aggregates composed of denatured cell membrane proteins and visible on slides stained with brilliant cresyl blue, occur in anemias caused by enzymatic defects. Malaria may also be diagnosed by examination of a peripheral blood smear.

2. Reticulocyte count. The presence of anemia and reticulocytosis should suggest a hemolytic process even in the absence of jaundice. Reticulocytosis disappears during aplastic crises in the hemolytic anemias.

3. Osmotic fragility

4. Serologic studies
   a. Test for blood group incompatibility if reaction follows transfusion
   b. Rh antibodies; ABO incompatibility in hemolytic disease of the newborn
   c. Coombs test. A positive direct result indicates the presence of an immunohemolytic anemia. The Coombs test is often positive in anemias caused by extracorpuscular mechanisms and almost always negative in those caused by intracorpuscular anomalies. Although the direct Coombs test is almost always positive in hemolytic disease of the newborn owing to Rh incompatibility, it is usually negative in those caused by ABO incompatibility.
   d. Autohemagglutinins: cold agglutinins, warm agglutinins
   e. Procedures utilizing trypsin-treated red blood cells and acidification of the patient's serum have been used to help demonstrate the presence of circulating antibodies in patients with acquired hemolytic anemia.
5. Antinuclear and anti-DNA antibodies
6. Screening examinations for the presence of infection, including blood cultures and chest roentgenogram
7. The serum bilirubin level may be increased in patients with hemolytic anemia. In the presence of good hepatic function, however, elevation of the serum bilirubin may be minimal or absent.
8. Hemoglobinuria is an indication of intravascular hemolysis.
9. Bilirubin may appear in the urine in some patients with hemolytic anemia caused by the development of regurgitation jaundice.
10. Hemoglobin electrophoresis is required when a hemoglobinopathy is suspected.
11. Screening test for G6PDH deficiency

## GENERAL REFERENCES

Baehner, R.L.: Anemia. *In* Green, M. and Haggerty, R.J. (eds.): *Ambulatory Pediatrics II*. Philadelphia, W. B. Saunders Co., 1977.

Nathan, D.G. and Oski, F.A. (eds.): *Hematology of Infancy and Childhood*. Philadelphia, W. B. Saunders Company, 1974.

## ETIOLOGIC CLASSIFICATION OF ANEMIA

CHAPTER **73**

# HEMORRHAGE AND PURPURA

Hemorrhage is an emergency symptom that requires prompt diagnosis and management. Bleeding may be due to either local causes, such as a Meckel's diverticulum, or to systemic disorders, such as thrombocytopenic purpura. In most instances, the cause of hemorrhage can readily be identified by the history, the physical examination and a few simple laboratory procedures. There are two major pathophysiologic processes involved in the pathogenesis of hemorrhagic disorders: an increase in capillary fragility (vascular factors) or a defect in the blood-clotting mechanism (intravascular factors). Systemic hemorrhagic disorders may range in severity from spontaneous hemorrhage or bleeding after insignificant trauma, a mild tendency to bleed noted only after dental extraction or tonsillectomy to recurrent epistaxis or easy bruising.

Epistaxis is discussed on page 72.

Hematemesis is discussed on page 289.

Hemoptysis is discussed on page 511.

Melena is discussed on page 342.

Hematuria is discussed on page 552.

Dysfunctional uterine bleeding is discussed on page 384.

## ETIOLOGIC CLASSIFICATION OF HEMORRHAGE AND PURPURA

I. Vascular factors

The factors that control or influence capillary fragility and the vascular factors in hemostasis are not well understood. Whatever the cause for hemorrhage, some defect in the vessel wall must always be postulated. The Rumpel-Leede test permits only a crude evaluation of capillary fragility. Diseases in which hemorrhage or purpura may be attributed to vascular factors are listed below.

The status of capillary fragility may be responsible for the presence or absence of bleeding in patients with thrombocytopenia.

A. Trauma or other physical cause for sudden rupture of a vessel
B. Infectious diseases may be accompanied by hemorrhagic manifestations as a result of bacterial emboli or other cause of endothelial damage. Hemorrhagic manifestations may occur in the acute exanthems, typhoid fever, infectious mononucleosis, bacterial endocarditis, the rickettsial diseases, congenital toxoplasmosis, septicemia and other disease processes. Meningococcemia must always be a diagnostic consideration in patients with acute, unexplained petechiae and purpura.
C. Drugs, chemicals, toxins
D. Scurvy
E. Allergic or anaphylactoid purpura (Henoch-Schönlein). The clinical manifestations may include a diagnostic rash with purpura (see p. 240); severe, cramping abdominal pain; painful, hot, swollen joints; localized edema; and possibly melena, epistaxis, hematemesis or hematuria. The renal sequelae of anaphylactoid purpura may be chronic. Allergic purpura may follow an acute infectious disease such as streptococcal pharyngitis, rheumatic fever, acute glomerulonephritis or periarteritis nodosa.
F. Irradiation
G. Metabolic diseases
1. Histiocytosis X in infants may be characterized by petechial skin lesions.
2. Cushing's syndrome
3. Cystic fibrosis

Soter, N.A., Mihm, M.C., Jr. and Colten, H.R.: Cutaneous necrotizing venulitis in patients with cystic fibrosis. *J. Pediatr. 95*:197, 1979.

H. Hereditary telangiectasia usually does not appear in young children but may be a rare cause of epistaxis in adolescents.
I. Ehlers-Danlos syndrome. Capillary hemorrhage and large hematomas may occur. The fragile skin breaks with slight trauma. Cutis hyperelastica and subcutaneous lipomas may be present.

II. Intravascular factors: defect in the blood-clotting mechanism

When the wall of a vessel is ruptured, reflex vasoconstriction and retraction temporarily prevent further blood loss. The platelets, in contact with the subendothelial collagen, release ADP (adenosine diphosphate), which causes development of a loose platelet plug as a result of platelet aggregation and adhesion. Simultaneously, the collagen fibers activate the intrinsic clotting mechanism, beginning with the conversion of proenzyme factor XII (Hageman) to the active enzyme XIIa. The cascade of enzymatic reactions continues, with XIIa acting on factor XI (PTA) as its substrate to produce XIa, which acts on factor IX (PTC or Christmas factor) to produce IXa, which converts factor X (Stuart) to Xa. This reaction is catalyzed when IXa forms a complex with factor VIII, phospholipid (contributed from platelets) and calcium. Factor X is also activated to Xa by tissue juice or thromboplastin, forming a complex with factor VII (stable factor) and calcium via the extrinsic pathway.

A complex of Xa, factor V (Labile factor), phospholipid and calcium then converts prothrombin (factor II) to thrombin, which converts fibrinogen (factor

I) to fibrin and activates fibrin-stabilizing factor XIII. Screening tests that permit identification of deficiencies in this hemostatic cascade include the partial thromboplastin time (PTT), prothrombin time (PT) and fibrinogen levels.

Circulating anticoagulants and fibrinolysins may occur. Prolongation of the whole blood clotting time is usually found.

The clinical states associated with intravascular deficiencies include the following:

A. Hemorrhagic diseases characterized by thrombocytopenia or qualitative platelet disorders

Gilchrist, G.S.: Platelet disorders. *Pediatr. Clin. N. Am. 19*:1047, 1972.

1. Thrombocytopenia
    a. Idiopathic thrombocytopenic purpura is a diagnosis made by the exclusion of known causes of thrombocytopenia. Idiopathic thrombocytopenic purpura often follows viral infection. Such illnesses, which occur one to six weeks before the onset of purpura, include upper respiratory tract infections, measles, rubella, mumps, chickenpox, infectious mononucleosis, hepatitis and cytomegalovirus infection. Measles vaccination is another known cause. Occasionally, idiopathic thrombocytopenic purpura occurs before or concomitantly with an autoimmune disorder such as hemolytic anemia. In other instances, there is no obvious preceding infection.

    In children, idiopathic thrombocytopenic purpura is usually a self-limited disorder, although intracranial hemorrhage may occur as a rare complication. While congenital thrombocytopenic purpura is often associated with maternal thrombocytopenia and/or purpura, the mother's platelet status may be normal. Maternal platelet antibody has been postulated to cross the placenta.

    In addition to the contribution of thrombocytopenia to the occurrence of hemorrhage, vascular changes are probably an even more important determinant of whether bleeding will occur. These bleeding or bruising tendencies may diminish even without an increase in the platelet count.

McClure, P.D.: Idiopathic thrombocytopenic purpura in children. *Pediatrics 55*:68, 1975.
Ozsoylu, S., Kanra, G. and Savas, G.: Thrombocytopenic purpura related to rubella infection. *Pediatrics 62*:567, 1978.

    b. Secondary thrombocytopenic purpura
        (1) Infections
            a. Systemic or local bacterial or viral infections are frequent causes of thrombocytopenic purpura. Infectious mononucleosis may rarely be complicated by thrombocytopenic purpura.

Overall, J.C., Jr. and Glasgow, L.A.: Virus infections of the fetus and newborn. *J. Pediatr. 77*:315, 1970.

            b. Disseminated intravascular coagulation
        (2) Drugs: sulfonamides, chloramphenicol, iodides, arsenicals, phenolphthalein
        (3) Poisons and toxins

(4) Irradiation

(5) Neoplasms, especially leukemia or neuroblastoma

(6) Congestive splenomegaly

(7) Lupus erythematosus

(8) Giant hemangiomas (Kasabach-Merritt syndrome)

(9) Storage diseases: histiocytosis X, Gaucher's disease, Niemann-Pick disease

(10) Exchange transfusion

(11) Hemolytic disease of the newborn owing to isoimmunologic factors

(12) Idiopathic hyperglycinuria

(13) Inborn metabolic errors

(14) Aplastic anemia

(15) Megaloblastic anemia with ineffective thrombopoiesis.

c. Wiskott-Aldrich syndrome, a sex-linked, recessive disorder characterized by thrombocytopenia, petechiae, bloody diarrhea, eczema, chronically draining ears and recurrent infections. Gross melena may be the initial manifestation in the newborn infant.

d. Familial hemophagocytic reticulosis is a fatal familial disease characterized by fever, hepatosplenomegaly, lymphadenopathy, pancytopenia, thrombocytopenia and hypofibrinogenemia.

McClure, P.D., Strachan, P. and Saunders, E.F.: Hypofibrinogenemia and thrombocytopenia in familial hemophagocytic reticulosis. *J. Pediatr. 85*:67, 1974.

e. Thrombotic thrombocytopenic purpura is characterized by hemorrhage, hemolytic anemia, fever, neurologic symptoms, and, often, azotemia.

Swaiman, K., Schaffhausen, M. and Krivit, W.: Thrombotic thrombocytopenic purpura. *J. Pediatr. 60*:823, 1962.

f. Bernard-Soulier syndrome, an autosomal recessive disorder, is characterized by giant platelets and shortened platelet survival.

g. Osteopetrosis

h. May-Hegglin syndrome is characterized by unusually large platelets, blue cytoplasmic inclusions in the neutrophils and, occasionally, thrombocytopenia.

2. Qualitative and functional platelet disorders are characterized by easy bruising, epistaxis, oozing after dental extraction, spontaneous petechiae and bleeding as a complication of surgery.

Hathaway, W.E.: Bleeding disorders due to platelet dysfunction. *Am. J. Dis. Child. 121*:127, 1971.

a. Glanzmann's thrombasthenia, a hemorrhagic disease transmitted as an autosomal recessive trait and usually symptomatic in infancy, is manifested by epistaxis, prolonged oozing, ecchymoses and petechiae that occur spontaneously in response to slight trauma or following surgery. Although normal in number, the platelets are physically or functionally abnormal. The bleeding time is prolonged, clot retraction is defective and platelet aggregation and adhesion decreased or absent.

Caen, J. P. et al.: Congenital bleeding disorders with long bleeding time and normal platelet count. I. Glanzmann's thrombasthenia (Report of fifteen patients). *Am. J. Med. 41*:4, 1966.

    b. von Willebrand's disease, usually transmitted as an autosomal dominant disorder, most frequently is associated with severe epistaxis. Menorrhagia may be another presenting symptom along with easy bruising and hemorrhage after trauma and surgery. Both sexes may be affected. In its severe form, all three functional components of the factor VIII system (clotting activity, antigen activity and the von Willebrand factor) are decreased. Since there are many variants, von Willebrand's disease is not ruled out by a normal amount of any one of these three factors. The best screening test depends upon the ability of the patient's plasma to support ristocetin-induced aggregation of normal platelets. The bleeding time is prolonged, the partial thromboplastin time abnormal and platelet adherence to glass beads decreased.

Gralnick, H.R., Sultan, Y. and Collier, B.S.: Von Willebrand's disease. Combined qualitative and quantitative abnormalities. *N. Engl. J. Med. 296*:1024, 1977.
Green, D. and Chediak, J.R.: Von Willebrand's disease: current concepts. *Am. J. Med. 62*:315, 1977.

    c. ADP release defect (thrombopathia, Portsmouth's disease). The platelet count and clot retraction are normal. Platelet adhesion and aggregation are decreased.
    d. PF3 release defect (thrombocytopathy). The platelet count, clot retraction, platelet adhesion and aggregation are normal, but PF3 release is decreased.
    e. Aspirin, antihistamines, phenothiazides, glycerol and glyceryl guiacolate interfere with the release of endogenous adenosine diphosphate and therefore prevent platelet aggregation and plug formation.

Schwartz, A.D. and Pearson, H.A.: Aspirin, platelets and bleeding. *J. Pediatr. 78*:558, 1971.

    f. Platelet dysfunction occurs in connective tissue disorders, glycogenosis type 1, uremia and cirrhosis.
    g. Wiskott-Aldrich syndrome is due, in part, to platelet dysfunction and shortened survival.

B. Inherited deficiencies of coagulation factors
    1. Deficiency of antihemophilic globulin (AGH, factor VIII) (hemophilia A) is the most frequent cause of hemophilia, an X-linked recessive disorder occurring in the male and transmitted through the female. About one half the patients with severe hemophilia have no family history of this disorder. While bleeding may occur after circumcision, hemophilia often does not become symptomatic until the toddler stage when the child bruises easily in response to slight trauma or bleeds from his mouth or frenulum of the tongue after a fall. The disorder is regarded as severe if the factor VIII level is less than 1 per cent and mild with a factor VIII

level over 1 to 5 per cent. Hemarthroses, which develop after the age of two or three years, always suggest hemophilia as the underlying cause.

There is no constant correlation between the whole blood coagulation time and hemorrhage. Although usually greatly prolonged, the clotting time may be normal in very mild disease. While the bleeding time is normal, bleeding may persist if too large a skin puncture is made. The partial thromboplastin time is increased, the thromboplastic generation test abnormal and the factor VIII level decreased.

2. Deficiency of factor IX or plasma thromboplastin component (hemophilia B or Christmas disease), transmitted as a sex-linked recessive disorder and clinically indistinguishable from hemophilia A, is responsible for about 15 per cent of cases of hemophilia. Laboratory findings are similar to those of hemophilia A except that the factor IX assay is decreased.

3. Hereditary deficiency of the other coagulation factors is much rarer than those of VIII and IX.

Strauss, H.S.: Diagnosis and treatment of inherited bleeding disorders. *Pediatr. Clin. N. Am. 19*:1009, 1972.

C. Acquired clotting factor deficiencies
   1. Disseminated intravascular coagulation (DIC) is characterized by the intravascular consumption of factors I, II, V, VIII and platelets; deposition of fibrin thrombi within the vascular system; and a generalized hemorrhagic state. Clinical manifestations include hemorrhage (purpura, oozing from venipuncture sites or other bleeding), thrombotic and embolic phenomena (hematuria, renal failure and thrombotic skin lesions); central nervous system symptoms such as convulsions or coma; gastrointestinal manifestations such as ileus, vomiting, diarrhea; and pallor, jaundice and shock. In addition to consumption of the clotting factors as just noted, laboratory findings include the presence of fibrin split products and microangiopathic hemolytic anemia. The PTT and PT are prolonged. Soluble fibrin is present in the plasma.

   Disseminated intravascular coagulation is a complication of bacterial sepsis, viral and rickettsial infections, burns, trauma, neonatal respiratory distress, malignancies, snake bite, purpura fulminans, cyanotic congenital heart disease, giant hemangiomas, shock and heat stroke. The differential diagnosis includes severe hepatocellular disease.

Abildgaard, C.F.: Recognition and treatment of intravascular coagulation. *J. Pediatr. 74*:163, 1969.
Corrigan, J.J.: Disseminated intravascular coagulopathy. *Pediatr. Rev. 1*:37, 1979.
Hathaway, W.E.: Care of the critically ill child: the problem of disseminated intravascular coagulation. *Pediatrics 46*:767, 1970.

   2. Vitamin K deficiency causes decreased levels of prothrombin and factors VII, IX and X. The prothrombin time and partial prothrombin time are greatly prolonged. The normal, physiologic deficiency of prothrombin between the second and tenth day may be prevented by vitamin K administration; otherwise, hemorrhagic disease of the newborn may occur. Acquired deficiency of vitamin K may occur with chronic diarrhea, malabsorption syndromes and coumarin administration. Hemorrhage usually does not occur unless the prothrombin time is less than 20 per cent of normal.

3. Liver disease such as hepatitis, Reye's syndrome or Wilson's disease may cause a fall in factors I, II, and V.
4. Uremia may be accompanied by thrombocytopenia and an increase in prothrombin time and fibrin split products.
5. Acyanotic and cyanotic congenital heart disease may be accompanied by a clotting disorder characterized by a tendency to bruise and to bleed excessively after trauma or surgery. A number of hemostatic abnormalities may occur.

Kontras, S.B., Sirak, H.D. and Newton, W.A., Jr.: Hematologic abnormalities in children with congenital heart disease. *JAMA 195*:611, 1966.
Naiman, J.L.: Clotting and bleeding in cyanotic congenital heart disease. *J. Pediatr. 76*:333, 1970.

## ETIOLOGIC CLASSIFICATION OF HEMORRHAGE OR PURPURA IN THE NEWBORN

I. Hemorrhagic disease of the newborn occurs on the second or third days of life owing to transient deficiencies of multiple coagulation factors such as prothrombin, factor VII, factor IX and factor X (Stuart).
II. Hemorrhagic manifestations at this time may also be due to congenital deficiency of such coagulation factors as V, VII, X, XI, XII.
III. Hemophilia
IV. Neonatal thrombocytopenic purpura. Petechiae in these infants occur in showers and involve the body generally.
  A. Fetal-maternal platelet antigen incompatibility, maternal idiopathic thrombocytopenic purpura or lupus erythematosus

Pearson, H.A., Shulman, N.R., Marder, V.J. and Cone, T.E., Jr.: Isoimmune neonatal thrombocytopenic purpura. Clinical and therapeutic considerations. *Blood 23*:154, 1964.

  B. Intrauterine infections: rubella, cytomegalovirus, toxoplasmosis and syphilis
  C. Sepsis
  D. Disseminated intravascular coagulation

Woods, W.G., Luban, N.L.C., Hilgartner, M.W. and Miller, D.R.: Disseminated intravascular coagulation in the newborn. *Am. J. Dis. Child. 133*:44, 1979.

  E. Megakaryocytic hypoplasia
  F. Wiskott-Aldrich syndrome may cause bloody diarrhea in the newborn male because of thrombocytopenia.
  G. Thrombocytopenia and absent radii (TAR syndrome)
  H. Hemolytic disease of the newborn
  I. Qualitative and functional platelet defects
  J. Congenital leukemia
  K. Suppression of platelet production by maternal drugs (e.g., thiazides)
  L. Congenital deficiency of thrombopoietin
V. Petechiae may occur around the head, neck or other presenting part in normal infants in the absence of thrombocytopenia. These disappear in a day or two.

Hathaway, W.E.: The bleeding newborn. *Semin. Hematol. 12*:175, 1975.

Hathaway, W.E. and Bonnar, J.: *Perinatal Coagulation*. New York, Grune and Stratton, 1978.

McIntosh, S., O'Brien, R.T., Schwartz, A.D. and Pearson, H.A.: Neonatal isoimmune purpura: response to platelet infusion. *J. Pediatr. 82*:1020, 1973.

Merenstein, G.B., O'Loughlin, E.P. and Plunket, D.C.: Effects of maternal thiazides on platelet counts of newborn infants. *J. Pediatr. 76*:766, 1970.

Oski, F.A. and Naiman, J.L.: *Hematologic Problems in the Newborn*. 2nd ed. Philadelphia, W.B. Saunders Co., 1972.

## PROCEDURES USEFUL IN DIAGNOSIS OF HEMORRHAGIC STATES

1. A careful history of an abnormal bleeding tendency in the child or the family (e.g., easy bruising or unusual bleeding after dental extraction or tonsillectomy) is a valuable screening tool. In the presence of a positive history, complete coagulation studies are indicated.

2. Selection of laboratory tests depends upon the facts of the history, physical examination and the results of screening laboratory tests.

   a. The Lee-White clotting time is as suitable as any other for determination of the clotting time, which normally is between 6 and 15 minutes.

   b. The bleeding time, normally between 1 and 5 minutes, depends upon the status of capillary contractility and platelet function as well as extravascular factors. The Ivy method, using the forearm with the blood pressure cuff inflated to 40 mm. of mercury, is preferred. The bleeding time may be prolonged with thrombocytopenic purpura, von Willebrand's disease and hypoprothrombinemia.

   c. Since clot retraction requires the presence of platelets, it correlates well with the number of platelets. Retraction is impaired or absent if the platelet count is less than 70,000 and poor in patients with thromboasthenia.

   d. Red blood cell count; hemoglobin; hematocrit; white blood cell count

   e. Platelet count

   f. The smear may be helpful in the diagnosis of infectious mononucleosis and leukemia. The presence of platelets in clumps tends to rule out thrombocytopenia.

   g. A petechial smear should be performed when meningococcemia is suspected. A petechial lesion is nicked moderately deeply with a Bard-Parker blade and a smear obtained, Gram-stained and examined for gram-negative intracellular diplococci.

   h. Examination of the bone marrow may be indicated to determine the status of the megakaryocytes and to rule out aplasia or leukemia. The presence of at least one megakaryocyte per low-power field in a cellular bone marrow is normal.

   i. Deficiencies in the intrinsic pathway (XII, XI, IX, VIII and X) show an abnormal partial prothrombin time, while prothrombin and fibrinogen levels are normal. Deficiencies in the extrinsic pathway (X, V, II, VII) show an abnormal partial prothrombin time and prothrombin time but normal fibrinogen level. With congenital absence of fibrinogen, clotting does not occur.

   j. Liver function tests

   k. A positive tourniquet result indicates the possible presence of a vascular defect; a negative result does not exclude such possibility.

## LABORATORY FINDINGS IN THROMBOCYTOPENIC PURPURA

1. Deficient clot reaction or absence of retraction
2. Lowered platelet count, usually under 75,000. The number of platelets and the patient's tendency to bleed may be poorly correlated.
3. Diminution or absence of platelets on peripheral blood smear. In idiopathic thrombocytopenic purpura, the young platelets are increased in size.
4. Bleeding time may be normal or increased. If the platelet count is under 60,000, the bleeding time is usually prolonged.
5. Coagulation time of whole blood is normal.
6. The capillary fragility may be increased. Since there is such a good correlation between capillary fragility and the patient's tendency to bruise and bleed, the tourniquet test may be a better guide in this respect than the platelet count.
7. The bone marrow should be examined for blast cells, neuroblastoma, other foreign cells and for aplasia. With idiopathic thrombocytopenic purpura, the megakaryocytes are normal or increased in number. In secondary thrombocytopenic purpura, they are normal, increased or absent.

## GENERAL REFERENCE

Baehner, R.L.: Bleeding. *In* Green, M. and Haggerty, R.J. (eds.): *Ambulatory Pediatrics II*. Philadelphia, W.B. Saunders Co., 1977.

## ETIOLOGIC CLASSIFICATION OF HEMORRHAGE AND PURPURA

I. Vascular factors, 575
  A. Trauma or other physical cause, 576
  B. Infectious diseases, 576
  C. Drugs, chemicals, toxins, 576
  D. Scurvy, 576
  E. Allergic or anaphylactoid purpura, 576
  F. Irradiation, 576
  G. Metabolic diseases, 576
    1. Histiocytosis X in infants
    2. Cushing's syndrome
    3. Cystic fibrosis
  H. Hereditary telangiectasia, 576
  I. Ehlers-Danlos syndrome, 576
II. Intravascular factors, 576
  A. Hemorrhagic diseases characterized by thrombocytopenia or qualitative platelet disorders, 577
    1. Thrombocytopenia
    2. Qualitative and functional platelet disorders
  B. Inherited deficiencies of coagulation factors, 579
    1. Deficiency of antihemophilic globulin (hemophilia A)
    2. Deficiency of factor IX (Hemophilia B or Christmas disease)
    3. Hereditary deficiency of other coagulation factors
  C. Acquired clotting factor deficiencies, 580
    1. Disseminated intravascular coagulation
    2. Vitamin K deficiency
    3. Liver disease
    4. Uremia
    5. Congenital heart disease

# ETIOLOGIC CLASSIFICATION OF HEMORRHAGE OR PURPURA IN THE NEWBORN

# APPENDIX

*Charts of Growth Statistics on*
*Boys and Girls from Birth to 18 Years**

*Courtesy of the National Center for Health Statistics, U.S. Government Department of Health, Education and Welfare, 1978.

# BOYS FROM BIRTH TO 36 MONTHS

## WEIGHT FOR AGE

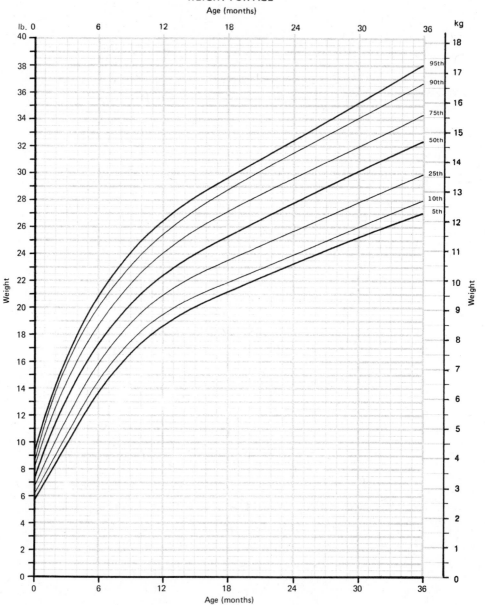

# BOYS FROM BIRTH TO 36 MONTHS

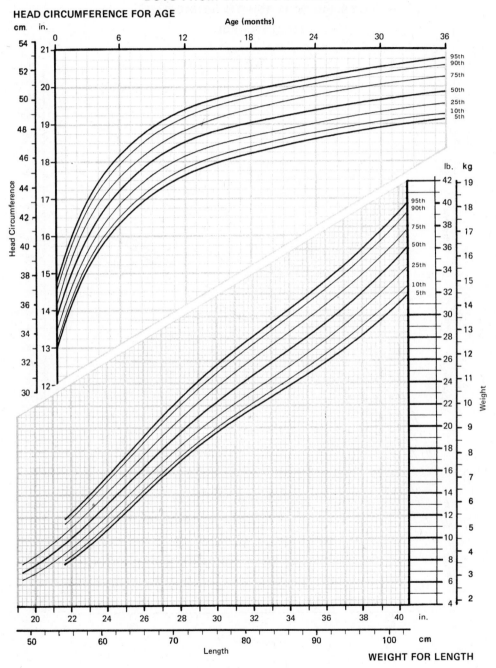

**HEAD CIRCUMFERENCE FOR AGE**

**WEIGHT FOR LENGTH**

# BOYS FROM BIRTH TO 36 MONTHS

## LENGTH FOR AGE

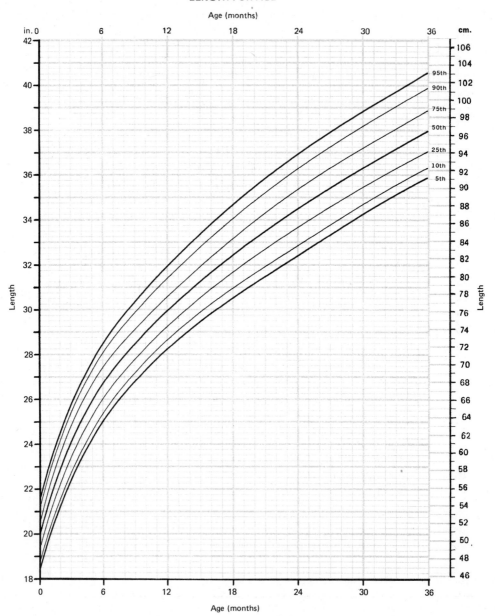

# BOYS FROM 2 TO 18 YEARS

## WEIGHT FOR AGE

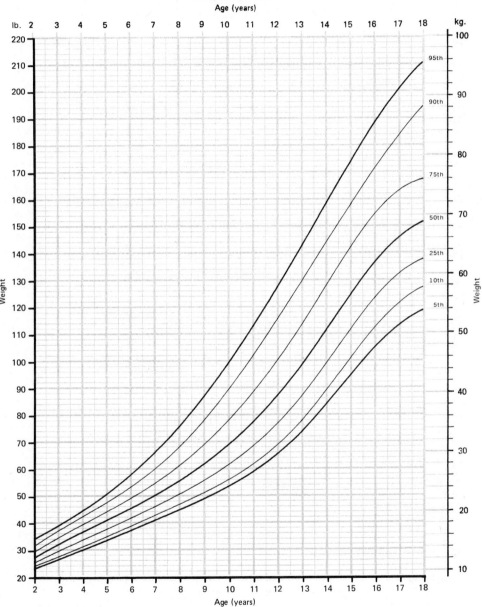

# PRE-PUBERTAL BOYS FROM 2 TO 11½ YEARS

## WEIGHT FOR STATURE

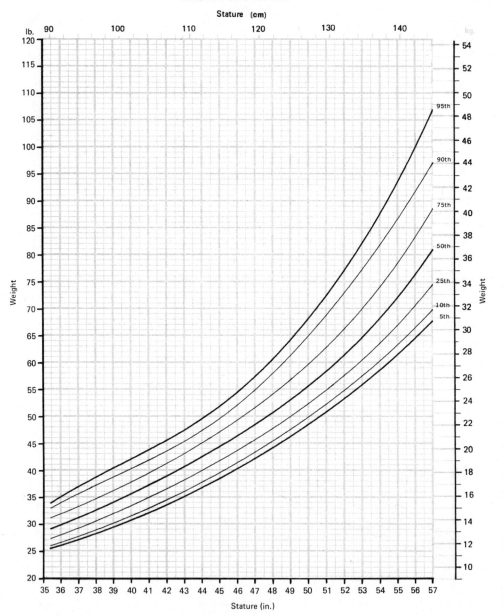

# BOYS FROM 2 TO 18 YEARS

## STATURE FOR AGE

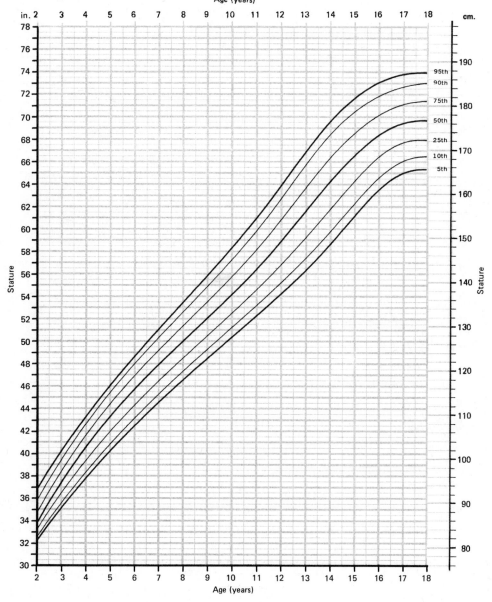

# GIRLS FROM BIRTH TO 36 MONTHS

## WEIGHT FOR AGE

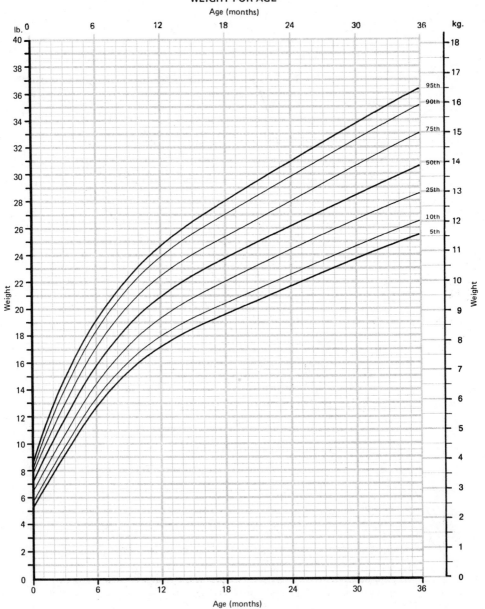

## GIRLS FROM BIRTH TO 36 MONTHS

HEAD CIRCUMFERENCE FOR AGE

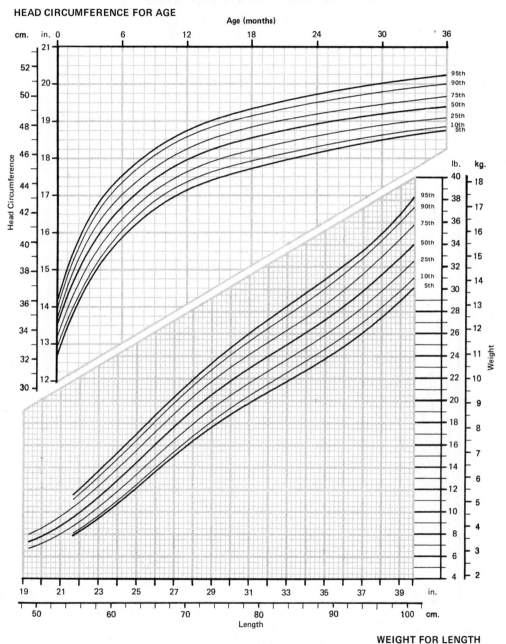

WEIGHT FOR LENGTH

# GIRLS FROM BIRTH TO 36 MONTHS

## LENGTH FOR AGE

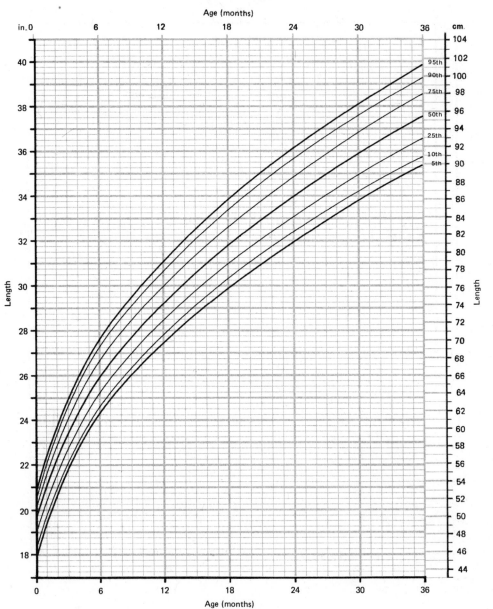

# GIRLS FROM 2 TO 18 YEARS

## WEIGHT FOR AGE

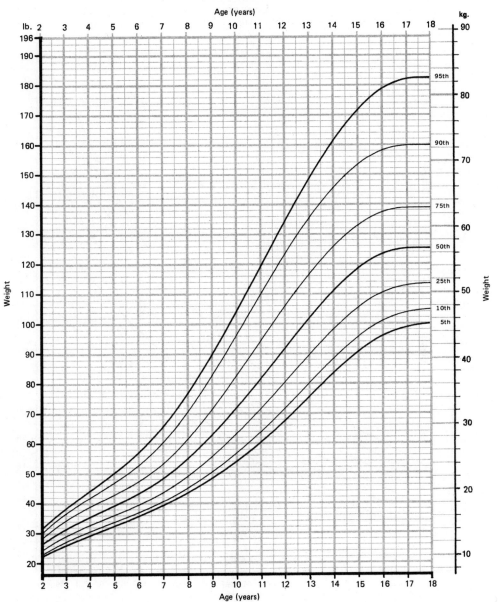

# PRE-PUBERTAL GIRLS FROM 2 TO 10 YEARS

## WEIGHT FOR STATURE

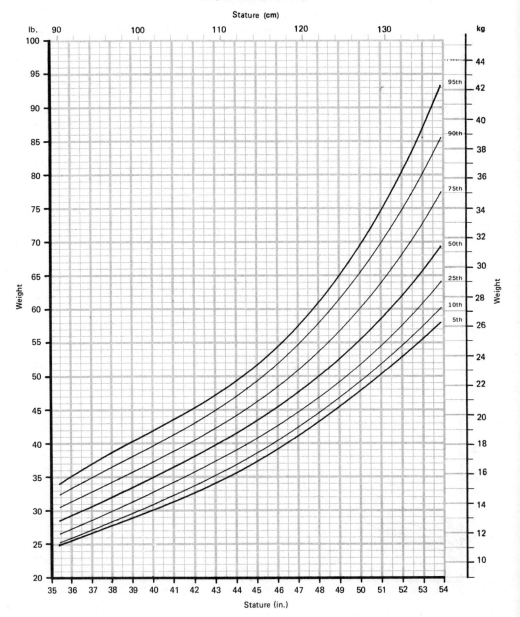

## GIRLS FROM 2 TO 18 YEARS

### STATURE FOR AGE

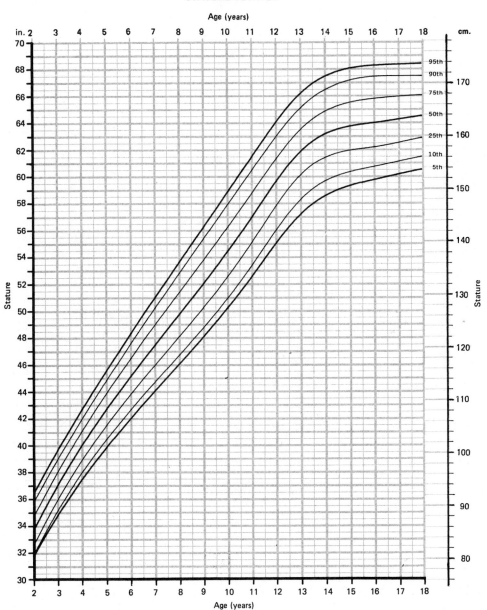

# INDEX

*Italic* numbers refer to illustrations; (t) indicates tables.

Confluence of eyebrows, in Waardenburg's
syndrome, 42
Confrontation test, as screening examination for
eye, 59
Congenital heart disease, bacterial endocarditis
in, 277
blood clotting disorder in, 581
cat's eye syndrome in, 51
cyanotic, 466–467
paroxysmal tachycardia in, 110
respiratory distress due to, 480
Congenital syphilis, cranial bossing in, 29
hair in, 32
jaundice due to, 354
osteochondritis due to, 200
rhagades due to, 76
skin signs of, 233
snuffles due to, 73
teeth in, 93
Congestion, nasal, 71
passive, and hepatomegaly, 140
venous, under tongue, 82
Congestive heart failure, cough due to, 508
cyanosis due to, 469
hepatojugular reflex in, 97
irritability in, 459
respiratory distress due to, 481
tachycardia in, 109
Conjugate movement of eyes, paralysis of, 57
Conjunctiva, examination of, 44–46
hemorrhage, due to blowout fracture, 41
infection, in orbital cellulitis, 40
telangiectasis, 45
Conjunctivitis, 44
chlamydia, 44
due to obstruction of nasolacrimal duct, 43
due to silver nitrate, 41
edema of eyelids due to, 41
inclusion, 44
vernal, 45
Conradi's disease, 49. See also *Chondrodysplasia
punctata.*
Consciousness. See also *Coma, Delirium,* etc.
lapses of, in petit mal epilepsy, 425
state of, alterations in, 440
Consistency, concept of, in child development,
164
Constant strabismus, 58
Constipation, 312–322
abdominal pain due to, 329
etiologic classification of, 316–322
fissures and excoriations due to, 146
stools in, 312
Constitution, understature due to, 376
Consultant, speech and language, indications for,
83
Contact dermatitis, 246
Continuous murmur, 117–118
Continuous thrill, 108
Contraction, of orbicularis muscle, due to
flashing light, 35
of pupil, unilateral, 47
premature, cardiac irregularity due to, 110
spasmodic, in myoclonic epilepsy, 425

Contracture, ischemic, Volkmann's, 217
joint, in dermatomyositis, 259
Convergence of eyes, 36
Convergent concomitant squint, 58
Convergent strabismus, 36
Conversion hysteria, headache due to, 456
Convulsions. See also *Seizures.*
Convulsions, 423–437
febrile, 424
incontinence due to, 550
in newborn, 434–435
Cooing, in speech development, 83
Cooley's anemia, 569
Coombs test, 350
in anemia, 574
Copper deficiency, anemia due to, 564
distended scalp veins due to, 34
Cord, spermatic. See *Spermatic cord.*
umbilical. See *Umbilicus.*
Cornea, clouding of, 47
examination of, 46–47
hypesthesia of, 47
in congenital glaucoma, 46
reflex of, 174
ulcer, 47
epiphora in, 43
Corns, 208
Coronal sutures, premature closure of, in Apert's
syndrome, 29
Corticosteroid therapy, cataracts due to, 49
papilledema in, 55
Cortisone, bradycardia due to, 109
Costochondral junctions, deformities of, 102
Coughing, chest pain due to, 514
clinical considerations of, 505–506
diagnosis of, 510–511
ear and, 510
etiologic classification of, 506–510
in viral pneumonia, 502
reflex, 506
syncope due to, 449
tic, in Gilles de la Tourette syndrome, 510
vomiting due to, 293
Cow milk, allergy, irritability due to, 460
respiratory distress due to, 482
anemia due to, 563–564
Coxa vara, 220
Coxsackie virus, infantile hemiplegia due to, 188
lymphadenopathy due to, 523
Craniofacial dysostosis, diagnosis of,
interpupillary distance in, 42
nose in, 71
prominent forehead in, 30
Craniofenestria, 26
Craniometaphyseal dysostosis, ocular
hypertelorism in, 42
Craniopharyngiomas, and understature, 375
Craniosynostosis, 26
in cranial growth, 28, 29
Craniotabes, 26
Cranium. See also *Brain, Head,* etc.
basilar impression of, 192
bifidum, 193
bossing, 29–30